THERAPEUTIC BLOOD LEVELS OF PSYCHOTROPIC DRUGS (continued)

Generic Name	Therapeutic Level	Toxic Level
Antidepressants (continued)		
nortriptyline	50–150 ng/ml	> 500 ng/ml
protriptyline	50–150 ng/ml	> 200 ng/ml
trazodone	500–2,500 ng/ml	> 4,000 ng/ml
Antimigraine Drugs		
propranolol	50–100 ng/ml	> 150 ng/ml
timolol	3–55 ng/ml	> 60 ng/ml
Antipsychotic Drugs		
chlorpromazine	50–300 ng/ml	> 750 ng/ml
haloperidol	5–15 ng/ml	> 50 ng/ml
prochlorperazine	50–300 ng/ml	> 1,000 ng/ml
thioridazine	100–600 ng/ml	> 2,000 ng/ml
trifluoperazine	50–300 ng/ml	> 1,000 ng/ml
Opioid Agonists		
methadone	100–400 ng/ml	> 2,000 ng/ml
Sedative-Hypnotics		
amobarbital	1–5 mcg/ml	> 15 mcg/ml
butabarbital	1–2 mcg/ml	> 10 mcg/ml
chloral hydrate	2–12 mcg/ml	> 20 mcg/ml
ethchlorvynol	2–8 mcg/ml	> 20 mcg/ml
flurazepam	20–110 ng/ml	> 1,500 ng/ml
pentobarbital	1–5 mcg/ml	> 10 mcg/ml
secobarbital	2–5 mcg/ml	> 15 mcg/ml

Nurse's
Handbook of
Behavioral and Mental Health Drugs

Nurse's Handbook of
Behavioral and Mental Health Drugs

Third Edition

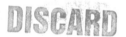

JONES AND BARTLETT PUBLISHERS
Sudbury, Massachusetts
BOSTON   TORONTO   LONDON   SINGAPORE

World Headquarters
Jones and Bartlett Publishers
40 Tall Pine Drive
Sudbury, MA 01776
978-443-5000
info@jbpub.com
www.jbpub.com

Jones and Bartlett Publishers
Canada
6339 Ormindale Way
Mississauga, Ontario L5V 1J2
Canada

Jones and Bartlett Publishers
International
Barb House, Barb Mews
London W6 7PA
United Kingdom

Jones and Bartlett's books and products are available through most bookstores and online book-sellers. To contact Jones and Bartlett Publishers directly, call 800-832-0034, fax 978-443-8000, or visit our website www.jbpub.com.

Substantial discounts on bulk quantities of Jones and Bartlett's publications are available to corporations, professional associations, and other qualified organizations. For details and specific discount information, contact the special sales department at Jones and Bartlett via the above contact information or send an email to special-sales@jbpub.com.

Production Credits
Publisher: Kevin Sullivan
Acquisitions Editor: Emily Ekle
Acquisitions Editor: Amy Sibley
Associate Editor: Patricia Donnelly
Editorial Assistant: Rachel Shuster
Supervising Production Editor: Carolyn F. Rogers
Associate Marketing Manager: Ilana Goddess
Manufacturing Buyer: Therese Connell

Clinical Reviewer: Marlene Ciranowicz-Steenburg, RN, MSN, CDE
Composition: Catherine E. Harold
Interior Illustrations: Rolin Graphics, Inc.
Cover Design: Kristin E. Ohlin
Cover Image: © ajt/ShutterStock, Inc.
Printing and Binding: Malloy, Inc.
Cover Printing: Malloy, Inc.

6048

Printed in the United States of America
12 11 10 09 08   10 9 8 7 6 5 4 3 2 1

CONTENTS

INDIVIDUAL DRUGS (organized alphabetically)

APPENDICES

Advisors

Steven L. Baumann, RN,CS, PhD, NPP, GNP
Associate Professor
Hunter College
New York, NY

Doris E. Bell, RN,BC, PhD, APRN
Professor of Nursing
Southern Illinois University
Edwardsville, IL

Katherine Berckman, RN,CS, DNSc
Associate Professor
College of Nursing
Valdosta State University
Valdosta, GA

Michelle Byrne, PharmD
Clinical Pharmacist Practitioner
Lahey Clinic
Burlington, MA
Adjunct Professor of Clinical Pharmacy
Massachusetts College of Pharmacy and Health Sciences
Boston, MA

Carlton K. Erickson, PhD
Professor of Pharmacology
College of Pharmacy
University of Texas
Austin, TX

Patrick R. Finley, PharmD, BCPP
Associate Clinical Professor
Psychopharmacology and Behavioral Health
Dept. of Clinical Pharmacy
University of California
San Francisco, CA

JoAnne D. Joyner, RN,CS, DNSc
Facility Service Line Manager, Acting
Mental Health Service Line
Dept. of Veteran Affairs Medical Center
Washington, DC

S. Casey Laizure, PharmD
Associate Professor
University of Tennessee
Memphis, TN

Peggy A. Szwabo, RN,CS, MSW, PhD, APN
Associate Professor
St. Louis University Medical School
St. Louis, MO
Consultant, Aging and Family
Szwabo & Assoc.
St. Louis, MO

Ronald Thomas, PhD
Assistant Professor
College of Pharmacy and Pharmaceutical Sciences
Florida A & M University
Tallahassee, FL

Reviewers and Clinical Consultants

Kimberly Anne Boykin Couch, PharmD
Clinical Specialist
Christiana Care Health System
Newark, DE
Adjunct Faculty
School of Nursing
University of Delaware
Newark, DE

Mark J. Cziraky, PharmD
Executive Vice President and Chief Operating Officer
Health Core
Newark, DE
Adjunct Assistant Professor
Philadelphia College of Pharmacy
University of the Sciences in Philadelphia
Philadelphia, PA

John P. Gatto, BS Pharm
Clinical Pharmacist
Owego, NY

Lisa A. Jensen, RN,CS, MS
Advanced Practice Registered Nurse
Salt Lake VA Healthcare System
Salt Lake City, UT

Patrick McDonnell, PharmD
Assistant Professor of Clinical Pharmacy
School of Pharmacy
Temple University
Philadelphia, PA

Susan L. Ravnan, PharmD
Assistant Professor
Thomas J. Long School of Pharmacy and Health Sciences
University of the Pacific
Stockton, CA

Michael J. Rice, RN,CSB, PhD, ARNP
Associate Professor
Intercollegiate Center for Nursing Education
Washington State University
Spokane, WA

P. Anne Roberts, RN,CS, MSN, ARNP, CARN
Instructor
College of Nursing
University of Kentucky
Lexington, KY

How to Use This Book

Jones and Bartlett's Nurse's Handbook of Behavioral and Mental Health Drugs, Third Edition, gives you what today's nurses working in the field of behavioral and mental health need: accurate, concise, and reliable facts. This book emphasizes the vital information you need to know before, during, and after drug administration. And as always, the information is presented in easy-to-understand language and organized alphabetically, so you can find what you need quickly.

What's Special

In addition to the drug information you expect to find in each entry (see "Drug Entries" for details), *Nurse's Handbook of Behavioral and Mental Health Drugs* boasts these special features:

- **Practical trim size and good-size type** give you a book that's easy to carry, easy to read, and easy to handle. You can hold the book in one hand, see complete pages at a glance, and use your other hand to document or perform other activities.
- **Colorful illustrations** throughout the text help you visualize selected mechanisms of action by showing how drugs work at the cellular, tissue, and organ levels. In addition, an appendix features a chart listing all the drugs whose mechanisms of action are illustrated, as well as other drugs with the same mechanisms of action.
- **No-nonsense writing style** that speaks everyday language and uses the terms and abbreviations you typically encounter in your practice. (See *Abbreviations* appendix.) And to avoid sexist language, we alternate between male and female pronouns throughout the book.
- **Up-to-date drug information,** including the latest FDA-approved drugs, new and changed indications, new warnings, and newly reported adverse reactions.
- **Dosage adjustment,** highlighted in color, alerts you to expected dosage changes for a patient with a specific condition or disorder, such as advanced age or renal impairment.
- **Warning,** highlighted in color, calls attention to important facts that you need to know before, during, and after drug administration. For example, in the amantadine hydrochloride entry, a warning informs you to monitor your patient for the signs and symptoms of neuroleptic malignant syndrome, a potentially life-

threatening condition, which may occur when the dosage is reduced or the drug discontinued.

- **Easy-to-use tables** for route, onset, steady state, peak, half-life, and duration and other tables in the appendices provide a time-saving way to track and check information. (See pages xv and xvi for details on route, onset, steady state, peak, half-life, and duration tables.)
- **Useful appendices** give an overview of the most important drug facts and nursing considerations related to behavioral and mental health nursing.

Drug Entries

Nurse's Handbook of Behavioral and Mental Health Drugs, Third Edition, clearly and concisely presents all the vital facts on the drugs that you'll typically administer. To help you find the information you need quickly, drug entries are organized alphabetically by generic drug name—from acamprosate to zonisamide. For ease of use, every drug entry follows a consistent format.

Generic and Trade Names

First, each entry identifies the drug's main generic name as well as alternate generic names. (For drugs prescribed by trade name, you can quickly check the comprehensive index, which refers you to the appropriate generic name and page.) Next, the entry lists the most common U.S. trade names for each drug. It also includes common trade names available only in Canada, marked (CAN).

Class, Category, and Schedule

Each entry lists the drug's chemical and therapeutic classes. With this information, you can compare drugs in the same chemical class but in different therapeutic classes and vice versa.

The entry also lists the FDA's pregnancy risk category, which categorizes drugs based on their potential to cause birth defects. (For details, see *FDA pregnancy risk categories.*) Where appropriate, the entry also includes the drug's controlled substance schedule. (For details, see *Controlled substance schedules,* page xvi.)

Indications and Dosages

This section lists FDA-approved indications specific to behavioral mental health. For each indication, you'll find the applicable drug form or route, age-group (adults, adolescents, or children), and dosage (which includes amount per dose, timing, and duration).

FDA PREGNANCY RISK CATEGORIES

Each drug may be placed in a pregnancy risk category based on the FDA's estimate of risk to the fetus. If the FDA hasn't provided a category, the *Nurse's Handbook of Behavioral and Mental Health Drugs* notes that the drug is "Not rated." The categories range from A to X, signifying least to greatest fetal risk.

A Controlled studies show no risk

Adequate, well-controlled studies with pregnant women have failed to demonstrate a risk to the fetus in any trimester of pregnancy.

B No evidence of risk in humans

Adequate, well-controlled studies with pregnant women haven't shown increased risk of fetal abnormalities despite adverse findings in animals, or—in the absence of adequate human studies—animal studies show no fetal risk. The chance of fetal harm exists but is remote.

C Risk can't be ruled out

Adequate, well-controlled human studies are lacking, and animal studies are lacking as well or have demonstrated a risk to the fetus. A chance of fetal harm exists if the drug is administered during pregnancy, but the potential benefits may outweigh the potential risk.

D Positive evidence of risk

Studies in humans, or investigational or post-marketing data, have demonstrated fetal risk. Nevertheless, potential benefits from the drug's use may outweigh potential risks. For example, the drug may be acceptable if needed in a life-threatening situation or serious disease for which safer drugs can't be used or are ineffective.

X Contraindicated in pregnancy

Studies in animals or humans, or investigational or post-marketing reports, have demonstrated positive evidence of fetal abnormalities or risks; these risks clearly outweigh any possible benefit to the patient.

Route, Onset, Steady State, Peak, Half-Life, and Duration

Quick-reference tables show you the drug's onset, steady state, peak, half-life, and duration (when known) for each administration route. The *onset of action* is the time a drug takes to be absorbed, reach a therapeutic blood level, and elicit an initial therapeutic response.

CONTROLLED SUBSTANCE SCHEDULES

The Controlled Substances Act of 1970 mandated that certain prescription drugs be categorized in schedules based on their potential for abuse. The greater their abuse potential, the greater the restrictions on their prescription. The controlled substance schedules range from I to V, signifying highest to lowest abuse potential.

I High potential for abuse

No accepted medical use exists for Schedule I drugs, which include heroin and lysergic acid diethylamide (LSD).

II High potential for abuse

Use may lead to severe physical or psychological dependence. Prescriptions must be written in ink or typewritten and must be signed by the prescriber. Oral prescriptions must be confirmed in writing within 72 hours and may be given only in a genuine emergency. No renewals are permitted.

III Some potential for abuse

Use may lead to low-to-moderate physical dependence or high psychological dependence. Prescriptions may be oral or written. Up to five renewals are permitted within 6 months.

IV Low potential for abuse

Use may lead to limited physical or psychological dependence. Prescriptions may be oral or written. Up to five renewals are permitted within 6 months.

V Subject to state and local regulation

Abuse potential is low; a prescription may not be required.

The *steady state* is achieved when the amount of drug that's excreted is equal to the amount of drug that's available. The *peak therapeutic effect* occurs when a drug reaches its highest blood concentration and the greatest amount of drug reaches the site of action, thus producing the maximum therapeutic response. The *half-life* is the amount of time required for half of the drug to be eliminated from the body. The *duration of action* is the amount of time that a drug remains at a blood concentration that produces a therapeutic response.

Mechanism of Action

Set off by a box, this section concisely describes how a drug achieves its therapeutic effects at the cellular, tissue, and organ levels, as appropriate. Illustrations of selected mechanisms of action lend exceptional detail and clarity to sometimes complex processes.

Incompatibilities

This section alerts you to drugs or solutions that are incompatible with the topic drug when mixed in a syringe or solution or infused through the same I.V. line.

Contraindications

An alphabetical list details the conditions and disorders that preclude administration of the topic drug.

Interactions

This section in each entry presents the drugs, foods, and activities (such as alcohol use and smoking) that can cause important, problematic, or life-threatening interactions with the topic drug. For each interacting drug, food, or activity, you'll learn the effects of the interaction.

Adverse Reactions

Organized by body system, this section highlights common, serious, and life-threatening adverse reactions in alphabetical order.

Overdose

This section alerts you to the signs and symptoms of overdose to help you recognize potential life-threatening adverse reactions. And you'll be informed of the medical and nursing interventions you can expect to take in response to the overdose so that you'll be prepared to administer care during an emergency situation.

Nursing Considerations

Warnings, general precautions, and key information that you must know before, during, and after drug administration are detailed in this section. Examples include whether or not a pill can be crushed and how to properly reconstitute, dilute, store, handle, or dispose of a drug.

Patient teaching information is also included here. You'll find important guidelines for patients, such as how and when to take each prescribed drug, how to spot and manage adverse reactions, which cautions to observe, when to call the prescriber, and more. To save you time, however, this section doesn't repeat basic patient-teaching points.

(For a summary of those, see *Teaching Your Patient About Behavioral and Mental Health Drug Therapy*.)

Other Therapeutic Uses

This section lists other FDA-approved therapeutic indications used outside the field of behavioral mental health for the topic drug.

In short, *Nurse's Handbook of Behavioral and Mental Health Drugs* is designed expressly to give you more of what you need. It puts vital drug information at your fingertips.

TEACHING YOUR PATIENT ABOUT BEHAVIORAL AND MENTAL HEALTH DRUG THERAPY

Your teaching about behavioral and mental health drug therapy will vary with your patient's needs and your practice setting. To help guide your teaching, each drug entry provides key information that you must teach your patient about that drug. For all patients, however, you should also:

☑ Teach the generic and trade name for each prescribed drug that he'll take after discharge—even if he took the drug before admission.

☑ Clearly explain why each drug was prescribed, how it works, and what it's supposed to do. To help your patient understand the drug's therapeutic effects, relate its action to her disorder or condition.

☑ Review the drug form, dosage, and route with the patient. Tell him whether the drug is a tablet, suppository, spray, aerosol, or other form, and explain how to administer it correctly. Also, tell him how often to take the drug and for what length of time. Emphasize that he should take the drug exactly as prescribed.

☑ Describe the drug's appearance and explain that scored tablets can be broken in half for safe, accurate dosing. Warn against breaking unscored tablets because doing so may alter the dosage. If your patient has trouble swallowing capsules, explain that she can open those that contain sprinkles and take them with food or a drink but that she shouldn't open capsules that contain powder. Also, warn her not to crush or chew enteric-coated, extended-release, or sustained-release drug forms.

☑ Teach the patient about common adverse reactions that may occur. Advise him to notify the prescriber at once if a dangerous adverse reaction, such as syncope, occurs.

(continued)

TEACHING YOUR PATIENT ABOUT BEHAVIORAL AND MENTAL HEALTH DRUG THERAPY *(continued)*

☑ Warn her not to suddenly stop taking a drug if she's bothered by unpleasant adverse reactions, such as a rash and mild itching. Instead, encourage her to discuss the reactions with her prescriber, who may adjust the dosage or substitute a drug that causes fewer adverse reactions.

☑ Warn the patient that some adverse reactions, such as dizziness and drowsiness, can impair his ability to operate machinery, drive a car, or perform other activities that require alertness. Help him develop a dosing schedule that prevents adverse reactions from interfering with such activities.

☑ Inform the patient which adverse reactions resolve with time.

☑ Teach the patient how to store the drug properly. Let him know if the drug is sensitive to light or temperature and how to protect it from these elements.

☑ Instruct the patient to store the drug in its original container, if possible, with the drug's name and dosage clearly printed on the label.

☑ Inform the patient which devices to use—and which ones to avoid—for drug storage or administration. For example, warn him not to take liquid paraldehyde with a plastic cup or utensils.

☑ Teach the patient what to do if she misses a dose. Generally, she should take a once-daily drug as soon as she remembers—provided that she remembers within the first 24 hours. If 24 hours have elapsed, she should take the next scheduled dose, but not double the dose. If she has questions or concerns about missed doses, tell her to contact the prescriber.

☑ Provide information that's specific to the prescribed drug. For example, if a patient takes an antidepressant, such as imipramine, urge him to avoid alcohol because of the risk for increased CNS depression. Or, if the patient takes a selective 5-hydroxytryptamine$_1$ (5-HT$_1$) receptor agonist, such as almotriptan, to treat acute migraine attacks, inform the patient that he shouldn't take the drug to treat non-migraine headaches.

☑ Advise the patient to refill prescriptions promptly, unless she no longer needs the drug. Also instruct her to discard expired drugs because they may become ineffective or even dangerous over time.

☑ Warn the patient to keep all drugs out of the reach of children at all times.

FOREWORD

Jones and Bartlett's Nurse's Handbook of Behavioral and Mental Health Drugs, Third Edition, is a nursing drug reference designed to help you provide safe, effective drug therapy—one of your most important responsibilities. It gives you the latest drug information and presents that information in easy-to-use and consistently organized drug entries that are sequenced alphabetically. This handbook will save you time and focus your efforts on giving the best patient care.

Meeting Your Needs

Nurse's Handbook of Behavioral and Mental Health Drugs is designed for nurses working in critical and acute care, home care, long-term care, and other health care settings, such as psychiatric hospitals, drug and alcohol rehabilitation facilities, outpatient centers, and emergency departments, as well as for clinical nurse specialists and nursing students.

The handbook has been developed, written, edited, and checked by experienced practicing nurses. Expert consultants, reviewers, and advisors—nurses and pharmacists—have helped to ensure the accuracy and reliability of the information covered in each entry. What's more, every fact is verified against the most prominent drug references today, including the *American Hospital Formulary Service Drug Information, Drug Facts and Comparisons, The Physicians' Desk Reference,* and the US PDI's *Drug Information for the Health Care Professional.*

Nurse's Handbook of Behavioral and Mental Health Drugs emphasizes the vital information you need to know before, during, and after drug administration. Each drug entry contains the latest FDA information on newly approved drugs and changes to existing drugs, including new indications, dosages, and adverse reactions. Beyond the drug facts, you'll also find sections that contain valuable nursing information, including:

• the nurse's role in delivering behavioral and mental health drug therapy
• key components of the nurse–patient relationship for successful drug therapy
• tips on assessing a patient with a behavioral or mental health disorder

• the safety concerns and nursing considerations you'll need to provide drug therapy to your patients with special needs.

Getting More from Your Drug Reference

The knowledge and skills to administer drugs safely and effectively are essential to your best patient care. You need to know how a drug is classified, its mechanism of action, how it's metabolized, and its intended effect. You also need to know the nursing considerations and patient teaching that are specific to each drug. *Nurse's Handbook of Behavioral and Mental Health Drugs* gives you all that and more. In the appendices, you'll find:

• Seizure classification
• Cytochrome P450 enzyme system
• Commonly abused drugs
• Common sources of caffeine
• Common sources of tyramine
• Drugs that cause serotonin syndrome
• Psychotropic herbal remedies
• Treating drug overdose
• Body mass index calculation
• Mechanism of action illustrations table
• Weights and equivalents
• Abbreviations

The approach to treating behavioral and mental health patients has changed dramatically over the past few decades, and much of that change can be attributed to pharmacologic advances. Drugs developed specifically to treat these disorders have opened doors otherwise closed for some patients and improved the quality of life for many.

With the introduction of a new drug comes the added responsibility of knowing how it works so that you can recognize important adverse reactions and monitor your patient for a therapeutic or unintended change. Also with new drugs come new drug combinations, so you need to know how drugs interact and how one drug may affect the metabolism of another. As a nurse, you are the professional your patient depends on to monitor his or her response to drug therapy.

With so much research and information available, you need a reference that gives you accurate, concise, and reliable drug facts to help you deliver the best and safest care possible. For this reason, you'll want your own copy of *Jones and Bartlett's Nurse's Handbook of Behavioral and Mental Health Drugs.* It gives you all this and more.

Thomas L. Hardie, RN,CS, EdD, NP
Associate Professor
Department of Nursing
University of Delaware
Newark, DE

Michelle Byrne, PharmD
Clinical Pharmacist Practitioner
Lahey Clinic
Burlington, MA
Adjunct Professor of Clinical Pharmacy
Massachusetts College of Pharmacy
    and Health Sciences
Boston, MA

HOW BEHAVIORAL AND MENTAL HEALTH DRUGS WORK

To understand how behavioral and mental health drugs work in the body, you'll need to recall how the nervous system functions. The following overview of the structure and function of the nervous system shows the connection between a drug's mechanism of action and its therapeutic response.

The Nervous System

The nervous system is the body's highly complex communication system that helps to maintain the balance among the other systems. It does this through status reports of chemical balances and imbalances sent from each body system to the brain through sensory (afferent) neurons and through commands, instructions, and responses from the brain sent back to each body system through motor (efferent) neurons.

The nervous system has two parts: the central nervous system (CNS) and the peripheral nervous system. The CNS consists primarily of the brain, brain stem, and spinal cord. The peripheral nervous system is comprised of all nerve fibers, nerve endings, and related nervous tissue throughout the body. The sensory nerves of the peripheral nervous system detect changes in the body's homeostasis, as well as all manner of sensory data such as light, sound, touch, heat and cold, odors, aromas, tastes, internal or external pain, physical comfort or discomfort, and virtually any identifiable emotion. The afferent neurons sense the stimulus and carry an impulse through a nerve fiber pathway to particular centers in the brain that analyze the data and form a response. This response is then carried back to the body by the efferent nerves and may command a muscle to move or a gland to secrete.

Neurons

The neurons of the nervous system have two important functions: to provide a link between adjacent neurons and receptors and to form proteins and amino acids for the production of chemical messages called *neurotransmitters.*

A neuron's structure is straightforward, if not exactly simple. The central area of a neuron is a body of cytoplasm that contains a nucleus and the endoplasmic reticulum and the Golgi apparatus, all of which are involved in synthesizing proteins and amino acids to be used as neurotransmitters.

A neuron has a unique cell structure, with dendrites branching out in asymmetrical directions. These are the neural connections to other similar cells. Dendrites receive neuronal impulses from adjacent cells and fibers and relay the impulse to the cell body. The cell body then produces and synthesizes the organic chemicals and compounds that will carry a chemoelectric impulse through the neuron so that it can be transmitted to adjacent neural tissues and sites.

The impulse travels through the cell body into a portion of the cell known as the axon. The axon is longer and larger than the dendrites, and it ends with paddle-like nerve endings called *axon terminals.* The function of the axon is to transport neurotransmitters to the axon terminals, where they're released into the synaptic cleft to bind with receptor sites on the membranes of adjacent cells. Thus, through this process of neuronal transmission, the nerve impulse is sent to the next neuron—one link in a chain of literally billions of cells.

By its structure, the neuron can only move impulses in one direction—from the dendrites, through the cell body, and through the axon terminals. An individual neuron mirrors the nervous system in this way; impulses may travel in only one direction through the nervous system, with sensory neurons always transmitting impulses toward the brain and motor neurons always transmitting information and commands from the brain to muscles, glands, and organs.

Nerve Impulse Conduction

Neurons have a cell membrane that is selectively permeable to various chemicals and nutrients and to ions such as sodium, potassium, and chloride, which give the membrane an electrical charge. In fact, there is a constantly operating system of balance between sodium and potassium ions across the neuronal membrane. With slightly more sodium ions on the outside of the cell membrane, the neuron has a positive charge, which is its resting membrane potential.

Sodium ions outside the neuron and potassium ions inside the neuron are exchanged through channels in the membrane and by way of the sodium-potassium pump. At rest, most of the sodium channels are closed and the potassium channels are open. The sodium-potassium pump actively transports three sodium ions out of the cell across the cell membrane and brings two potassium ions into the cell to maintain the positive charge on the outside of the cell.

Stimulation of the neuron causes the sodium channels to open, and sodium rushes inside the cell. With an influx of sodium ions and a depletion of potassium ions, the neuron becomes increasingly depolarized. When the influx of sodium ions peaks, the neuron reaches an action potential. It is electrically unstable and ready to fire an impulse.

The ebb and flow of potassium and sodium ions through the neuronal membrane is a self-propagating series of polarizations and depolarizations that continues as long as impulses are being received. Thus, after an impulse has been conducted, potassium ions will again be concentrated inside the membrane and sodium ions outside the membrane, and the process of achieving an action potential begins again.

Synapses

Neurons communicate with each other and with receptor cells across synapses, which are the junctions across which impulses are transmitted. Between synapses are synaptic clefts, which provide an insulating barrier between neurons and receptor cells. An impulse will not cross a synaptic cleft unless it has sufficient strength to stimulate the action of neurotransmitters stored in vesicles within the axon terminal. When the neurotransmitter is released into the synaptic cleft, it travels to the adjacent cell's membrane and binds to compatible receptor sites. When these receptor sites become occupied, the impulse is transmitted into the new cell. If the receptor cell happens to be a neuron, the signal continues through it to the next axon terminal. If the receptor happens to be a muscle cell or a glandular cell, then the impulse may trigger physical movement, a contraction, or a glandular secretion.

Receptors

Membrane receptors are a vital component of synaptic transmission. When neurotransmitters are released from the presynaptic (sending) neuron and travel across the synaptic cleft, they must make contact with a receptor embedded in the postsynaptic (receiving) cell's membrane to transmit their information. Most receptors are made up of transmembrane glycoprotein chains, and the binding of a neurotransmitter with a receptor initiates a change in the makeup of the protein. This molecular and structural change signals the transfer of information from one cell to another.

Receptors offer clues about the potency of the neurotransmitter bound to them. The relative effectiveness of a neurotransmitter can be seen by comparing its actual effect with the maximum level of change possible. The type of effect possible may be determined by the type of receptors and the neurotransmitters they respond to. For example, cholinergic neurotransmitters bind to cholinergic receptors, and catecholamine neurotransmitters bind to adrenergic receptors. Like locks, membrane receptors will open only to the key that fits.

Neurotransmitters

As described above, neurotransmitters conduct impulses across synaptic clefts as part of neuronal transmission. Whether a neuron resides adjacent to a finger and transmits a sensory impulse that was triggered by touch or it resides in the limbic system and transmits an impulse that causes an emotional response, the basic mechanism of neuronal transmission is the same. (See *Defining a Neurotransmitter: Three Essential Criteria.*)

The body uses various groups of organic chemicals to provide the language of neuronal transmission. These different groups of neurotransmitters appear to have certain influences within the body. Their balances are delicate, and the potential for neurological dysfunction is always present, especially in the contexts of nutrition, ingestion of drugs, and other external variables.

An important distinction among various neurotransmitters is molecular size. The size of the molecule determines the speed of neuronal transmission and offers clues as to how the neurotransmitter is synthesized. Small-molecule neurotransmitters—such as dopamine and norepinephrine—transmit impulses rapidly and directly. This rapid speed occurs because the neurotransmitter typically causes only an ion channel to open, which changes the membrane's polarity and transmits an impulse. Large-molecule neurotransmitters—such as the neuropeptides—transmit their impulse more slowly and are harder to synthesize. They usually must bind with another substance in the receptor cell, not simply a channel, and this chemical action sends out a second substance inside the postsynaptic cell to trigger various cellular responses. However, neuronal transmission that's stimulated by a neuropeptide sometimes can involve a single step, such as when the intended receptor site is an ion channel. In such instances, the neurotransmission is about as fast as that initiated by a small-molecule neurotransmitter.

All neurotransmitters are synthesized within the neuron. Usually, small-molecule neurotransmitters are synthesized in the cytoplasm of the neuron and then transported to the axon terminal in synaptic vesicles, or containers, formed by the Golgi apparatus. These neurotransmitters can also be synthesized within the maturing vesicles as they're transported through the axon to the axon

DEFINING A NEUROTRANSMITTER: THREE ESSENTIAL CRITERIA

In order to qualify as a neurotransmitter, a chemical substance must meet the following criteria:

- *Localization*—The chemical substance must be present in the presynaptic terminal of the neuron.
- *Release*—The chemical substance must be released from the neuron when it's stimulated and simultaneous with the neuron's depolarization. Thus, not only is the neurotransmitter released, but it also transmits a chemoelectric charge.
- *Identity*—The chemical substance must have the same effect on a target cell as stimulation of a nerve impulse would produce.

terminal. Large-molecule neurotransmitters undergo a more complex synthesis, which begins in the cell's ribosomes and proceeds through the endoplasmic reticulum. After this, they're packaged into large vesicles, processed by the Golgi apparatus, and repackaged into vesicles that are ready for transport to the synaptic site.

When a nerve impulse reaches the axon terminal and the vesicle has fused with the presynaptic cell's membrane, the neurotransmitter is released into the synaptic cleft to bind with compatible receptor sites on the postsynaptic cell's membrane. Then a chemical reaction occurs—possibly a change in molecular structure—that sends a chemical message into the receptor cell. The response might be excitatory (replicating or enhancing the impulse) or inhibitory (effectively blocking an impulse).

Basically, neurotransmitters stimulate the opening or closing of ion channels in the membrane of the postsynaptic cell and either cause it to polarize or depolarize. Excitatory neurotransmitters may open channels for sodium and potassium ions to depolarize the membrane. Inhibitory neurotransmitters may open channels for potassium and chloride ions to polarize the membrane. Ultimately, however, the receptors of the postsynaptic cell determine whether a response is to be excitatory or inhibitory. A neurotransmitter might have either effect, depending on the type of receptor. (See *Comparing Neurotransmitters,* pages xxx and xxxi.)

Various neurotransmitters have different functions and chemical structures. Grouped below by their chemical structures, they are: acetylcholine, amino acids, monoamines, and neuropeptides.

COMPARING NEUROTRANSMITTERS

Neurons use neurotransmitters to communicate with each other, facilitating our thoughts, feelings, and actions. The following table shows the effects and characteristics of selected neurotransmitters.

Neurotransmitter	Effect	Characteristics
Acetylcholine	Excitatory or inhibitory	• Located in CNS and peripheral nervous system • Regulates sleep cycle, memory, muscle activity • Decreased amounts in Alzheimer's disease
Amino Acids Aspartate and glutamate	Excitatory	• Located in CNS • Glutamate may have a role in Alzheimer's disease, Huntington's disease, Parkinson's disease, cognition, and memory
GABA and glycine	Inhibitory	• Located in CNS • Drugs that increase GABA regulate anxiety and sleep by inhibiting excitatory response
Monoamines Dopamine	Excitatory or inhibitory	• Located in brain • Regulates cognition, emotions, motor function, and motivation • A lack of dopamine found in Parkinson's disease; an excess of dopamine found in schizophrenia
Norepinephrine	Excitatory or inhibitory	• Located in CNS and autonomic nervous system • Stimulates the heart and skeletal muscles; facilitates vasoconstriction • Regulates attention and mood • Plays a role in anxiety and depressive disorders
Epinephrine	Excitatory or inhibitory	• Located in CNS and autonomic nervous system • Causes anxiety, increased alertness, tachycardia, tachypnea, and vasodilation

COMPARING NEUROTRANSMITTERS *(continued)*

Neurotransmitter	Effect	Characteristics
Monoamines (continued)		
Histamine	Excitatory	• Located in blood vessels, bronchial smooth muscles, CNS, GI mucosa, and skin • First line of defense against bodily injury; regulates biorhythms, emotions, temperature and water balance
Serotonin	Inhibitory	• Located in CNS and GI tract • Regulates sleep cycle, mood, pain, and temperature • A lack of serotonin found in patients with depression
Neuropeptides Endorphins and enkephalins	Inhibitory	• Located in CNS, GI tract, and retina • Blocks pain sensation
Substance P	Excitatory	• Located in CNS • Regulates transmission of pain information; promotes memory • Metabolism of substance P may be altered in Alzheimer's disease

Acetylcholine

Acetylcholine is formed by the union of acetylcoenzyme A and choline in the presynaptic axon terminals, and it is stored in vesicles located near the cell membrane. Its primary function is to inhibit or mediate synaptic activity in the nervous system. When acetylcholine is released from the presynaptic axon terminal, it traverses the synaptic cleft and binds to either nicotinic or muscarinic receptors. Nicotinic receptors are found on the postsynaptic myoneural junction. When acetylcholine binds with these receptors, it allows sodium ions to enter the cell, causing depolarization. Muscarinic receptors are found primarily in the parasympathetic nervous system. The binding of acetylcholine to muscarinic receptors signals a secondary response inside the cell, so these reactions take longer to have an effect.

Acetylcholine functions within the parasympathetic nervous system to balance the dopaminergic effects of the sympathetic nervous system. These two systems actually enervate many of the same organs and provide excitatory and inhibitory impulses to regulate their functioning. The parasympathetic nervous system functions to conserve energy and restore body resources. In contrast, the sympathetic nervous system is poised for action, ready to expend energy and body resources in response to emergency situations or stressors.

Amino Acids

Amino acids are the essential building blocks of proteins. Over a hundred different amino acids occur in nature, twenty of which provide the structural basis of all proteins, peptides, and polypeptides.

Aspartate (aspartic acid) and glutamate (glutamic acid) function as excitatory neurotransmitters in the CNS. Glutamate binds to the N-methyl-D-aspartate (NMDA) receptor and causes a chain of events related to many biological functions. It also may have a role in Alzheimer's disease, Huntington's disease, and Parkinson's disease.

Gamma-aminobutyric acid (GABA) and glycine are inhibitory amino acid neurotransmitters. GABA receptors are found throughout the nervous system. When GABA binds to its receptors, it increases membrane permeability to chloride ions, causing hyperpolarization and inhibiting the excitatory response. Excess GABA in the synaptic cleft is probably removed by the glial cells to prevent buildup. Glycine is found mostly in the spinal cord. It's a fast acting neurotransmitter that, like GABA, causes hyperpolarization and inhibits the excitatory response.

Monoamines

The monoamine system consists of compounds with a molecular structure of a single nitrogen atom. Monoamines that function as neurotransmitters include histamine, serotonin, and the catecholamines—dopamine, epinephrine, and norepinephrine. The catecholamines are found throughout the nervous system.

In the neurons, tyrosine is converted to levodopa and then to dopamine, and it's stored in the presynaptic vesicles where it may then be converted to norepinephrine. Dopamine exerts a slow inhibitory action on CNS neurons. It's located in the brain and autonomic nervous system, where it modulates emotions and moods and regulates motor function. Dopamine is important in the treatment of Parkinson's disease and schizophrenia. The symptoms of Parkinson's disease may be caused by a lack of dopamine in the brain of these patients, while patients with schizophrenia may have an excess of dopamine in the brain.

Norepinephrine is found in the CNS and in the sympathetic branch of the autonomic nervous system. It has numerous receptor sites within the body and functions to balance or counteract para-sympathetic neuronal impulses. Consequently, neurologic functions associated with rest and digestion are shut down, and those functions related to preparing the body for strenuous physical action are activated. Norepinephrine stimulates the heart to beat faster, facilitates vasoconstriction, and stimulates skeletal muscles. A lack of norepinephrine at the synapse may occur in depression.

Epinephrine, also known as adrenalin, is the "emergency use" neurotransmitter. It elicits similar effects as norepinephrine, such as increasing the heart rate, but it also strengthens contractions of the heart muscle. Other effects of epinephrine include anxiety, increased alertness, tachypnea, and vasodilation—all of which are necessary for emergency and stress-related movement.

Histamine is the first line of defense against bodily injury caused by ingested or inhaled agents or tactile contact with agents that cause an inflammatory or allergic response. Histamines are found in the bloodstream, gastrointestinal mucosa, CNS, and skin, along small blood vessels in connective tissue, and in the tissues of the bronchial smooth muscle cells. Histamine has an excitatory function, and it also may help to regulate biorhythms, emotions, and temperature.

Serotonin, which is also known as 5-hydroxytryptamine (5-HT), comes from tryptophan, an amino acid found in animal and fish products, and it's metabolized by the enzyme monoamine oxidase. It's located in the CNS, stomach, and upper small intestine. Serotonin has several receptor types to which it binds, and its function is mostly inhibitory. It's known to interact with and influence other drugs and disease conditions. For instance, serotonin supplies part of the chemical framework for normal sleep patterns, which includes brain-active and brain-inactive sleep in several cycles throughout a typical night's rest. A depletion of serotonin has been observed to cause prolonged wakefulness in animals. Also, a lowered level of serotonin in the brain increases a person's sensitivity to pain. As a person's tolerance toward morphine develops, the production of serotonin nearly doubles, although the accumulation of serotonin doesn't. There may be a correlation between low serotonin levels in the brain and depression.

Neuropeptides
The neuropeptide neurotransmitters have a large and complex molecular structure. They're synthesized in the cell body and transported to active zones. Usually, they're slower acting than the small-molecule neurotransmitters because a second-messenger substance

within the postsynaptic cell typically will be involved in the transmission sequence. Also, the neuropeptide usually binds with another substance—such as a protein—at the receptor site, which takes more time than opening an ion channel.

Neuropeptides are located in the CNS, gastrointestinal tract, and the retina. Their function, which may be excitatory or inhibitory, is to regulate behavior, cardiovascular and respiratory function, digestive processes, emotions, food intake, growth, memory, reproduction, and salt and water metabolism. In relation to behavioral and mental health therapy, the neuropeptide neurotransmitters that function in the CNS include the opioid peptides and substance P.

The endogenous opioid neuropeptides (those synthesized within the body) include the endorphins and the enkephalins. They are called *opioids* because they have morphinelike effects and their molecular structure is similar to morphine. Opioid neuropeptides increase the polarization level of the neuronal membrane and disrupt the successful firing of an impulse at the strength that's necessary for it to bridge the synaptic cleft. The opioids are also capable of inhibiting neurotransmitter release.

Because pain is a composite of many complex neurologic and physiologic processes, the control of pain by endogenous opioids is also complex. The endorphins apparently can only affect the sensation of pain. If endorphins are repeatedly released or administered, the body develops a tolerance to them, and sudden withdrawal produces symptoms similar to withdrawal from morphine.

The enkephalins are derived from proenkephalin (found in the adrenal gland and reproductive system) and are widely distributed in the brain, especially the pituitary gland, thalamus, and hypothalamus. When axon terminals release enkephalins, they have a depressant effect upon the CNS, and they function to control and regulate pain at the spinal neuronal pathways and beyond. They may inhibit other neurotransmitters and reduce the emotional and physiologic perception of pain intensity. They're quickly degraded in the tissues and in circulation; thus, they are only short-term painkillers. The opioid neuropeptides, along with other neuropeptides, may be involved with the development of psychopathologic behavior.

Substance P, another neuropeptide, was first isolated from extracts of intestine and from brain tissue, and since it was in powdered form, the discoverers labeled it substance P. Because this neuropeptide figures so highly in the perception of pain, the label is even more appropriate now than at the time of its discovery. Substance P is widely distributed in the CNS, especially in areas where the endogenous pain control systems are located. It functions as a pain neurotransmitter from the periphery. Substance P also regulates processes related to visual, olfactory, and auditory perception. Its distribution follows neuronal pathways that parallel those of the enkephalins, so these neuropeptides together may provide neurotransmitter control to switch on or inhibit the sensation of pain as it's presented to the body. As a neurotransmitter, substance P triggers a low and long-lasting depolarization in the axon terminals of the primary sensory nerves of the spinal cord. It has also been found to inhibit some of the action of acetylcholine and modulate neurotransmission involving excitatory amino acids and aspartate in the brain.

Substance P can promote memory and also improve functional recovery of certain types of brain lesions, which may make substance P a suitable model for the development of drugs that mimic these effects. And because the metabolism of substance P is altered in Alzheimer's disease, the disease and the neuropeptide may be linked.

Therapeutic Classes

Here are some examples of the therapeutic classes you'll find in *Nurse's Handbook of Behavioral and Mental Health Drugs.*

Antialcohol Drugs

This class of drugs helps maintain abstinence from alcohol, which, when consumed long-term in excessive amounts, may disrupt the balance of neuronal excitation and inhibition and may cause liver damage and potentially life-threatening cirrhosis. Alcoholism is a major societal problem in the United States and Canada.

Two drugs classified as antialcohol drugs are disulfiram and acamprosate. Disulfiram supports the treatment of chronic alcoholism by producing an acute sensitivity to alcohol. Unlike disulfiram, acamprosate does not cause alcohol aversion nor does it cause a disulfiram-like reaction as a result of alcohol intake. Although its mechanism of action has not been clearly determined, it may support alcohol abstinence by interacting with glutamate and GABA neurotransmitter systems in the central nervous system to restore the balance between neuronal excitation and inhibition.

Antianxiety Drugs

The cause of anxiety is unknown, but the limbic system and cortical area of the brain contain specific receptors that may help to regulate anxiety. The main inhibitory neurotransmitter is GABA, and when it's released from the presynaptic nerve ending, it binds with the GABA receptor that's embedded in the postsynaptic cell membrane. This causes the chloride channel within the receptor to open, allowing chloride ions to flow into the cell and causing hyperpolarization and inhibition of the excitatory impulse. Benzodiazepines and other drugs, such as zaleplon and zolpidem, engage with the GABA receptor by interacting with its benzodiazepine binding site. This enhances the action of GABA, causing the chloride channels to open more frequently and leading to hyperpolarization. The increased inhibition relieves anxiety.

Buspirone is an example of a drug that acts selectively at serotonin receptors in the brain. Buspirone has a high affinity for the serotonin 5-hydroxytryptamine$_{1A}$ (5-HT$_{1A}$) receptor. When the drug interacts with presynaptic 5-HT$_{1A}$ receptors, it decreases the firing rate of the neuron so that less serotonin is released into the synapse. The drug may also act as a partial agonist at the postsynaptic 5-HT$_{1A}$ receptors, blocking the effects of serotonin.

Anticonvulsants

Seizures are caused by the abnormal discharge of neurons in the CNS. Anticonvulsants prevent seizures by three main mechanisms: affecting the voltage-dependent sodium ion channels, enhancing GABA-induced inhibition, and reducing excitatory transmission.

Sodium is needed for conduction of nerve impulses. Normally, when sodium channels are open in the neuronal cell membrane, sodium moves into the cell, which causes depolarization and conduction of the nerve impulse. Drugs such as carbamazepine and oxcarbazepine keep sodium out of the cell by blocking sodium channels, which slows nerve impulse transmission and neuron firing. Lamotrigine may stabilize neuron membranes by blocking sodium channels, preventing release of excitatory neurotransmitters, such as glutamate and aspartate. Phenytoin and other hydantoin derivatives regulate voltage-dependent sodium and calcium channels in neurons.

Although gabapentin is a drug that's similar to endogenous GABA, it probably doesn't act on GABA receptors. Its exact mechanism of action is unknown, but it may cause altered GABA metabolism or reuptake, which inhibits the rapid firing of neurons that are normally associated with seizures. Other drugs such as benzodiazepines prevent seizures by potentiating the effects of GABA and stopping the spread of seizure activity caused by seizure-producing foci in the cortex, thalamus, and limbic structures. Tiagabine and valproic acid inhibit neuronal reuptake of GABA, leaving more available in the synapse to open chloride channels. This results in hyperpolarization and prevents the transmission of nerve impulses. Topiramate increases the availability of GABA by blocking voltage-sensitive sodium channels, which promotes the movement of chloride ions into neurons.

Drugs that elevate the seizure threshold reduce the frequency of seizure attacks by depressing the motor cortex, making the CNS less responsive to convulsive stimuli. Ethosuximide and the barbiturate phenobarbital may act in this way. Primidone prevents seizures by decreasing the excitability of neurons and increasing the motor cortex's threshold of electrical stimulation.

Antidepressants

Depression may occur when a person has a synaptic lack of the monoamine neurotransmitters dopamine, norepinephrine, or serotonin. Several categories of drugs with different mechanisms of action are used to treat depression, including tricyclic antidepressants, MAO inhibitors, selective serotonin reuptake inhibitors (SSRIs), and newer drugs that are more specific to certain receptors.

The tricyclic antidepressants, such as amitriptyline, block norepinephrine and serotonin reuptake by the adrenergic nerve terminals. Normally, when these neurotransmitters are released, they bind with receptor sites on the postsynaptic cell membrane. Then the neurotransmitters are taken back into the nerve and stored for future use. By blocking the reuptake mechanism, norepinephrine and serotonin levels are increased, which may elevate mood and reduce depression.

Normally, the enzyme monoamine oxidase (MAO), breaks down monoamine neurotransmitters, such as serotonin, and the catecholamines dopamine, epinephrine, and norepinephrine. An MAO inhibitor, such as phenelzine, blocks the action of this enzyme and increases the level of these neurotransmitters in the synapse, making more available to engage with receptors on the postsynaptic cell membrane. After continuous therapy of 2 to 4 weeks, the serotonin receptors become desensitized or less active, which may explain why the therapeutic effects of an MAO inhibitor take several weeks and why the effects are prolonged after the drug is discontinued.

An SSRI, such as fluoxetine, selectively inhibits the reuptake of serotonin by CNS neurons, making more serotonin available in the synapse. An elevated serotonin level may elevate the patient's mood and reduce depression.

Nefazodone is an example of an antidepressant that's more selective in its mechanism of action. It inhibits the reuptake of serotonin at the presynaptic neuron, which increases the level of serotonin. It also may antagonize the postsynaptic serotonin receptor, further increasing the level of serotonin at the synapse.

Antidyskinetics

Dopamine is synthesized and released by neurons in the brain leading from the substantia nigra to the basal ganglia. It functions as an inhibitory neurotransmitter, balancing the excitatory effects of acetylcholine. Patients with Parkinson's disease have progressive degeneration of these neurons, which reduces the supply of intrasynaptic dopamine, and results in an excessive amount of stimuli going to the voluntary muscles, which is why patients with Parkinson's disease have muscle rigidity, a shuffling gait, and tremors of the head and extremities.

Levodopa, the precursor of dopamine, is used to supplement a low level of endogenous dopamine, very little of which gets across the blood-brain barrier. Levodopa crosses the blood-brain barrier where it's converted to dopamine in the neurons. Carbidopa is usually given with levodopa because it inhibits the peripheral distribution of levodopa, making more available for transport across the blood-brain barrier into the CNS.

Amantadine is used to treat Parkinson's disease because it may cause dopamine to accumulate in the basal ganglia by increasing the release of dopamine or by blocking its reuptake into presynaptic neurons. It may also stimulate dopamine receptors or cause postsynaptic receptors to be more sensitive to dopamine.

Benztropine, biperiden, procyclidine, and trihexyphenidyl may block the action of acetylcholine at cholinergic receptor sites, restoring the normal balance of dopamine and acetylcholine and relaxing muscle movement. These drugs also may inhibit dopamine reuptake, thereby prolonging the action of dopamine.

Patients with Parkinson's disease also may lack the enzymes necessary for synthesizing dopamine. Bromocriptine, pergolide, pramipexole, and ropinirole are dopamine agonists. They compensate for the loss of dopamine by directly stimulating the postsynaptic dopamine receptors. The enzyme monoamine oxidase (type B) metabolizes dopamine; its action is inhibited by selegiline, increasing the amount of dopamine that's available to treat the signs and symptoms of Parkinson's disease. Another enzyme that metabolizes dopamine is catechol-O-methyltransferase (COMT). Drugs such as entacapone and tolcapone inhibit COMT. When given with levodopa, these drugs prolong the plasma half-life of levodopa, making more available for diffusion into the CNS, where it's converted to dopamine.

Antipsychotic Drugs

Antipsychotic drugs may be used to treat a variety of disorders from anxiety to vomiting, but they're most commonly used to treat psychosis, especially schizophrenia. The signs and symptoms of psychosis may be caused by increased dopamine activity in the areas of the brain—such as the cerebral cortex, hypothalamus, and limbic system—that are involved with emotional behavior, voluntary movement, and the inhibition of prolactin secretion.

Most antipsychotic drugs block postsynaptic dopamine receptors, which alters central dopamine metabolism and function. For example, the phenothiazines, such as perphenazine, haloperidol, and pimozide block D_2 receptors; clozapine blocks D_4 receptors; and olanzapine and risperidone block both dopamine and serotonin receptors. As a result, antipsychotic drugs control agitation, delusions, and hallucinations. However, they may also cause serious adverse effects for which you'll need to monitor your patient. (See *Common Side Effects of Antipsychotic Drugs,* pages xl to xlii.)

Sedative-hypnotics

The drugs classified as sedative-hypnotics are used primarily to produce drowsiness and sedation, and they include a variety of drugs with different therapeutic classifications.

Some benzodiazepines, such as estazolam and flurazepam, and nonbenzodiazepine drugs, such as zaleplon and zolpidem, engage with benzodiazepine binding sites on GABA receptors in the limbic and cortical areas of the brain. They potentiate the inhibitory effects of the neurotransmitter GABA, thereby producing sedation.

Barbiturates also interact with GABA receptors, but at different binding sites, and these drugs may potentiate or mimic the effects of GABA. Barbiturates also depress the reticular activating system and interfere with impulse transmission from the periphery to the cerebral cortex. The reticular activating system is a network of neurons that relay excitatory messages from the spinal cord to the cerebral cortex, thus maintaining consciousness. The ability of a barbiturate to produce varying levels of sedation, from mild relief of anxiety to deep coma, depends on the dose, route of administration, and the patient's response.

Diphenhydramine crosses the blood-brain barrier and blocks histamine receptors, depressing the CNS and producing sedation. Promethazine, a phenothiazine derivative, blocks receptor sites in the CNS, reducing stimuli to the brain, and causing relief of anxiety and sedation.

COMMON SIDE EFFECTS OF ANTIPSYCHOTIC DRUGS

Antipsychotic drugs block dopamine receptors in areas of the brain that control emotions and behavior, relieving the signs and symptoms of psychosis. However, these drugs also block dopamine receptors in other areas of the brain, such as in the extrapyramidal tracts—groups of motor nerves responsible for the control of voluntary movements. This action disrupts the normal balance of neurotransmitters and may cause extrapyramidal symptoms (EPS). During antipsychotic drug therapy, monitor your patient for the presence of the following EPS and notify her prescriber if they occur.

Akathisia
Akathisia is the most common EPS, and it may be related to the administration of a high-potency antipsychotic drug, such as haloperidol. This EPS usually occurs within the first three months of therapy. Monitor your patient for signs and symptoms of akathisia, such as fidgeting, restlessness, rhythmic leg movements, rocking back and forth, or shifting his weight from side to side.

Determine if these symptoms are new because akathisia may be misdiagnosed as psychotic agitation. Anticipate that the patient will require a dose reduction or change in her drug (possibly to an atypical antipsychotic drug, such as clozapine or risperidone), or treatment with an anticholinergic drug, a benzodiazepine, or propranolol. Expect that akathisia may lead to noncompliance, so question your patient about this, and monitor her therapeutic response.

Dystonia
Dystonia may occur after the first week of therapy with an antipsychotic drug, so monitor your patient for signs and symptoms, such as abnormal eye movements; difficulty breathing, speaking, or swallowing; muscle spasms of the head, neck, and extremities that cause unusual body positions, twisting movements, or resemble a seizure; and ticlike movements. Be aware that these signs and symptoms are more common in men, and they'll usually resolve in two weeks.

Be prepared to administer an anticholinergic drug, such as benztropine or diphenhydramine, as prescribed. If your patient develops laryngospasm, expect to administer the anticholinergic drug intravenously. If your patient is considered to be at risk for developing an EPS, anticipate that he may also be given prophylactic treatment with an anticholinergic when antipsychotic therapy begins. A patient who is at high risk is one who has a history of

COMMON SIDE EFFECTS OF ANTIPSYCHOTIC DRUGS *(continued)*

developing an EPS and is noncompliant, a young male, and has been prescribed a high-potency antipsychotic, such as haloperidol.

Pseudoparkinsonism

Because antipsychotic drugs block dopamine receptors in the brain, your patient may develop signs and symptoms that mimic Parkinson's disease, which is also characterized by a lack of dopamine. Monitor her for signs and symptoms such as akinesia (absence or slowness of movement), difficulty speaking or swallowing, drooling, loss of balance, mask-like facies, shuffling gait, stiffness of the extremities, and tremor.

Pseudoparkinsonism may occur weeks to several months after therapy begins. It's more common in women and elderly patients. Be aware that if your patient is elderly, these signs and symptoms may actually represent Parkinson's disease and may also be confused with depression or some of the abnormal movements that occur with schizophrenia. Anticipate the use of an antidyskinetic drug, such as amantadine, benztropine, or trihexyphenidyl, to treat pseudoparkinsonism.

Tardive dyskinesia

Tardive dyskinesia (TD) is a long-term side effect of antipsychotic drugs. It's caused by prolonged blockade of the dopamine receptors, which causes them to become supersensitive. Up to 50% of patients receiving long-term therapy develop TD, but most of these cases are mild. It usually develops after years of therapy but may occur after only four months. Patients who are more at risk for developing TD include those on high dose long-term therapy, those receiving anticholinergic therapy for an EPS, elderly patients, and women. Monitor your patient for signs and symptoms, such as involuntary movements of the extremities, face, and trunk, including cheek puffing, lip smacking, pelvic thrusting, random limb movements, shoulder shrugging, squirming, and tongue protrusions. Expect that these abnormal movements may be mild, disabling, or permanent. Sometimes they appear when a patient's dose has been reduced or discontinued or if an anticholinergic drug is given with an antipsychotic drug.

Notify the patient's prescriber immediately if you observe the signs and symptoms of TD, and anticipate that the antipsychotic drug dose will be lowered and the anticholinergic drug (if prescribed) will

(continued)

COMMON SIDE EFFECTS OF ANTIPSYCHOTIC DRUGS *(continued)*

be discontinued. All antipsychotic drugs are capable of causing TD, but the atypical antipsychotic drugs, such as risperidone, may have a lower risk because they block dopamine and serotonin receptors.

Neuroleptic Malignant Syndrome

Neuroleptic malignant syndome (NMS) is an uncommon but potentially fatal reaction to antipsychotic drugs. It occurs most commonly in the first month of therapy or after a patient's dose has been increased or his antipsychotic drug has been changed. NMS may occur more frequently in frail elderly patients; young male patients; patients with dehydration or organic brain disease; those treated with fluphenazine, haloperidol, multiple drugs, or the depot form of drugs; and those on long-term antipsychotic therapy.

Monitor your patient for signs and symptoms of NMS, including altered mental status, autonomic dysfunction (diaphoresis, hypertension, tachycardia), hyperthermia, and muscle rigidity that progress rapidly over 1 to 3 days. Expect your patient also to have an elevated creatine kinase level, elevated liver enzyme test results, and leukocytosis. Be aware that NMS is a serious condition; notify your patient's prescriber immediately if signs and symptoms appear, and expect to discontinue the drug. Maintain his airway, administer I.V. fluids, and treat hyperthermia with a cooling blanket, as prescribed. Anticipate the use of bromocriptine or dantrolene, as needed. If the antipsychotic drug is restarted, monitor the patient for a recurrence of NMS because he may be more at risk for developing it again.

THE ROLE OF THE NURSE IN BEHAVIORAL AND MENTAL HEALTH DRUG THERAPY

To ensure that an accurate diagnosis is made and that the most appropriate drugs are selected to treat a patient who has a behvioral or mental health disorder, you'll need to start by performing a thorough assessment.

First, you'll need to establish a therapeutic relationship with your patient. The quality of this relationship can have a direct impact on the quality of the assessment you're able to make. Provide for your patient's comfort, be empathic and nonjudgmental, and strive for a high level of trust. A private, uninterrupted clinical setting is essential.

Conducting an Assessment Interview

You may need to include the patient's relatives or friends in the interview, particularly if the patient is a child, an older adult with cognitive deficits, someone who is experiencing significant psychotic symptoms, or one who is uncooperative with the interview process. Although note taking is optional and can be distracting, many patients see it as an indication that you're concerned and attentive to their problems.

During the interview, ask open-ended questions that will help you obtain the information that you need to complete your assessment. At the same time, maintain a certain amount of focus during the interview. Avoid asking leading questions that could limit the information you're trying to obtain. Typically, the information obtained during the interview will include the patient's psychiatric history, affect, appearance, behavior, and cognition.

Psychiatric History

Begin your assessment by obtaining a psychiatric history. First, determine the chief complaint—your patient's own words to describe why he's seeking help at this time. Ask the patient to talk about what has been going on in his life. Give him time to describe the difficulties he's experiencing. A patient who has been referred to you may state that he doesn't know the reason he's been sent for help. Use empathetic communication skills with your patient. Ask relevant questions at appropriate points to clarify the history that's presented. By allowing your patient to tell his own story, you'll acquire the most information and build a trusting therapeutic relationship.

Record the history of the presenting illness; it's the part of the history that's the most useful in formulating a diagnosis because it will help you establish how your patient's symptoms developed. Include information about your patient's current symptoms, the onset of the episode or symptoms, and any precipitating events. Expected symptoms or negative findings should also be documented. For example, if your patient describes manic behavior but tells you he's sleeping regularly, make a note of this.

To find out how your patient's symptoms are affecting his life, you'll need to know the details about how his illness impacts his work and relationships. Descriptions of problems noticed by other people close to the patient are helpful, as are the interventions your patient has attempted on his own and what he's found to be useful in dealing with his symptoms.

Include your patient's psychiatric history in your assessment. Ask him about past psychiatric diagnoses and specific details regarding these diagnoses. Include specific symptoms your patient is experiencing. For example, if he tells you about the presence of auditory hallucinations, ask him if he recognizes the voice, if there is more than one voice, and if the voices talk to each other. List any previous hospitalizations with such details as the precipitating event, length of stay, and the treatment he received. Also, record information pertaining to outpatient treatment with specific details about the type of treatment, his response to the treatment, and the length of time that the treatment was provided.

As part of your assessment, also record any psychiatric drugs your patient is receiving and summarize his response to the drugs. If your patient tells you that a drug wasn't helpful, determine what response, if any, was achieved. Then decide if an adequate trial of the drug was administered to the patient. To do so, find out how long the drug was given, along with the dosage that was used. Document any side effects your patient experienced. Anecdotal information from the patient regarding specific drugs is also significant. If possible, obtain records from past treatments, both inpatient and outpatient, and review them.

Patients may have had past episodes of their illness that went untreated. Find out all you can about these episodes. Did your patient attend any type of self-help group? What coping mechanisms did he find to be most helpful? This is all important information that you should include in your assessment.

Document any family history of psychiatric problems and the treatment that was received. Your patient may describe symptoms that a family member has experienced, and you can ask the patient how the family member was treated. Details of this sort are helpful in formulating an accurate diagnosis. The response to a psychotropic drug by any biological relative is an important piece of information because this may be a predictor of response in your patient.

Your patient's social history plays an important part in your assessment. It begins with a childhood history. Include information about your patient's parents, the number of children in the family, and the relationships between the parents and the various family members while growing up and at the present time. Was the patient raised by his parents, or were other caregivers involved? If he was raised by some other caregivers, find out the reason for this and the extent of their involvement in his upbringing. Questions about the developmental phases of the patient should also be addressed. For instance, did the patient have any special childhood problems?

School history is also important. Did the patient enjoy school as a child? What grades did he achieve, and what were his favorite subjects? Document the highest level of the patient's education and whether his education included vocational training or university courses. Find out what the patient did with his free time, such as his involvement in extracurricular activities and whether he had a part-time job. Also find out who he spent his free time with during his childhood and the types of friends he had in and out of school.

Describe the marital and relationship history, and include the development of the relationship, the status of the marriage, and whether the patient has any children. Note any problems that arose in the marriage and whether the marriage ended in divorce. Also include the current status of the relationship.

Other items in the psychiatric history include the patient's current living situation, how he supports himself, and whether he receives disability. Does the patient have or has he had any legal problems? This includes any arrests and jail or prison terms. Document your patient's religious background while growing up and what his current religious beliefs are. Find out if your patient has a military history, whether he was involved in combat, whether he was ever wounded, and whether he has current difficulties because of his military experience.

Affect

Mood is the emotion through which your patient sees his world. Affect is your patient's current emotional responsiveness. Generally, the patient reports the mood, and the interviewer intuits the affect. (See *Describing Your Patient's Affect*.) The predominant mood the patient reports and the affect presented in the interview are both meaningful. Document whether your patient identifies his mood spontaneously, or if you must ask him how he's feeling. Note whether or not the mood and affect are congruent. Discord between the two may be indicative of a disordered thought process or a personality disorder.

DESCRIBING YOUR PATIENT'S AFFECT

Affect, which can vary individually and by cultural norms, is displayed by facial expressions, hand gestures, tone of voice, and displays of emotion, such as laughter. Use the criteria below to ensure an accurate and consistent description of your patient's affect.

Affect	Description
Full	Demonstrates facial expression, body movements, inflection, and tone of voice that are typical of most people.
Constricted	Demonstrates mild decrease in the intensity of emotional expression. The patient may move his eyebrows, have a slight smile on his face, and some variation in his voice when talking about a pleasurable event.
Blunted	Demonstrates severe reduction in the intensity of emotional expression. The patient may have a slight smile, but no other facial expression, and talk in a monotone.
Flat	Shows no sign of emotion. The patient's face may be expressionless, his body fixed, and his voice a monotone.
Inappropriate	Displays emotion that doesn't match the situation. The patient may describe a sad event, yet laugh when doing so.
Labile	Displays emotion that changes easily and rapidly.

Your patient may have difficulty labeling his mood, particularly if he's not very psychologically minded. Thus, your observations are important in determining his overall affect. You may find it helpful to use a simple rating scale that has a range from 1 to 10, and ask your patient to rate his own mood. Be sure to instruct him how to use the scale, and document whether 1 is a low mood or a high mood. This simple tool can then be used in future interviews to assess your patient's response to treatment.

A depressed patient will usually have a saddened affect and a mood that can be described as being blue, depressed, down, or sad. A depressed patient also may be irritable. The psychotic patient may have a blunted or flattened affect, showing little or no emotion. The bipolar disordered patient will report an affect based on where he is in his mood cycle. Thus, in a depressed phase, he may appear down or sad, and in a manic or hypomanic phase, he'll exhibit an expansive and grandiose mood. He may also have an irritable affect. A patient with mixed bipolar disorder will report moods that fluctuate, or he may report feeling down but agitated and restless at the same time.

Appearance

Your patient's physical appearance provides important information in determining the diagnosis. A patient who is depressed may neglect his appearance. This could result from a low level of energy or lack of motivation that renders him unable to complete activities of daily living. Such patients may have a disheveled appearance, soiled clothing, and hair that is uncombed and unwashed. In short, the patient may look as if he has paid little or no attention to the details of his appearance.

A patient who is exhibiting manic behavior will likely dress inappropriately for his appointment. Whether it's extremely bright colors, extravagant jewelry, or excessive make-up, the appearance will usually be flamboyant. The patient may be dressed in a provocative or seductive manner, particularly if the provider is of the opposite sex, or he may be dressed too formally for the clinical setting.

A thought-disordered or psychotic patient will also most likely have a unique presentation. As with the depressed patient, his appearance may indicate that he has neglected the details. He may be disheveled or have soiled clothing. His choice of attire may be inappropriate for the season. For example, during warm summer months, he may come to the appointment wearing a stocking cap and a winter jacket. Conversely, during cold weather, he may be wearing no coat at all or be wearing summer-weight clothing. He may also wear an odd combination of clothing, such as nonmatching shoes.

Behavior

The behavior your patient exhibits during the interview can provide information that's useful in making a diagnosis. Displays of hostile or angry behavior may be the result of suspiciousness or paranoid thoughts. A depressed patient may sit slumped in the chair with his head down, making little eye contact. You may also detect tearfulness in a depressed patient. A thought-disordered patient may exhibit suspiciousness, looking about the room carefully. You may find clues in his behavior that he's experiencing auditory hallucinations, such as hesitation in answering questions, mumbling as if in answer to voices, or turning his head as if listening to a voice.

Look closely at your patient's actions during the interview. Depression may cause psychomotor retardation in your patient, which you'll observe as slowed gait and movements. In a patient with an agitated depression, you'll observe the opposite behavior, such as hand wringing and pacing. An anxious patient will often fidget while sitting in the chair, tapping his feet and legs and demonstrating difficulty with sitting through the interview. A bipolar patient in a manic phase will be highly distractible, responding to cues in the environment around him. He may be restless and have trouble focusing on the conversation, with his speech rambling to topics unrelated to the discussion.

Other behaviors you should note and document include gestures, mannerisms, and tics. Observe your patient for combativeness, rigidity, or stereotyped behaviors. A patient who is unable to sit in his chair and paces about the room may be experiencing akathisia, a side effect of antipsychotic drugs. Keep in mind that a patient's behavior could be a response to his drug therapy.

When describing characteristics of your patient's speech, observe the rate, quality, and quantity of his speech. For example, his speech should be specified in terms of speed: whether it's rapid or slow, pressured or hesitant. You may describe the patient as articulate, reluctant to offer information, spontaneous in his conversation, or talkative. Also note demonstrations of speech that are dramatic, highly emotional, loud, monotonous, or whispered, and any impairment in your patient's speech, such as lisping or stuttering.

Document whether your patient was passive during the interview, briefly answering questions but not initiating information without being prompted, or conversely, taking control of the interview and guiding the discussion. Note the level of cooperativeness, and whether he was reluctant to answer questions and participate in the interview.

Cognition

Examine and define your patient's thought processes, which are generally divided into two parts: the form of his thoughts and the content of his thoughts. He may demonstrate a lack of thoughts or ideas or an excess of thoughts, which he may experience as racing thoughts. The patient with an excess of ideas will have rapid thinking, which if it's extreme, could be described as a flight of ideas. Patients who jump from topic to topic with little comprehensible connection demonstrate loose associations. Your patient's ideas may be presented in a rambling pattern or one that is blocked or interrupted before completion. Tangentiality may be seen in a patient who loses his train of thought, moving from topic to topic, which is similar to loose associations but with more connection between his ideas.

A patient with disturbed content of thought may demonstrate delusions, which are fixed, false beliefs about his world. Delusions can have a persecutory or paranoid theme; they can also be grandiose in nature, somatic, or bizarre. Describe with detail whether your patient has obsessional thoughts or any phobias or thoughts of doing harm to himself or others. Ideas of reference, in which your patient believes he gets messages from the media, or thought insertion, in which he believes thoughts are put into his mind, are all demonstrations of disturbed thought content.

Be aware that impaired cognition can be caused by a number of different behavioral mental health disorders. To evaluate your patient's perception of long-term memory, ask him about events in his distant past, such as from his childhood. To measure more recent memory, ask him to recall events from the past few months. Your patient may have a dementia disorder or a high level of anxiety, which could contribute to his impaired cognition. Patients who are acutely psychotic will generally demonstrate cognitive difficulties. An individual with severe depression may demonstrate a pseudodementia, which may respond to treatment with an antidepressant drug. If you have any doubt regarding your patient's cognitive function, expect that a physical work-up will be initiated to rule out any possible organic causes.

Evaluate your patient's abstract thinking process by asking him to explain similarities or give meaning to simple proverbs, such as "people who live in glass houses shouldn't throw stones." His answers may be overly concrete or abstract, which you should document, along with the appropriateness of his answers. Expect to evaluate your patient's judgment and insight by asking specific questions, such as, "What would you do if you found a stamped, addressed envelope lying on the sidewalk?" Insight is your patient's ability to recognize his illness and understand the necessity of getting treatment. Thus, your patient may demonstrate a denial of his illness, an awareness of his illness but place blame for it on someone else, or an admission of his illness and recognition of the need for a change in his behavior.

Safety Considerations

Certain patient populations require special safety considerations you need to keep in mind when providing behavioral and mental health drug therapy. These groups of patients include battered patients, children and adolescents, elderly patients, pregnant patients, and suicidal patients.

Battered Patients

Battered patients may include women who have been abused by a partner. They also may be children, adolescents, and elderly men and women who may have been abused. Be especially attentive with this group of patients to provide an environment in which they'll be comfortable and relaxed, with their privacy and confidentiality maintained.

A battered patient may be fearful of interacting with you. This fear could be based on past experiences in which health care providers weren't seen as helpful. A battered or abused patient who unsuccessfully sought help in the past may be hesitant to seek help again. The patient may also have sought help and had an overzealous provider who notified authorities, resulting in further abuse. Another factor is whether the batterer is still involved in the patient's life. The batterer may not support treatment of the patient, and this can be expressed through an unwillingness to pay for drugs or by hindering the patient's access to these drugs or to follow-up appointments. Or the batterer may accompany the patient to the appointment, insist on being present for the interview, and answer questions for the patient. Whenever possible in such situations, conduct the interview privately.

A battered patient may be fearful of taking drugs. She may be concerned that she won't be able to think clearly and that she'll be slowed down, unable to protect herself or her children. Her concerns are certainly valid because some psychotropic drugs, such as an antianxiety drug, may cause initial confusion. Your patient also may not believe she's suffering from a behavioral or mental health illness; she may instead attribute her symptoms to her dangerous living situation.

Carefully assess the risk for suicide with the battered patient. Depression is a common diagnosis among abused women. Such a patient may have a limited social support system and view suicide as a viable solution to her problems. Thus, she could be at high risk for overdose or other types of suicide attempts. Be sure to address and explore this possibility and take necessary precautions to ensure the safety of the patient.

Some abused women suffer from emotional difficulties related to the abuse. As mentioned, depression is a common problem. Anxiety disorders are also common, and medical problems may be exacerbated, as well; so be sure to explore these possibilities.

Be aware that a battered patient's drugs may not be secure in her home environment. For example, if a woman is still living with her abuser, he may take her drugs from her. His motivation could be to further harm her by denying her treatment, or he might attempt to sell the drugs on the street, particularly if one is an antianxiety drug, such as a benzodiazepine.

Remember that you'll need to have a safe, confidential place for assessing a battered patient. Convey a sense of trustworthiness to the patient. Be familiar with the resources available in the community for a battered patient, and be prepared to refer her as needed. And remember to evaluate your patient's risk of suicide with each visit.

Children and Adolescents

Treating children and adolescents with behavioral and mental health drug therapy presents several safety concerns. Typically, these patients don't present themselves for treatment. Rather, their parents or a school system refers them. Consequently, they may not see the importance of treatment, and they may not cooperate in the treatment.

Conducting an interview with a child is different from working with an adult. First, explain the reason for the interview. Then find out the child's perception of his illness, how he gets along with his family and friends, and whether he likes school. Keep in mind that a child may be less able to describe his symptoms, response to a drug, and any adverse reactions to it. Make sure you compliment the child naturally and thank him for participating in the interview.

When evaluating a child for thought disorders, keep his developmental stage in mind. For example, in a young child, magical thinking is common and shouldn't be considered abnormal. The child may not be able to distinguish fantasy from reality. Also, he may not think abstractly. Keep in mind that a mood stabilizer, such as lithium, may adversely affect cognition in the child.

Perform an initial baseline assessment before beginning drug therapy, which gives you a reference to evaluate his future response. Monitoring a child's behavior and cognitive functioning can be difficult because of changes as he grows.

The child may need help with adverse reactions to a drug. Use a systematic approach for assessing his reactions. Rating scales and checklists can be especially useful, and physical examinations and laboratory tests are also important in ongoing assessments. Remember that the child is not just a small adult, so expect to use the lowest dose that's effective for the shortest time to prevent possible long-term consequences of the drug therapy.

A child's lack of compliance with drug therapy may be a significant barrier to his treatment. A child who comes from a dysfunctional family with poor communication skills is more prone to noncompliance. Other factors that result in noncompliance include adverse effects and parents who may be dissatisfied with the treatment their child is receiving. The attitudes of the parents can influence their child's use of drugs, too. Parents may be reluctant to use a drug if the primary referral is from school personnel. They may be hesitant to use drugs in general and, thus, won't be supportive. Conversely, the parents may abuse the drug or administer it on a schedule different from one that's prescribed. A child who witnesses this parental behavior may adapt his behavior accordingly. If the drug is administered at school, the child may think he is different and may not take the drug.

Successful drug therapy begins with an alliance that you've built with the family, school personnel, and other treatment providers for the child. Expect to involve the parents and school staff in the treatment planning and educate them about the drug, the responses that are expected, and any possible adverse reactions.

Interviewing an adolescent patient presents other unique challenges. Confidentiality is particularly important to a teen, and he may not speak openly. A teen may be hostile or angry. He may sense that being asked by his parents to come to the session is challenging his independence. However, the adolescent may relax if he senses that you aren't going to be punitive or judgmental.

You may want to interview the entire family when formulating a diagnosis. Such interviews can be informative because you can observe how the family interacts and communicates. In such an interview, especially if other children in the family aren't labeled ill or problematic, use caution to avoid scapegoating the patient.

Adolescents are particularly susceptible to extrapyramidal symptoms from antipsychotic drugs. Advise the adolescent patient and his parents about this possibility. Teens are prone to trying out one another's drugs (which often occurs on inpatient units), so observe the patient for the development of adverse reactions to a drug that he may not be prescribed. If this occurs, you should conduct a careful inquiry of where he may have obtained the drug.

Another common side effect of some psychotropic drugs is weight gain, which teens find particularly upsetting. Be aware that an adolescent may refuse to take such drugs regularly.

Because symptoms of a behavioral or mental health disorder can change rapidly during adolescence, assess your patient frequently for the continued need for drug therapy, the need to switch drugs, or the need to combine drugs.

Safety considerations for both children and adolescents include safe management of the drug therapy. (See *Ensuring Safe Drug Administration,* page liv.) Help your patient and his parents decide who is responsible for managing and administering the drug. With children, a parent will most often give the child his drug, with the school nurse taking the responsibility for doses administered during the school day. With an adolescent patient, you should carefully determine whether the teen can administer his own drug. Giving a reliable teen this responsibility may result in greater compliance due to an increased sense of independence. However, be aware that it could also result in noncompliance or possible overdose if the teen is prone to acting-out behavior or has a low level of maturity. (See *Handling Adolescent Noncompliance,* page lv.)

Elderly Patients

An elderly patient may be less likely to visit a psychiatric profes-

ENSURING SAFE DRUG ADMINISTRATION

To administer drugs safely to children and adolescents, follow these safety guidelines:

- Obtain informed consent from the responsible family member along with the agreement of the child or adolescent, if appropriate.
- Teach the patient or family member to take or administer the drug as it's prescribed and not adjust the dose.
- Assess the reliability of the family member who will be giving the drug, especially if the drug is a stimulant.
- Be alert to the possibility that a family member may ingest the drug or try to sell it.
- Assess the patient's risk for suicide.

sional because of a denial of emotional problems or mental illness. She may be more stoic and less willing to admit she needs help. She may also doubt that a mental health professional can help. For these reasons, a nurse in any clinical practice setting is the logical person to be involved with treating behavioral and mental health illnesses in an older patient.

Interviewing an elderly patient is similar to interviewing an adult patient. Try to make her comfortable. Keep in mind that an elderly patient may need more time to answer questions. Also, she may spend more time alone, so allow for some time during the interview to interact with her socially and help her relax. You may need to obtain information from collateral sources when assessing an elderly patient who experiences cognitive difficulties. Reports from family, friends, and caregivers may be necessary to make an accurate diagnosis.

Be sure to document an elderly patient's current medical condition. This information is important for determining the appropriate drug therapy. You may be able to obtain this information through an interview with the patient or through a review of the patient's medical records. The patient may take a large number of drugs for specific medical ailments, so you'll need to be alert for potential drug interactions. Carefully review the drugs she's taking, including any OTC medications or herbal preparations, because an older patient may rely heavily on the use of these. Assess her level of un-

HANDLING ADOLESCENT NONCOMPLIANCE

Adolescent patients have a high rate of noncompliance with behavioral and mental health drug therapy. Common reasons for noncompliance include the following:

- fear of being labeled mentally ill
- avoidance of undesirable adverse reactions
- resentment of the need to take medication
- concern about drug abuse or becoming dependent
- peer pressure.

Here are five practical tips to help you effectively deal with a noncompliant adolescent:

1. Encourage expression of feelings and teach the adolescent about his illness. Explain to him that having a behavioral or mental health disorder no longer carries a negative stigma.
2. Listen to his concerns about adverse reactions. Notify the prescriber, as appropriate, and make every attempt to alleviate the drug's adverse effects.
3. Explain why drug therapy is necessary and involve the adolescent in decisions about his drug therapy to promote independence and decrease his feelings of resentment.
4. Allow your patient to discuss concerns about drug abuse or dependence. For each prescribed drug, as appropriate, explain why the drug should not be discontinued abruptly or taken in greater amounts than prescribed. Be sure to differentiate between physical and psychological abuse or dependence. Reinforce why the drug is necessary to control the patient's symptoms.
5. Suggest that he attend group therapy sessions with other adolescents.

derstanding about why she takes each drug, and educate her about the therapeutic goal for each, which will improve compliance with any new prescription.

Expect an elderly patient to begin drug therapy at a reduced dosage that's titrated on an individual basis. The older adult is at risk for toxicity from medications for a number of reasons. She may have reduced liver function, which may result in a higher drug blood level. She may have increased adipose tissue; since many psychotropic drugs are fat soluble, this can lead to longer elimination times. Also, she may have a decreased serum albumin level, which leads to less drug binding and increases the amount of the drug that's available in her system. Be aware that drugs need to be given an adequate trial to determine whether they're effective. An elderly patient may need a longer trial period than a younger patient because of differences in metabolism. In general, an elderly patient will experience a higher concentration of a psychotropic drug than a younger patient, resulting in an increased therapeutic and toxic response to the drug.

Consider the potential side effects when administering drugs to this patient. For example, expect to monitor your patient's blood pressure if she receives venlafaxine because this drug may increase her blood pressure. In this instance, the extended-release form of venlafaxine may be preferable to avoid possible dose-related hypertension.

Monitor the patient taking a tricyclic antidepressant for arrhythmias, prolonged conduction time, and tachycardia. Trazodone may cause orthostatic hypotension, which increases your patient's potential for falls. Orthostatic hypotension can be particularly common at night, when she may get up to urinate. Patient teaching about this potential side effect is crucial.

Many drugs are available to treat the depressed elderly patient, so expect to use a drug that has the least risk of side effects. A tricyclic antidepressant can cause anticholinergic side effects, such as cognitive impairment, constipation, drowsiness, dry mouth, urine retention, and weight gain—all of which should be avoided with an elderly patient. Because a tricyclic antidepressant can result in cardiac toxicity, the drug of choice may be a serotonin reuptake inhibitor (SSRI). There's also a lower risk of overdose with an SSRI. Be aware that your elderly patient may forget she's taken her drug and may take an additional dose, which could lead to an unintentional overdose.

An elderly patient who has atypical depression that hasn't responded to an SSRI may be prescribed a monoamine oxidase (MAO) inhibitor because it lacks cardiac side effects and has a low incidence of anticholinergic side effects. However, an MAO inhibitor may require dietary restrictions and cause orthostatic hypotension and sleep disturbances.

Antipsychotic drugs may be used to treat an elderly patient who has a history of agitation or anxiety or a psychotic disorder such as paranoia, schizoaffective disorder, or schizophrenia. The elderly patient may benefit from one of the newer, atypical antipsychotic drugs because the side effect profile of these medications is more favorable and these drugs may be more effective at treating the negative symptoms of schizophrenia. However, clozapine, an atypical antipsychotic, isn't recommended for use in an elderly patient because of its unique risk of causing agranulocytosis. Be aware that you should monitor your patient taking an older, typical antipsychotic drug for anticholinergic side effects (similar to those seen with a tricyclic antidepressant) and extrapyramidal symptoms (such as tardive dyskinesia).

Benzodiazepines may be used to treat acute agitation and anxiety in an elderly patient. Be aware that these drugs should only be used for a short time because of the risk for dependency. However, benzodiazepines that don't have an active metabolite—such as alprazolam, lorazepam, oxazepam, and temazepam—are recommended for older adults.

If your patient receives a benzodiazepine, monitor her for possible cognitive impairment and sedation. Be aware that a benzodiazepine can cause paradoxical agitation in some patients and also interfere with the sleep cycle. A benzodiazepine may cause ataxia, which may result in falls, and it can cause incontinence in the elderly. Long-term use of a benzodiazepine may result in chronic sedation. Older people who are chronically sedated may become agitated, belligerent, and confused. Sedation can also exacerbate symptoms of dementia so that these patients may become more agitated, disoriented, or forgetful. Thus, long-term benzodiazepine therapy should be used very cautiously, if not avoided, in the elderly. When a benzodiazepine is discontinued, expect to taper the drug slowly because abruptly stopping it may cause withdrawal signs and symptoms and seizures.

Mood stabilizers may be effective for treating bipolar illness in an elderly patient. Lithium may be prescribed, but it's not the drug of choice because of the potential for side effects and the need to frequently monitor the drug blood level. If lithium is used, expect the prescriber to titrate your elderly patient's dose to a lower blood level than the level that's therapeutic in younger patients. Valproic acid can be used safely in the elderly patient to manage mood swings and behavioral problems, as well as to manage a bipolar mood disorder.

Remember that an elderly patient may have some difficulty swallowing her drug. One solution may be to use a liquid form of the drug. Other drugs, such as olanzapine, are available in a disintegrating tablet that dissolves under the patient's tongue, thus allowing for easier administration. If the elderly patient is cared for in her home, teach the caregiver about proper drug administration techniques to ensure proper dosing. Encourage the patient to use a medication box to help avoid missing doses or taking additional doses. An older patient living in an extended care facility may require supervision with her drug therapy or have her drug administered to her. Be aware that drug administration to a confused or demented elderly patient needs to be supervised.

Pregnant Patients

With a pregnant patient, the safest option for the fetus would be to avoid drugs during any part of the pregnancy. (See *Pregnancy and Drug Therapy: Protecting Your Patient.*) However, this isn't always possible because chronic psychiatric problems could complicate the pregnancy if left untreated. Before administering any drug to a female patient of childbearing age, determine if she could be pregnant or could become pregnant, and share your concerns with her prescriber.

If a pregnant patient experiences symptoms of a psychiatric disorder and she's not taking an antipsychotic drug, expect the prescriber to make every attempt to manage her symptoms without drugs, but this isn't always possible. For example, a severely depressed and suicidal woman may need an antidepressant to ensure her safety and that of her unborn child. A psychotic pregnant woman's behavior may make her too disorganized to keep appointments to check the progress of her pregnancy. She may be unable to follow an appropriate diet and may not get the rest she needs. If she is paranoid and fears being poisoned, she may become reluctant to take drugs, such as prenatal vitamins. She may cause physical harm to herself or the fetus. For such patients, the prescriber will perform a risk–benefit analysis to determine whether the risk of exposure to the drug is greater than the consequences of leaving a psychiatric disorder untreated.

If the prescriber decides to initiate or continue a psychotropic drug, he'll typically select the safest drug. Unfortunately, limited information is available about the effects on the fetus of traditional antipsychotic drugs or the newer atypical antipsychotic drugs. The available research suggests that high potency antipsychotics, such as haloperidol, pose no teratogenic effects. A low dose antipsychotic drug may have a higher risk of congenital malformations after the first trimester, although no data exists for treatment related adverse effects on neonates in utero.

A woman may present with a new onset depressive disorder during her pregnancy. She may also be taking a maintenance drug for depression at the time of her pregnancy. Research suggests that taking a tricyclic antidepressant during the first trimester doesn't increase the risk of congenital malformations. However, reports confirm tricyclic antidepressant withdrawal syndrome in infants following delivery. Although tricyclic antidepressants pose little danger to the pregnant patient, these drugs are seldom used because of their side effects. If a tricyclic antidepressant is used, expect the prescriber to choose one that causes the least amount of orthostatic hypotension, such as desipramine or nortriptyline, to reduce the risk of falls.

The newer SSRIs are used more often today to treat depressive disorders, but little information exists about the safety of these drugs during the first trimester of pregnancy. If a woman being treated for mild to moderate depression becomes pregnant or chooses to conceive, expect her prescriber to taper her off the antidepressant drug and manage her depression with nonpharmacologic therapy. If she suffers from severe depression or develops a depressive episode during her pregnancy that doesn't respond to nonpharmacologic therapy, drug therapy may be necessary. In these cases, expect her prescriber to choose fluoxetine, since more information is available about that drug and its use during pregnancy, unlike MAO inhibitors, which are not typically used.

Be aware that a pregnant patient with a history of depression or who develops depression during pregnancy has an increased risk of postpartum depression. Monitor such patients closely following the birth for new or recurring depressive symptoms. Women with severe recurrent depression or prior episodes of postpartum depression may benefit from antidepressant drug therapy during the third trimester of their pregnancy.

The treatment of bipolar disorders typically involves the use of mood stabilizers. Advise a woman with bipolar disorder who's being treated with a drug to plan her pregnancy so that her drug can be safely and slowly tapered off before she becomes pregnant. Be aware that lithium administered during the first trimester may cause congenital cardiovascular malformations in neonates. Also, neonatal toxicity can occur with exposure to lithium, causing "floppy baby" syndrome. Neonates exposed to lithium in the second and third trimester have not had any physical deficits.

For a pregnant bipolar patient with a history of rapid cycling disorder, the prescriber may not be able to taper the drug and effectivly manage the patient's mania. Mania can be potentially dangerous to both the mother and the fetus. With mania, any accompanying psychosis may further impair the pregnant patient's judgment. In these cases, anticipate the use of lithium or low-dose valproic acid. A pregnant bipolar disorder patient experiencing psychotic symptoms may need to be treated with an antipsychotic drug. Expect to use a low dose.

Anticonvulsants are used extensively to treat behavioral mental health disorders. Fetal exposure to carbamazepine or valproic acid during the first trimester may cause neural tube defects and orofacial clefts. Because of these risks, anticonvulsants should be avoided in pregnant women, particularly during the first trimester.

Be aware that benzodiazepines used to treat an anxiety or panic disorder in a pregnant patient during the first trimester may increase the risk of cleft palate in the neonate. Adverse effects may also occur in infants exposed to a benzodiazepine during the last trimester. Be aware that a patient with an anxiety disorder who wishes to become pregnant should be tapered off benzodiazepine and managed with cognitive behavioral therapy or other nonpharmacologic therapies. Sometimes, the prescriber may order a tricyclic antidepressant or fluoxetine, but these drugs increase the risk of cleft abnormalities.

Remember that you should advise your pregnant patient about the risks to the neonate if she takes a psychotropic drug during pregnancy. Urge a patient of childbearing age who is taking a psychotropic drug to use birth control. Regularly assess a pregnant woman with a history of psychosis because she may decompensate quickly. If she becomes paranoid or delusional, she may cause harm to herself or the fetus.

Suicidal Patients

During your treatment of patients with behavioral and mental health disorders, you're likely to be involved with the management of potentially suicidal patients. You may not be able to predict which patients are likely to attempt or commit suicide or determine who has a risk of suicidal behavior. However, here are some generalizations about who may be at greater risk, based on information from or about patients who have attempted to commit or succeeded at committing suicide.

Patients with affective disorders, such as major depression and bipolar disorder, represent the highest risk for suicide. Individuals with panic disorders are the next highest group at risk, along with young adult males who have experienced their first psychotic break and a resulting diagnosis of schizophrenia. Within this latter group, the risk is further increased in those who are better educated, unemployed, and who have never lived alone. Assess all of your patients for suicidal behavior, especially the groups just mentioned (see *Warning Signs of Suicide*, page lxii).

Some patients have more risk factors for suicide. One major risk factor is the patient who presents with a specific plan for suicide, particularly one that involves the use of a lethal weapon and with access to the weapon. A patient who lives alone, is unemployed,

WARNING SIGNS OF SUICIDE

Suicide is the 8th leading cause of death in the United States. The rate of suicide is highest among young adults and the very old. However, you should assess all your patients for the warning signs of suicide and be prepared to intervene, as appropriate.

Warning Signs of Suicide
- Verbal threat with a specific plan
- Ready access to lethal weapons
- Impulsive behavior
- Mood disturbances
- Sense of hopelessness
- Giving away valued possessions
- Sudden increase in energy with improved mood

Nursing Interventions
- Consider the context of the threat; ask the patient about recent stressors.
- Determine if the patient has a plan for a suicide attempt and the means to carry it out, such as access to a gun.
- Question the patient about recent substance abuse.
- Encourage the expression of feelings, and help the patient identify coping strategies to manage stress.
- Focus on the long-term consequences of behavior.
- Determine if the patient can control his behavior; be prepared to notify the health care provider because immediate hospitalization may be required.

and has little or no social support in place is also at risk. Patients with impulsive behavior, those who have experienced a recent loss, and those with a sense of hopelessness and no ability to see solutions to problems all have significant risk factors.

A patient who has a family history of suicide, one who has witnessed a suicide or a violent death, or one with a history of alcohol or drug abuse has an increased risk of suicidal behavior. Be aware that suicide can occur in people of all age-groups, but the risk may actually increase in the elderly, especially in people who are over age 85.

Interventions in the field of behavioral and mental health have traditionally included the use of suicide contracts. Although the usefulness of such contracts is debatable, a provider who chooses to use a no-harm contract should establish it within the context of a therapeutic relationship. Know however, that while a contract may relieve some anxiety on the part of the health care provider, it doesn't completely abolish the risk.

Focus on the long-term consequences of suicide when treating a suicidal patient. Help him to imagine the effect such an act could have on his family. Don't agree with him that suicide is a viable option to his situation. Instead, explain that people attempt suicide because of unhappiness and that, while most people are unhappy at some point in their lives, many have developed coping skills for dealing with their unhappiness.

Teaching your patient about the risks of suicide is one of your most important and useful interventions. Encourage your patient to talk about any thoughts or plans of suicide, then discuss treatment alternatives with him. Ideally, he should be an active partner in choosing which treatment solution to employ.

Sociocultural Considerations

Your professional and personal values may not always be the same as those of your patient. To achieve a mutual and shared therapeutic relationship between you and your patient, begin by communicating acceptance and understanding. Respect the individual culture of your patient. Familiarize yourself with the specifics of his culture, especially how he views illness and health care.

During your assessment, remember that manners of communication may differ among cultures. For example, a Japanese patient may say *yes* to be polite, but he isn't necessarily agreeing with you; a Chinese patient may laugh or smile when he is embarrassed; and a Native American doesn't look directly at you because making eye contact is viewed as disrespectful by his culture.

Patients may be unwilling to take medications because of existing cultural differences. Certain religions may discourage their members from taking medications. Some cultures may believe that an illness is caused by higher beings and see prayer as the route to healing. Different cultures may describe illness in different ways. For example, in describing depression, a Latino patient may tell you he's having a problem with *nerves,* while an Asian patient may use terms such as *weakness* and *fatigue.*

A lack of adequate finances may be a barrier to your patient's receiving treatment. Many of the newer psychotropic drugs are expensive. If your patient has a limited income or is without health insurance, he may be unable to find the financial resources to pay for his drugs. You'll need to be resourceful and creative when helping this patient. Ask the prescriber to order a generic preparation, if appropriate. Be aware of the pharmaceutical companies that offer indigent programs to provide medications to patients with low incomes.

The prevalence of behavioral and mental health disorders may differ among socioeconomic classes. Anxiety disorders may be more common among individuals with a lower socioeconomic status, as may be sleep disturbances, perhaps because of poor overall health, an unhealthy lifestyle, or limited access to health care.

Be aware that your patient may be hesitant to go to a behavioral or mental health professional. Mental illness continues to hold a stigma in our culture, which is difficult for many people to overcome. Consequently, behavioral and mental health disorders are often diagnosed in the primary care setting.

Be aware that ethnicity can affect the way a drug is metabolized. In general, people of Asian descent have a slower metabolism, and they may need lower doses of drugs. The same is true for women and elderly patients. Patients with a higher rate of metabolism will require a higher dose of a drug to achieve the same effect as a patient with a lower rate of metabolism. However, despite these generalizations, expect each of your patients to respond differently to the drug therapy. If possible, measure drug blood levels to help determine effectiveness, but be sure to monitor your patient's therapeutic response because that's the best way to determine how well a drug is working.

Psychotherapy Considerations

Drug therapy has proven to be very useful to many patients suffering from a behavioral or mental health illness. In most cases, however, drug therapy alone cannot completely treat the illness. (See *Long-term Psychotherapies.*) Other therapies and interventions play an important role in the management of the illness. Individual and group therapy can be particularly helpful.

In today's world, where finances often drive treatment, short-term or brief therapy has become popular. This type of treatment has a pre-determined number of sessions, with specific goals agreed upon up front by the therapist and patient. Brief therapy is useful in obtaining symptom relief. It can be particularly beneficial for depressive episodes related to situational crises. This type of therapy

LONG-TERM PSYCHOTHERAPIES

Here are several types of long-term psychotherapy. A psychotropic drug may be indicated to treat the underlying illness in a patient undergoing any of these therapies. For example, a patient involved in long-term therapy may be suffering from a type of depression, so expect that an antidepressant will be used.

- *Psychoanalytic psychotherapy*—The emphasis is on current interpersonal and intrapsychic dynamics. The goals are analysis of defenses used by the patient and transference observed and played out in therapy, with limited reconstruction of the past and past issues. This type of therapy can last for several years.
- *Object-relations therapy*—The therapist uses the therapeutic relationship between the patient and the therapist to bring about a change in the patient. The focus is on the here-and-now, as well as on critical relationships in the life of the patient.
- *Insight-oriented therapy*—The therapist helps the patient look at lifelong patterns of behavior. The focus is on the dynamics of the patient's feelings, responses, and behaviors in current relationships with others, as well as with the therapist.
- *Supportive psychotherapy*—Typically shorter in duration, this therapy's goals are to provide ego support to the patient, support reality testing, and maintain or reestablish an adequate level of functioning. This type of therapy is usually used following a crisis in the patient's life.

may offer some character changes, but it's mainly used to teach the patient new coping skills. The therapist is usually very active in this type of therapy, and medications are a useful adjunct. Cognitive behavioral therapy is effective for dealing with anxiety disorders. Patients learn how their thinking patterns can control their response to situations, and they learn to become proactive rather than reactive in stressful situations. The relationship among thoughts, feelings, and behaviors is explored in this type of therapy. The patient is taught new coping skills that can be used in anxiety-provoking situations. Behavioral rewards are often used, and homework is assigned between sessions. A drug may be indicated when cognitive behavioral therapy is being used to assist the patient while she learns new coping skills.

Cognitive behavioral therapy is also effective when treating social phobias. Patients are slowly exposed to various situations that have been frightening to them. They learn how to reframe their thinking and correct misinterpretations. SSRI therapy combined with cognitive behavioral therapy may be used to treat social phobias.

Patients dealing with phobic disorders may work with a therapist in a type of therapy known as exposure therapy, in which the patient is taught relaxation techniques and then increasingly exposed to the fearful situation or object. The goal is for the patient to become desensitized to the experience over time. The short-term use of an antianxiety drug may be useful while the patient is learning new coping strategies.

Group therapy is commonly used to treat a behavioral or mental health disorder. Group therapy offers many advantages and curative factors. Patients discover that other people suffer from problems similar to their own, perhaps even worse than their own, and they have an opportunity to help others in the group. Members who are coping well serve as role models to others, and patients learn new coping skills from other members of the group.

Several types of therapy can be used in a group setting. Groups may be open-ended—in which new members can be added at any time, or closed—in which a set number of patients begin the group and aren't replaced if a member drops out. Open-ended groups are usually ongoing, with no specific beginning or end point. Closed groups ordinarily run for a specific number of sessions.

Process-oriented groups focus on the process of the group, rather than the content. Participants learn first hand about their interaction patterns and how their behaviors affect others. The group becomes a microcosm of the patient's world and can be a beneficial learning experience for all of the members.

Groups may be psychoeducational, similar to a class, with specific didactic learning and limited time for discussion among group members. Other psychoeducational groups may offer a portion of the session as education and an equal portion for the group to process what has been presented and discuss its application in their lives. Self-help or support groups consist of members who have something in common, such as a struggle with some form of substance abuse. A professional leader may participate. Discussion in these groups focuses on how members can cope with their common issues and symptoms rather than focusing on interpersonal issues or changes.

Nurses may form groups on inpatient units or in outpatient clinics to educate patients about their drug therapy. Be aware that confidentiality may be a factor that limits participation in groups. If you're involved in such a group, encourage group participation and discussion because the power of the group comes from the contribution of its members. If a patient claims to be having difficulty dealing with a side effect of her drug therapy, encourage the group to offer suggestions. Find out the common problems, and let the group come up with the solutions.

BEHAVIORAL AND MENTAL HEALTH DRUGS

(organized alphabetically)

acamprosate calcium
Campral

Class and Category
Chemical class: Synthetic endogenous amino acid homotaurine, gamma-aminobutyric acid (GABA) analogue
Therapeutic class: Anti-alcoholic
Pregnancy category: C

Indications and Dosages
▶ *To maintain abstinence from alcohol for alcohol-dependent patients who are abstinent at the start of treatment*
E.R. TABLETS
Adults. 666 mg t.i.d.
DOSAGE ADJUSTMENT For patients with moderate renal impairment (creatinine clearance of 30 to 50 ml/min/1.73 m^2), 333 mg t.i.d.

Route	Onset	Peak	Duration
P.O.	Unknown	3 to 8 hr	Unknown

Contraindications
Hypersensitivity to acamprosate or its components, severe hepatic (Child-Pugh class C) or renal impairment

Interactions
DRUGS
antidepressants: Increased weight gain
tetracyclines: Decreased tetracycline absorption

Adverse Reactions
CNS: Abnormal thinking, amnesia, anxiety, asthenia, chills, depression, dizziness, headache, insomnia, paresthesia, somnolence, suicidal ideation, syncope, tremor
CV: Chest pain, hypertension, palpitations, peripheral edema, vasodilation
EENT: Abnormal vision, dry mouth, pharyngitis, rhinitis, taste perversion

Mechanism of Action

Chronic alcoholism may alter the balance between excitation and inhibition in neurons in the brain; acamprosate restores it.

When the neurotransmitter gamma-aminobutyric acid (GABA) binds to its receptors in the CNS, it opens the chloride ion channel and releases chloride (Cl^-) into the cell (below left), thereby reducing neuronal excitability by inhibiting depolarization. By interacting with GABA receptor sites, acamprosate prevents GABA from binding (below right).

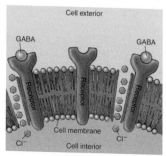
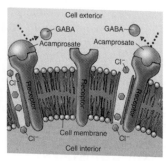

When glutamate binds to its receptors, it closes the chloride ion channel, increasing neuronal excitability by promoting depolarization (below left). This imbalance fosters a craving for alcohol. By interacting with glutamate receptor sites, acamprosate prevents glutamate from binding (below right).

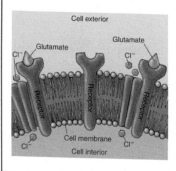
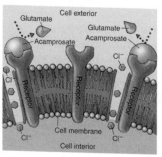

GI: Abdominal pain, anorexia, constipation, diarrhea, flatulence, increased appetite, indigestion, nausea, vomiting
GU: Acute renal failure, decreased libido, impotence
HEME: Leukopenia, lymphocytosis, thrombocytopenia
MS: Arthralgia, back pain, myalgia
RESP: Bronchitis, cough, dyspnea

SKIN: Diaphoresis, pruritus, rash
Other: Flulike symptoms, infection, weight gain

Overdose
Acamprosate overdose has no specific antidote. Information about acamprosate overdose is limited, and the only symptom reported with acute overdoses up to 56 grams is diarrhea. Chronic overdose may lead to hypercalcemia.

Expect to give symptomatic and supportive care, as needed. Institute suicide precautions according to facility policy, and anticipate psychiatric re-evaluation.

Nursing Considerations
• Be aware that acamprosate therapy should start as soon as possible after the patient has undergone alcohol withdrawal and achieved abstinence.
• Continue to give acamprosate even during alcohol relapse.

PATIENT TEACHING
• Instruct patient to take acamprosate exactly as prescribed, even if a relapse occurs, and to seek help for a relapse.
• Warn the patient that acamprosate won't reduce the symptoms of alcohol withdrawal if relapse occurs followed by cessation.
• Urge caregivers to monitor patient for evidence of depression (lack of appetite or interest in life, fatigue, excessive sleeping, difficulty concentrating) or suicidal tendencies because a small number of patients taking acamprosate have attempted suicide.
• Advise patient to use caution when performing hazardous activities until the drug's adverse CNS effects are apparent.
• Tell female patients to notify the prescriber if they become pregnant or intend to become pregnant while taking acamprosate; the drug may need to be stopped because fetal risks are unknown.
• Because drug may cause fetal abnormalities, urge her to notify prescriber if pregnancy is suspected or occurs.

acetazolamide
Acetazolam (CAN), Ak-Zol, Apo-Acetazolamide (CAN), Dazamide, Diamox, Storzolamide

acetazolamide sodium
Diamox

Class and Category
Chemical class: Sulfonamide derivative

Therapeutic class: Anticonvulsant
Pregnancy category: C

Indications and Dosages

▶ *To treat absence, generalized tonic-clonic, mixed, myoclonic, and simple partial seizures*

TABLETS, I.V. OR I.M. INJECTION

Adults and children. 8 to 30 mg/kg daily in divided doses. *Optimal:* 375 to 1,000 mg daily. When used with other anticonvulsants, 250 mg daily.

Route	Onset	Steady State	Peak	Half-Life	Duration
P.O.	60 to 90 min	Unknown	2 to 4 hr	10 to 15 hr	8 to 12 hr
I.V.	2 min	Unknown	15 min	Unknown	4 to 5 hr

Mechanism of Action

Inhibits the enzyme carbonic anhydrase, which normally appears in the brain's choroid plexes. In the brain, inhibition may delay abnormal, intermittent, and excessive discharge from neurons that cause seizures. Beneficial effects may also result from systemic metabolic acidosis caused by acetazolamide.

Contraindications

Chronic noncongestive angle-closure glaucoma; cirrhosis; hyperchloremic acidosis; hypersensitivity to acetazolamide; hypokalemia; hyponatremia; severe adrenocortical, hepatic, or renal impairment; severe pulmonary obstruction

Interactions

DRUGS

amphetamines, methenamine, phenobarbital, procainamide, quinidine: Decreased excretion and possibly toxicity of these drugs
corticosteroids: Increased risk of hypokalemia
cyclosporine: Increased blood cyclosporine level, possibly nephrotoxicity or neurotoxicity
lithium: Increased excretion and decreased effectiveness of lithium
primidone: Decreased blood and urine primidone levels
salicylates: Increased risk of salicylate toxicity

Adverse Reactions

CNS: Ataxia, confusion, depression, disorientation, dizziness, drowsiness, fatigue, fever, flaccid paralysis, headache, lassitude, malaise, nervousness, paresthesia, seizures, tremor, weakness

EENT: Altered taste, tinnitus, transient myopia
GI: Anorexia, constipation, diarrhea, hepatic dysfunction, melena, nausea, vomiting
GU: Crystalluria, decreased libido, glycosuria, hematuria, hyperuricemia, impotence, nephrotoxicity, phosphaturia, polyuria, renal calculi, renal colic, urinary frequency
HEME: Agranulocytosis, hemolytic anemia, leukopenia, pancytopenia, thrombocytopenia, thrombocytopenic purpura
SKIN: Photosensitivity, pruritus, rash, Stevens-Johnson syndrome, urticaria
Other: Acidosis, hypokalemia, weight loss

Overdose

Monitor patient for signs and symptoms of overdose, including anorexia, ataxia, dizziness, drowsiness, nausea, paresthesia, tinnitus, tremor, and vomiting.

Be prepared to institute supportive measures such as inducing vomiting or performing gastric lavage. Anticipate the use of bicarbonate to correct hyperchloremic acidosis, and be aware that potassium supplementation may be required.

Nursing Considerations

- Use acetazolamide cautiously in patients with calcium-based renal calculi, diabetes mellitus, gout, or respiratory impairment.
- Know that acetazolamide may increase risk of hepatic encephalopathy in patients with hepatic cirrhosis.
- Reconstitute each 500-mg vial with at least 5 ml of sterile water for injection. Use within 24 hours; drug has no preservative.
- To avoid painful I.M. injections (caused by alkaline solution), administer acetazolamide by mouth or I.V. injection if possible.
- Monitor blood test results during acetazolamide therapy to detect electrolyte imbalances.

PATIENT TEACHING
- Urge patient to take drug exactly as prescribed. Tell him to take a missed dose as soon as he remembers and not to double it.
- Tell patient that tablets may be crushed and suspended in chocolate or other sweet syrup. Alternatively, one tablet may be dissolved in 10 ml of hot water and added to 10 ml of honey or syrup.
- Advise patient to avoid potentially hazardous activities if dizziness or drowsiness occurs.
- Warn patient who takes a high dosage of a salicylate to notify prescriber immediately if signs or symptomsof salicylate toxicity—such as anorexia, lethargy, and tachypnea—occur.

Other Therapeutic Uses
Acetazolamide is also indicated for the following:
- To treat chronic simple (open-angle) glaucoma
- For short-term therapy, to treat secondary glaucoma and preoperatively to treat acute congestive (angle-closure) glaucoma
- To induce diuresis in patients with heart failure
- To treat drug-induced edema
- To prevent or relieve evidence of acute mountain sickness

almotriptan malate
Axert

Class and Category
Chemical class: Selective 5-hydroxytryptamine$_1$ (5-HT$_1$) receptor agonist
Therapeutic class: Antimigraine drug
Pregnancy category: C

Indications and Dosages
▶ *To treat acute migraine*
TABLETS
Adults. *Initial:* 6.25 to 12.5 mg as a single dose, repeated in 2 hr as needed. *Maximum:* 2 doses/24 hr or four migraine treatments/mo.
DOSAGE ADJUSTMENT Initial dose reduced to 6.25 mg with a maximum daily dose of 12.5 mg for patients with renal or hepatic impairment.

Route	Onset	Steady State	Peak	Half-Life	Duration
P.O.	Unknown	Unknown	Unknown	3 to 4 hr	Unknown

Mechanism of Action
May stimulate 5-HT$_1$ receptors on intracranial blood vessels and sensory nerves in the trigeminal-vascular system. By activating these receptors, almotriptan selectively constricts inflamed and dilated cranial blood vessels and inhibits the production of proinflammatory neuropeptides. The drug also interrupts the transmission of pain signals to the brain.

Contraindications
Basilar or hemiplegic migraine; cerebrovascular or peripheral vascular disease or coronary artery disease (CAD) (ischemic or

vasospastic); hypersensitivity to almotriptan or its components; hypertension (uncontrolled); use within 24 hours of other serotonin-receptor agonists or ergotamine-containing or ergot-type drugs

Interactions
DRUGS
ergotamine-containing drugs: Prolonged vasospastic reactions
erythromycin, itraconazole, ketoconazole, ritonavir: Possibly increased blood almotriptan level
MAO inhibitors, verapamil: Increased blood almotriptan level
selective serotonin reuptake inhibitors: Increased risk of hyperreflexia, lack of coordination, and weakness

Adverse Reactions
CNS: Dizziness, headache, paresthesia, somnolence, syncope
CV: Coronary artery vasospasm, hypertension, ischemia, MI, palpitations, vasodilation, ventricular fibrillation, ventricular tachycardia
EENT: Dry mouth
GI: Nausea

Overdose
Monitor patient for evidence of overdose, including hypertension and serious cardiovascular reactions. Monitor vital signs, and expect to continue ECG monitoring for at least 20 hours.

Be prepared to perform gastric lavage, followed by administration of activated charcoal, as prescribed. Be aware that the effect of hemodialysis or peritoneal dialysis on the blood almotriptan level is unknown.

Nursing Considerations
- Be prepared to give the first dose of almotriptan in a medical facility for patients who have risk factors for CAD but have no known cardiovascular abnormatilites.
- Obtain an ECG immediately after the first dose, as ordered, in patients with risk factors for CAD because cardiac ischemia can occur without clinical symptoms.
- **WARNING** Because almotriptan therapy can cause coronary artery vasospasm, monitor patient with CAD for signs and symptoms of angina. Because drug may also cause peripheral vasospastic reactions, such as ischemic bowel disease, monitor patient for abdominal pain and bloody diarrhea.
- Expect to give a lower dosage to patients with hepatic or renal dysfunction because of impaired drug metabolism or excretion.

- Monitor blood pressure regularly during therapy in patients with hypertension because almotriptan may produce a transient increase in blood pressure.

PATIENT TEACHING

- Inform patient that almotriptan is used to treat acute migraine attacks and that he shouldn't take the drug to treat nonmigraine headaches.
- Advise patient to consult prescriber before taking any OTC or prescription drugs.
- Advise patient not to take more than maximum prescribed dosage during any 24-hour period.
- Caution patient that drug may cause adverse CNS reactions, and advise him to avoid potentially hazardous activities until he knows how the drug affects him.
- Instruct patient to seek emergency care immediately if he develops cardiac symptoms—such as heaviness, pain, pressure, or tightness in the chest, jaw, neck, or throat—after taking almotriptan.

alprazolam

Alprazolam Intensol, Apo-Alpraz (CAN), Niravam, Novo-Alprazol (CAN), Nu-Alpraz, Xanax, Xanax XR

Class, Category, and Schedule

Chemical class: Benzodiazepine
Therapeutic class: Antianxiety drug
Pregnancy category: D
Controlled substance schedule: IV

Indications and Dosages

▶ *To control anxiety disorders, relieve anxiety (short-term therapy), or treat anxiety associated with depression*

ORAL SOLUTION, ORALLY DISINTEGRATING TABLETS, TABLETS

Adults. *Initial:* 0.25 to 0.5 mg t.i.d., adjusted to patient's needs. *Maximum:* 4 mg daily in divided doses.

DOSAGE ADJUSTMENT In elderly or debilitated patients or patients with advanced hepatic disease, initial dosage reduced to 0.25 mg b.i.d. or t.i.d. and increased gradually, as needed and tolerated.

▶ *To treat panic attacks*

ORAL SOLUTION, ORALLY DISINTEGRATING TABLETS, TABLETS

Adults. *Initial:* 0.5 mg t.i.d., increased every 3 to 4 days by no more than 1 mg daily, based on patient response. *Maximum:* 10 mg daily in divided doses.

E.R. TABLETS
Adults. *Initial:* 0.5 to 1 mg daily in morning, increased every 3 to 4 days by no more than 1 mg daily, based on patient response. *Maximum:* 10 mg daily as a single dose in morning.

Route	Onset	Steady State	Peak	Half-Life	Duration
P.O.	Unknown	2 to 3 days	Unknown	6 to 27 hr	Unknown

Mechanism of Action
May increase the effects of gamma-aminobutyric acid (GABA) and other inhibitory neurotransmitters by binding to specific benzodiazepine receptors in the limbic and cortical areas of the CNS. GABA inhibits excitatory stimulation, which helps control emotional behavior. The limbic system contains many benzodiazepine receptors, which may help explain the drug's antianxiety effects.

Contraindications
Acute angle-closure glaucoma; hypersensitivity to alprazolam, its components, or other benzodiazepines; itraconazole or ketoconazole therapy

Interactions
DRUGS
antacids: Possibly altered rate of absorption of alprazolam
cimetidine, disulfiram, fluoxetine, isoniazid, metoprolol, oral contraceptives, propoxyphene, propranolol, valproic acid: Possibly decreased elimination and increased effects of alprazolam
CNS depressants: Possibly increased CNS effects of both drugs
digoxin: Possibly increased blood digoxin level, causing digitalis toxicity
itraconazole, ketoconazole: Possibly profoundly inhibited metabolism of alprazolam
levodopa: Possibly decreased effects of levodopa
neuromuscular blockers: Possibly potentiated or antagonized effects of these drugs
phenytoin: Possibly increased blood phenytoin level, causing phenytoin toxicity
probenecid: Possibly faster onset or prolonged effects of alprazolam
ranitidine: Possibly reduced absorption of alprazolam

ACTIVITIES

alcohol use: Increased adverse CNS effects of alprazolam

Adverse Reactions

CNS: Agitation, akathisia, confusion, depression, dizziness, drowsiness, fatigue, hallucinations, headache, insomnia, irritability, lack of coordination, light-headedness, memory loss, nervousness, paresthesia, rigidity, speech problems, syncope, tremor, weakness

CV: Chest pain, edema, hypotension, nonspecific ECG changes, palpitations, tachycardia

EENT: Blurred vision, decreased or increased salivation, dry mouth, nasal congestion, tinnitus

ENDO: Galactorrhea, gynecomastia, hyperprolactinemia

GI: Abdominal discomfort, anorexia, constipation, diarrhea, elevated liver function test results, hepatitis, hepatic failure, nausea, vomiting

GU: Decreased or increased libido, urinary hesitancy

MS: Dysarthria, muscle rigidity and spasms

RESP: Hyperventilation, upper respiratory infection

SKIN: Dermatitis, diaphoresis, pruritus, rash, Stevens-Johnson syndrome

Other: Weight gain or loss

Overdose

Monitor patient for signs and symptoms of overdose, including bradycardia, coma, confusion, dyspnea, hyporeflexia, seizures, severe drowsiness, shakiness, slurred speech, staggering, and weakness.

Maintain an open airway, institute continuous cardiac monitoring, and administer continuous I.V. fluids, as prescribed, to maintain blood pressure and promote diuresis. Institute seizure precautions according to facility protocol.

To decrease alprazolam absorption in a conscious patient who isn't at risk for coma or seizures, be prepared to induce vomiting or perform gastric lavage. Expect to also give oral activated charcoal.

For an unconscious patient, anticipate assisting with insertion of an endotracheal tube and then performing gastric lavage. The inflated cuff of the endotracheal tube will help prevent aspiration of gastric contents into the lungs.

Anticipate the use of a benzodiazepine receptor antagonist such as flumazenil to reverse the sedative effects. Be aware that flumazenil may induce seizures, especially in a patient who has been taking benzodiazepines for a long time or who has also ingested a cyclic antidepressant. If excitation occurs, be aware that a barbiturate shouldn't be used because it may increase excitement and prolong CNS depression. Dialysis is ineffective for treating benzodiazepine overdose. Institute suicide precautions according to facility policy, and anticipate psychiatric re-evaluation.

Nursing Considerations

- Expect to administer a higher dosage to a patient with a history of panic attacks that occur unexpectedly or, for example, while driving.
- Because alprazolam use can lead to dependency and because abrupt discontinuation of therapy can lead to withdrawal signs and symptoms, expect to reduce dosage gradually when tapering off the drug.

PATIENT TEACHING

- Instruct patient or caregiver to measure the alprazolam oral solution with the dropper that's provided with the drug. Instruct him to mix the drug with a liquid (such as water or soda) or a semisolid food (such as applesauce or pudding) just before taking it.
- If alprazolam is prescribed to treat panic attacks, tell patient that drug isn't intended to relieve everyday stress.
- Warn patient not to stop taking the drug abruptly because withdrawal signs and symptoms may occur.
- Instruct patient never to increase the prescribed dosage because of the increased risk of dependency.
- Urge patient to avoid drinking alcohol during alprazolam therapy.
- Advise patient to avoid driving and activities that require alertness until he knows how the drug affects him.
- Instruct female patient of childbearing age to notify prescriber immediately if she is or could be pregnant because drug isn't recommended during pregnancy.

alprostadil (intracavernosal injection)

Caverject, Edex

alprostadil (urogenital suppository)

Muse

Class and Category

Chemical class: Prostaglandin E_1
Therapeutic class: Anti-impotence drug
Pregnancy category: C

Indications and Dosages

▶ *To treat erectile dysfunction caused by vascular or psychogenic issues or both*

INTRACAVERNOUS INJECTION

Adults. *Initial:* 2.5 mcg. Dosage increased to 5 mcg if partial response is apparent or 7.5 mcg if no response is apparent, followed by incremental increases of 5 to 10 mcg until erection suitable for intercourse, not exceeding 1-hr duration, is achieved. No more than 2 doses, separated by 1 hr, should be given on a single day during initial titration phase. *Maximum:* 3 doses/week; each dose separated by 24 hr.

URETHRAL SUPPOSITORY

Adults. *Initial:* 125 to 250 mcg. If no response, dosage increased in stepwise increments to 500 or 1,000 mcg until erection suitable for intercourse, not exceeding 1-hr duration, is achieved. *Maximum:* 2 doses/24 hr.

▶ *To treat erectile dysfunction caused by spinal cord injury*

INTRACAVERNOUS INJECTION

Adults. *Initial:* 1.25 mcg. Dosage increased to 2.5 mcg if patient has partial response; then increased to 5 mcg and in 5-mcg increments until erection is achieved that is suitable for intercourse but does not exceed 1 hour in duration. No more than 2 doses, separated by 1 hr, should be given on a single day during initial titration phase. *Maximum:* 3 doses/week; each dose separated by 24 hr.

Route	Onset	Steady State	Peak	Half-Life	Duration
Intracavernous injection	5 to 20 min	Unknown	Unknown	Unknown	60 min
Intraurethral suppository	5 to 10 min	Unknown	Unknown	30 sec to 10 min	30 to 60 min

Contraindications

Anuria, balanitis (inflammation of the head of the penis), cavernosal fibrosis, children, hypersensitivity to alprostadil or its components, hyperviscosity syndrome, indwelling urethral catheter, leukemia, men for whom sexual activity is contraindicated, men prone to developing venous thrombosis, multiple myeloma, penile angulation, penile implants, Peyronie's disease, polycythemia, severe hypospadius (urethral opening on the underside of the penis), sickle cell anemia or trait, thrombocythemia, urethral obstruction or stricture, urethritis, women

Mechanism of Action

Alprostadil causes penile erection by increasing blood flow to the penis through relaxation of trabecular smooth muscles and dilation of cavernosal arteries.

A naturally occurring prostaglandin, alprostadil interacts with specific membrane-bound receptors in the corpora cavernosa cells of the penis. This action activates intracellular adenyl cyclase, which in turn converts adenosine triphosphate (ATP) to cyclic adenosine monophosphate (cAMP). Increased intracellular levels of cAMP activate protein kinase, an enzyme that activates other enzymes to initiate a cascade of chemical reactions. These chemical reactions cause the trabecular smooth muscles to relax and the cavernosal arteries to dilate. Blood flow to the penis is then increased, which distends the penile lacunar spaces and compresses the veins, trapping blood in the penis and causing it to become enlarged and rigid.

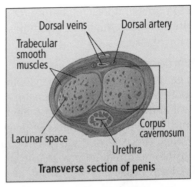

Transverse section of penis

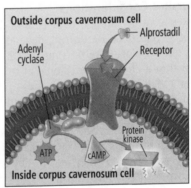

Interactions
DRUGS
anticoagulants: Possibly increased risk of bleeding
cyclosporine: Possibly decreased blood cyclosporine level

Adverse Reactions
CNS: Dizziness, headache, syncope
CV: Hypertension, hypotension, tachycardia, vasodilation
EENT: Nasal congestion, sinusitis
GU: Disorders of the penis, including edema, fibrosis, pain, and rash; pelvic pain; priapism; prolonged erection; prostatic pain or

enlargement; urethral abrasions; urethral bleeding
MS: Back pain
RESP: Cough, upper respiratory tract infection
Other: Flulike symptoms, injection site bruising or hematoma, needle breakage

Overdose

Monitor patient for signs and symptoms of overdose, including hypotension, persistent penile pain, and priapism. Priapism, an erection that lasts longer than 6 hours, can result in permanent penile tissue damage and loss of potency. Monitor patient until all systemic effects have resolved or detumescence (decline of erection) has occurred. Be prepared to treat systemic effects as ordered and needed.

Nursing Considerations

- Reconstitute solution with 1 ml of diluent, for a concentration of 5, 10, 20, or 40 mcg/ml, depending on vial strength. Gently swirl contents of reconstituted vial. Use reconstituted solution within 24 hours when stored at room temperature. Don't use any vials containing precipitates or discoloration. Discard unused portion of reconstituted solution.
- Using a ½-inch 27G to 30G needle, inject drug at a 90-degree angle into the proximal third of the spongy tissue that runs the length of the dorsolateral aspect of the penis, avoiding any visible veins. Rotate injection sites by alternating sides of the penis used for injection.
- Carefully examine the penis for signs and symptoms of penile fibrosis. Expect to discontinue treatment if patient develops cavernosal fibrosis, penile angulation, or Peyronie's disease (hardening of the corpora cavernosa that causes the penis to become distorted when erect) during therapy.
- **WARNING** Assess patient for prolonged erection after drug administration. Notify prescriber and be prepared to treat patient for priapism if erection lasts longer than 4 hours.
- If patient is receiving an anticoagulant, such as warfarin or heparin, monitor him for bleeding at injection site because alprostadil may inhibit platelet aggregation.

PATIENT TEACHING
- Inform patient that initial alprostadil therapy must be performed in the office setting. Teach him how to correctly administer intracavernous injection or urethral suppositories. Explain that the goal is to produce an erection that lasts no longer than 1 hour.

- Advise patient to use alprostadil for injection no more than 3 times weekly and to separate doses by 24 hours. Inform patient using urethral suppositories not to use more than 2 doses in a 24-hour period.
- Instruct patient to inform prescriber immediately of the development of nodules or hard tissue in the penis; an erection that persists for more than 4 hours; any new or worsened penile pain; or persistent curvature, redness, swelling, or tenderness of the erect penis.
- Inform patient that common adverse effects are mild to moderate pain immediately after injection and burning after the suppository is inserted.
- Inform patient of possibility of needle breakage. Encourage him to handle injection device properly and to follow prescriber instructions precisely. If needle breaks during injection and patient can see the broken end, tell him to remove it and contact the prescriber. If he cannot see or grasp the broken end, he should contact the prescriber immediately.
- Instruct patient using suppository form of drug to urinate just before inserting suppository and to insert the suppository with the applicator supplied with the drug. Tell the patient to hold the penis upright after insertion and to roll it firmly between his hands to distribute the drug.
- Tell the patient to sit, stand, or walk for 10 minutes after inserting the suppository to increase blood flow, which enhances erection.
- Inform patient that he can expect an erection to occur within 5 to 20 minutes after injecting the drug or about 10 minutes after inserting the suppository.
- Advise patient not to change drug dosage without consulting his prescriber and to keep regularly scheduled follow-up appointments to monitor progress.
- Warn patient that alprostadil offers no protection from sexually transmitted diseases. Urge him not to reuse or share needles or syringes. Explain proper procedure for sharps disposal. Urge him to use a condom to decrease risk of blood-borne diseases. Explain that injection may cause minor bleeding at the injection site.
- Warn patient taking the suppository form not to engage in sexual intercourse with a pregnant woman unless a condom is used because the effect of the drug on pregnancy is unknown.
- Advise patient who plans to travel not to check the drug with airline baggage or store it in a closed car.

Other Therapeutic Uses

Alprostadil is also indicated for the following:

• As adjunct to tests to diagnose erectile dysfunction
• As palliative therapy to temporarily maintain patency of ductus arteriosus in neonates who have congenital heart defects

amantadine hydrochloride (adamantanamine hydrochloride)

Endantadine (CAN), Gen-Amantadine (CAN), Symmetrel

Class and Category

Chemical class: Adamantane derivative
Therapeutic class: Antidyskinetic
Pregnancy category: C

Indications and Dosages

▶ *To manage symptoms of primary Parkinson's disease, postencephalitic parkinsonism, arteriosclerotic parkinsonism, and parkinsonism caused by CNS injury from carbon monoxide intoxication*

CAPSULES, SYRUP, TABLETS

Adults. *Initial:* 100 mg b.i.d. *Maximum:* 400 mg daily in divided doses.

▶ *To treat drug-induced extrapyramidal reactions*

CAPSULES, SYRUP, TABLETS

Adults. *Initial:* 100 mg b.i.d. *Maximum:* 300 mg daily in divided doses.

DOSAGE ADJUSTMENT For elderly patients, patients taking high doses of other antidyskinetics, and patients with a serious medical condition (such as heart failure, epilepsy, or psychosis), initial dosage reduced to 100 mg daily, with gradual titration to 100 mg b.i.d. after 1 to several wk. For patients with impaired renal function, dosage adjusted to 200 mg on day 1 and then 100 mg daily if creatinine clearance is 30 to 50 ml/min/1.73 m^2; 200 mg on day 1 and then 100 mg every other day if creatinine clearance is 15 to 29 ml/min/1.73 m^2; and 200 mg every wk if creatinine clearance is less than 15 ml/min/1.73 m^2 or if patient is receiving hemodialysis.

Route	Onset	Steady State	Peak	Half-Life	Duration
P.O.	In 48 hr	2 to 3 days	Unknown	11 to 15 hr*	Unknown

* For patients with normal renal function. Half-life is 24 to 29 hr for elderly patients, 18 to 81 hr for patients with severe renal function impairment, and 8 days for those receiving hemodialysis.

Mechanism of Action

May cause dopamine to accumulate in the basal ganglia by increasing release or blocking reuptake of dopamine into presynaptic neurons of the CNS. Dopamine, a neurotransmitter synthesized and released by neurons leading from substantia nigra to basal ganglia, is essential for normal motor function. In Parkinson's disease, progressive degeneration of these neurons substantially reduces the supply of intrasynaptic dopamine. Amantadine may also stimulate dopamine receptors or make postsynaptic receptors more sensitive to dopamine. These actions help control alterations in involuntary muscle movements, such as tremors and rigidity, in Parkinson's disease.

Contraindications

Angle-closure glaucoma, hypersensitivity to amantadine or its components

Interactions

DRUGS

anticholinergics or other drugs with anticholinergic activity, other antidyskinetics, antihistamines, phenothiazines, tricyclic antidepressants: Possibly increased anticholinergic effects and risk of paralytic ileus
carbidopa-levodopa, levodopa: Increased effectiveness of these drugs
CNS stimulants: Excessive CNS stimulation, possibly causing arrhythmias, insomnia, irritability, nervousness, or seizures
hydrochlorothiazide, triamterene: Possibly decreased amantadine clearance and increased risk of toxicity
live-virus vaccines: Possibly interference with vaccine effectiveness
quinidine, quinine, trimethoprim-sulfamethoxazole: Increased blood amantadine level

ACTIVITIES

alcohol use: Possibly increased risk of CNS effects—including confusion, dizziness, and light-headedness—and orthostatic hypotension

Adverse Reactions

CNS: Agitation, anxiety, confusion, dizziness, drowsiness, fatigue, hallucinations, insomnia, irritability, light-headedness, mental impairment, nervousness, nightmares, suicidal ideation, syncope
CV: Orthostatic hypotension, peripheral edema
EENT: Blurred vision; dry mouth, nose, or throat
GI: Constipation, diarrhea, nausea
GU: Dysuria
HEME: Agranulocytosis, leukopenia, neutropenia
SKIN: Livedo reticularis (purplish, netlike rash)

Overdose

Amantadine overdose has no specific antidote. Monitor patient for signs and symptoms of overdose, including arrhythmias, pulmonary edema, seizures, status epilepticus, and toxic psychosis characterized by aggressive and violent behavior and hallucinations. Monitor vital signs, fluid intake and output, serum electrolyte levels, and urine pH.

Initiate seizure precautions according to facility protocol and cardiac monitoring to assess patient for arrhythmias. Anticipate the use of I.V. fluids to prevent or treat hypotension. If drug ingestion was recent, expect to perform gastric lavage or give activated charcoal, as prescribed. Vomiting shouldn't be induced because of the risk of seizures. Anticipate giving an antiarrhythmic and an antihypotensive, as prescribed. Use caution when giving an adrenergic, such as isoproterenol, because amantadine overdose may result in severe arrhythmias. Institute suicide precautions according to facility policy, and anticipate psychiatric re-evaluation.

Nursing Considerations

- Monitor patients who have a history of psychiatric illness or substance abuse because amantadine may worsen these conditions. Be aware that some patients taking amantadine have attempted suicide or had suicidal ideation.
- If patient has a history of heart failure or peripheral edema, monitor weight gain and assess patient for edema because drug may cause a redistribution of body fluid.
- Be aware that the drug may increase seizure activity in patients with a history of seizures.
- **WARNING** Monitor patient for evidence of neuroleptic malignant syndrome during dosage reduction or discontinuation of therapy. These include fever, hypertension or hypotension, involuntary motor activity, mental changes, muscle rigidity, tachycardia, and tachypnea. Be prepared to provide supportive treatment and additional drug therapy, as prescribed.
- Patients receiving more than 200 mg daily are more likely to experience adverse or toxic reactions.
- Monitor patient for decreased drug effectiveness over time. If he demonstrates a decreased therapeutic response, expect drug to be increased or discontinued temporarily.

PATIENT TEACHING

- Instruct patient to take amantadine exactly as prescribed and not to stop taking it abruptly. Advise patient to notify prescriber if drug becomes less effective.

- **WARNING** Advise patient or family members to notify prescriber immediately if thoughts of suicide occur.
- Encourage patient to avoid alcohol ingestion during amantadine therapy because alcohol may increase risk of confusion, dizziness, light-headedness, and orthostatic hypotension.
- Advise patient to avoid driving and other activities that require a high level of alertness until he knows how the drug affects him because it may cause blurred vision and mental impairment.
- Advise patient to change position slowly to minimize effects of orthostatic hypotension.
- Tell patient to use ice chips or sugarless candy or gum to relieve dry mouth.
- Caution patient to resume physical activities gradually as signs and symptoms improve.

Other Therapeutic Uses
Amantadine hydrochloride is also indicated for the following:
- To prevent influenza A
- To treat infection caused by influenza A

amitriptyline hydrochloride
Apo-amitriptyline (CAN), Endep, Levate (CAN), Novotriptyn (CAN)

Class and Category
Chemical class: Dibenzocycloheptadiene derivative
Therapeutic class: Antidepressant
Pregnancy category: D

Indications and Dosages
▶ *To relieve depression, especially when accompanied by anxiety and insomnia*
TABLETS
Adults and children over age 12. *Outpatient:* 75 mg daily in divided doses, increased to 150 mg daily, if needed. *Inpatient:* 100 mg daily, gradually increased to 300 mg daily, if needed. *Maintenance:* 40 to 100 mg daily at bedtime.
DOSAGE ADJUSTMENT Maintenance dosage reduced to 10 mg t.i.d. plus 20 mg at bedtime for adolescent and elderly patients.

Route	Onset	Steady State	Peak	Half-Life	Duration
P.O.	14 to 21 days	4 to 10 days	Unknown	31 to 46 hr	Unknown

Mechanism of Action

Normally, when an impulse reaches adrenergic nerves, the nerves release serotonin and norepinephrine from their storage sites. Some serotonin and norepinephrine reaches receptor sites on target tissues. Most is taken back into the nerves and stored by the reuptake mechanism, as shown below.

   Amitriptyline, a tricyclic antidepressant, blocks serotonin and norepinephrine reuptake by adrenergic nerves. By doing this, it raises serotonin and norepinephrine levels at nerve synapses, as shown below. This action may elevate mood and reduce depression.

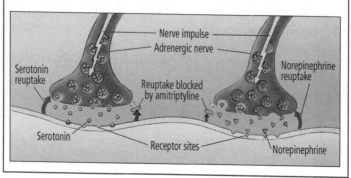

Contraindications

Acute recovery phase after an MI, hypersensitivity to amitriptyline, MAO inhibitor therapy within 14 days

Interactions

DRUGS

anticholinergics, epinephrine, norepinephrine: Increased effects of these drugs

barbiturates: Decreased blood amitriptyline level

carbamazepine: Decreased blood amitriptyline level; increased blood carbamazepine level, which increases the therapeutic and toxic effects of carbamazepine

cimetidine, disulfiram, fluoxetine, fluvoxamine, haloperidol, H₂-receptor antagonists, methylphenidate, oral contraceptives, paroxetine, phenothiazines, sertraline: Increased blood amitriptyline level

cisapride: Possibly prolonged QT interval, increased risk of arrhythmias

clonidine, guanethidine, and other antihypertensives: Decreased antihypertensive effects

dicumarol: Increased anticoagulant effect of dicumarol

levodopa: Decreased levodopa absorption; sympathetic hyperactiv-

ity, sinus tachycardia, hypertension, agitation
MAO inhibitors: Possibly seizures and death
thyroid replacement drugs: Arrhythmias, increased antidepressant effects
ACTIVITIES
alcohol use: Enhanced CNS depression
smoking: Decreased effects of amitriptyline

Adverse Reactions

CNS: Anxiety, ataxia, coma, chills, delusions, disorientation, drowsiness, extrapyramidal signs and symptoms, fatigue, fever, headache, insomnia, neuroleptic malignant syndrome, nightmares, peripheral neuropathy, tremor
CV: Arrhythmias (including prolonged AV conduction, cardiomyopathy, heart block, and tachycardia), hypertension, MI, nonspecific ECG changes, orthostatic hypotension, palpitations
EENT: Abnormal taste, black tongue, blurred vision, dry mouth, increased salivation, nasal congestion, tinnitus
ENDO: Gynecomastia, altered serum glucose level, increased serum prolactin level, syndrome of inappropriate ADH secretion
GI: Abdominal cramps, constipation, diarrhea, flatulence, ileus, increased appetite, nausea, vomiting
GU: Impotence, libido changes, menstrual irregularities, testicular swelling, urinary hesitancy, urine retention
HEME: Agranulocytosis, bone marrow depression, eosinophilia, leukopenia, thrombocytopenia
SKIN: Alopecia, flushing, purpura
Other: Weight gain

Overdose

Monitor patient for signs and symptoms of overdose, including agitation, arrhythmias, confusion, disturbed concentration, drowsiness, dyspnea, fever, hallucinations, irregular heartbeat, mydriasis, restlessness, seizures, unusual fatigue, weakness, and vomiting.

Maintain an open airway, and closely observe patient's blood pressure, respiratory rate, and temperature. Institute continuous ECG monitoring and seizure precautions according to facility protocol. Be prepared to use supportive measures, such as performing gastric lavage to decrease drug absorption. Expect to administer activated charcoal followed by a bowel stimulant to enhance drug elimination. Anticipate possible digitalization to prevent heart failure. Be prepared to treat arrhythmias with lidocaine and sodium bicarbonate, as prescribed.

Be aware that use of I.V. physostigmine isn't routinely recommended, but it may be prescribed for patients in a coma with respiratory depression, serious arrhythmias, severe hypertension, or uncontrollable seizures to reverse the anticholinergic effects of amitriptyline.

Be prepared to institute emergency measures, including administering anticonvulsant therapy and at least 5 days of continuous cardiac monitoring. Tricyclic antidepressants are highly protein-bound; therefore, dialysis, exchange transfusions, and forced diuresis are ineffective for treating overdose. Institute suicide precautions according to facility policy, and anticipate psychiatric reevaluation.

Nursing Considerations

- Monitor patient closely for evidence of neuroleptic malignant syndrome, a rare but possibly fatal disorder, when starting amitriptyline therapy or increasing dosage. Evidence includes altered mental status, tachycardia, diaphoresis, tremor, fever, and muscle rigidity.
- Because of amitriptyline's atropine-like effects, use it cautiously in patients with a history of angle-closure glaucoma, seizures, or urine retention.
- **WARNING** Don't administer an MAO inhibitor within 14 days of amitriptyline because of the risk of seizures and death.
- Closely monitor patient with cardiovascular disorder because amitriptyline may cause arrhythmias, such as sinus tachycardia and prolonged conduction times.
- Monitor blood pressure, and assess patient for hypotension or hypertension.
- Stay alert for behavior changes, such as decreased interest in personal appearance and obvious hallucinations. Be aware that schizophrenic patients may develop psychosis, and paranoid patients may develop exaggerated symptoms.
- Avoid abrupt withdrawal of amitriptyline after prolonged therapy; otherwise, headache, nausea, nightmares, and vertigo may occur.

PATIENT TEACHING

- Instruct patient to take amitriptyline at bedtime to avoid daytime drowsiness.
- Instruct patient to avoid using alcohol or OTC drugs containing alcohol during amitriptyline therapy because alcohol enhances the drug's CNS depressant effects.

amobarbital sodium

Amytal, Novamobarb (CAN)

Class, Category, and Schedule

Chemical class: Barbiturate
Therapeutic class: Anticonvulsant, sedative-hypnotic
Pregnancy category: D
Controlled substance schedule: II

Indications and Dosages

▶ *To produce sedation*

CAPSULES, ELIXIR, TABLETS, I.V. OR I.M. INJECTION

Adults. 30 to 50 mg b.i.d. or t.i.d. and may range from 15 to
120 mg b.i.d or t.i.d. *Maximum I.V.:* 1,000 mg/dose. *Maximum I.M.:*
500 mg/dose.

Children over age 6. 2 mg/kg daily in 4 divided doses.

▶ *To treat insomnia*

CAPSULES, ELIXIR, TABLETS

Adults. 65 to 200 mg at bedtime for up to 2 wk.

▶ *To induce a hypnotic state*

CAPSULES, ELIXIR, TABLETS, I.V. OR I.M. INJECTION

Adults. 65 to 200 mg/dose. *Maximum I.V.:* 1,000 mg/dose. *Maximum I.M.:* 500 mg/dose.

Children age 6 and over. 65 to 500 mg I.V. per dose; 2 to 3 mg/
kg I.M. per dose.

Children up to age 6. 2 to 3 mg/kg I.M. per dose.

▶ *To manage seizures*

I.V. OR I.M. INJECTION

Adults. *Usual:* 65 to 500 mg. *Maximum:* 1,000 mg. The dosage for
acute seizures is determined by response. Doses of 200 to 500 mg
are typically required to control seizures.

Children age 6 and over. 65 to 500 mg I.V.

Children up to age 6. 3 to 5 mg/kg/dose.

WARNING Use I.V. route only when other routes aren't appropriate. For I.V. injection, use I.M. dose and inject slowly at a
rate of 50 mg/min or less to prevent sudden apnea, laryngospasm, hypotension, or respiratory depression.

Route	Onset	Steady State	Peak	Half-Life	Duration
P.O.*	60 min	Unknown	Unknown	Unknown	10 to 12 hr
I.V.	45 to 60 min	Unknown	Unknown	16 to 40 hr	6 to 8 hr
I.M.	45 to 60 min	Unknown	Unknown	16 to 40 hr	6 to 8 hr

* For capsules, elixir, and tablets.

Mechanism of Action

Nonselectively acts on the CNS to depress the sensory cortex, decrease motor activity, alter cerebral function, and produce drowsiness, hypnosis, and sedation. Appears to reduce wakefulness and alertness by acting in the thalamus, where it depresses the reticular activating system and interferes with impulse transmission from the periphery to the cortex. Produces CNS depressant effects ranging from mild sedation and anxiety reduction to anesthesia and coma, depending on the dosage, route, and individual patient's response.

Incompatibilities

Don't mix amobarbital in solution with other drugs.

Contraindications

Alcoholism, hepatic or renal disease, history of barbiturate or sedative addiction, history of porphyria, hypersensitivity to barbiturates, severe respiratory disease, sleep apnea, suicidal tendency, uncontrolled pain

Interactions

DRUGS

acetaminophen: Increased metabolism and decreased effectiveness of acetaminophen; risk of hepatotoxicity

antihistamines, CNS depressants, phenothiazines, tranquilizers: Increased CNS depression

beta blockers, carbamazepine, clonazepam, corticosteroids, doxycycline, estrogens, griseofulvin, metronidazole, oral anticoagulants, oral contraceptives, phenylbutazones, quinidine, theophyllines, tricyclic antidepressants: Decreased blood levels and effects of these drugs

chloramphenicol: Inhibited amobarbital metabolism, enhanced chloramphenicol metabolism

MAO inhibitors: Increased blood level and sedative effects of amobarbital

methoxyflurane: Increased nephrotoxicity

phenytoin: Altered effects of phenytoin

rifampin: Decreased blood level and effects of amobarbital

valproic acid: Increased effects of amobarbital

ACTIVITIES

alcohol use: Increased blood level of amobarbital, additive CNS depressant effects

Adverse Reactions

CNS: Agitation, anxiety, ataxia, CNS depression, confusion, dizziness, hallucinations, hangover, headache, hyperkinesia, insomnia, nervousness, nightmares, paradoxical stimulation, permanent neurologic deficit (with injection near nerve), psychiatric disturbance, somnolence, syncope, vertigo

CV: Bradycardia, hypotension, shock

EENT: Laryngospasm

GI: Constipation, diarrhea, epigastric pain, nausea, vomiting

RESP: Apnea, bronchospasm, hypoventilation, respiratory depression

SKIN: Exfoliative dermatitis, rash, Stevens-Johnson syndrome, urticaria

Other: Angioedema, gangrene of arm or leg from accidental injection into artery, injection site tissue damage and necrosis, physical and psychological dependence, potentially fatal withdrawal syndrome, tolerance

Overdose

Monitor patient for evidence of overdose, including bradycardia, Cheyne-Stokes respiration, coma, confusion, decreased or absent reflexes, dyspnea, fever, hypothermia, miosis or mydriasis, oliguria, severe drowsiness, severe weakness, shock, slurred speech, staggering, tachycardia, and unusual eye movements. Consider chronic overdose if such signs and symptoms as continued irritability, insomnia, poor judgment, and severe confusion occur.

Maintain an open airway, and carefully monitor temperature and blood pressure.

If the patient is conscious, be prepared to administer ipecac syrup, as prescribed, to induce vomiting. Expect to administer 30 to 60 g of activated charcoal with water or sorbitol to prevent further absorption and to enhance drug elimination.

If the patient is unconscious, be prepared to assist with insertion of an endotracheal tube and then to perform gastric lavage. The inflated cuff of the endotracheal tube will help prevent aspiration of gastric contents into the patient's lungs. Be prepared to administer drugs to promote urine alkalization to increase drug elimination. Administer I.V. fluids and a vasopressor, as prescribed. For severe cases, hemodialysis or hemoperfusion may be needed.

Be aware that, in cases of extreme barbiturate overdose, the patient may have a flat EEG because all electrical activity in the brain has ceased; however, this effect may be reversible. Institute suicide precautions according to facility policy, and anticipate psychiatric re-evaluation.

Nursing Considerations

• Use amobarbital cautiously in patients with cardiac disease, debilitation, diabetes mellitus, fever, hyperthyroidism, severe anemia, shock, status asthmaticus, or uremia.

• For I.M. use, inject deep into muscle, preferably a large one.

• During I.V. use, closely monitor blood pressure, pulse, and respirations. Keep emergency equipment and drugs nearby in case of respiratory depression.

• **WARNING** Don't administer solution after 30 minutes of exposure to air. Solution quickly becomes unstable because amobarbital sodium hydrolyzes in it.

• To prevent withdrawal signs and symptoms—such as diaphoresis, insomnia, irritability, nightmares, and tremors—expect to taper amobarbital dosage gradually after long-term use, especially for epileptic patients.

• **WARNING** To prevent tissue damage and necrosis at I.M. injection site, don't administer more than 5 ml of this highly alkaline drug at any one site. Know that accidental arterial injection may cause gangrene of the arm or leg.

PATIENT TEACHING

• Advise patient to use caution when driving or performing tasks that require alertness.

• Instruct patient not to use alcohol or other CNS depressants (unless prescribed) because they increase amobarbital's effects.

• Warn patient not to stop taking drug abruptly because withdrawal signs and symptoms can occur.

• Instruct patient to report if he experiences severe dizziness, persistent drowsiness, rash, or skin lesions.

• Advise patient that amobarbital's effects, such as drowsiness, may become less pronounced after a few days and when drug is taken with food.

Other Therapeutic Uses

Amobarbital sodium is also indicated for the following:
• To produce preanesthesia sedation

amoxapine
Asendin

Class and Category

Chemical class: Dibenzoxazepine derivative
Therapeutic class: Antidepressant
Pregnancy category: C

Indications and Dosages

▶ *To relieve depression, including endogenous (long-term) depression and depression associated with anxiety and agitation*

TABLETS

Adults and children age 16 and over. *Initial:* 50 mg b.i.d. or t.i.d., increased to 100 mg b.i.d. or t.i.d. by end of first wk, if tolerated. *Maintenance:* If 300-mg daily dose is ineffective after 2-wk trial period, dosage increased to a maximum of 400 mg daily in divided doses. Inpatients may receive up to a maximum of 600 mg daily in divided doses. When effective dosage is achieved, a single dose may be given at bedtime, not to exceed 300 mg.

DOSAGE ADJUSTMENT Dosage reduced for elderly patients. *Initial:* 25 mg b.i.d. or t.i.d., increased to 50 mg b.i.d. or t.i.d. by end of first wk. *Maintenance:* 100 to 150 mg daily in divided doses, carefully increased to 300 mg daily as tolerated. When effective dosage is achieved, a single dose may be given at bedtime, not to exceed 300 mg.

Route	Onset	Steady State	Peak	Half-Life	Duration
P.O.	1 to 2 wk	2 to 7 days	Unknown	8 hr*	Unknown

Mechanism of Action

A tricyclic antidepressant that blocks serotonin and norepinephrine reuptake by adrenergic nerves. By doing this, it raises serotonin and norepinephrine levels at nerve synapses. This action may elevate mood and reduce depression.

Normally, when an impulse reaches adrenergic nerves, the nerves release serotonin and norepinephrine from their storage sites. Some serotonin and norepinephrine reaches receptor sites on target tissues. Much is taken back into the nerves and stored by the reuptake mechanism. Amoxapine and its metabolites also exert a potent postsynaptic dopamine-blocking effect, which may cause the patient to experience extrapyramidal signs and symptoms.

Contraindications

Acute recovery phase after an MI, hypersensitivity to amoxapine or its components, MAO inhibitor therapy within 14 days

Interactions

DRUGS

anticholinergics, epinephrine, norepinephrine: Increased effects of these drugs

---

* 6½ hr for 7-hydroxyamoxapine metabolite; 30 hr for 8-hydroxyamoxapine metabolite.

barbiturates: Decreased blood amoxapine level
carbamazepine: Decreased blood amoxapine level; increased blood carbamazepine level, which increases the therapeutic and toxic effects of carbemazepine
cimetidine, disulfiram, fluoxetine, fluvoxamine, haloperidol, H_2-receptor antagonists, methylphenidate, oral contraceptives, paroxetine, phenothiazines, sertraline: Increased blood amoxapine level
clonidine, guanethidine, other antihypertensives: Decreased antihypertensive effects
dicumarol: Increased anticoagulant effect of dicumarol
levodopa: Decreased levodopa absorption; agitation, hypertension, sinus tachycardia, sympathetic hyperactivity
MAO inhibitors: Possibly seizures and death
thyroid replacement drugs: Arrhythmias, increased antidepressant effects
ACTIVITIES
alcohol use: Increased CNS depression
smoking: Decreased effects of amoxapine

Adverse Reactions

CNS: Agitation, anxiety, ataxia, chills, confusion, CVA, dizziness, drowsiness, excitement, extrapyramidal signs and symptoms, fatigue, fever, headache, insomnia, nervousness, nightmares, paresthesia, restlessness, sedation, seizures, syncope, tremor, weakness
CV: Atrial arrhythmias, heart block, heart failure, hypertension, hypotension, MI, palpitations, tachycardia
EENT: Blurred vision, dry mouth, increased salivation, nasal congestion, taste perversion, tinnitus
ENDO: Altered serum glucose level, elevated serum prolactin level, gynecomastia, syndrome of inappropriate ADH secretion
GI: Anorexia, constipation, diarrhea, elevated liver function test results, excessive appetite, flatulence, nausea, vomiting
GU: Impotence, libido changes, menstrual irregularities, testicular swelling, urinary hesitancy, urine retention
HEME: Agranulocytosis, leukopenia
SKIN: Diaphoresis, flushing, photosensitivity, pruritus, rash
Other: Weight gain or loss; withdrawal signs and symptoms, such as headache, nausea, nightmares, and vertigo

Overdose

Monitor patient for signs and symptoms of overdose, including agitation, arrhythmias, confusion, disturbed concentration, drowsiness, dyspnea, fever, hallucinations, irregular heartbeat, mydriasis, restlessness, seizures, unusual fatigue, vomiting, and weakness.

Maintain an open airway, institute continuous ECG monitoring, and closely observe the patient's blood pressure, respiratory rate, and temperature. Be prepared to institute supportive measures such as gastric lavage to decrease drug absorption. Expect to administer activated charcoal followed by a bowel stimulant to increase drug elimination. Anticipate possible digitalization to prevent heart failure. Be prepared to treat arrhythmias with lidocaine and sodium bicarbonate, as prescribed.

Be aware that I.V. physostigmine is contraindicated in amoxapine overdose because of the risk of seizures, which may be severe in amoxapine overdose and lead to acute tubular necrosis or rhabdomyolysis. Be prepared to take emergency measures, including anticonvulsant therapy and at least 5 days of continuous cardiac monitoring. Tricyclic antidepressants are highly protein bound, making dialysis, exchange transfusions, and forced diuresis ineffective for overdose. Take suicide precautions according to facility policy, and anticipate psychiatric re-evaluation.

Nursing Considerations
- **WARNING** Don't administer an MAO inhibitor within 14 days of amoxapine.
- Expect to taper drug gradually before discontinuing to prevent withdrawal signs and symptoms.

PATIENT TEACHING
- Suggest taking amoxapine at bedtime if daytime sedation occurs.
- Instruct patient not to stop taking drug abruptly because withdrawal signs and symptoms can occur.
- Encourage patient to avoid alcohol because it can potentiate amoxapine's effects.
- Tell patient to report if he experiences difficulty urinating, dizziness, dry mouth, nausea, or palpitations.
- Instruct patient to take drug with food to prevent GI upset.
- Warn patient to avoid driving and other tasks that require alertness until he knows how the drug affects him.

amphetamine and dextroamphetamine
Adderall, Adderall XR

Class, Category, and Schedule
Chemical class: Phenylisopropalamine
Therapeutic class: CNS stimulant
Pregnancy category: C
Controlled substance schedule: II

Indications and Dosages

▶ *To treat attention deficit hyperactivity disorder (ADHD)*
TABLETS
Children age 6 and over. *Initial:* 5 mg once or twice daily. Dosage increased by 5 mg daily every wk until desired response occurs. *Maximum:* 40 mg daily.
Children ages 3 to 6. *Initial:* 2.5 mg daily. Dosage increased by 2.5 mg daily every wk until desired response occurs. *Maximum:* 40 mg daily.
E.R. CAPSULES
Adults. 20 mg daily.
Adolescents ages 13 to 18. *Initial:* 10 mg daily. Increased to 20 mg daily after 1 wk if needed.
Children age 6 and older. *Initial:* 10 mg daily. Increased by 10 mg daily every wk until desired response occurs. *Maximum:* 30 mg daily.
▶ *To treat narcolepsy*
TABLETS
Adults and children age 12 and over. *Initial:* 10 mg daily. Dosage increased by 10 mg daily every wk until desired response occurs. *Maximum:* 60 mg daily for adults.
Children ages 6 to 12. *Initial:* 5 mg daily, increased by 5 mg daily each wk until desired response occurs. *Maximum:* 40 mg daily.

Route	Onset	Steady State	Peak	Half-Life	Duration
P.O. (amphetamine)	Unknown	Unknown	Unknown	10 to 30 hr	Unknown
P.O. (dextro-amphetamine)	Unknown	Unknown	Unknown	10 to 12 hr*	Unknown

Mechanism of Action

May produce CNS stimulation by facilitating norepinephrine release at adrenergic nerve terminals and blocking its reuptake and by directly stimulating alpha and beta receptors in the peripheral nervous system. Drug also causes release and blocks reuptake of dopamine in limbic regions of the brain. Drug's main action appears to be in the cerebral cortex and, possibly, the reticular activating system. Also, dextroamphetamine may stimulate inhibitory autoreceptors in the brain. These actions decrease drowsiness, fatigue, and motor restlessness and increase mental alertness. Peripheral actions include increased blood pressure, mild bronchodilation, and respiratory stimulation.

---

* For adults. Half-life is 6 to 8 hr for children.

Contraindications

Advanced arteriosclerosis; agitation; glaucoma; history of drug abuse; hypersensitivity to amphetamine, dextroamphetamine, or any of their components; hyperthyroidism; MAO inhibitor therapy within 14 days; moderate to severe hypertension; structural cardiac abnormalities; symptomatic cardiovascular disease

Interactions

DRUGS

anesthetics (inhaled): Increased risk of severe ventricular arrhythmias

antacids (calcium- and magnesium-containing), carbonic anhydrase inhibitors, citrates, sodium bicarbonate, urinary alkalinizing agents such as acetazolamide, thiazides: Increased effects of amphetamine

antihypertensives, diuretics: Possibly decreased hypotensive effects

beta blockers: Increased risk of hypertension or excessive bradycardia, possibly heart block

CNS stimulants: Additive CNS stimulation

digoxin, levodopa: Possibly arrhythmias

ethosuximide, phenobarbital, phenytoin: Delayed intestinal absorption of these drugs

glutamic acid hydrochloride; urinary acidifiers, such as ammonium chloride and sodium acid phosphate: Increased excretion and decreased blood levels and effects of amphetamine

haloperidol, loxapine, molindone, phenothiazines, pimozide, thioxanthenes: Reduced antipsychotic effectiveness of these drugs, inhibited CNS stimulant effects of amphetamine and dextroamphetamine

MAO inhibitors: Potentiated effects of amphetamine, possibly hypertensive crisis

meperidine: Increased analgesia

metrizamide: Increased risk of seizures

norepinephrine: Possibly increased adrenergic effect of norepinephrine

propoxyphene: Increased CNS stimulation, risk of fatal seizures

sympathomimetics: Increased cardiovascular effects of both drugs

thyroid hormones: Enhanced effects of both drugs

tricyclic antidepressants: Possibly increased cardiovascular effects

FOODS

ascorbic acid, fruit juices: Decreased absorption and effects of amphetamine

Adverse Reactions

CNS: Agitation, anxiety, CVA, depression, dizziness, drowsiness, emotional lability, fatigue, fever, headache, insomnia, irritability, light-headedness, mania, motor tics, nervousness, psychoses, seizures, tremor

CV: Arrhythmias, hypertension, MI, sudden death, tachycardia

EENT: Accommodation abnormality, blurred vision, dry mouth, taste perversion

GI: Abdominal pain, anorexia, constipation, diarrhea, dyspepsia, nausea, vomiting

GU: Decreased libido, UTI

RESP: Dyspnea

SKIN: Diaphoresis, rash, Stevens-Johnson syndrome, toxic epidermal necrolysis

Other: Angioedema, anaphylaxis, weight loss

Overdose

Amphetamine and dextroamphetamine overdose has no specific antidote. Monitor patient for signs and symptoms of overdose, including abdominal cramps, arrhythmias, chest pain, confusion, delirium, diaphoresis, diarrhea, dizziness, dyspnea, flushing, hallucinations, hyperpyrexia, hypertension or hypotension, irregular heartbeat, nausea, pallor, palpitations, panic reaction, paranoia, photosensitive mydriasis, polypnea, psychotic reactions, rhabdomyolysis, shock, syncope, tachypnea, toxic psychosis, tremor, unusual fatigue, vomiting, and weakness. If possible, physically isolate the patient to limit external stimuli.

Expect to provide symptomatic and supportive treatment, including gastric lavage and induced vomiting. Anticipate giving I.V. fluids to manage hypotension, as needed. Expect to give drugs and fluids to enhance diuresis, as prescribed. Be aware that drug treatment to acidify urine may also be prescribed to increase drug excretion, except in patients with hemoglobinemia, myoglobinuria, or rhabdomyolysis because these patients have an increased risk of renal failure. Be prepared to give drugs such as a barbiturate or chlorpromazine to control CNS stimulation and phentolamine to manage hypertension. Institute emergency supportive measures, and protect patient from self-injury. Take suicide precautions according to facility policy, and anticipate psychiatric re-evaluation.

Nursing Considerations

- Keep in mind that, when signs and symptoms of ADHD occur with acute stress reactions or with structural cardiac abnormalities, treatment with amphetamines usually isn't indicated because the reaction may worsen or sudden death may occur.

- Give first dose of tablet form when patient awakens and additional doses at 4- to 6-hour intervals. Give E.R. capsule form when patient awakens.
- If patient takes divided doses of tablet form, he may be switched to the E.R. capsule form at the same daily dose, to be taken once in the morning.
- **WARNING** If the patient suddenly stops taking the drug after long-term, high-dose therapy, watch for evidence of withdrawal, such as abdominal pain, depression, nausea, tremor, unusual fatigue, vomiting, and weakness. Expect to restart therapy and gradually taper dosage, as prescribed.
- Monitor pulse rate and blood pressure in patients who have hypertension, including even mild hypertension, because drug may increase blood pressure and cause arrhythmias, including tachycardia. Report abnormal findings, including exertional chest pain, unexplained syncope and other symptoms suggestive of cardiac disease, to prescriber.
- Monitor growth and development in children because drug may adversely affect growth.
- Assess patient for potential dependence, drug-seeking behavior, or drug tolerance. Be alert for signs and symptoms of long-term amphetamine abuse characterized by hyperactivity, irritability, marked insomnia, personality changes, and severe dermatoses.
- Assess patient with history of Tourette's syndrome, motor or vocal tics, or psychological disorders for worsening of these conditions during amphetamine therapy.
- Monitor children and adolescents for first-time manifestation of psychotic or manic symptoms. If present, notify prescriber and expect drug to be discontinued.

PATIENT TEACHING
- Stress importance of taking drug exactly as prescribed because misuse of this drug may cause serious adverse cardiovascular reactions, including sudden death.
- Advise patient to take amphetamine and dextroamphetamine with food or after a meal because anorexia may occur.
- Advise patient not to take drug with acidic fruit juice because it may decrease drug absorption.
- Tell patient or caregiver that E.R. capsules may be taken whole or opened and sprinkled on applesauce, then swallowed immediately without chewing.
- Urge patient to avoid potentially hazardous activities until he knows how the drug affects him.

- Inform patient of abuse potential of drug and stress importance of not altering dosage unless prescribed.
- Inform parents or caregivers that child may be placed on drug-free weekend and holiday schedule, as prescribed, if signs and symptoms of ADHD are controlled.

amphetamine sulfate

Class, Category, and Schedule

Chemical class: Phenylisopropylamine
Therapeutic class: CNS stimulant
Pregnancy category: C
Controlled substance schedule: II

Indications and Dosages

▶ *To treat attention deficit hyperactivity disorder (ADHD)*
TABLETS
Children age 6 and over. 5 mg once or twice daily; then increased by 5 mg daily at 1-wk intervals until desired response occurs. *Usual:* 0.1 to 0.5 mg/kg daily.
Children ages 3 to 5. 2.5 mg daily; then increased by 2.5 mg/day at 1-wk intervals until desired response occurs. *Usual:* 0.1 to 0.5 mg/kg daily.
▶ *To treat narcolepsy*
TABLETS
Adults and children age 12 and over. *Initial:* 10 mg daily, then increased by 10 mg daily at 1-wk intervals until desired response occurs.
Children ages 6 to 12. 2.5 mg b.i.d.; then increased by 5 mg/day at 1-wk intervals until desired response occurs or adult dosage is reached to a maximum of 60 mg daily.

Route	Onset	Steady State	Peak	Half-Life	Duration
P.O.	Unknown	Unknown	Unknown	10 to 30 hr	Unknown

Contraindications

Advanced arteriosclerosis, agitation (for narcolepsy treatment), glaucoma, history of drug abuse, hypersensitivity or idiosyncratic reaction to sympathomimetic amines, hyperthyroidism, MAO inhibitor therapy within 14 days, moderate to severe hypertension, structural cardiac abnormalities, symptomatic cardiovascular disease

Mechanism of Action

May produce its CNS stimulant effects by facilitating the release and blocking the reuptake of norepinephrine at the adrenergic nerve terminals and by
directly stimulating alpha and beta receptors in the peripheral nervous system. The drug also releases and blocks the reuptake of dopamine in limbic
regions of the brain. The drug's main action appears to be in the cerebral
cortex and, possibly, the reticular activating system. These actions cause decreased drowsiness, fatigue, and motor restlessness and increased alertness.
The drug's peripheral actions include increased blood pressure and mild bronchodilation and respiratory stimulation.

Interactions

DRUGS

adrenergic blockers: Inhibited adrenergic blockade
alkalizers, such as sodium bicarbonate; acetazolamide; some thiazides: Increased blood level and effects of amphetamine
antihistamines: Possibly reduced sedation from antihistamine
antihypertensives: Possibly decreased antihypertensive effects
chlorpromazine: Inhibited CNS stimulant effects of amphetamine
ethosuximide: Possibly delayed absorption of ethosuximide
GI acidifiers, such as ascorbic acid; reserpine: Decreased absorption of
amphetamine
guanethidine: Decreased antihypertensive effect and decreased absorption of amphetamine
haloperidol: Decreased CNS stimulation
lithium carbonate: Possibly decreased anorectic and stimulant effects of amphetamine
MAO inhibitors: Potentiated effects of amphetamine, possibly hypertensive crisis
meperidine: Increased analgesia
methenamine: Increased urine excretion of amphetamine, which
decreases its effects
norepinephrine: Possibly increased adrenergic effect of norepinephrine
phenobarbital, phenytoin: Synergistic anticonvulsant action
propoxyphene: Increased CNS stimulation, potentially fatal seizures
tricyclic antidepressants: Possibly enhanced effects of antidepressant,
decreased effects of amphetamine
urine acidifiers, such as ammonium chloride and sodium acid phosphate:

Increased excretion and decreased blood level and effects of amphetamine

veratrum alkaloids: Decreased hypotensive effect
FOODS
acidic fruit juices: Decreased absorption of amphetamine

Adverse Reactions

CNS: Agitation, anxiety, CVA, dizziness, dyskinesia, dysphoria, emotional lability, euphoria, exacerbation of motor and phonic tics and Tourette's syndrome, fever, hallucinations, headache, insomnia, mania, nervousness, overstimulation, paranoia, psychotic episodes, restlessness, seizures, tremor

CV: Cardiomyopathy, hypertension, MI, palpitations, sudden death, tachycardia

EENT: Accommodation abnormaility, blurred vision, dry mouth, unpleasant taste

GI: Anorexia, constipation, diarrhea, dyspepsia

GU: Impotence, libido changes, UTI

SKIN: Rash, Stevens-Johnson syndrome, toxic epidermal necrolysis, urticaria

Other: Angioedema, anaphylaxis, weight loss

Overdose

Amphetamine overdose has no specific antidote. Monitor patient for signs and symptoms of overdose, including abdominal cramps, arrhythmias, chest pain, confusion, delirium, diaphoresis, diarrhea, dizziness, dyspnea, faintness, flushing, hallucinations, hyperpyrexia, hypertension or hypotension, irregular heartbeat, nausea, pallor, palpitations, panic reaction, paranoia, photosensitive mydriasis, polypnea, psychotic reactions, rhabdomyolysis, shock, syncope, tachypnea, toxic psychosis, tremor, unusual fatigue, vomiting, and weakness. Monitor the patient for cardiac and respiratory changes. If possible, isolate the patient to limit external stimuli.

Expect to provide symptomatic and supportive treatment, including performing gastric lavage or inducing vomiting. Anticipate the use of I.V. fluids to manage hypotension, as needed. Expect to administer drugs and fluids to enhance diuresis, as prescribed. Be aware that drug treatment to induce urine acidification may also be prescribed to increase drug excretion, except for patients with hemoglobinemia, myoglobinuria, or rhabdomyolysis because of increased risk of renal failure. Be prepared to administer drugs such as a barbiturate or chlorpromazine to control CNS stimulation and phentolamine to manage hypertension. Institute emergency supportive measures, and protect patient from self-injury. Institute suicide precautions according to facility policy, and anticipate psychiatric re-evaluation.

Nursing Considerations

- Keep in mind that, when signs and symptoms of ADHD occur with acute stress reactions or with pre-existing structural cardiac abnormalities, treatment with amphetamines usually isn't indicated because the reaction may worsen or sudden death may occur.
- **WARNING** To prevent hypertensive crisis, don't administer amphetamine during MAO inhibitor therapy or for up to 14 days after it.
- Give first dose when patient awakens and additional doses at 4- to 6-hour intervals.
- Monitor growth and development in children because drug use may adversely affect growth.
- **WARNING** If patient suddenly stops drug after long-term, high-dose regimen, monitor him for withdrawal signs and symptoms, including abdominal pain, depression, nausea, tremor, unusual fatigue, vomiting, and weakness. Anticipate restarting drug therapy and gradually tapering dosage as prescribed.
- Monitor pulse rate and blood pressure in patients who have hypertension, including even mild hypertension, because drug may increase blood pressure and cause arrhythmias, including tachycardia. Report abnormal findings, including exertional chest pain, unexplained syncope, or other symptoms suggestive of cardiac disease, to prescriber.
- If patient experiences bothersome adverse reactions, such as insomnia and anorexia, expect to decrease dosage. To minimize insomnia, administer drug earlier in day.
- Be alert for signs and symptoms of long-term amphetamine abuse, such as hyperactivity, irritability, marked insomnia, personality changes, and severe dermatoses.
- Assess patient with a history of Tourette's syndrome, motor or vocal tics, or psychological disorders for worsening of these conditions during amphetamine therapy.
- Monitor children and adolescents for first-time manifestation of psychotic or manic symptoms. If present, notify prescriber and expect drug to be discontinued.

PATIENT TEACHING
- Stress importance of taking this drug exactly as prescribed be-

cause misuse may cause serious adverse cardiovascular reactions, including sudden death.

• Instruct breast-feeding patient to avoid breast-feeding during amphetamine therapy because drug is excreted in breast milk.

• Teach patient to take first dose on awakening and subsequent doses at 4- to 6-hour intervals. Tell him not to take last dose late in evening because insomnia may occur.

• Advise patient to take amphetamine with food or after a meal because anorexia may occur.

• Tell patient to avoid potentially hazardous activities until he knows how the drug affects him.

• Tell patient not to take amphetamine with acidic fruit juice because it decreases drug absorption.

• Inform parent or caregiver that child may be placed on drug-free weekend and holiday schedule, as prescribed, if signs and symptoms of ADHD are controlled.

• Inform patient of drug's abuse potential, and stress importance of not altering dosage unless prescribed.

apomorphine hydrochloride
Apokyn

Class and Category
Chemical class: Nonergoline dopamine agonist
Therapeutic class: Hypomobilic antiparkinsonian
Pregnancy category: C

Indications and Dosages
▶ *To treat hypomobility "off" episodes (end-of-dose wearing off and unpredictable on/off episodes) in advanced Parkinson's disease*
SUBCUTANEOUS INJECTION
Adults. *Initial:* 0.2 ml (2 mg) p.r.n. Dosage adjusted as needed in 0.1-ml (1-mg) increments every few days. *Maximum:* 0.6 ml (6 mg).

DOSAGE ADJUSTMENT For patients who tolerate 0.2 ml (2 mg) but have no response, a 0.4-ml (4-mg) dose may be given under medical supervision, with standing and supine blood pressure checked every 20 minutes for 1 hour at the next observed "off" period, as long as it is at least 2 hours after the initial 0.2-ml (2-mg) test dose was given. If tolerated, a dose 0.1 ml (1 mg) lower may be given p.r.n. and increased in 0.1-ml (1-mg) increments every few days as needed to a maximum dose of 0.6 ml (6 mg).

If patient doesn't tolerate a 0.4-ml (4-mg) test dose, a 0.3-ml (3-mg) test dose may be given under medical supervision, with standing and supine blood pressure checked every 20 minutes for 1 hour at the next observed "off" period, as long as it's at least 2 hours after the initial 0.4-ml (4-mg) test dose. If tolerated, a 0.2-ml (2-mg) dose can be started p.r.n. and increased no to higher than 0.3 ml (3 mg) if needed after a few days.

For patients with mild to moderate renal impairment, the initial dose should be reduced to 0.1 ml (1 mg).

Route	Onset	Peak	Duration
SubQ	10 to 60 min	Unknown	Unknown

Mechanism of Action

Probably stimulates postsynaptic dopamine D2 receptors in the caudate-putamen of the brain. As a result, apomorphine improves motor function and activity levels in patients with Parkinson's disease.

Contraindications

Concurrent therapy with 5HT$_3$ antagonists, such as alosetron, dolasetron, granisetron, ondansetron, and palonosetron; hypersensitivity to apomorphine or its components, including sodium metabisulfite

Interactions

DRUGS

5HT$_3$ antagonists: Increased risk of profound hypotension and loss of consciousness

antihypertensives, vasodilators: Increased risk of serious adverse reactions, such as hypotension, MI, and bone or joint injuries

dopamine antagonists (such as butyrophenones, metoclopramide, phenothiazines, thioxanthenes): Decreased apomorphine effectiveness

drugs that prolong QT interval: Increased risk of torsades de pointes

entacapone, tolcapone: Increased risk of tachycardia, hypertension, and arrhythmias

ACTIVITIES

alcohol use: Increased risk of hypotension

Adverse Reactions

CNS: Aggravated Parkinson's disease, anxiety, confusion, depression, dizziness, drowsiness, dyskinesia, euphoria, fatigue, hallucinations, headache, insomnia, somnolence, weakness, yawning

CV: Angina, chest pain, congestive heart failure, edema, MI, orthostatic hypotension, prolonged QT interval
EENT: Rhinorrhea
GI: Constipation, diarrhea, nausea, vomiting
GU: UTI
MS: Arthralgia, back or limb pain
RESP: Dyspnea, pneumonia, tachypnea
SKIN: Contact dermatitis, diaphoresis, ecchymosis, flushing, pallor
Other: Dehydration; injection site bruising, granuloma, or pruritus

Overdose

Apomorphine overdose has no specific antidote. Monitor patient for signs and symptoms of overdose, including severe nausea and vomiting, life-threatening hypotension, QT-interval prolongation, and loss of consciousness.

Maintain an open airway, and monitor vital signs and cardiac monitor for arrhythmias, especially torsades de pointes. Expect to give symptomatic and supportive care, as needed.

Give an antiemetic to combat severe nausea and vomiting, and insert a nasogastric tube, as prescribed. Give I.V. fluids and a vasopressor, as prescribed, to combat hypotension.

Take suicide precautions according to facility policy, and anticipate psychiatric re-evaluation.

Be prepared to assist with artificial respiration, as needed.

Nursing Considerations

- Use apomorphine cautiously in patients with hepatic or renal insufficiency.
- Be aware that an antiemetic, such as tri-methobenzamide 300 mg t.i.d., should be started 3 days before apomorphine therapy starts and continue for at least the first 2 months of therapy. Apomorphine may cause severe nausea and vomiting, even with an antiemetic.
- Monitor patient's blood pressure closely because apomorphine can cause severe orthostatic hypotension.
- Administer a 0.2-ml (2-mg) test dose of apomorphine, as prescribed, and then monitor patient's supine and standing blood pressure 20, 40, and 60 minutes later.
- Monitor patient closely if he has an increased risk of prolonged QT interval, as from hypokalemia, hypomagnesemia, bradycardia, use of certain drugs, or genetic predisposition. QT-interval prolongation may lead to torsades de pointes.

- Monitor patient for evidence of abuse. Although rare, drug may cause psychosexual stimulation and increased libido, which may cause patient to use it more often than needed for Parkinson's disease symptoms.

PATIENT TEACHING
- Tell patient that an antiemetic will be prescribed starting 3 days before first apomorphine dose. Instruct patient to take the antiemetic exactly as prescribed. Explain that it will be needed for 2 months or longer during apomorphine therapy.
- Explain that a test dose will be needed to determine response and drug's effects on blood pressure before patient can go home with drug.
- Teach patient how to use dosing pen and how to give drug subcutaneously.
- Emphasize that apomorphine doses are expressed as milliliters, not milligrams. Tell patient to draw up each dose carefully to reduce the chance of dosage error.
- Instruct patient to rotate apomorphine injection sites in a systematic manner.
- Stress importance of taking apomorphine only as prescribed because serious adverse reactions may occur.
- Advise patient to avoid potentially hazardous activities until drug's CNS effects are known. In particular, caution patient that apomorphine increases the risk of falling asleep suddenly, without feeling sleepy.

aripiprazole
Abilify, Abilify Discmelt

Class and Category
Chemical class: Dihydrocarbostyril
Therapeutic class: Atypical antipsychotic
Pregnancy category: C

Indications and Dosages
▶ *To treat schizophrenia; to maintain stability in patients with schizophrenia*
ORALLY DISINTEGRATING TABLETS, ORAL SOLUTION, TABLETS
Adults. *Initial:* 10 or 15 mg daily. Increased to 30 mg daily, as needed, with dosage adjustments at 2-wk intervals.
Adolescents ages 13 to 17. *Initial:* 2 mg daily for 2 days; then increased to 5 mg daily for 2 days; then increased to 10 mg daily, as needed.

▶ *To treat acute manic and mixed episodes in bipolar disorder; as adjunct to lithium or valproate to treat acute manic and mixed episodes in bipolar I disorder*
ORALLY DISINTEGRATING TABLETS, ORAL SOLUTION, TABLETS
Adults. *Initial:* 15 mg daily. Increased to 30 mg daily, as needed.
Children age 10 and over. *Initial:* 2 mg daily for 2 days; then increased to 5 mg daily for 2 days; then increased to 10 mg daily.
▶ *To maintain stability in patients with bipolar I disorder who have had a recent manic or mixed episode and who have been stabilized and then maintained for at least 6 wk*
ORALLY DISINTEGRATING TABLETS, ORAL SOLUTION, TABLETS
Adults. 30 mg daily. Decreased to 15 mg daily, as clinically indicated.
Children age 10 and over. 10 mg daily.
▶ *As adjunct therapy for acute treatment of a major depressive disorder*
ORALLY DISINTEGRATING TABLETS, ORAL SOLUTION, TABLETS
Adults. 2 to 5 mg daily. Increased in increments of up to 5 mg daily every 7 days as needed.
▶ *To treat agitation in schizophrenia or bipolar mania*
I.M. INJECTION
Adults. *Initial:* Depending on severity of agitation, 5.25 to 15 mg. May be repeated 2 or more hr later, as needed. *Maximum:* 30 mg daily.
DOSAGE ADJUSTMENT Dosage reduced to half of normal dose when given with fluoxetine, itraconazole, ketoconazole, paroxetine, or quinidine. Dosage doubled when given with carbamazepine.

Mechanism of Action

May produce antipsychotic effects through partial agonist and antagonist actions. Aripiprazole acts as a partial agonist at dopamine—especially D2—receptors and serotonin—especially 5-HT_{1A}—receptors. The drug acts as an antagonist at 5-HT_{2A} serotonin receptor sites.

Contraindications
Breast-feeding, hypersensitivity to aripiprazole or its components

Interactions
DRUGS
anticholingerics: Increased risk for potentially fatal elevation of body temperature

carbamazepine and other CYP3A4 inducers: Possibly increased clearance and decreased blood level of aripiprazole
CNS depressants: Increased CNS depression
fluoxetine, paroxetine, quinidine, and other CYP2D6 inhibitors; ketoconazole and other CYP3A4 inhibitors: Possibly inhibited elimination and increased blood aripiprazole level
ACTIVITIES
alcohol use: Increased CNS depression

Adverse Reactions

CNS: Abnormal gait, agitation, akathisia, anxiety, asthenia, cognitive and motor impairment, confusion, CVA (elderly), delusions, depression, dizziness, dream disturbances, dystonia, extrapyramidal reactions, fatigue, fever, gait disturbance, hallucinations, headache, hostility, insomnia, intracranial hemorrhage, lethargy, lightheadedness, mania, nervousness, neuroleptic malignant syndrome, paranoia, restlessness, schizophrenic reaction, seizures, somnolence, suicidal ideation, tardive dyskinesia, transient ischemic attack (elderly), tremor
CV: Angina, arrhythmias, bradycardia, cardiopulmonary arrest, chest pain, circulatory collapse, deep vein thrombosis, elevated serum CK levels, heart failure, hypertension, MI, orthostatic hypotension, peripheral edema, prolonged QT interval, tachycardia
EENT: Blurred vision, conjunctivitis, dry mouth, increased salivation, laryngospasm, nasal congestion, oropharyngeal spasm, pharyngitis, rhinitis, sinusitis
ENDO: Hyperglycemia
GI: Abdominal discomfort, constipation, decreased appetite, diarrhea, difficulty swallowing, GI bleeding, hepatitis, indigestion, intestinal obstruction, irritable bowel syndrome, jaundice, loose stools, nausea, pancreatitis, vomiting
GU: Renal failure, urinary incontinence
HEME: Anemia, leukopenia, thrombocytopenia
MS: Arthralgia, elevated creatinine phosphokinase level, muscle spasms, myalgia, neck and pelvic pain, neck and limb rigidity, rhabdomyolysis
RESP: Apnea, aspiration, asthma, cough, dyspnea, pneumonia, pulmonary edema or embolism, respiratory failure
SKIN: Diaphoresis, dry skin, ecchymosis, pruritus, rash, ulceration, urticaria
Other: Anaphylaxis, angioedema, dehydration, flulike symptoms, heat stroke, weight gain

Overdose

Aripiprazole overdose has no specific antidote. Monitor patient for evidence of overdose, including vomiting; changes in level of consciousness from lethargy or confusion to coma; tremor; aggression; seizures that may evolve into status epilepticus; hypertension or hypotension; arrhythmias, such as bradycardia, tachycardia, atrial fibrillation, and prolonged QRS or QT interval; acidosis; and respiratory arrest.

Maintain an open airway, and be prepared to assist with endotracheal intubation if patient develops respiratory depression. Monitor vital signs, institute continuous ECG monitoring, and assess capillary refill, peripheral pulses, skin sensation, and warmth. Administer oxygen therapy and possibly mechanical ventilation, as needed. Expect to treat seizures with a barbiturate, a benzodiazepine or other anticonvulsant, as prescribed. Treat acidosis as prescribed.

To decrease drug absorption, be prepared to give activated charcoal, as prescribed. Hemodialysis is unlikely to be effective since aripiprazole is highly bound to plasma proteins.

Give I.V. fluids or volume expanders as needed and prescribed to treat hypotension. Provide additional symptomatic and supportive therapy as indicated.

Take suicide precautions according to facility policy, and anticipate psychiatric re-evaluation.

Nursing Considerations

- Know that aripiprazole shouldn't be given to elderly patients with dementia-related psychosis because drug increases the risk of death.
- Use cautiously in patients with cardiovascular disease, cerebrovascular disease, or conditions that would predispose them to hypotension. Also use cautiously in those with a history of seizures or with conditions that lower seizure threshold, such as Alzheimer's disease.
- Also use cautiously in elderly patients because of increased risk of serious adverse cerebrovascular effects, such as CVA and transient ischemic attack.
- Be aware that oral solution may be given on a milligram-per-milligram basis in place of tablets up to 25 mg. For example, if patient needs 30 mg in tablet form and is switched to oral solution, expect to give 25 mg of solution.
- Inject parenteral form slowly, deep into muscle mass; never inject intravenously or subcutaneously.

- If patient (particularly a child or an adolescent) takes aripiprazole for depression, watch closely for evidence of suicidal tendencies, especially when therapy starts or dosage changes.
- Monitor patient for difficulty swallowing or excessive somnolence, which could predispose him to accidental injury or aspiration.
- **WARNING** Be aware that aripiprazole rarely may cause neuroleptic malignant syndrome, tardive dyskinesia, and seizures. Monitor patient closely throughout therapy, and take safety precautions as needed.
- Monitor patient's blood glucose level routinely because aripiprazole may increase risk of hyperglycemia.

PATIENT TEACHING

- If patient will take orally disintegrating tablets tell him not to open the blister pack until ready to take the tablet. Tell him to peel back the foil to expose the tablet; explain that pushing the tablet through the foil could damage the tablet. Instruct him to remove the tablet immediately with dry hands and place the tablet on his tongue. Explain that it will dissolve rapidly in saliva without additional fluid. Caution patient not to chew, crush, or split the tablet.
- If patient (particularly a child or an adolescent) takes aripiprazole for depression, urge caregivers to watch closely for suicidal tendencies, especially when therapy starts or dosage changes.
- Advise patient to get up slowly from a lying or sitting position to minimize orthostatic hypotension during therapy.
- Urge patient to avoid alcohol during aripiprazole therapy.
- Instruct patient to avoid hazardous activities until drug's effects are known.
- Caution patient to avoid activities that may suddenly increase his body temperature, such as strenuous exercise or exposure to extreme heat, and to compensate for situations that may lead to dehydration, such as vomiting or diarrhea.
- Instruct patient to inform all prescribers of any drugs he's taking, including OTC drugs, because of a potential for interactions.
- Advise female patient of childbearing age to notify prescriber if she is, could be, or plans to become pregnant during aripiprazole therapy.
- Instruct diabetic patient taking the oral solution to monitor blood glucose levels closely because each milliliter of solution contains 400 mg of sucrose and 200 mg of fructose.

armodafinil
Nuvigil

Class and Category
Chemical class: Diphenylmethyl sulfinylacetamide
Therapeutic class: CNS stimulant
Pregnancy category: C

Indications and Dosages
▶ *To treat narcolepsy or as adjunct to standard therapy for excessive daytime sleepiness in obstructive sleep apnea/hypopnea syndrome*
TABLETS
Adults. 150 or 250 mg once daily in the morning.
▶ *To improve daytime wakefulness in patients with excessive sleepiness from circadian rhythm disruption (shift-work sleep disorder)*
TABLETS
Adults. 150 mg once daily about 1 hr before start of work shift.
DOSAGE ADJUSTMENT Decreased dosage recommended for patients who are elderly, have severe hepatic impairment, or take steroidal contraceptives.

Route	Onset	Peak	Duration
P.O.	Unknown (fasting) 4 to 6 hr (with food)	2 hr	Unknown

Mechanism of Action
May produce CNS-stimulant effects by binding to the dopamine transporter in the brain and inhibiting dopamine reuptake in the limbic region. These actions increase alertness and reduce drowsiness and fatigue.

Contraindications
Hypersensitivity to armodafinil, modafinil, or their components

Interactions
DRUGS
amitriptyline, citalopram, clomipramine, diazepam, imipramine, propranolol, tolbutamide, topiramate: Possibly prolonged elimination time and increased blood levels of these drugs
barbiturates (such as phenobarbital, primidone), dexamethasone, rifabutin, rifampin: Possibly decreased blood level and effectiveness of armodafinil
carbamazepine: Possibly decreased armodafinil effectiveness and

decreased blood carbamazepine level

cimetidine, clarithromycin, erythromycin, fluconazole, fluoxetine, fluvoxamine, itraconazole, ketoconazole, nefazodone, sertraline: Possibly inhibited metabolism, decreased clearance, and increased blood level of armodafinil

clozapine: Possibly increased clozapine level from decreased secondary hepatic metabolism

contraceptive-containing implants or devices: Possibly contraceptive failure

cyclosporine: Possibly decreased blood cyclosporine level and increased risk of organ transplant rejection

dextroamphetamine, methylphenidate: Possibly 1-hour delay in armodafinil absorption when these drugs are given together

fosphenytoin, mephenytoin, phenytoin: Possibly decreased effectiveness of armodafinil, increased blood phenytoin level, and increased risk of phenytoin toxicity

midazolam, triazolam: Possibly decreased effectiveness of triazolam or midazolam

oral contraceptives: Possibly decreased contraceptive effectiveness

theophylline: Possibly decreased theophylline blood level and effectiveness

warfarin: Possibly decreased warfarin metabolism and increased risk of bleeding

FOODS

all foods: 2- to 4-hour delay for armodafinil to reach peak levels and possibly delayed onset of action

caffeine: Increased CNS stimulation

grapefruit juice: Possibly decreased armodafinil metabolism

ACTIVITIES

alcohol use: Possibly adverse CNS effects

Adverse Reactions

CNS: Agitation, anxiety, attention disturbance, depression, dizziness, fatigue, fever, headache (including migraine), insomnia, nervousness, paresthesia, suicidal ideation, thirst, tremor

CV: Increased heart rate, palpitations

EENT: Dry mouth

GI: Abdominal pain (upper), anorexia, constipation, decreased appetite, diarrhea, dyspepsia, loose stools, nausea, vomiting

GU: Polyuria

RESP: Dyspnea

SKIN: Contact dermatitis, hyperhydrosis, rash

Other: Angioedema, flulike illness

Overdose

Monitor patient for signs and symptoms of overdose, including agitation, excitation, hypertension, insomnia, and tachycardia. Maintain an open airway, and monitor cardiovascular function.

To decrease drug absorption, be prepared to induce vomiting or perform gastric lavage. The effectiveness of dialysis or drugs that change urine pH on modafinil overdose is unknown.

Institute suicide precautionary measures according to facility policy, and anticipate psychiatric re-evaluation.

Nursing Considerations

- Be aware that armodafinil shouldn't be given to patients with mitral valve prolapse syndrome or a history of left ventricular hypertrophy because drug may cause ischemic changes.
- **WARNING** If patient has a history of alcoholism, stimulant abuse, or other substance abuse, monitor him for compliance with armodafinil therapy. Watch for signals of misuse or abuse, including frequent prescription refill requests, increased frequency of doses, and drug-seeking behavior. Also watch for evidence of excessive armodafinil use, including agitation, anxiety, diarrhea, nausea, nervousness, palpitations, sleep disturbances, and tremor.
- Be aware that armodafinil, like other CNS stimulants, may alter mood, perception, thinking, judgment, feelings, and motor skills and may produce signs that the patient needs sleep.
- If giving drug to patient with a history of psychosis, emotional instability, or psychological illness with psychotic features, be prepared to perform baseline behavioral assessments or frequent clinical observation.

PATIENT TEACHING

- Inform patient that armodafinil can help, but not cure, narcolepsy and that drug's full effects may not occur right away.
- Advise patient to avoid taking armodafinil within 2 hours of eating because food may delay the time to peak drug effect and onset of action. If patient drinks grapefruit juice, encourage him to drink a consistent amount daily.
- Inform patient that drug can affect his concentration and function and can hide signs of fatigue. Urge him not to drive or perform activities that require mental alertness until drug's full CNS effects are known.
- Because alcohol may decrease alertness, advise patient to avoid ingesting it during armodafinil therapy.
- Encourage a regular sleeping pattern.

- Caution patient to avoid excessive intake of caffeine-containing foods, beverages, and over-the-counter drugs because caffeine may lead to increased CNS stimulation.
- Inform female patient that armodafinil can decrease the effectiveness of certain contraceptives, including birth control pills and implanted hormonal contraceptives. If she uses such contraceptives, urge her to use an alternate birth control method during armodafinil therapy and for up to 1 month after she stops taking the drug.
- Advise patient to keep follow-up appointments with prescriber so that her progress can be monitored.

atomoxetine hydrochloride

Strattera

Class and Catgegory

Chemical class: Selective norepinephrine reuptake inhibitor
Therapeutic class: Anti–attention deficit hyperactivity agent
Pregnancy category: C

Indications and Dosages

▶ *To treat attention deficit hyperactivity disorder (ADHD)*
CAPSULES
Adults and children weighing 70 kg (154 lb) or less. *Initial:* 0.5 mg/kg daily, increased after a minimum of 3 days to 1.2 mg/kg daily given either as a single dose in the morning or in evenly divided doses in the morning and late afternoon or early evening, as needed. *Maximum:* 1.4 mg/kg or 100 mg daily, whichever is less.
Adults and children weighing more than 70 kg. *Initial:* 40 mg daily, increased after a minimum of 3 days to 80 mg daily given either as a single dose in the morning or in evenly divided doses in the morning and late afternoon or early evening. After 2 to 4 additional wk, dosage may be increased to 100 mg daily if optimal response hasn't been achieved. *Maximum:* 100 mg daily.
▶ *To maintain stability once achieved in the treatment of ADHD*
CAPSULES
Children ages 6 to 15. 1.2 to 1.8 mg/kg daily.
DOSAGE ADJUSTMENT For patients with moderate (Child-Pugh Class B) hepatic impairment, dosage reduced by 50%. For patients with severe (Child-Pugh Class C) impairment, dosage reduced by 75%. For patients weighing 70 kg or less and tak-

ing strong CYP2D6 inhibitors, such as paroxetine, fluoxetine, or quinidine, initial dosage of 0.5 mg/kg daily should be increased to 1.2 mg/kg daily only if symptoms fail to improve after 4 wk. For patients weighing more than 70 kg and taking strong CYP2D6 inhibitors, initial dosage of 40 mg daily should be increased to 80 mg daily only if symptoms fail to improve after 4 wk.

Mechanism of Action

Selectively inhibits presynaptic norepinephrine transport in the nervous system to increase attention span and produce a calming effect.

Contraindications

Angle-closure glaucoma, hypersensitivity to atomoxetine or its components, use within 14 days of MAO inhibitor therapy

Interactions

DRUGS

albuterol and other beta₂ agonists: May potentiate action of albuterol and other beta₂ agonists on cardiovascular system
CYP2D6 inhibitors (such as fluoxetine, paroxetine, and quinidine): Increased blood atomoxetine level
MAO inhibitors: Possibly induced hypertensive crisis
pressor agents: Possibly altered blood pressure

Adverse Reactions

CNS: Aggressiveness, crying, CVA, depression, dizziness, early morning awakening, fatigue, headache, hostility, insomnia, irritability, lethargy, mood changes, paresthesia, peripheral coldness, pyrexia, rigors, sedation, sleep disturbance, somnolence, suicidal ideation (children and adolescents), syncope, tremor, unusual dreams
CV: Chest pain, hypertension, orthostatic hypotension, MI, palpitations, QT-interval prolongation, Raynaud's phenomenon, tachycardia
EENT: Dry mouth, ear infection, mydriasis, nasal congestion, nasopharyngitis, pharyngitis, rhinorrhea, sinus congestion
GI: Abdominal pain (upper), anorexia, constipation, diarrhea, elevated liver function test results, flatulence, gastroenteritis (viral), indigestion, nausea, severe hepatic dysfunction, vomiting
GU: Decreased libido, dysmenorrhea, ejaculation disorders, erectile dysfunction, impotence, menstrual irregularities, orgasm

abnormality, priapism, prostatitis, urinary hesitancy, urine retention

MS: Arthralgia, back pain, myalgia

RESP: Cough, upper respiratory tract infection

SKIN: Dermatitis, diaphoresis, pruritus, rash, urticaria

Other: Angioedema, hot flashes, influenza, weight loss

Overdose

Atomoxetine overdose has no specific antidote. Monitor patient for signs and symptoms of overdose, including CNS changes such as somnolence, agitation, disorientation, hallucinations, hyperactivity, abnormal behavior; GI symptoms such as nausea and vomiting; sympathetic nervous system activation such as mydriasis, tachycardia, and dry mouth; and cardiac changes such as QT-interval prolongation.

Maintain an open airway, and monitor vital signs and cardiac monitor for prolonged QT interval. Expect to give symptomatic and supportive care, as needed.

To decrease drug absorption in a conscious patient, be prepared to perform gastric lavage. Expect that oral activated charcoal may follow to limit absorption. Be aware that dialysis isn't likely to be useful in eliminating drug because atomoxetine is highly protein bound.

Take suicide precautions according to facility policy, and anticipate psychiatric re-evaluation.

Nursing Considerations

- Use atomoxetine cautiously in patients with cerebrovascular or CV disease (especially hypertension or tachycardia) because drug may increase blood pressure and heart rate. Also use cautiously in those prone to orthostatic hypotension and those with serious structural cardiac abnormalities or other serious cardiac problems because drug may increase the risk of sudden death from these conditions.
- **WARNING** Monitor children and adolescents closely for evidence of suicidal thinking, suicidal behavior, and such psychotic or manic symptoms as hallucinations, delusional thinking, or mania because atomoxetine increases the risk of psychosis, mania, and suicidal ideation in these age-groups.
- Obtain baseline blood pressure and heart rate before starting therapy. Monitor patient's vital signs after dosage increases and periodically during therapy.

• Monitor patient closely for allergic reactions. If these occur, notify prescriber.
• Monitor child's or adolescent's growth and weight. Expect to interrupt therapy, as prescribed, if patient isn't growing or gaining weight appropriately.
• Monitor patient's liver function studies, as ordered. Notify prescriber immediately if enzyme levels are elevated or patient has signs or symptoms of hepatic dysfunction, such as jaundice, dark urine, pruritus, right upper quadrant tenderness, or unexplained flulike symptoms. Expect atomoxetine to be stopped permanently.

PATIENT TEACHING
• Remind patient not to open capsules. If a capsule comes open, tell him to wash his hands and any other contaminated surface promptly. If drug gets into his eye, he should flush the eye immediately with water and seek medical attention.
• Instruct patient or parent to immediately report to prescriber any adverse reactions to atomoxetine therapy, such as facial swelling, itching, or rash.
• **WARNING** Urge parents to watch their child or adolescent closely for evidence of abnormal thinking, abnormal behavior, or increased aggression or hostility. If unusual changes occur, stress need to notify prescriber.
• Urge patient to tell prescriber immediately about yellowing of his skin or eyes, itchiness, right upper abdominal pain, dark urine, or flulike symptoms.
• Caution patient to assume sitting or standing position slowly because of drug's potential effect on blood pressure.
• Advise patient to report urinary hesitancy or urine retention to prescriber.
• Remind patient of the importance of alerting all prescribers to any OTC drugs, dietary supplements, or herbal remedies he's taking.
• Caution patient to avoid potentially hazardous activities until drug's CNS effects are known.
• Reassure patient or parent that drug doesn't cause physical or psychological dependence.
• Instruct patient or parent to monitor weight during therapy.
• Advise male patient to seek medical attention immediately if a penile erection becomes overly sustained or painful.

belladonna alkaloids

Class and Category
Chemical class: Tertiary amine
Therapeutic class: Anticholinergic, antimuscarinic
Pregnancy category: C

Indications and Dosages
▶ *To treat idiopathic and postencephalitic parkinsonism*
TABLETS
Adults. 0.25 to 0.5 mg t.i.d.
Children over age 6. 0.125 to 0.25 mg t.i.d.
TINCTURE
Adults. 0.6 to 1 ml t.i.d. or q.i.d.
Children. 0.03 ml/kg (0.8 ml/m^2) t.i.d.

Route	Onset	Steady State	Peak	Half-Life	Duration
P.O.	1 to 2 hr	Unknown	Unknown	Unknown	4 hr

Mechanism of Action
Inhibits acetylcholine's muscarinic actions at postganglionic parasympathetic receptor sites, including smooth muscles, secretory glands, and CNS. These actions relax smooth muscles and diminish GI, GU, and biliary tract secretions. Belladonna alkaloids also selectively depress certain central motor actions in the CNS, which helps to control muscle tone and movement in parkinsonism.

Contraindications
Angle-closure glaucoma, hepatic disease, hypersensitivity to anticholinergics or scopolamine, ileus, myasthenia gravis, myocardial ischemia, obstructive condition of GI or GU tract, renal disease, severe ulcerative colitis, tachycardia, toxic megacolon, unstable cardiovascular status in patients with acute hemorrhage

Interactions
DRUGS
amantadine: Increased adverse anticholinergic effects

atenolol, digoxin: Possibly increased therapeutic and adverse effects of these drugs
phenothiazines: Possibly decreased effectiveness of phenothiazine, increased adverse effects of belladonna alkaloids
tricyclic antidepressants: Possibly increased adverse anticholinergic effects

Adverse Reactions

CNS: CNS stimulation (with high doses), confusion, dizziness, drowsiness, headache, insomnia, nervousness, weakness
CV: Bradycardia, palpitations, tachycardia
EENT: Altered taste, blurred vision, dry mouth, increased intraocular pressure, mydriasis, nasal congestion, photophobia
GI: Bloating, constipation, dysphagia, heartburn, ileus, nausea, vomiting
GU: Impotence, urinary hesitancy, urine retention
SKIN: Decreased sweating, flushing, urticaria
Other: Anaphylaxis

Overdose

Monitor patient for signs and symptoms of overdose, including changes in near vision; clumsiness; continuing blurred vision; dizziness; dyspnea; fever; hallucinations; irritability; nervousness; restlessness; seizures; severe drowsiness; severe dryness of mouth, nose, or throat; severe fatigue; severe muscle weakness; slurred speech; tachycardia; unsteady gait; unusual excitement; and unusually dry, flushed, warm skin.

Maintain an open airway, and institute emergency supportive measures. Expect to provide symptomatic and supportive treatment, including performing gastric lavage with 4% tannic acid solution, as prescribed, or inducing vomiting. Anticipate administering activated charcoal.

Expect to administer physostigmine, 0.5 to 2 mg, I.V. at no more than 1 mg/minute, up to a maximum of 5 mg in adult, to reverse anticholinergic effects. Or, be prepared to administer neostigmine methylsulfate, 0.5 to 1 mg, I.M. or I.V., as needed and prescribed. Be aware that small doses of a short-acting barbiturate, a benzodiazepine, or a rectal infusion of 2% chloral hydrate may be prescribed to control excitement or delirium. Anticipate I.V. infusion of drugs such as norepinephrine or metaraminol and I.V. fluids to maintain blood pressure, as prescribed.

Institute suicide precautions according to facility policy, and anticipate psychiatric re-evaluation.

Nursing Considerations

• Avoid giving high doses of belladonna alkaloids in patients with ulcerative colitis because these drugs may inhibit intestinal motility and precipitate or aggravate toxic megacolon. Also, avoid using high doses in patients with hiatal hernia and reflux esophagitis because these drugs may also aggravate esophagitis.

• Use belladonna alkaloids cautiously in patients with allergies, arrhythmias, asthma, autonomic neuropathy, coronary artery disease, debilitating chronic lung disease, heart failure, hypertension, hyperthyroidism, or prostatic hyperplasia.

• Administer drug 30 to 60 minutes before patient eats.

• **WARNING** Monitor elderly patients for agitation, confusion, drowsiness, and excitement, even with small doses. Elderly patients are more sensitive to the effects of the drug and are more likely to develop these adverse reactions. If they develop, the dosage may need to be decreased.

• Take safety precautions to protect patient from falling.

PATIENT TEACHING

• Instruct patient to take belladonna alkaloids 30 to 60 minutes before eating.

• Tell patient to notify prescriber of constipation, difficulty urinating, or persistent or severe diarrhea.

• Caution patient to avoid driving and similar activities until she knows how belladonna alkaloids affect her.

• **WARNING** Urge patient to avoid extremely hot or humid conditions because heatstroke may occur.

Other Therapeutic Uses

Belladonna alkaloids are also indicated for the following:

• To treat diarrhea, diverticulitis, dysmenorrhea, functional digestive disorders (including mucous, spastic, and ulcerative colitis), motion sickness, nausea and vomiting of pregnancy, nocturnal enuresis, pancreatitis, and peptic ulcer disease

benzphetamine hydrochloride

Didrex

Class, Category, and Schedule

Chemical class: Phenylalkylamine
Therapeutic class: Appetite suppressant
Pregnancy category: X
Controlled substance schedule: III

Indications and Dosages

▶ *As adjunct to treat exogenous obesity with caloric restriction, exercise, and behavior modification*

TABLETS

Adults and children age 16 and over. 25 to 50 mg daily. Dosage increased, as needed and tolerated, up to 25 to 50 mg t.i.d. *Maximum:* 150 mg daily.

Route	Onset	Steady State	Peak	Half-Life	Duration
P.O.	Unknown	Unknown	Unknown	6 to 12 hr	Unknown

Mechanism of Action

Stimulates the release of dopamine and norepinephrine from adrenergic nerve terminals in the lateral hypothalamic feeding center of the cerebral cortex and reticular activating system, thus reducing appetite. By stimulating the CNS, drug may produce other effects, including decreasing gastric acid production and increasing metabolism, which may be effective in treating obesity.

Contraindications

Advanced arteriosclerosis; agitation; cerebral ischemia; glaucoma; history of drug or alcohol abuse; hypersensitivity to benzphetamine, other sympathomimetic amines, or any of their components; hyperthyroidism; MAO inhibitor therapy within 14 days; moderate to severe hypertension; symptomatic cardiovascular disease

Interactions

DRUGS

antacids (calcium- and magnesium-containing), carbonic anhydrase inhibitors, citrates, sodium bicarbonate: Increased blood benzphetamine level

antidiabetic drugs (insulin or oral): Altered serum glucose level

amphetamines, other appetite suppressants, selective serotonin reuptake inhibitors: Possibly increased risk of cardiac valve dysfunction

anesthetics (inhaled): Increased risk of arrhythmias

antihypertensives (especially clonidine, guanadrel, guanethidine, methyldopa, rauwolfia alkaloids): Decreased hypotensive effect

CNS stimulants, thyroid hormones: Additive CNS stimulation

MAO inhibitors: Potentiated effects of benzphetamine, possibly hypertensive crisis

phenothiazines: Reduced anorectic effect of benzphetamine
tricyclic antidepressants: Possibly potentiated adverse cardiovascular effects
urinary acidifiers (including ammonium chloride, potassium, and sodium phosphates): Decreased blood benzphetamine level
vasopressors (especially catecholamines): Possibly potentiated vasopressor effect of these drugs
FOODS
ascorbic acid: Decreased blood benzphetamine level
ACTIVITIES
alcohol: Increased adverse CNS effects

Adverse Reactions

CNS: Cerebral ischemia, CNS stimulation, depression, dizziness, headache, insomnia, light-headedness, mania, nervousness, psychosis, syncope, tremor
CV: Chest pain, hypertension, palpitations, peripheral edema
EENT: Dry mouth
GI: Abdominal pain, constipation, nausea, vomiting
GU: Dysuria
RESP: Dyspnea
SKIN: Hives, rash
Other: Exercise intolerance

Overdose

Appetite suppressant overdose has no specific antidote. Monitor patient for signs and symptoms of overdose, including abdominal cramps, arrhythmias, coma, confusion, diarrhea, dyspnea, hallucinations, hostility, hyperreflexia, hyperthermia, labile blood pressure, nausea, panic reaction, restlessness, seizures, shock, tachypnea, tremor, and vomiting. Expect fatigue and depression to follow CNS excitement.

Maintain an open airway, monitor vital signs, and protect patient from self-injury. Expect to provide symptomatic and supportive treatment, as needed. Perform gastric lavage or induce vomiting, then administer activated charcoal, as prescribed, to decrease drug absorption. Expect to administer a drug to promote urine acidification and I.V. fluids, as prescribed, to increase drug excretion. Be prepared to possibly administer a barbiturate, diazepam, or phenytoin to control CNS stimulation and seizures. Anticipate administering such drugs as lidocaine to control arrhythmias, phentolamine or a nitrate to manage hypertension, and a beta blocker to control tachycardia. Be aware that the effectiveness of hemodialysis or peritoneal dialysis is unknown. Institute suicide precautions according to facility policy, and anticipate psychiatric re-evaluation.

Nursing Considerations

- **WARNING** Expect to taper drug gradually before discontinuing to prevent withdrawal and increased rebound appetite. Monitor patient for withdrawal signs and symptoms, including abdominal cramps, depression, insomnia, nausea, nightmares, severe fever, and tremor. Notify prescriber immediately if they persist or worsen.
- Be aware that drug may cause physical and psychological dependence. Monitor patient for effects of drug abuse, including hyperactivity, insomnia, personality changes, psychosis, severe dermatoses, and severe irritability.
- Monitor patient for chest pain, dyspnea, exercise intolerance, peripheral edema, or syncope, which may indicate cardiac valve dysfunction or pulmonary hypertension.

PATIENT TEACHING

- Advise patient to notify prescriber immediately of chest pain, dyspnea, exercise intolerance, peripheral edema, or syncope.
- Instruct patient to take last dose at least 4 to 6 hours before bedtime to prevent insomnia.
- Instruct patient to take drug exactly as prescribed because of risk of addiction. Caution her that tolerance to drug effects may develop in a few weeks and that long-term drug use may cause psychological or physical dependence. Tell her that the drug will be gradually reduced to avoid withdrawal signs and symptoms.
- Explain to patient that changes in eating and activity behaviors are necessary for long-term weight loss. Stress the importance of maintaining a reduced caloric intake and routine exercise program.
- Instruct patient to avoid alcohol because of the risk of increased confusion, dizziness, light-headedness, and syncope.
- Advise patient to avoid potentially hazardous activities until she knows how the drug affects her.
- Tell patient to relieve dry mouth by sucking on ice chips or sugarless candy or gum.
- Caution patient that drug may cause a false-positive result in urine drug screen for amphetamines.
- Advise patient to notify prescriber immediately of known or suspected pregnancy. Caution patient against breast-feeding while taking benzphetamine.

benztropine mesylate

Apo-Benztropine (CAN), Cogentin, PMS Benztropine (CAN)

Class and Category

Chemical class: Tertiary amine
Therapeutic class: Antidyskinetic
Pregnancy category: C

Indications and Dosages

▶ *As adjunct, to treat all forms of Parkinson's disease*
TABLETS, I.V. OR I.M. INJECTION
Adults and adolescents with Parkinson's disease. 1 to 2 mg daily (usual dosage) with a range of 0.5 to 6 mg daily.
Adults and adolescents with idiopathic Parkinson's disease. *Initial:* 0.5 to 1 mg at bedtime. *Maximum:* 4 to 6 mg daily.
Adults and adolescents with postencephalitic Parkinson's disease. 2 mg daily in one or more doses; may begin with 0.5 mg at bedtime and increase as needed.
▶ *To control extrapyramidal symptoms (except tardive dyskinesia) caused by phenothiazines and other neuroleptic drugs*
TABLETS, I.V. OR I.M. INJECTION
Adults and adolescents. 1 to 4 mg once or twice daily.
▶ *To treat acute dystonic reactions*
TABLETS, I.V. OR I.M. INJECTION
Adults. *Initial:* 1 to 2 ml (1 to 2 mg total dose) I.V. or I.M. *Maintenance:* 1 to 2 mg P.O. b.i.d. to prevent recurrence.

Route	Onset	Steady State	Peak	Half-Life	Duration
P.O.	1 to 2 hr	Unknown	Unknown	Unknown	24 hr
I.V., I.M	In min	Unknown	Unknown	Unknown	24 hr

Mechanism of Action

Blocks acetylcholine's action at cholinergic receptor sites. This restores the brain's normal dopamine and acetylcholine balance, which relaxes muscle movement and decreases drooling, rigidity, and tremor. Benztropine also may inhibit dopamine reuptake and storage, which prolongs dopamine's action.

Contraindications

Achalasia, bladder neck obstruction, duodenal or pyloric obstruction, glaucoma, hypersensitivity to benztropine mesylate or its components, megacolon, myasthenia gravis, prostatic hyperplasia, stenosing peptic ulcer

Interactions
DRUGS

amantadine: Possibly increased adverse anticholinergic effects
digoxin: Possibly increased blood digoxin level
haloperidol: Possibly increased schizophrenic signs and symptoms, decreased blood haloperidol level, development of tardive dyskinesia
levodopa: Possibly decreased effectiveness of levodopa
phenothiazines: Possibly reduced phenothiazine effects, increased psychiatric signs and symptoms

Adverse Reactions
CNS: Agitation, confusion, delirium, delusions, depression, disorientation, dizziness, drowsiness, euphoria, excitement, fever, hallucinations, headache, light-headedness, listlessness, memory loss, nervousness, paranoia, psychosis, weakness
CV: Hypotension, mild bradycardia, orthostatic hypotension, palpitations, tachycardia
EENT: Angle-closure glaucoma, blurred vision, diplopia, dry mouth, increased intraocular pressure, mydriasis, suppurative parotitis
GI: Constipation, duodenal ulcer, epigastric distress, ileus, nausea, vomiting
GU: Dysuria, urinary hesitancy, urine retention
MS: Muscle spasms, muscle weakness
SKIN: Decreased sweating, dermatoses, flushing, rash, urticaria

Overdose
Monitor patient for evidence of overdose, including clumsiness; dyspnea; hallucinations; insomnia; seizures; severe drowsiness; severe dryness of mouth, nose, and throat; tachycardia; toxic psychoses; unsteadiness; and unusually dry, flushed, warm skin.

Maintain an open airway, and institute emergency supportive measures, as needed. Expect to induce vomiting or perform gastric lavage to decrease drug absorption, as prescribed, except in patients who may be convulsive, precomatose, or psychotic.

If patient is an adult, expect to administer 1 to 2 mg of physostigmine salicylate I.M. or I.V., repeated in 2 hours, as needed, to reverse cardiovascular and CNS toxic effects. Be prepared to administer a short-acting barbiturate or diazepam, as prescribed, to control excitement. Be aware that pilocarpine 0.5% may be prescribed to treat mydriasis.

Institute suicide precautions according to facility policy, and anticipate psychiatric re-evaluation.

Nursing Considerations

• Expect to administer benztropine by I.V. or I.M. route to a patient who needs more rapid response than oral drug can provide. Be aware that I.M. route is commonly used because it provides effects in about the same amount of time as I.V. route. Watch for improvement a few minutes after administration. If parkinsonian signs and symptoms reappear, expect to repeat dose.

• Know that because benztropine has a cumulative action, therapy generally begins with a low dose followed by gradual increases of 0.5 mg every 5 to 6 days.

• Assess muscle rigidity and tremor as a baseline. Then monitor them frequently for improvement, which indicates benztropine's effectiveness.

• Give drug before or after meals based on patient's need and response. If patient has increased salivation, expect to give drug after meals; if patient has dry mouth, give it before meals unless nausea develops.

• **WARNING** When administering benztropine to patient with drug-induced extrapyramidal reactions, be alert for exacerbation of psychiatric signs and symptoms.

• Know that high-dose benztropine therapy may cause weakness and inability to move specific muscle groups. If this occurs, expect to reduce the dose.

PATIENT TEACHING

• Warn patient that benztropine has a cumulative effect, increasing risk of adverse reactions and overdose.

• Caution patient to avoid driving and similar activities until she knows how the drug affects her, because it may cause blurred vision, dizziness, or drowsiness.

• **WARNING** Because benztropine decreases diaphoresis, urge patient to avoid extremely hot or humid conditions to reduce risk of heatstroke and severe hyperthermia. This is especially important for elderly patients and those who abuse alcohol or have chronic illness or CNS disease.

• Stress the importance of periodic ocular examinations and intraocular pressure measurements because benztropine may cause angle-closure glaucoma and may increase intraocular pressure.

biperiden hydrochloride
Akineton

biperiden lactate
Akineton Lactate

Class and Category
Chemical class: Tertiary amine
Therapeutic class: Antidyskinetic
Pregnancy category: C

Indications and Dosages
▶ *As adjunct to treat all forms of Parkinson's disease*
TABLETS
Adults and adolescents. 2 mg t.i.d. or q.i.d. up to 16 mg daily.
▶ *To control extrapyramidal symptoms (except tardive dyskinesia) caused by phenothiazines and other neuroleptic drugs*
TABLETS
Adults and adolescents. 2 mg one to three times daily.
I.V. OR I.M. INJECTION
Adults. 2 mg repeated every 30 min until signs and symptoms resolve or maximum of 4 consecutive doses in 24 hr is reached.

Route	Onset	Steady State	Peak	Half-Life	Duration
I.V.	In min	Unknown	Unknown	Unknown	1 to 8 hr
I.M.	10 to 30 min	Unknown	Unknown	Unknown	Unknown

Mechanism of Action
Blocks acetylcholine's action at cholinergic receptor sites. This action restores the brain's normal dopamine and acetylcholine balance, which relaxes muscle movement and decreases rigidity and tremors. Biperiden also may inhibit dopamine reuptake and storage, which prolongs dopamine's action.

Contraindications
Angle-closure glaucoma, achalasia, bladder neck obstruction, duodenal or pyloric obstruction, hypersensitivity to biperiden, myasthenia gravis, prostatic hyperplasia, stenosing peptic ulcer, toxic megacolon

Interactions
DRUGS
amantadine: Possibly increased adverse anticholinergic effects
digoxin: Possibly increased blood digoxin level

haloperidol: Possibly increased schizophrenic signs and symptoms, decreased serum haloperidol level, development of tardive dyskinesia

levodopa: Possibly decreased effectiveness of levodopa

phenothiazines: Possibly reduced phenothiazine effects, increased psychiatric signs and symptoms

Adverse Reactions

CNS: Agitation, confusion, delirium, delusions, depression, disorientation, dizziness, drowsiness, euphoria, excitement, fever, hallucinations, headache, light-headedness, listlessness, memory loss, nervousness, paranoia, psychosis, weakness

CV: Hypotension, mild bradycardia, orthostatic hypotension, palpitations, tachycardia

EENT: Angle-closure glaucoma, blurred vision, diplopia, dry mouth, increased intraocular pressure, mydriasis, suppurative parotitis

GI: Constipation, duodenal ulcer, epigastric distress, ileus, nausea, vomiting

GU: Dysuria, urinary hesitancy, urine retention

MS: Muscle spasms, muscle weakness

SKIN: Decreased sweating, dermatosis, flushing, rash, urticaria

Overdose

Monitor patient for signs and symptoms of overdose, including clumsiness; dyspnea; hallucinations; insomnia; seizures; severe drowsiness; severe dryness of mouth, nose or throat; tachycardia; toxic psychoses; unsteadiness; and unusually dry, flushed, warm skin.

Maintain open airway, and institute emergency supportive measures, as needed. Expect to induce vomiting or perform gastric lavage to decrease absorption of drug, as prescribed, except in patients who may be convulsive, precomatose, or psychotic. If the patient is an adult, expect to administer physostigmine salicylate, 1 to 2 mg, I.M. or I.V., repeated in 2 hours, as needed, to reverse cardiovascular and CNS toxic effects. Be prepared to administer a short-acting barbiturate or diazepam, as prescribed, to control excitement. Be aware that pilocarpine 0.5% may be prescribed to treat mydriasis. Institute suicide precautions according to facility policy, and anticipate psychiatric re-evaluation.

Nursing Considerations

- Expect to administer I.V. or I.M. biperiden when patient needs more rapid response than oral drug can provide.

- Assess muscle rigidity and tremor as baseline. Then monitor them frequently for improvement, which indicates biperiden's effectiveness.
- **WARNING** When administering biperiden to a patient with drug-induced extrapyramidal reactions, be alert for exacerbation of psychiatric signs and symptoms.

PATIENT TEACHING

- Caution patient to avoid driving and other activities that require alertness until she knows how the drug affects her.
- **WARNING** Because biperiden decreases sweating, urge patient to avoid extremely hot and humid conditions to reduce risk of heatstroke and severe hyperthermia. This is especially important for elderly patients and those who abuse alcohol or have chronic illness or CNS disease.
- Stress the importance of periodic ocular examinations and intraocular pressure measurements because biperiden therapy may cause angle-closure glaucoma and may increase intraocular pressure.

bromocriptine mesylate

Alti-Bromocriptine (CAN), Apo-Bromocriptine (CAN), Parlodel, Parlodel SnapTabs

Class and Category

Chemical class: Ergot alkaloid derivative
Therapeutic class: Antidyskinetic, dopamine agonist
Pregnancy category: B

Indications and Dosages

▶ *To treat Parkinson's disease*

CAPSULES, TABLETS

Adults. *Initial:* 1.25 mg daily at bedtime with a snack or b.i.d. with meals. Increased by 2.5 mg every 14 to 28 days, if needed. *Maintenance:* 2.5 to 40 mg daily in divided doses with meals.

Route	Onset	Steady State	Peak	Half-Life	Duration
P.O.	30 to 90 min	Unknown	2 hr	4 to 4.5 hr*	Unknown

Contraindications

Hypersensitivity to bromocriptine, other ergot alkaloids, or their components; severe ischemic heart disease or peripheral vascular disease

---

* For alpha phase. Half-life is 15 hr for terminal phase.

Mechanism of Action

Decreases dopamine turnover in the CNS, depleting dopamine or blocking dopamine receptors in the brain. This alleviates dyskinesia.

Interactions

DRUGS

antihypertensives: Increased hypotensive effects

clarithromycin, erythromycin, troleandomycin: Increased risk of bromocriptine toxicity

ergot alkaloids or derivatives: Increased risk of hypertension

haloperidol, loxapine, MAO inhibitors, methyldopa, metoclopramide, molindone, phenothiazines, pimozide, reserpine, risperidone, thioxanthenes: Decreased effectiveness of bromocriptine

levodopa: Additive effects requiring levodopa dosage reduction

ritonavir: Increased blood bromocriptine level

ACTIVITIES

alcohol use: Possibly disulfiram-like reaction

Adverse Reactions

CNS: Confusion, dizziness, drowsiness, dyskinesia, fatigue, hallucinations, headache, light-headedness, narcolepsy, neuroleptic malignant syndrome, somnolence, syncope

CV: Constrictive pericarditis, hypertension, hypotension, orthostatic hypotension, pericardial effusions, Raynaud's phenomenon

EENT: Dry mouth, nasal congestion

GI: Abdominal cramps, anorexia, constipation, diarrhea, GI bleeding, indigestion, nausea, retroperitoneal fibrosis, vomiting

RESP: Pleural effusions, pleural and pulmonary fibrosis

Overdose

Monitor patient for signs and symptoms of overdose, including nausea, severe hypotension, and vomiting.

Anticipate the need to empty the stomach by aspiration and lavage. Institute supportive measures, and expect to treat hypotension with I.V. fluids, as prescribed.

Nursing Considerations

- Use bromocriptine cautiously if patient has a history of psychosis or cardiovascular disease, especially after an MI with residual arrhythmia.
- Expect to give bromocriptine with levodopa if patient is being treated for Parkinson's disease.

- Assess patient for hypotension (when therapy starts) and hypertension (typically during 2nd week). Monitor blood pressure frequently if patient takes another drug with hypertensive effects.
- If patient has a history of peptic ulcer or GI bleeding, monitor for signs and symptoms of new bleeding.
- Take safety precautions, such as keeping the bed in low position with side rails up, because bromocriptine can cause dizziness, drowsiness, light-headedness, and syncope.

PATIENT TEACHING

- Tell patient to take each dose with a meal, milk, or a snack to minimize nausea.
- Advise patient against stopping bromocriptine abruptly because, although rare, a very serious condition called neuroleptic malignant syndrome may occur.
- Alert patient that sudden sleep episodes may occur during activities of daily living. Caution patient to avoid engaging in any hazardous activities, such as driving, while taking drug.
- Caution patient that drug may cause dizziness, drowsiness, and light-headedness.
- Advise patient to avoid sudden position changes to minimize the effects of orthostatic hypotension.
- Warn patient to avoid alcohol while taking bromocriptine because it may cause disulfiram-like reactions, such as blurred vision, chest pain, confusion, diaphoresis, a fast or pounding heartbeat, facial flushing, nausea, a throbbing headache, vomiting, and severe weakness.
- Tell patient to take a missed dose as soon as she remembers it, unless it's almost time for the next dose. In that case, tell her to wait until the next scheduled dose. Warn her not to double the dose. Advise her to contact prescriber if she misses more than one dose.
- Tell patient who takes large doses of bromocriptine to schedule regular dental checkups because the drug can decrease salivary flow, which may encourage dental caries, discomfort, oral candidiasis, and periodontal disease.

Other Therapeutic Uses

Bromocriptine mesylate is also indicated for the following:

- To treat amenorrhea, galactorrhea, infertility from hyperprolactinemia, and male hypogonadism
- To treat prolactin-secreting adenoma
- To treat acromegaly

bupropion hydrochloride
Wellbutrin, Wellbutrin SR, Wellbutrin XL, Zyban

bupropion hydrobromide
Aplenzin

Class and Category
Chemical class: Aminoketone derivative
Therapeutic class: Antidepressant, smoking cessation adjunct
Pregnancy category: C

Indications and Dosages
▶ *To treat depression*
E.R. TABLETS (WELLBUTRIN SR)
Adults. *Initial:* 150 mg daily in the morning for 3 days; then 150 mg b.i.d. and, after several wk, 200 mg b.i.d., as needed and tolerated. *Maximum:* 400 mg daily or 200 mg/dose.
E.R. TABLETS (WELLBUTRIN XR)
Adults. *Initial:* 150 mg daily in the morning for at least 3 days; then 150 mg daily and, after 4 wk, 450 mg daily, as needed and tolerated. *Maximum:* 450 mg daily.
TABLETS
Adults. *Initial:* 100 mg b.i.d., increased after 3 or more days to 100 mg t.i.d., as needed. *Maximum:* 450 mg daily or 150 mg/dose.
E.R. TABLETS (APLENZIN)
Adults. *Initial:* 174 mg once daily in the morning for at least 3 days; then 348 mg once daily in the morning and, after 4 wk, 522 mg once daily in the morning, as needed. *Maximum:* 522 mg daily.
▶ *To prevent seasonal major depressive episodes in patients with seasonal affective disorder*
E.R. TABLETS (WELLBUTRIN XR)
Adults. *Initial:* Starting in autumn before the onset of depression symptoms, 150 mg daily in the morning, increased after 1 wk to 300 mg daily in the morning if well tolerated. In early spring, decreased to 150 mg daily in the morning 2 weeks before stopping therapy. If 300 mg daily is not well tolerated, dosage reduced to 150 mg daily and discontinued in early spring.
▶ *To aid smoking cessation*
E.R. TABLETS
Adults. *Initial:* 150 mg daily for 3 days and then 150 mg b.i.d. for 7 to 12 wk. *Maximum:* 300 mg daily or 150 mg/dose.
DOSAGE ADJUSTMENT For patients with severe hepatic cirrhosis, dosage shouldn't exceed 75 mg daily for Wellbutrin,

100 mg daily or 150 mg every other day for Wellbutrin SR, and 150 mg every other day for Wellbutrin XL and Zyban. For patients with renal impairment, dose or frequency will be decreased.

Route	Onset	Steady State	Peak	Half-Life	Duration
P.O.	1 to 3 wk	5 to 8 days	Unknown	8 to 24 hr	Unknown
P.O. (E.R.)	Unknown	Unknown	Unknown	21 hr	Unknown

Mechanism of Action

May inhibit norepinephrine, serotonin, and dopamine uptake by neurons. Such inhibition significantly relieves signs and symptoms of depression, improving the patient's sense of well-being and mood. Also, as nicotine levels drop with abstinence, the firing rates of noradrenergic neurons in the CNS increase, causing withdrawal signs and symptoms. Bupropion decreases these firing rates, which causes a reduction in these signs and symptoms.

Contraindications

Anorexia, bulimia, concurrent treatment with another form of bupropion, hypersensitivity to bupropion or its components, seizure disorder, treatment requiring abrupt discontinuation of alcohol or sedatives (including benzodiazepines), use within 14 days of an MAO inhibitor

Interactions

DRUGS

Amantadine, levodopa: Increased adverse reactions to bupropion
carbamazepine, cimetidine, phenobarbital, phenytoin: Increased metabolism of bupropion
clozapine, fluoxetine, haloperidol, lithium, loxapine, maprotiline, molindone, phenothiazines, thioxanthenes, trazodone, tricyclic antidepressants: Increased risk of major motor seizures
MAO inhibitors: Increased risk of acute bupropion toxicity
nicotine: Possibly increased blood pressure

ACTIVITIES

alcohol use, recreational drug abuse: Lowered seizure threshold

Adverse Reactions

CNS: Agitation, akathisia, anxiety, asthenia, CNS stimulation, coma, confusion, CVA, decreased concentration or memory, delusions, dizziness, euphoria, fever, general or migraine headache, hallucinations, hostility, hot flashes, insomnia, irritability, nerv-

ousness, paranoia, paresthesia, seizures, somnolence, suicidal
ideation, syncope, tremor, vertigo
CV: Arrhythmias, complete AV block, hypertension, MI, orthostatic hypotension, phlebitis, tachycardia, vasodilation
EENT: Altered taste, amblyopia, auditory disturbances, diplopia,
blurred vision, deafness, dry mouth, pharyngitis, sinusitis, tinnitus
ENDO: Hyperglycemia, hypoglycemia, syndrome of inappropriate
antidiuretic hormone
GI: Abdominal pain, anorexia, constipation, diarrhea, dysphagia,
flatulence, GI hemorrhage, hepatitis, increased appetite, intestinal
perforation, nausea, pancreatitis, stomach ulcer, vomiting
GU: Decreased libido, urinary frequency and urgency, UTI, vaginal hemorrhage
HEME: Anemia, leukocytosis, leukopenia, lymphadenopathy,
pancytopenia, thrombocytopenia
MS: Arthralgia, arthritis, muscle twitching, myalgia, rhabdomyolysis
RESP: Bronchospasm, cough, pulmonary embolism
SKIN: Diaphoresis, exfoliative dermatitis, flushing, pruritus, rash,
urticaria
Other: Angioedema, generalized pain, infection, serum sickness,
weight loss

Overdose
Monitor patient for signs and symptoms of overdose, including
hallucinations, loss of consciousness, nausea, seizures, tachycardia,
and vomiting.

Maintain an open airway, and be prepared to participate in
emergency resuscitation measures, as required. Also, be aware
that seizures are common, occurring in about one-third of all
overdose cases. Be prepared to perform gastric lavage within initial 12 hours of ingestion to decrease absorption of drug. For an
unconscious patient, anticipate assisting with the insertion of an
endotracheal tube and then performing gastric lavage. The inflated cuff of the endotracheal tube will help prevent aspiration of
gastric contents into the lungs. Anticipate administering activated
charcoal every 6 hours during initial 12 hours, as prescribed. Be
aware that ipecac syrup shouldn't be used to induce vomiting because of risk of seizures.

Expect to use I.V. benzodiazepines to treat seizure activity, as
prescribed. Plan to perform continuous cardiac monitoring for at
least 48 hours. Bupropion and its metabolites diffuse slowly from
tissue to plasma, so diuresis, dialysis, and hemoperfusion are inef-

fective for treating overdose. Institute suicide precautions according to facility policy, and anticipate psychiatric re-evaluation.

Nursing Considerations

- Use cautiously in patients with renal impairment because drug is excreted by the kidneys.
- Monitor depressed patient closely for worsened depression and suicide risk, especially in a child or an adolescent and especially when therapy starts or dosage changes.
- Be aware that 522 mg bupropion hydrobromide is equivalent to 450 mg bupropion hydrochloride; 348 mg of bupropion hydrobromide is equivalent to 300 mg bupropion hydrochloride; and 174 mg bupropion hydrobromide is equivlanet to 150 mg bupropion hydrochloride.
- To reduce the risk of seizures, allow at least 4 hours between doses of tablets and 8 to 24 hours (depending on product prescribed) between doses of E.R. tablets.
- Use seizure precautions, especially in patients who take OTC stimulants or anorectics; use excessive alcohol or sedatives; are addicted to opioids, cocaine, or stimulants; take drugs that lower the seizure threshold; have a history of seizures, head trauma, or CNS tumors; have severe hepatic cirrhosis; or take insulin or an oral antidiabetic.
- Although a nicotine transdermal system may be used with bupropion to treat nicotine dependence, the combination may cause hypertension. Monitor blood pressure frequently.

PATIENT TEACHING

- Advise patient who uses bupropion for smoking cessation to take it for 7 or more days before stopping smoking. Encourage her to join a smoking cessation support program.
- Tell patient to swallow E.R. tablets whole and not to crush, break, or chew them.
- Tell patient to take bupropion with food to minimize GI distress.
- Advise patient to take the last dose early in the evening to avoid insomnia.
- Advise patient to avoid potentially hazardous activities until she knows how the drug affects her.
- Urge patient to minimize or avoid alcohol because it can lower the seizure threshold when combined with bupropion. Also urge patient to avoid stopping alcohol or sedative abruptly during bupropion therapy; serious adverse reactions may result.
- Tell patient to skip a missed dose and resume the regular dosing schedule but not to double the dose.

- To reduce the risk of seizures from drug interactions, tell patient to inform all prescribers that she takes bupropion.
- Tell patient to report bothersome or severe adverse reactions.
- Urge caregivers to monitor depressed patient closely for worsened depression, especially when therapy starts or dosage changes.

buspirone hydrochloride
BuSpar, BuSpar DIVIDOSE, Bustab (CAN)

Class and Category
Chemical class: Azaspirodecanedione
Therapeutic class: Antianxiety drug
Pregnancy category: B

Indications and Dosages
▶ *To manage anxiety*
TABLETS
Adults. *Initial:* 5 mg t.i.d. or 7.5 mg b.i.d. increased by 5 mg daily at 2- to 3-day intervals until desired response occurs. *Maintenance:* 20 to 30 mg daily (usual therapeutic range). *Maximum:* 60 mg daily.
DOSAGE ADJUSTMENT When used with nefazodone, dosage decreased to 2.5 mg daily.

Route	Onset	Steady State	Peak	Half-Life	Duration
P.O.	1 to 4 wk	Unknown	3 to 6 wk	2 to 3 hr	Unknown

Mechanism of Action
May act as a partial agonist at serotonin 5-hydroxytryptamine$_{1A}$ receptors in the brain, producing antianxiety effects.

Contraindications
Hypersensitivity to buspirone or its components

Interactions
DRUGS
erythromycin, itraconazole, nefazodone: Increased blood level and adverse effects of buspirone
haloperidol: Increased blood haloperidol level
MAO inhibitors: Increased risk of hypertension

Adverse Reactions

CNS: Akathisia, anger, ataxia, cogwheel rigidity, confusion, decreased concentration, depression, dizziness, dream disturbances, drowsiness, dystonia, dyskinesia, excitement, extrapyramidal symptoms, fatigue, headache, hostility, insomnia, lack of coordination, light-headedness, nervousness, numbness, paresthesia, parkinsonism, restless legs syndrome, restlessness, serotonin syndrome, tremor, weakness
CV: Chest pain, palpitations, tachycardia
EENT: Blurred vision, dry mouth, nasal congestion, pharyngitis, tinnitus
GI: Abdominal or gastric distress, constipation, diarrhea, nausea, vomiting
GU: Urine retention
MS: Myalgia
SKIN: Diaphoresis, rash, urticaria
Other: Angioedema

Overdose

Buspirone overdose has no specific antidote. Monitor patient for signs and symptoms of overdose including dizziness, light-headedness, loss of consciousness, miosis, nausea, severe drowsiness, and vomiting. Monitor vital signs frequently, and assess the patient for extrapyramidal signs and symptoms, mania, and panic.

Be prepared to institute supportive measures such as gastric lavage within 1 to 1½ hours of ingestion to decrease absorption of the drug. Institute suicide precautions according to facility policy, and anticipate psychiatric re-evaluation.

Nursing Considerations

- Use buspirone cautiously in patients with hepatic or renal impairment.
- Take safety precautions because the drug may cause adverse CNS reactions.

PATIENT TEACHING

- Reassure patient that buspirone isn't addictive.
- Inform patient that 1 to 2 weeks of therapy may be needed before she notices drug's antianxiety effect.
- Stress importance of not taking more buspirone than prescribed.
- Advise patient to avoid potentially hazardous activities until she knows how the drug affects her.
- Tell patient to take a missed dose as soon as possible unless the next scheduled dose is soon. Warn against doubling the dose.

butabarbital sodium
Busodium, Butalan, Butisol, Sarisol No. 2

Class, Category, and Schedule
Chemical class: Barbiturate
Therapeutic class: Sedative-hypnotic
Pregnancy category: D
Controlled substance schedule: III

Indications and Dosages
▶ *To provide daytime sedation*
ELIXIR, TABLETS
Adults. 15 to 30 mg t.i.d. or q.i.d.
▶ *To treat insomnia*
ELIXIR, TABLETS
Adults. 50 to 100 mg daily at bedtime.
DOSAGE ADJUSTMENT Dosage reduced in patients with impaired hepatic or renal function and in elderly or debilitated patients because they may be more sensitive to drug.

Route	Onset	Steady State	Peak	Half-Life	Duration
P.O.	45 to 60 min	Unknown	Unknown	66 to 140 hr	6 to 8 hr

Mechanism of Action
Inhibits the upward conduction of nerve impulses in the brain's reticular formation, which disrupts impulse transmission to the cortex. As a result, butabarbital depresses the CNS and produces drowsiness, hypnosis, and sedation.

Contraindications
History of addiction to sedative or hypnotic drug, hypersensitivity to butabarbital or its components, porphyria, severe hepatic or respiratory disease

Interactions
DRUGS
acetaminophen: Increased metabolism and decreased effectiveness of acetaminophen; risk of hepatotoxicity
activated charcoal: Reduced absorption of butabarbital
aminophylline, oxtriphylline, theophylline: Decreased blood level and effects of these drugs
carbamazepine: Decreased blood carbamazepine level

chloramphenicol, corticosteroids: Increased metabolism and decreased effects of these drugs
clonazepam: Increased clearance and decreased effectiveness of clonazepam
CNS depressants, including OTC hypnotics and sedatives: Additive CNS depression
doxycycline: Shortened half-life and decreased effects of doxycycline
fenoprofen: Reduced bioavailability and effects of fenoprofen
griseofulvin: Reduced absorption of griseofulvin
hydantoins, such as phenytoin: Unpredictable effects on barbiturate metabolism
MAO inhibitors: Prolonged barbiturate effects
meperidine: Prolonged CNS depressant effects of meperidine
methadone: Reduced methadone action
methoxyflurane: Increased risk of nephrotoxicity
metronidazole: Decreased antimicrobial effect of metronidazole
oral anticoagulants: Decreased anticoagulant effect
oral contraceptives with estrogen: Decreased contraceptive effect
phenylbutazone: Reduced elimination half-life of phenylbutazone
rifampin: Decreased effectiveness of butabarbital
sodium valproate, valproic acid: Decreased metabolism and increased adverse CNS effects of butabarbital
ACTIVITIES
alcohol use: Additive CNS depression

Adverse Reactions

CNS: Agitation, anxiety, ataxia, clumsiness, CNS depression, confusion, depression, dizziness, drowsiness, fever, hallucinations, headache, hyperkinesia, insomnia, irritability, nervousness, nightmares, psychiatric disturbance, sleep-driving, somnolence, syncope
CV: Hypertension
EENT: Laryngospasm
GI: Constipation, hepatic dysfunction, nausea, vomiting
MS: Rickets
RESP: Apnea, bronchospasm, respiratory depression
SKIN: Exfoliative dermatitis, Stevens-Johnson syndrome
Other: Anaphylaxis, angioedema, drug tolerance, physical and psychological dependence

Overdose

Monitor patient for signs and symptoms of overdose, including bradycardia, Cheyne-Stokes respiration, coma, confusion, decreased or absent reflexes, dyspnea, fever, hypothermia, miosis or mydriasis, oliguria, severe drowsiness, severe weakness, shock, slurred speech, staggering, tachycardia, and unusual eye movements. Consider chronic overdose if such signs and symptoms as continued irritability, insomnia, poor judgment, and severe confusion occur. Maintain an open airway, and carefully monitor temperature and blood pressure.

If patient is conscious, be prepared to administer ipecac syrup, as prescribed, to induce vomiting. Expect to administer 30 to 60 g of activated charcoal with water or sorbitol to prevent further absorption and to enhance drug elimination.

For an unconscious patient, anticipate assisting with insertion of an endotracheal tube and then performing gastric lavage. The inflated cuff of the endotracheal tube will help prevent aspiration of gastric contents into the lungs.

Be prepared to administer drugs to promote urine alkalization to enhance drug elimination. Administer I.V. fluids and a vasopressor, as prescribed. For severe cases, anticipate the need for hemodialysis or hemoperfusion. Be aware that, in cases of extreme barbiturate overdose, the patient may have a flat EEG because all electrical activity in the brain has ceased; however, this effect may be reversible. Institute suicide precautions according to facility policy, and anticipate psychiatric re-evaluation.

Nursing Considerations

- Use butabarbital cautiously, if at all, in patients with depression, hepatic dysfunction, history of drug abuse, or suicidal tendency. Don't administer drug to patients with premonitory signs or symtoms of hepatic coma.
- **WARNING** Monitor patient closely after butabarbital ingestion because anaphylaxis or angioedema, although rare, may occur with first dose or later doses. Notify prescriber immediately, and provide supportive emergency care.
- Monitor patient for worsening of insomnia or emergence of new thinking or behavior abnormalities because butabarbital may unmask them. If so, patient may need a more extensive work-up.
- Expect to give drug for no more than 2 weeks to treat insomnia because, like all barbiturates, it loses effectiveness for sleep induction and sleep maintenance after 2 weeks.
- Monitor butabarbital intake closely during long-term use because tolerance and psychological and physical dependence may develop.

- Avoid abrupt withdrawal of butabarbital to prevent withdrawal signs and symptoms.
- Monitor elderly and debilitated patients closely because drug may cause marked confusion, depression, and excitement in them.
- If patient in pain receives butabarbital, monitor her closely for paradoxical excitement.
- If pregnant patient took butabarbital during last trimester, monitor infant for withdrawal symptoms.

PATIENT TEACHING

- Stress the importance of taking butabarbital exactly as prescribed because it can be addictive. Warn against adjusting the dosage without consulting prescriber.
- Tell patient to avoid alcohol and OTC hypnotics and sedatives during butabarbital therapy because of additive CNS effects.
- Urge patient to avoid potentially hazardous activities until she knows how the drug affects her.
- Advise female patient not to rely on oral contraceptives during butabarbital therapy.
- Advise patient to notify prescriber if insomnia persists despite more than 7 days of butabarbital therapy.
- Tell family to report any sleep-driving episodes, in which patient drives while not fully awake and usually has no recall of the event.

Other Therapeutic Uses

Butabarbital sodium is also indicated for the following:
- To provide preoperative sedation

carbamazepine

Apo-Carbamazepine (CAN), Atretol, Carbatrol, Epitol, Equetro, Novo-Carbamaz (CAN), Tegretol, Tegretol Chewtabs (CAN), Tegretol-XR

Class and Category

Chemical class: Tricyclic iminostilbene derivative
Therapeutic class: Anticonvulsant
Pregnancy category: C

Indications and Dosages

▶ *To treat epilepsy*

E.R. CAPSULES (CARBATROL), E.R. TABLETS (TEGRETOL-XR)

Adults and children age 12 and over. *Initial:* 200 mg b.i.d. Increased weekly by 200 mg daily, if needed. *Maximum:* 1,600 mg daily in adults; 1,200 mg daily in children age 16 and older; and 1,000 mg daily in children ages 12 to 16.

Children ages 6 to 12. *Initial:* 100 mg b.i.d. Increased weekly by 100 mg daily, if needed. *Maximum:* 1,000 mg daily.

ORAL SUSPENSION

Adults and children age 12 and over. *Initial:* 100 mg q.i.d. Increased weekly by 200 mg daily, if needed, given in divided doses t.i.d. or q.i.d. *Maximum:* 1,600 mg daily in adults; 1,200 mg daily in children age 16 and older; and 1,000 mg daily in children ages 12 to 16.

Children ages 6 to 12. *Initial:* 50 mg q.i.d. Increased weekly by 100 mg daily, if needed, given in divided doses t.i.d. or q.i.d. *Maximum:* 1,000 mg daily.

Children up to age 6. *Initial:* 10 to 20 mg/kg daily in divided doses q.i.d. *Maximum:* 35 mg/kg daily.

CHEWABLE TABLETS, TABLETS

Adults and children age 12 and over. *Initial:* 200 mg b.i.d. Increased weekly by 200 mg daily, if needed, given in divided doses t.i.d. or q.i.d. *Maximum:* 1,600 mg daily in adults; 1,200 mg daily in children age 16 and older; and 1,000 mg daily in children ages 12 to 16.

Children ages 6 to 12. *Initial:* 100 mg b.i.d. Increased weekly by 100 mg daily, if needed, given in divided doses t.i.d. or q.i.d. *Maximum:* 1,000 mg daily.

Children up to age 6. *Initial:* 10 to 20 mg/kg daily in divided doses b.i.d. or t.i.d. Increased weekly, if needed, divided and given t.i.d. or q.i.d. *Maximum:* 35/kg daily.

▶ *To treat acute manic and mixed episodes in bipolar disorder*
E.R. CAPSULES (EQUETRO)
Adults. *Initial:* 200 mg b.i.d. increased, as needed, in 200-mg increments. *Maximum:* 1,600 mg daily.

Route	Onset	Steady State	Peak	Half-Life	Duration
P.O.	In 1 mo	Unknown	Unknown	8 to 29 hr*	Unknown

Mechanism of Action

Normally, sodium moves into a neuronal cell by passing through a gated sodium channel in the cell membrane. Carbamazepine may prevent or halt seizures by closing or blocking sodium channels, as shown, thus preventing sodium from entering the cell. Keeping sodium out of the cell may slow nerve impulse transmission, thus slowing the rate at which neurons fire.

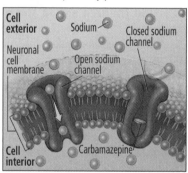

Contraindications

History of bone marrow depression; hypersensitivity to carbamazepine, tricyclic compounds, or their components; MAO inhibitor or nefazodone therapy

Interactions
DRUGS

acetaminophen, alprazolam, amitriptyline, bupropion, buspirone, citalopram, clobazam, clonazepam, clozapine, cyclosporine, delavirdine, desipramine, diazepam, dicumarol, doxycycline, ethosuximide, felbamate, felodipine, glucocorticoids, haloperidol, itraconazole, lamotrigine, levothy-

---

* For subsequent doses. Half-life is 25 to 65 hr for initial dose.

roxine, lorazepam, methadone, methsuximide, midazolam, mirtazapine, nortriptylline, olanzapine, oral contraceptives, oxcarbazepine, phenytoin, praziquantel, protease inhibitors, quetiapine, risperidone, theophylline, topiramate, tiagabine, tramadol, trazodone, triazolam, valproate, warfarin, ziprasidone, zonisamide: Decreased blood levels of these drugs
acetazolamide, azole antifungals, cimetidine, clarithromycin, dalfopristin, danazol, delavirdine, diltiazem, erythromycin, fluconazole, fluoxetine, fluvoxamine, isoniazid, itraconazole, ketoconazole, loratadine, nefazadone, niacinamide, nicotinamide, propoxyphene, protease inhibitors, quinine, quinupristin, terfenadine, troleandomycin, valproate, verapamil, zileuton: Increased blood carbamazepine level
chloroquine, mefloquine: Possibly antagonized action of carbamazepine
cisplatin, doxorubicin, methsuximide, phenobarbital, phenytoin, primidone, rifampin, theophylline: Decreased blood carbamazepine level
clomipramine, phenytoin, primidone: Increased blood levels of these drugs
felbamate: Decreased blood level of carbamazepine or felbamate
isoniazid: Increased risk of carbamazepine toxicity and isoniazid hepatotoxicity
lithium: Increased risk of CNS toxicity
oral anticoagulants: Increased metabolism and decreased effectiveness of anticoagulant
nefazodone: Decreased nefazodone effectiveness and increased carbamazepine blood level
nondepolarizing neuromuscular blockers: Possibly reduced duration or decreased effectiveness of neuromuscular blocker
ACTIVITIES
alcohol use: Possibly enhanced CNS effect
FOODS
grapefruit juice: Increased blood carbamazepine level

Adverse Reactions
CNS: Chills, confusion, dizziness, drowsiness, fatigue, fever, headache, syncope, talkativeness, unsteadiness, visual hallucinations
CV: Arrhythmias, including AV block; edema; heart failure; hypertension; hypotension; thromboembolism; thrombophlebitis; worsened coronary artery disease
EENT: Blurred vision, conjunctivitis, dry mouth, glossitis, nystagmus, oculomotor disturbances, stomatitis, tinnitus, transient diplopia
ENDO: Syndrome of inappropriate ADH secretion, water intoxication

GI: Abdominal pain, anorexia, constipation, diarrhea, dyspepsia, elevated liver function test results, hepatitis, nausea, pancreatitis, vomiting

GU: Acute urine retention, albuminuria, azotemia, glycosuria, impotence, oliguria, renal failure, urinary frequency

HEME: Acute intermittent porphyria, agranulocytosis, aplastic anemia, bone marrow depression, eosinophilia, leukocytosis, leukopenia, pancytopenia, thrombocytopenia

MS: Arthralgia, leg cramps, myalgia

RESP: Pulmonary hypersensitivity (dyspnea, fever, pneumonia, or pneumonitis)

SKIN: Aggravation of disseminated lupus erythematosus, alopecia, altered skin pigmentation, diaphoresis, erythema multiforme, erythema nodosum, exfoliative dermatitis, jaundice, Lyell's syndrome, photosensitivity reactions, pruritic and erythematous rash, purpura, Stevens-Johnson syndrome, toxic epidermal necrolysis, urticaria

Other: Adenopathy, lymphadenopathy

Overdose

Monitor patient for signs and symptoms of overdose, including anuria, oliguria, or urine retention; ataxia; athetoid movements; conduction abnormalities; dysmetria; hyperreflexia, then hyporeflexia; hypertension or hypotension; muscle twitching; mydriasis; nausea; opis-thotonos; respiratory depression; restlessness; seizures; severe dizziness or drowsiness; shock; tachycardia; tremor; and vomiting.

Maintain an open airway, monitor vital signs and pupillary reactions, and institute emergency supportive measures, as needed. Expect to induce vomiting or perform gastric lavage and administer activated charcoal or a laxative, as prescribed, to reduce absorption. Administer I.V. fluids to promote diuresis.

Anticipate administering a vasopressor and a plasma volume expander to treat hypotension and shock. Be prepared to give a benzodiazepine or a barbiturate, as prescribed, for seizures, unless the patient has ingested an MAO inhibitor in the previous 14 days.

Dialysis may be considered if the overdose is associated with renal failure, and small children may require replacement transfusion. Expect to monitor the patient's vital signs, pupillary reflexes, and renal function for several days. Institute suicide precautions according to facility policy, and anticipate psychiatric re-evaluation.

Nursing Considerations

• Carbamazepine shouldn't be used in patients with a history of hepatic porphyria because drug may precipitate acute attacks.

• **WARNING** Find out if patients of Asian ancestry have been evaluated for a genetic allelic variant, HLA-B 1502, before they start carbamazepine therapy. Patients with this variant shouldn't receive carbamazepine because they have ten times the risk of serious, sometimes fatal, dermatologic reactions.

• Use carbamazepine cautiously in patients with impaired hepatic function because it's mainly metabolized in the liver. Monitor results of liver function tests, as directed.

• Use carbamazepine cautiously in patients with increased intraocular pressure; drug may have mild anticholinergic action.

• Monitor patient closely for adverse reactions; many are serious.

• Periodically monitor blood carbamazepine level to assess for therapeutic and toxic levels; a blood level of 6 to 12 mcg/ml is optimal for anticonvulsant effects.

• **WARNING** Monitor WBC and platelet counts monthly for first 2 months. Decreased counts may indicate bone marrow depression.

• Monitor patient's total cholesterol, LDL, and HDL levels, as ordered, because they may increase in some patients carbamazepine or other anticonvulsants.

• Withdraw carbamazepine therapy gradually, as prescribed, to minimize the risk of seizures.

PATIENT TEACHING

• Tell patient to take carbamazepine with food (except oral suspension, which shouldn't be taken with other liquid drugs or diluents).

• Explain that drug may cause blurred vision, dizziness, and unsteadiness.

• Inform patient that the coating of E.R. tablets isn't absorbed and may appear in stool.

• Tell patient not to crush or chew E.R. capsules or tablets. If he can't swallow capsules, have him open them and sprinkle contents on food. Tell him that chewable tablets are also available.

• If patient has a seizure diorder, warn him not to stop carbamazepine abruptly; life-threatening status epilepticus may result.

• Instruct patient to wear sunscreen and protective clothing to prevent photosensitivity reactions.

• Tell patient to notify prescriber of unusual bleeding or bruising, fever, mouth ulcers, or rash.

• Warn female patient that drug decreases oral contraceptive effectiveness, and urge her to use another form of contraception. Because drug may cause fetal abnormalities, urge her to notify prescriber if she is or could be pregnant.

Other Therapeutic Uses
Carbamazepine is also indicated for the following:
• To relieve pain in trigeminal neuralgia

carbidopa and levodopa
Apo-Levocarb (CAN), Atamet, Sinemet, Sinemet CR

Class and Category
Chemical class: Hydralazine analogue of levodopa (carbidopa), levorotatory isomer of dihydroxyphenylalanine (levodopa)
Therapeutic class: Antidyskinetic
Pregnancy category: C

Indications and Dosages
▶ *To relieve symptoms of Parkinson's disease*
E.R. TABLETS
Adults not taking levodopa. *Initial:* 1 tablet (25 mg carbidopa and 100 mg levodopa or 50 mg carbidopa and 200 mg levodopa) b.i.d. with doses spaced at least 6 hr apart. Dose increased or decreased every 3 days or more, if needed, based on patient's response to drug therapy. *Maintenance:* 400 to 1,600 mg levodopa daily in divided doses every 4 to 8 hr. *Maximum:* 2,400 mg levodopa daily.
Adults taking levodopa, regardless of dosage. 1 tablet (25 mg carbidopa and 100 mg levodopa or 50 mg carbidopa and 200 mg levodopa) b.i.d. at least 12 hr after levodopa is discontinued. *Maximum:* 2,400 mg levodopa daily.
Adults taking conventional carbidopa and levodopa. If patient takes 300 to 400 mg levodopa in combination product, regimen switched to 1 E.R. tablet (200 mg levodopa) b.i.d. given 4 to 8 hr apart. If he takes 500 to 600 mg levodopa in combination product, regimen switched to 1 E.R. tablet (300 mg levodopa) b.i.d. or t.i.d. given 4 to 8 hr apart. If he takes 700 to 800 mg levodopa in combination product, regimen switched to 4 E.R. tablets (800 mg levodopa) daily divided into 3 doses and given 4 to 8 hr apart. *Maximum:* 2,400 mg levodopa daily.
TABLETS
Adults not taking levodopa. *Initial:* 1 tablet (25 mg carbidopa

and 100 mg levodopa) t.i.d. or 1 tablet (10 mg carbidopa and 100 mg levodopa) t.i.d. or q.i.d. Increased by 1 tablet daily or every other day, if needed, up to maximum dosage. *Maximum:* 200 mg carbidopa and 2,000 mg levodopa daily.

Adults taking more than 1,500 mg levodopa. 1 tablet (25 mg carbidopa and 250 mg levodopa) t.i.d. or q.i.d. at least 12 hr after levodopa is discontinued. *Maximum:* 200 mg carbidopa and 2,000 mg levodopa daily.

Adults taking less than 1,500 mg levodopa. 1 tablet (25 mg carbidopa and 100 mg levodopa or 10 mg carbidopa and 100 mg levodopa) t.i.d. or q.i.d. at least 12 hr after levodopa therapy is discontinued. *Maximum:* 200 mg carbidopa and 2,000 mg levodopa daily.

ORALLY DISINTEGRATING TABLETS

Adults. *Initial:* 1 tablet (25 mg carbidopa and 100 mg levodopa) t.i.d. increased, as needed, by 1 tablet daily or every other day. Or, 1 tablet (10 mg carbidopa and 100 mg levodopa) t.i.d. or q.i.d. increased, as needed, by 1 tablet daily or every other day. *Maximum:* 8 tablets (25 mg carbidopa and 100 mg levodopa or 10 mg carbidopa and 100 mg levodopa) daily.

Route	Onset	Steady State	Peak	Half-Life	Duration
P.O.	Unknown	0.5 to 0.7 hr	Unknown	0.75 to 1.5 hr*; 1 to 2 hr†	Unknown
P.O. (E.R.)	Unknown	2.1 to 2.4 hr	Unknown	Unknown	Unknown

Mechanism of Action

When carbidopa and levodopa are adiminstered together, carbidopa inhibits peripheral distribution of levodopa, making more levodopa available for transport to the brain. In extracerebral tissues, levodopa is converted to dopamine. Then it's transported to the CNS, where it replenishes depleted dopamine stores, which are thought to cause Parkinson's disease, thus helping to improve muscle control and normalize body movements.

Contraindications

Angle-closure glaucoma; concurrent MAO inhibitor therapy; history of melanoma; hypersensitivity to carbidopa, levodopa, or their components; suspicious undiagnosed skin lesions

---

* For levodopa.
† For carbidopa.

Interactions
DRUGS
antihypertensives: Increased risk of symptomatic orthostatic hypotension
benzodiazepines, droperidol, haloperidol, hydantoin anticonvulsants, loxapine, metoclopramide, metyrosine, molindone, papaverine, phenothiazines, rauwolfia alkaloids, thioxanthenes: Decreased effects of carbidopa-levodopa
bromocriptine: Additive effects of carbidopa and levodopa
iron salts: Decreased absorption, blood level, and effectiveness of levodopa
MAO inhibitors: Increased risk of severe orthostatic hypotension
methyldopa: Altered antidyskinetic effects of levodopa, additive CNS toxic effects
pyridoxine: Reversed effects of levodopa
tricyclic antidepressants: Increased risk of adverse reactions to carbidopa-levodopa
FOODS
high-protein food: Possibly delayed or reduced drug absorption

Adverse Reactions
CNS: Anxiety, confusion, depression, headache, insomnia, mood or mental changes, nervousness, neuroleptic malignant syndrome, nightmares, tiredness, uncontrolled movements, weakness
CV: Arrhythmias, orthostatic hypotension
EENT: Blurred vision, darkened saliva, dry mouth, eyelid spasm, ptosis
GI: Anorexia, constipation, diarrhea, nausea, vomiting
GU: Darkened urine, dysuria
MS: Muscle twitching
SKIN: Darkened sweat, flushing

Overdose
An early symptom of overdose is blepharospasm, so monitor patient for increased blinking or spasms of the eyelids. Overdose of carbidopa and levodopa has no specific antidote.

Maintain an open airway, institute ECG monitoring, and assess patient for arrhythmias. Expect to use gastric lavage to decrease drug absorption. Administer I.V. fluids and an antiarrhythmic, as prescribed.

Institute suicide precautionary measures according to facility policy, and anticipate psychiatric re-evaluation.

Nursing Considerations
- Use carbidopa and levodopa cautiously in patients with history of psychoses because drug can cause mental disturbances. Carefully monitor all patients for depression and suicidal tendencies.
- Also, use carbidopa and levodopa cautiously in patients with bronchial asthma; endocrine, hepatic, or renal disease; history of MI and residual atrial, nodal, or ventricular arrhythmias; history of peptic ulcer; or severe cardiovascular or pulmonary disease. Monitor patient closely, especially when therapy begins and dosage is adjusted.
- **WARNING** Avoid giving carbidopa and levodopa within 2 weeks of an MAO inhibitor because doing so could cause suddenly extremely high blood pressure.
- Assess patient for neuroleptic malignant syndrome during dosage reduction or drug discontinuation, especially if he also receives a neuroleptic drug. This uncommon syndrome is life-threatening and causes altered level of consciousness, autonomic dysfunction, diaphoresis, fever, high or low blood pressure, involuntary movement, muscle rigidity, tachycardia, and tachypnea. If these signs and symptoms occur, notify prescriber immediately.

PATIENT TEACHING
- If patient can't swallow E.R. tablet whole, tell him to break it in half for swallowing but not to crush or chew it.
- If patient takes orally disintegrating form, tell him to gently remove tab from bottle with dry hands, place it on top of his tongue, let it dissolve (which takes seconds), and swallow it with saliva. Explain that no other liquids are needed.
- Remind patient that he may need to take drug for several weeks or months before full effects occur.
- Stress need to take carbidopa and levodopa regularly and in exact dosage prescribed. Altering the dosage may increase the risk of adverse reactions or decrease drug effectiveness.
- Tell patient to notify prescriber if involuntary movements appear or worsen during therapy because dosage may need to be adjusted.
- Inform patient who is switching from regular to E.R. tablets that the onset of effect may be delayed for up to 1 hour after the first morning dose, compared with the effect usually obtained from the regular tablet. If this delay poses a problem, tell patient to notify prescriber.

carbidopa, levodopa, and entacapone
Stalevo

Class and Category
Chemical class: Hydralazine analogue of levodopa (carbidopa),
levorotatory isomer of dihydroxyphenylalanine (levodopa),
catechol-O-methyltransferase (COMT) inhibitor (entacapone)
Therapeutic class: Antidyskinetic
Pregnancy category: C

Indications and Dosages
▶ *To treat idiopathic Parkinson's disease*
TABLETS
Adults. Highly individualized and used only as a substitute for
patients already stabilized on equivalent doses of carbidopa, levodopa, and entacapone. *Maintenance:* Highly individualized. When
less levodopa is needed, strength or frequency of dosage can be
decreased; when more levodopa is needed, dosage frequency can
be increased or next higher strength can be given. *Maximum:*
1 tablet of equivalent strength (12.5 mg carbidopa, 50 mg levodopa, and 200 mg entacapone; 25 mg carbidopa, 100 mg levodopa, and 200 mg entacapone; or 37.5 mg carbidopa, 150 mg
levodopa, and 200 mg entacapone) per dosing interval; 8 tablets
daily.

Mechanism of Action
Carbidopa inhibits peripheral distribution of levodopa, making more levodopa
available in the brain. Entacapone inhibits peripheral catechol-O-methyltransferase (COMT), the major metabolizing enzyme for levodopa. During
levodopa metabolism, COMT produces a levodopa metabolite that reduces
levodopa effectiveness. By inhibiting COMT, entacapone increases blood levels of levodopa, making more available for diffusion into the CNS. Levodopa
is transported to the CNS, where it replenishes depleted dopamine, which is
thought to cause Parkinson's disease, thus helping to improve muscle control
and normalize body movements.

Contraindications
Angle-closure glaucoma; history of melanoma; hypersensitivity to
carbidopa, levodopa, entacapone, or their components; suspicious,
undiagnosed skin lesions; use within 14 days of an MAO inhibitor

Interactions
DRUGS
carbidopa, levodopa, and entacapone
alpha-methyldopa, apomorphine, bitolterol, dobutamine, dopamine, epi-nephrine, isoetharine, isoproterenol, norepinephrine, other COMT metab-olizers: Possibly increased heart rate, arrhythmias, and extreme changes in blood pressure
antihypertensives: Possibly symptomatic orthostatic hypotension
iron salts: Possibly reduced bioavailability of carbidopa, levodopa, and entacapone
MAO inhibitors: Possibly inhibited catecholamine metabolism
selegiline: Possibly severe orthostatic hypotension
tricyclic antidepressants: Possibly hypertension and dyskinesia
levodopa component
dopamine D2-receptor antagonists (such as butyrophenones, isoniazid, phenothiazines, and risperidone): Possible reduced effectiveness of levodopa
metoclopramide: Increased bioavailability but decreased effective-ness of levodopa
papaverine, phenytoin: Possible reversed effects of levodopa in Parkinson's disease
entacapone component
ampicillin, cholestyramine, erythromycin, probenecid, rifampin: Possible interference with biliary excretion of entacapone
FOODS
high-protein food: Possibly delayed or reduced drug absorption

Adverse Reactions
CNS: Activation of latent Horner's syndrome, aggravation of Parkinson's disease symptoms, agitation, anxiety, asthenia, ataxia, bradykinetic episodes, confusion, decreased mental acuity, delu-sions, dementia, depression, disorientation, dizziness, dyskinesia, euphoria, fatigue, gait abnormalities, hallucinations, headache, hyperkinesia, hypokinesia, insomnia, malaise, memory loss, nerv-ousness, neuroleptic malignant syndrome, nightmares, paranoia, paresthesia, peripheral neuropathy, sense of stimulation, somno-lence, syncope, tremor increase, trismus
CV: Arrhythmias; chest pain; edema; hypotension, including or-thostatic; hypertension; MI; palpitations; phlebitis
EENT: Blepharospasm, blurred vision, darkened saliva, dilated pupils, diplopia, dry mouth, excessive salivation, hoarseness, ocu-logyric crisis, taste disturbance, tongue burning

ENDO: Hyperglycemia

GI: Abdominal pain, elevated function test results, anorexia, bruxism, constipation, diarrhea, duodenal ulcer, dysphagia, flatulence, gastritis, GI bleeding, GI pain, hiccups, indigestion, nausea, vomiting

GU: Bacteria, blood, glucose, or protein in urine, darkened urine; elevated BUN and serum creatinine levels; elevated uric acid levels; elevated WBC count in urine; increased libido; urinary frequency, incontinence, or retention; UTI

HEME: Agranulocytosis, decreased hemoglobin and hematocrit, hemolytic and non-hemolytic anemia, leukopenia, positive Coombs' test, thrombocytopenia

MS: Back, leg, and shoulder pain; muscle cramps or twitching; rhabdomyolysis

RESP: Abnormal breathing patterns, dyspnea, upper respiratory tract infection

SKIN: Alopecia, bullous lesions, darkened sweat, diaphoresis, flushing, malignant melanoma, pruritus, purpura, rash, urticaria

Other: Angioedema, hot flashes, hypokalemia, weight gain or loss

Overdose

Carbidopa, levodopa, and entacapone overdose has no specific antidote. Pyridoxine isn't effective in reversing it. Monitor patient for evidence of overdose. An early indication is blepharospasm, or eyelid spasm, caused by levodopa; monitor patient for increased blinking or spasms of the eyelids. Also monitor patient for CNS disturbances, arrhythmias, hypotension, tachycardia, abdominal pain, diarrhea, and psychiatric changes. Be aware that, although rare, rhabdomyolysis and transient renal insufficiency have occurred with levodopa overdose.

Maintain an open airway, institute ECG monitoring, and assess patient for arrhythmias. Expect to perform gastric lavage to decrease drug absorption and administer repeated doses of charcoal over time to hasten the elimination of the drug. Administer I.V. fluids and an antiarrhythmic, as prescribed. Provide symptomatic and supportive care, as prescribed. Be aware that the effectiveness of hemodialysis is unknown.

Institute suicide precautionary measures according to facility policy, and anticipate psychiatric re-evaluation.

Nursing Considerations

• Use drug cautiously in patients with past or current psychosis because drug may cause depression and suicidal tendencies.

- Use cautiously in patients with severe CV or pulmonary disease; biliary obstruction; bronchial asthma; or renal, hepatic, or endocrine disease.
- If patient has chronic open-angle glaucoma, make sure intraocular pressure is well controlled because drug may lead to increased intraocular pressure.
- If patient has a history of MI with residual atrial, nodal, or ventricular arrhythmias, expect to make initial dosage adjustment in a facility with intensive cardiac care.
- Monitor patient closely for adverse CNS effects. Such adverse effects as dyskinesia may occur at lower dosages and more quickly with the use of carbidopa, levodopa, and entacapone tablets than when levodopa is used alone. If dyskinesia occurs, notify prescriber and expect to decrease dosage.
- Closely monitor patient with a history of peptic ulcer because drug may increase risk of GI hemorrhage.
- If drug must be stopped, taper it slowly to prevent high fever or severe rigidity.
- Assess patient for neuroleptic malignant syndrome during dosage reduction or drug discontinuation, especially in a patient who also receives a neuroleptic drug. This uncommon syndrome is life-threatening and causes altered level of consciousness, autonomic dysfunc tion, diaphoresis, fever, high or low blood pressure, involuntary movement, muscle rigidity, tachycardia, and tachypnea. If these occur, notify prescriber immediately.

PATIENT TEACHING

- To provide uniform drug effect, stress importance of taking carbidopa, levodopa, and entacapone at regular intervals according to the prescribed schedule.
- Advise patient to avoid a high-protein diet and iron salts (such as those found in many multivitamin tablets) because protein and iron may delay absorption of the levodopa component of drug and reduce the amount available for the body to use to control the symptoms of Parkinson's disease.
- Alert patient to the possibility of nausea, especially at the beginning of therapy. Tell him that this adverse reaction usually resolves with continued therapy.
- Tell patient to notify prescriber if he's taking any other medication, including OTC and herbal preparations, because of potential drug interactions.

- Inform patient that drug's effect may sometimes appear to wear off at the end of a dosing interval. If this occurs, instruct him to notify his prescriber to see if a dosage adjustment is needed.
- Caution patient that hallucinations may occur; advise him to avoid hazardous activities until drug's CNS effects are known.
- Advise patient to rise slowly after sitting or lying down to avoid a sudden drop in blood pressure.
- Instruct patient to notify prescriber if dyskinesia occurs.
- Tell patient that body fluids such as saliva, urine and sweat may turn a dark color, such as red, brown, or black. Reassure him that this effect is harmless but that fluids may stain clothing.
- Advise female patients of childbearing age to notify prescriber immediately about known or suspected pregnancy because changes to drug therapy may be required.
- Inform diabetic patient that drug may cause false-positive result for urinary ketones using a test tape and a false-negative result for urine glucose using a glucose-oxidase method. Encourage patient to monitor blood glucose levels and seek medical attention if he suspects ketonuria.

chloral hydrate

Aquachloral Supprettes, Novo-Chlorhydrate (CAN), PMS-Chloral Hydrate (CAN)

Class, Category, and Schedule

Chemical class: Chloral derivative
Therapeutic class: Sedative-hypnotic
Pregnancy category: C
Controlled substance schedule: IV

Indications and Dosages

▶ *To prevent or suppress alcohol withdrawal signs and symptoms*
CAPSULES, SYRUP, SUPPOSITORIES
Adults. 250 mg t.i.d. after meals. *Maximum:* 2,000 mg.
▶ *To produce nocturnal sedation*
CAPSULES, SYRUP, SUPPOSITORIES
Adults. 0.5 to 1 g 30 min before bedtime. *Maximum:* 2 g.

Route	Onset	Steady State	Peak	Half-Life	Duration
P.O.	½ to 1 hr	Unknown	Unknown	7 to 10 hr*	4 to 8 hr
P.R.	Unknown	Unknown	Unknown	Unknown	4 to 8 hr

* For trichloroethanol, the principal active metabolite.

Mechanism of Action
Produces CNS depression by an unknown mechanism involving trichloro-ethanol, the drug's active metabolite.

Contraindications
Gastritis; hypersensitivity or idiosyncrasy to chloral hydrate or its components; severe cardiac, hepatic, or renal disease

Interactions
DRUGS
CNS depressants: Increased CNS effects of chloral hydrate
furosemide (I.V.): Increased incidence of adverse reactions when ad-ministered after chloral hydrate
phenytoin: Increased excretion and subsequent decreased effective-ness of phenytoin
warfarin: Transient increase in anticoagulant effect
ACTIVITIES
alcohol use: Increased CNS effects of chloral hydrate

Adverse Reactions
CNS: Ataxia, disorientation, hangover, incoherence, paranoia, somnolence
GI: Gastric irritation, nausea, vomiting
SKIN: Rash, urticaria
Other: Drug dependence

Overdose
Monitor patient for evidence of overdose, including albuminuria, areflexia, arrhythmias, coma, esophagitis, gastric necrosis and per-foration, GI bleeding, hypotension, hypothermia, jaundice, miosis, muscle flaccidity, respiratory depression, and vomiting.

Maintain an open airway, and monitor partient's temperature and circulation. If patient is conscious, expect to perform gastric lavage or induce vomiting. If he's unconscious, anticipate assisting with the insertion of an endotracheal tube and then performing gastric lavage. The inflated cuff of the endotracheal tube will help prevent aspiration of gastric contents into the lungs. Administer activated charcoal to prevent drug absorption, as prescribed. Hemodialysis may enhance elimination of trichloroethanol, the active metabolite of chloral hydrate. Institute suicide precautions according to facility policy, and anticipate psychiatric re-evalua-tion.

Nursing Considerations
• Administer drug with full glass of water or juice to minimize GI distress from chloral hydrate capsules. Dilute syrup in a half-glass of water, ginger ale, or fruit juice.
• **WARNING** If patient has a history of tartrazine sensitivity, monitor him carefully for hypersensitivity reaction.
• Suspect physical or psychological dependence if disontinuation of chloral hydrate therapy produces confusion, hallucinations, nausea, nervousness, restlessness, stomach pain, tremor, unusual excitement, or vomiting.

PATIENT TEACHING
• Teach patient to take capsules with a full glass of water or juice or to mix syrup in a half-glass of water, ginger ale, or fruit juice.
• Advise patient to avoid potentially hazardous activities until he knows how the drug affects him.
• Caution patient that drug may be habit forming. Advise taking it exactly as prescribed and not to stop taking it abruptly because withdrawal signs and symptoms could occur.
• Instruct patient to immediately notify prescriber about unusual stomach pains or tarry stools.

Other Therapeutic Uses
Chloral hydrate is also indicated for the following:
• As adjunct to opioids and analgesics to control postoperative pain
• To produce preoperative sedation
• To provide sedation before dental or medical procedure

chlordiazepoxide and amitriptyline hydrochloride
Limbitrol, Limbitrol DS

Class and Category
Chemical class: Benzodiazepine (chlordiazepoxide), dibenzocyclo-heptadiene derivative (amitriptyline hydrochloride)
Therapeutic class: Antianxiety drug, antidepressant
Pregnancy category: Not rated

Indications and Dosages
▶ *To treat moderate to severe depression with anxiety*
TABLETS (5 MG CHLORDIAZEPOXIDE AND 12.5 MG AMITRIPTYLINE HYDROCHLORIDE)
Adults and adolescents 12 and over. *Initial:* 3 to 4 tablets daily in divided doses.

DOUBLE-STRENGTH TABLETS (10 MG CHLORDIAZEPOXIDE AND 25 MG AMITRIPTYLINE HYDROCHLORIDE)

Adults and adolescents 12 and over. *Initial:* 2 to 4 tablets daily in divided doses. *Maximum:* 6 tabs daily.

Route	Onset	Steady State	Peak	Half-Life	Duration
P.O.	Unknown*; 14 to 21 days[†]	5 to 14 days*; 4 to 10 days[†]	Unknown*; unknown[†]	5 to 30 hr*; 31 to 46 hr[†]	Unknown*; unknown[†]

Mechanism of Action

Act together on the CNS. Chlordiazepoxide may potentiate the effects of gamma aminobutyric acid (GABA) and other inhibitory neurotransmitters by binding to specific benzodiazepine receptors in the limbic and cortical areas of the CNS. Binding to these receptors increases inhibitory effects of GABA and blocks cortical and limbic arousal, which helps control emotional behavior. Amitriptyline, a tricyclic antidepressant, blocks serotonin and norepinephrine reuptake by adrenergic nerves, which raises serotonin and norepinephrine levels at nerve synapses, resulting in mood elevation and reduced depression.

Contraindications

Acute recovery phase after an MI, hypersensitivity to either amitriptyline or chlordiazepoxide, MAO inhibitor therapy within 14 days.

Interactions

DRUGS

CNS depressants: Increased CNS effects

cimetidine, flecainide, other antidepressants, phenothiazines, propafenone, quinidine, selective serotonin reuptake inhibitors: Decreased metabolism of amitriptyline and possibly increased toxicity

guanethidine: Decreased antihypertensive effect

ACTIVITIES

alcohol use: Enhanced CNS depression

Adverse Reactions

CNS: Confusion, dizziness, drowsiness, fatigue, lethargy, restlessness, suicidal thoughts, tremor, unusual dreams, weakness
EENT: Blurred vision, dry mouth, nasal congestion
GI: Anorexia, bloating, constipation, hepatic dysfunction

---

* For chlordiazepoxide.
[†] For amitriptyline.

GU: Impotence
HEME: Granulocytopenia
SKIN: Jaundice

Overdose

Because drug is a combination product, treatment of overdose must address both the chlordiazepoxide and amitriptyline components. Monitor patient for signs and symptoms of overdose, including agitation; arrhythmias; CNS depression; coma; confusion; decreased concentration; drowsiness; ECG changes, especially in the axis or width of the QRS complex; hallucinations; hyperreflexia or hyporeflexia; hyperthermia or hypothermia; hypotension; muscle rigidity; mydriasis; seizures; stupor; and vomiting.

Maintain an open airway, obtain ECG, institute continuous cardiac monitoring, and establish I.V. access. Expect to perform gastric lavage and then to administer activated charcoal, as prescribed. Administer sodium bicarbonate, as prescribed, for serum alkalization, and initiate hyperventilation, as needed, in patient with arrhythmias or QRS widening. Observe patient for signs and symptoms of CNS or respiratory depression, and expect early intubation because his condition may deteriorate rapidly.

Hemoperfusion may be beneficial in patient who has acute refractory cardiac instability; however, dialysis, exchange transfusions, and forced diuresis are generally ineffective. Be aware that the benzodiazepine antagonist flumazenil is contraindicated because of the amitriptyline component (a tricyclic antidepressant) of the drug. Institute suicide precautions according to facility policy, and anticipate psychiatric re-evaluation.

Nursing Considerations

- Expect dosage to be adjusted according to severity of patient's signs and symptoms and his response to drug. The therapeutic goal is to find the smallest dose possible to maintain remission.
- Monitor depressed patient closely for worsened depression and suicide risk, especially when therapy starts and dosage changes.
- Be aware that, in patients with a history of angle-closure glaucoma or urine retention, the drug's atropine-like effects may aggravate these conditions.
- Closely monitor patient with cardiovascular disorder because amitriptyline component may cause arrhythmias, such as prolonged conduction times and sinus tachycardia.
- Assess elderly patients for increased sensitivity to drug's effects, including ataxia, confusion, and oversedation.
- **WARNING** Be aware that chlordiazepoxide may cause birth

defects in developing fetus. Expect drug to be discontinued at least during the first trimester of pregnancy to prevent severe adverse effects on fetal organ development.

- Monitor liver function and CBC test results during long-term therapy.

PATIENT TEACHING

- Advise patient not to change his dosage or stop taking chlordiazepoxide and amitriptyline without consulting his prescriber because withdrawal signs and symptoms may occur.
- Advise patient to take the larger portion of the daily dosage at bedtime.
- Instruct patient to avoid performing hazardous activities because the drug may impair mental alertness.
- Instruct patient to avoid using alcohol or OTC drugs containing alcohol because they enhance the drug's CNS depressant effects.
- Instruct female patient to notify prescriber immediately if pregnant or if planning a pregnancy.

chlordiazepoxide hydrochloride

Apo-Chlordiazepoxide (CAN), Librium, Novo-Poxide (CAN)

Class, Category, and Schedule

Chemical class: Benzodiazepine
Therapeutic class: Antianxiety drug, sedative-hypnotic
Pregnancy category: Not rated
Controlled substance schedule: IV

Indications and Dosages

▶ *To provide short-term management of mild anxiety*
CAPSULES, TABLETS
Adults. 5 to 10 mg t.i.d. or q.i.d.
Children over age 6. 5 mg b.i.d. to q.i.d. increased as needed to 10 mg b.i.d. or t.i.d., or 0.5 mg/kg daily in equally divided doses every 6 to 8 hr.
▶ *To provide short-term management of severe anxiety*
CAPSULES, TABLETS
Adults. 20 to 25 mg t.i.d. or q.i.d.
I.V. OR I.M. INJECTION
Adults. *Initial:* 50 to 100 mg. Then, 25 to 50 mg t.i.d. or q.i.d., p.r.n. *Maximum:* 300 mg daily.
I.M. INJECTION
Children age 12 and over. 0.5 mg/kg daily in equally divided doses every 6 to 8 hr.

▶ *To provide short-term treatment of acute alcohol withdrawal*
CAPSULES, TABLETS, I.V. OR I.M. INJECTION
Adults. *Initial:* 50 to 100 mg, usually given I.V. or I.M. Repeated in 2 to 4 hr followed by individualized oral dosage if needed to control signs and symptoms. *Maximum:* 300 mg daily.
DOSAGE ADJUSTMENT Dosage reduced to 5 mg P.O. b.i.d. to q.i.d. or 25 to 50 mg I.V. or I.M., p.r.n., for elderly or debilitated patients.

Route	Onset	Steady State	Peak	Half-Life	Duration
P.O.	Unknown	5 to 14 days	Unknown	5 to 30 hr	Unknown

Mechanism of Action
May potentiate the effects of gamma-aminobutyric acid (GABA) and other inhibitory neurotransmitters by binding to specific benzodiazepine receptors in the limbic and cortical areas of the CNS. By binding to these receptors, chlordiazepoxide increases GABA's inhibitory effects and blocks cortical and limbic arousal, which helps control emotional behavior. It also helps relieve signs and symptoms of alcohol withdrawal by causing CNS depression.

Contraindications
Hypersensitivity to chlordiazepoxide or its components

Interactions
DRUGS
antacids: Altered rate of chlordiazepoxide absorption
cimetidine, disulfiram, fluoxetine, isoniazid, ketoconazole, metoprolol, oral contraceptives, propoxyphene, propranolol, valproic acid: Increased blood chlordiazepoxide level
CNS depressants: Increased CNS effects
digoxin: Increased blood digoxin level and risk of digitalis toxicity
levodopa: Decreased efficacy of levodopa's antidyskinetic effects
neuromuscular blockers: Potentiated, counteracted, or diminished effects of neuromuscular blockers
phenytoin: Possibly increased phenytoin toxicity
probenecid: Shortened onset of action or prolonged effect of chlordiazepoxide
rifampin: Decreased effect of chlordiazepoxide
theophyllines: Antagonized sedative effects of chlordiazepoxide
ACTIVITIES
alcohol use: Increased CNS effects

Adverse Reactions

CNS: Ataxia, confusion, depression, drowsiness
CV: ECG changes, hypotension, tachycardia
GI: Hepatic dysfunction
HEME: Agranulocytosis
SKIN: Jaundice
Other: Injection site pain, redness, and swelling

Overdose

Monitor patient for signs and symptoms of overdose, including bradycardia, coma, confusion, dyspnea, hyporeflexia, seizures, severe drowsiness, shakiness, slurred speech, staggering, and weakness.

Maintain an open airway, initiate continuous cardiac monitoring, and administer continuous I.V. fluids, as prescribed, to maintain blood pressure and promote diuresis. Institute seizure precautions according to facility protocol. To decrease drug absorption in a conscious patient who isn't at risk for coma or seizures, be prepared to induce vomiting or perform gastric lavage. Expect that oral activated charcoal may also be prescribed.

For an unconscious patient, anticipate assisting with the insertion of an endotracheal tube and then performing gastric lavage. The inflated cuff of the endotracheal tube will help prevent aspiration of gastric contents into the lungs. Anticipate use of a benzodiazepine receptor antagonist such as flumazenil to reverse the sedative effects. Be aware that flumazenil may induce seizures, especially in a patient who has undergone long-term benzodiazepine therapy or one who has also ingested a cyclic antidepressant. If excitation occurs, be aware that a barbiturate shouldn't be used because it may increase excitement and prolong CNS depression. Dialysis is ineffective for treating benzodiazepine overdose. Institute suicide precautions according to facility policy, and anticipate psychiatric re-evaluation.

Nursing Considerations

- Use chlordiazepoxide cautiously in patients with hepatic or renal impairment or porphyria.
- **WARNING** Be aware that prolonged use of even a therapeutic dosage can lead to dependence.
- For I.V. use, reconstitute ampule contents with 5 ml of sterile water for injection or sodium chloride for injection. Agitate gently until completely dissolved. Give slowly over 1 minute.
- For I.M. use, reconstitute only with diluent provided by manufacturer.

- **WARNING** Don't use supplied diluent to prepare drug for I.V. use because air bubbles form on the surface.
- Don't give opalescent or hazy solution.
- Observe patient for signs and symptoms of phlebitis or thrombophlebitis after I.V. administration.
- Monitor liver function test results during therapy.
- If patient is a hyperactive, aggressive child or has a history of psychiatric disorders, monitor him for paradoxical reactions—such as acute rage, excitement, and stimulation—during first 2 weeks of therapy.

PATIENT TEACHING
- Warn patient that drug may cause drowsiness.
- Advise patient to avoid other CNS depressants during therapy.
- Warn patient not to take an antacid with drug.

Other Therapeutic Uses
Chlordiazepoxide hydrochloride is also indicated for the following:
- To provide perioperative relaxation and reduce apprehension and anxiety

chlorpromazine
Largactil (CAN), Thorazine
chlorpromazine hydrochloride
Chlorpromanyl (CAN), Novo-Chlorpromazine (CAN), Thorazine, Thorazine Spansule

Class and Category
Chemical class: Propylamine derivative of phenothiazine
Therapeutic class: Antipsychotic drug, tranquilizer
Pregnancy category: Not rated

Indications and Dosages
▶ *To manage symptoms of psychotic disorders or control manic manifestations of manic-depression in outpatients*
E.R. CAPSULES
Adults. 30 to 300 mg once to three times daily with dosage adjusted as needed. *Maximum:* 1 g daily.
ORAL CONCENTRATE, SYRUP, TABLETS
Adults. 10 mg t.i.d. or q.i.d., or 25 mg b.i.d. or t.i.d. After 1 to 2 days, dosage increased by 20 to 50 mg semiweekly until patient is calm. After 2 wk of calmness, dosage gradually reduced to maintenance level of 200 to 800 mg daily in equally divided doses.

▶ *To control acutely disturbed or manic hospitalized patients*
I.M. INJECTION
Adults. 25 mg. Repeated 25 to 50 mg in 1 hr, if needed. Increased gradually over several days up to 400 mg every 4 to 6 hr for severe cases until behavior is controlled. Then, regimen switched to oral form and outpatient dosage.
▶ *To treat severe behavioral problems in children*
ORAL CONCENTRATE, SYRUP, TABLETS
Children ages 6 months to 12 years. 0.55 mg/kg every 4 to 6 hr, p.r.n.
SUPPOSITORIES
Children ages 6 months to 12 years. 1 mg/kg every 6 to 8 hr, p.r.n.
I.M. INJECTION
Children ages 6 months to 12 years. 0.55 mg/kg every 6 to 8 hr. *Maximum:* 75 mg daily for children ages 5 to 12 years or weighing 50 to 100 lb (23 to 45 kg), except in unmanageable cases; 40 mg daily for children up to age 5 years or weighing up to 50 lb.
DOSAGE ADJUSTMENT Dosage possibly reduced for patients with hepatic dysfunction. Dosage reduced to one-third to one-half the normal adult dosage for elderly or debilitated patients.

Route	Onset	Steady State	Peak	Half-Life	Duration
P.O.	Up to several wk	4 to 7 days	6 wk to 6 mo	Unknown	Unknown

Mechanism of Action
Depresses areas of the brain that control activity and aggression, including the cerebral cortex, hypothalamus, and limbic system, by an unknown mechanism. It may relieve anxiety by causing indirect reduction in arousal and increased filtering of internal stimuli to the reticular activating system in the brain stem.

Incompatibilities
Don't mix chlorpromazine with atropine, solutions that don't have a pH of 4 to 5, or thiopental because a precipitate will form. Don't mix chlorpromazine injection with other drugs in a syringe.

Contraindications
Comatose states; hypersensitivity to chlorpromazine, phenothiazines, or their components; large amounts of CNS depressants

Interactions

DRUGS

amphetamines: Decreased amphetamine effectiveness, decreased antipsychotic effectiveness of chlorpromazine

antacids (aluminum hydroxide or magnesium trisilicate gel): Decreased absorption and effectiveness of chlorpromazine

barbiturates: Decreased blood level and, possibly, effectiveness of chlorpromazine

CNS depressants: Prolonged and intensified CNS depression

metrizamide: Possibly lowered seizure threshold

oral anticoagulants: Decreased anticoagulant effect

phenytoin: Interference with phenytoin metabolism, increased risk of phenytoin toxicity

propranolol: Increased blood levels of both drugs

thiazide diuretics: Possibly increased orthostatic hypotension

ACTIVITIES

alcohol use: Prolonged and intensified CNS depression

Adverse Reactions

CNS: Drowsiness, extrapyramidal signs and and symptoms (such as dystonia, fever, motor restlessness, pseudoparkinsonism, and tardive dyskinesia), neuroleptic malignant syndrome, seizures

CV: ECG changes, such as nonspecific, usually reversible Q- and T-wave changes; orthostatic hypotension; tachycardia

EENT: Blurred vision, dry mouth, nasal congestion, ocular changes (fine particle deposits in lens and cornea) with long-term therapy

ENDO: Gynecomastia, hyperglycemia, hypoglycemia, lactation, moderate breast engorgement

GI: Constipation, ileus, nausea

GU: Amenorrhea, ejaculation disorders, impotence, priapism, urine retention

HEME: Agranulocytosis, aplastic anemia, eosinophilia, hemolytic anemia, leukopenia, pancytopenia, thrombocytopenic purpura

SKIN: Exfoliative dermatitis, jaundice, photosensitivity, tissue necrosis, urticaria

Overdose

Monitor patient for signs and symptoms of overdose, including agitation, areflexia or hyperreflexia, arrhythmias, blurred vision, cardiac arrest, coma, confusion, disorientation, drowsiness, dry mouth, dyspnea, heart failure, hyperpyrexia, hypotension, hypothermia, mydriasis, pulmonary edema, QRS complex changes, respiratory depression, seizures, shock, stupor, tachycardia, ventricular fibrillation, and vomiting.

Maintain an open airway, monitor patient for arrhythmias, and maintain temperature. Institute seizure precautions according to facility protocol. Perform gastric lavage, and administer activated charcoal, as prescribed. Expect to administer saline cathartic if patient ingested E.R. form. Be aware that vomiting should not be induced because of the potential for impaired consciousness or dystonic reactions of the head and neck.

Expect to administer phenytoin to control arrhythmias, and norepinephrine or phenylephrine and I.V. fluids to treat hypotension, as prescribed. Epinephrine shouldn't be used because of risk of paradoxical hypotension. Anticipate digitalizing patient for heart failure, as prescribed. To manage seizures, expect to administer diazepam, followed by phenytoin. Avoid barbiturates because they may potentiate CNS and respiratory depression. Anticipate administering benztropine or diphenhydramine, as prescribed, to manage acute dyskinetic effects. Dialysis is ineffective for treating phenothiazine overdose.

Expect to continue ECG monitoring for at least 5 days, and continue to treat patient who has overdosed on E.R. form for as long as signs and symptoms remain. Be aware that phenothiazine tablets are visible on X-ray. Institute suicide precautions according to facility policy, and anticipate psychiatric re-evaluation.

Nursing Considerations
• Don't open or crush E.R. capsules.
• Use chlorpromazine cautiously in patients (especially children) with chronic respiratory disorders (such as severe asthma or emphysema) or acute respiratory tract infections because drug has CNS depressant effect. Also use cautiously in patients with cardiovascular, hepatic, or renal disease because of increased risk of developing arrhythmias, heart failure, and hypotension.
• Because of chlorpromazine's anticholinergic effects, use it cautiously in patients with glaucoma. Also use it cautiously in those who are exposed to extreme heat or organophosphorus insecticides and those receiving atropine or a related drug.
• Protect concentrate from light. Refrigeration isn't required.
• Dilute concentrate in at least 60 ml of diluent just before giving it. Use a carbonated beverage, coffee, fruit or tomato juice, milk, orange syrup, simple syrup, tea, water, or a semisolid food, such as pudding or soup.
• Protect parenteral solution from light. Solution should be clear

and colorless to pale yellow. Discard markedly discolored solution.

- Don't inject drug by subcutaneous route because it can cause severe tissue necrosis.
- Wear gloves when working with liquid or injectable form because parenteral solution may cause contact dermatitis.
- Give I.M. injection slowly and deep into upper outer quadrant of buttocks, such as in the gluteus maximus. To minimize hypotensive effects, keep patient lying flat, and monitor blood pressure for 30 minutes after injection.
- **WARNING** Stay alert for suppressed cough reflex, which increases the patient's risk of aspirating vomitus.
- If patient has a history of hepatic encephalopathy from cirrhosis, monitor him for increased sensitivity to chlorpromazine's CNS effects.
- **WARNING** If signs and symptoms of neuroleptic malignant syndrome—including altered mental status, autonomic instability, hyperpyrexia, and muscle rigidity—develop, notify prescriber immediately, and expect to discontinue drug and begin intensive medical treatment. If patient resumes antipsychotic drug therapy, monitor him carefully for recurrence.

PATIENT TEACHING

- Instruct patient to swallow E.R. capsules whole and not to crush, break, or chew them.
- Tell patient not to take drug within 2 hours of an antacid. Allow him to take drug with food or a full glass of milk or water.
- If patient takes the suppository form, instruct him to chill the suppository, moisten it with cold water, and insert it well inside the rectum.
- Tell patient to store oral concentrate at room temperature and away from light. Instruct him to measure it with the dropper provided and to dilute it in 4 ounces of fluid just before use.
- Because drug may cause blurred vision, dizziness, and drowsiness(especially during the first few days of therapy), advise the patient to avoid potentially hazardous activities until he knows how the drug affects him.
- Tell patient to avoid alcohol because it may cause additive effects and hypotension.
- Advise patient, especially if elderly, to rise slowly from a supine or seated position to avoid dizziness, fainting, and light-headedness.
- Tell patient to inform physicians and dentists that he's taking chlorpromazine before he undergoes surgery, medical tests, or dental work.

- Explain that drug may reduce the body's response to heat and cold; tell patient to avoid temperature extremes, as in a sauna, hot tub, or very cold or hot shower. Remind patient to dress warmly in cold weather.
- Warn patient not to take OTC drugs for a cold or an allergy; they can increase the risk of heatstroke and other adverse reactions.
- Inform patient that drug increases sensitivity to sunlight; tell him to stay out of the sun as much as possible or to protect his skin from exposure.
- If patient reports dry mouth, suggest sugarless chewing gum, hard candy, and fluids.
- Urge patient to report if he suddenly experiences sore throat or other signs and symptoms of infection.

Other Therapeutic Uses

Chlorpromazine is also indicated for the following:
- To treat nausea and vomiting
- To provide intraoperative control of nausea and vomiting
- To treat intractable hiccups
- To provide preoperative relaxation
- To treat acute intermittent porphyria
- To treat tetanus (usually as adjunct with a barbiturate)

citalopram hydrobromide

Celexa

Class and Category

Chemical class: Racemic, bicyclic phthalate derivative
Therapeutic class: Antidepressant
Pregnancy category: C

Indications and Dosages

▶ *To treat depression*

ORAL SOLUTION, ORALLY DISINTEGRATING TABLETS, TABLETS

Adults. *Initial:* 20 mg daily. Daily dosage increased by 20 mg at weekly intervals, as prescribed. *Usual:* 40 mg daily. *Maximum:* 60 mg daily.

DOSAGE ADJUSTMENT For elderly patients and those with hepatic impairment, maximum dosage is 40 mg daily.

Route	Onset	Steady State	Peak	Half-Life	Duration
P.O.	1 to 4 wk	7 days	Unknown	35 to 37 hr	Unknown

Mechanism of Action

Blocks serotonin reuptake by adrenergic nerves, which normally release this neurotransmitter from their storage sites when activated by a nerve impulse. This blocked reuptake increases serotonin levels at nerve synapses, which may elevate mood and reduce depression.

Contraindications

Hypersensitivity to citalopram or its components, MAO inhibitor therapy within 14 days

Interactions

DRUGS

amitriptyline, bromocriptine, buspirone, clomipramine, dextromethorphan, fluoxetine, fluvoxamine, furazolidone, imipramine, levodopa, lithium, meperidine, naratriptan, nefazodone, paroxetine, pentazocine, phenelzine, procarbazine, selegiline, sertraline, sibutramine, sumatriptan, tramadol, tranylcypromine, trazodone, venlafaxine, zolmitriptan: Possibly enhanced serotonergic effects of citalopram, resulting in agitation, confusion, diaphoresis, diarrhea, fever, hyperreflexia, hypomania, incoordination, myoclonus, shivering, or tremor

aspirin, NSAIDS, warfarin: Increased risk of upper GI bleeding

carbamazepine: Possibly increased clearance of citalopram

cimetidine: Possibly increased blood citalopram level

desipramine, metoprolol: Increased blood levels of these drugs

furazolidone, procarbazine, selegiline: Possibly hyperthermia, myoclonus, rigidity, and extreme agitation progressing to delirium and coma

itraconazole, ketoconazole, macrolide antibiotics, omeprazole: Possibly decreased clearance of citalopram

warfarin: Possibly increased PT

Adverse Reactions

CNS: Agitation, akathisia, anxiety, asthenia, delirium, dizziness, drowsiness, dyskinesia, fatigue, fever, insomnia, myoclonus, neuroleptic malignant syndrome, seizures, serotonin syndrome, suicidal thoughts, tremor

CV: chest pain, prolonged QT interval, thrombosis, ventricular arrhythmias

EENT: Blurred vision, dry mouth, rhinitis, sinusitis

GI: Abdominal pain, anorexia, diarrhea, GI bleeding, hepatic necrosis, indigestion, nausea, pancreatitis, vomiting

GU: Acute renal failure, anorgasmia, decreased libido, dysmenorrhea, ejaculation disorders, impotence, priapism
HEME: Abnormal bleeding, decreased PT, hemolytic anemia, thrombocytopenia
MS: Arthralgia, myalgia, rhabdomyolysis
RESP: Upper respiratory tract infection
SKIN: Diaphoresis, ecchymosis, erythema multiforme
Other: Angioedema, anaphylaxis, weight gain or loss

Overdose

Citalopram overdose has no specific antidote. Monitor patient for signs and symptoms of overdose, including amnesia, coma, confusion, cyanosis, diaphoresis, dizziness, drowsiness, ECG changes, hyperventilation, nausea, QT interval prolongation, rhabdomyolysis, seizures, tachycardia, torsades de pointes, tremor, ventricular arrhythmias, and vomiting.

Maintain an open airway, monitor vital signs, observe for ECG changes, and institute seizure precautions according to facility protocol. Prepare to perform gastric lavage and administer activated charcoal, as prescribed, to decrease drug absorption. Dialysis, exchange transfusions, forced diuresis, and hemoperfusion are ineffective for treating citalopram overdose. Institute suicide precautions according to facility policy, and anticipate psychiatric reevaluation.

Nursing Considerations

- For patients who have difficulty swallowing tablets, drug is available in oral solution or orally disintegrating tablet forms.
- **WARNING** Whenever citalopram dosage is increased, monitor for possible serotonin syndrome, characterized by agitation, confusion, diaphoresis, diarrhea, fever, hyperactive reflexes, poor coordination, restlessness, shaking, shivering, talking or acting with uncontrolled excitement, tremor, and twitching.
- Monitor patient closely for suicidal tendencies, especially a child or an adolescent and especially when therapy starts or dosage changes, because depression may worsen at these times.
- Be aware that effective antidepressant therapy may transform depression into mania in predisposed people. If your patient develops signs and symptoms of mania, notify prescriber immediately, and expect to discontinue drug.
- During initial drug therapy, monitor patient for suicidal ideation, and institute suicide precautions as appropriate, according to facility policy.

- Monitor patient with hepatic disease for increased adverse reactions because drug is extensively metabolized in the liver.
- Monitor elderly patients and those taking a diuretic for signs and symptoms of inappropriate secretion of ADH, including hyponatremia and increased serum and urine osmolarity.
- Monitor patient for changes in mental status because citalopram may impair judgment, thinking, and motor skills. Be prepared to institute safety precautions.
- If drug will be stopped, expect to taper dosage gradually to reduce the risk of serious adverse reactions.

PATIENT TEACHING
- Explain that citalopram's full effects may take up to 4 weeks.
- Caution patient not to stop citalopram abruptly because doing so may lead to serious adverse reactions.
- Advise patient to avoid potentially hazardous activities, such as driving, until he knows how the drug affects him.
- Urge caregivers to monitor patient closely for suicidal tendencies, especially a child or an adolescet and especially when therapy starts or dosage changes.
- Caution against taking OTC aspirin, NSAIDs, or other remedies (including herbal products, such as St. John's wort) while taking citalopram because they may increase the risk of bleeding.

clomipramine hydrochloride
Anafranil

Class and Category
Chemical class: Dibenzazepine derivative
Therapeutic class: Antiobsessional drug
Pregnancy category: C

Indications and Dosages
▶ *To treat obsessive-compulsive disorder*
CAPSULES, TABLETS
Adults. *Initial:* 25 mg daily. Gradually increased to 100 mg daily given in divided doses during first 2 wk and then to maximum of 250 mg daily in divided doses over next few weeks. Total daily dose may be given at bedtime when maximum dose is reached.
Children age 10 and over. *Initial:* 25 mg daily. Gradually increased to 3 mg/kg daily or 100 mg daily, whichever is less, given in divided doses during first 2 wk and then to maximum of 3 mg/kg daily or 200 mg daily, whichever is less. Total daily dose may be given at bedtime when maximum dose is reached.

Route	Onset	Steady State	Peak	Half-Life	Duration
P.O.	14 to 21 days	7 to 14 days	2 to 4 wk	19 to 37 hr	Unknown

Mechanism of Action

May inhibit neuronal reuptake of norepinephrine and serotonin, which may be a factor in normalizing neurotransmission in obsessive-compulsive behavior.

Contraindications

Acute recovery period after an MI, hypersensitivity to clomipramine or its components, MAO inhibitor therapy within 14 days

Interactions

DRUGS

anticholinergics: Increased anticholinergic effects

barbiturates: Decreased blood level and effects of clomipramine, additive CNS depression

bupropion, cimetidine, haloperidol, H$_2$-receptor antagonists, selective serotonin reuptake inhibitors, valproic acid: Increased blood level and therapeutic and adverse effects of clomipramine

carbamazepine: Decreased blood clomipramine level, increased blood carbamazepine level

clonidine: Severely increased blood pressure and risk of hypertensive crisis

CNS depressants: Increased CNS depression

dicumarol: Increased anticoagulant effect

grepafloxacin, quinolones, sparfloxacin: Increased risk of life-threatening arrhythmias

guanethidine: Antagonized antihypertensive effect of guanethidine

levodopa: Delayed absorption and decreased bioavailability of levodopa

MAO inhibitors: Increased risk of seizures, coma, and death

rifamycins: Decreased blood clomipramine level

sympathomimetics: Possibly potentiated cardiovascular effects

thyroid drugs: Increased effects of thyroid drugs and clomipramine

ACTIVITIES

alcohol use: Increased CNS depression

Adverse Reactions

CNS: Anxiety, confusion, depersonalization, depression, dizziness, drowsiness, emotional lability, fatigue, headache, insomnia, panic reaction, paresthesia, somnolence, suicidal thoughts, syncope, tremor, unusual dreams, yawning

CV: Orthostatic hypotension, palpitations, tachycardia

EENT: Blurred vision, dry mouth, epistaxis, pharyngitis, rhinitis, sinusitis, unpleasant taste

GI: Abdominal pain, anorexia, constipation, diarrhea, flatulence, increased appetite, indigestion, nausea, vomiting

GU: Dysmenorrhea, ejaculation failure, impotence, urinary hesitancy, urine retention

RESP: Bronchospasm

SKIN: Abnormal skin odor, acne, dermatitis, dry skin, photosensitivity, rash, urticaria

Other: Weight gain

Overdose

Monitor patient for signs and symptoms of overdose, including agitation, arrhythmias, confusion, disturbed concentration, drowsiness, dyspnea, fever, hallucinations, irregular heartbeat, mydriasis, restlessness, seizures, unusual fatigue and weakness, and vomiting.

Maintain an open airway, institute continuous ECG monitoring and seizure precautions, and closely observe patient's blood pressure, respiratory rate, and temperature. Be prepared to institute supportive measures such as performing gastric lavage to decrease drug absorption. Expect to administer activated charcoal followed by a bowel stimulant to enhance drug elimination. Anticipate that the patient may need possible digitalization to prevent heart failure. Be prepared to treat arrhythmias with lidocaine and sodium bicarbonate, as prescribed. Be aware that the use of I.V. physostigmine isn't routinely recommended, but it may be prescribed for patients in coma with respiratory depression, serious arrhythmias, severe hypertension, or uncontrollable seizures to reverse the anticholinergic effects of the drug.

Be prepared to institute emergency measures, including anticonvulsant therapy and at least 5 days of continuous cardiac monitoring. Tricyclic antidepressants are highly protein bound; therefore, dialysis, exchange transfusions, and forced diuresis are ineffective for treating overdose. Institute suicide precautions according to facility policy, and anticipate psychiatric re-evaluation.

Nursing Considerations

- Be aware that stopping clomipramine abruptly may cause withdrawal signs and symptoms and worsen disorder.
- **WARNING** Don't give drug within 14 days of an MAO in-

hibitor to avoid seizures, coma, or death.
- Monitor children and adolescents closely for suicidal thinking and behavior because clomipramine increases the risk of suicidal ideation in these age groups.

PATIENT TEACHING
- Tell patient not to use alcohol, barbiturates, or other CNS depressants; clomipramine increases their effects.
- Alert parents to watch their child or adolescent closely for abnormal thinking or behavior or an increase in aggression or hostility. If unusual changes occur, stress importance of notifying prescriber.
- Inform male patients about risk of sexual dysfunction while taking drug.
- Caution patient that drug may cause drowsiness, especially during initial dosage adjustment.
- Advise patient not to perform hazardous activities until adverse CNS effects are known.
- Warn patient not to stop taking drug abruptly.
- Instruct patient to take a missed dose as soon as he remembers unless it's almost time for the next scheduled dose, in which case he should skip the missed dose. Warn against doubling the dose.
- Teach patient how to prevent photosensitivity reactions.
- Tell patient to report any difficulty urinating, dizziness, dry mouth, mental changes, and sedation.

clonazepam

Apo-Clonazepam (CAN), Clonapam (CAN), Gen-Clonazepam (CAN), Klonopin, Rivotril (CAN)

Class, Category, and Schedule
Chemical class: Benzodiazepine
Therapeutic class: Anticonvulsant, antipanic drug
Pregnancy category: D
Controlled substance schedule: IV

Indications and Dosages
▶ *To treat Lennox-Gastaut syndrome (type of absence seizure disorder) and akinetic and myoclonic seizures*
TABLETS
Adults and children over age 10. 1.5 mg daily in divided doses t.i.d. Increased by 0.5 to 1 mg every 3 days, if needed, until seizures are controlled. *Maximum:* 20 mg daily.

Children age 10 and under or weighing less than 30 kg (66 lb). 0.01 to 0.03 mg/kg daily in divided doses b.i.d. or t.i.d. Increased by 0.25 to 0.5 mg every 3rd day up to maintenance dosage. *Maintenance:* 0.1 to 0.2 mg/kg daily, preferably in three equal doses, or if unequal, with largest dose given at bedtime.

▶ *To treat panic disorder*
TABLETS
Adults. *Initial:* 0.25 mg b.i.d. Increased, if needed, to 1 mg daily after 3 days. If more than 1 mg daily is required, dosage increased in increments of 0.125 to 0.25 mg b.i.d. every 3 days until panic disorder is controlled or adverse reactions make additional increases undesirable. This maintenance dosage may be given as a single dose at bedtime. *Maximum:* 4 mg daily.

Route	Onset	Steady State	Peak	Half-Life	Duration
P.O.	Unknown	5 to 14 days	Unknown	18 to 50 hr	Unknown

Mechanism of Action
Produces CNS depression by potentiating the effects of gamma-aminobutyric acid (GABA), which is an inhibitory neurotransmitter. Suppresses the spread of seizure activity caused by seizure-producing foci in the cortex, thalamus, and limbic structures.

Contraindications
Acute angle-closure glaucoma, hepatic disease, hypersensitivity to benzodiazepines or their components

Interactions
DRUGS
antianxiety drugs, barbiturates, MAO inhibitors, opioids, phenothiazines, tricyclic antidepressants: Increased CNS depression
ACTIVITIES
alcohol use: Increased CNS depression

Adverse Reactions
CNS: Ataxia, confusion, depression, dizziness, drowsiness, emotional lability, fatigue, headache, memory loss, nervousness, reduced intellectual ability
CV: Palpitations
EENT: Blurred vision, eyelid spasm, increased salivation, loss of taste, pharyngitis, rhinitis, sinusitis
GI: Abdominal pain, anorexia, constipation

GU: Difficult ejaculation, dysmenorrhea, dysuria, enuresis, impotence, nocturia, urine retention, UTI
HEME: Anemia, eosinophilia, leukopenia, thrombocytopenia
MS: Dysarthria, myalgia
RESP: Bronchitis, cough
Other: Allergic reaction

Overdose

Monitor patient for signs and symptoms of overdose, including bradycardia, coma, confusion, dyspnea, hyporeflexia, seizures, severe drowsiness, shakiness, slurred speech, staggering, and weakness.

Maintain an open airway, initiate continuous cardiac monitoring, and administer continuous I.V. fluids, as prescribed, to maintain blood pressure and promote diuresis. Institute seizure precautions according to facility protocol. For a conscious patient who isn't at risk for coma or seizures, be prepared to induce vomiting or perform gastric lavage to decrease drug absorption. Expect that oral activated charcoal may also be prescribed.

For an unconscious patient, anticipate assisting with insertion of an endotracheal tube and then performing gastric lavage. The tube's inflated cuff will help prevent aspiration of gastric contents. Anticipate giving a benzodiaze-pine receptor antagonist such as flumazenil to reverse sedative effects. Be aware that flumazenil may induce seizures, especially in a patient who has been undergoing long-term benzodiazepine therapy or one who has ingested a cyclic antidepressant. If excitation occurs, be aware that a barbiturate shouldn't be used because it may increase excitement and prolong CNS depression. Dialysis is ineffective for treating benzodiazepine overdose. Institute suicide precautions according to facility policy, and anticipate psychiatric re-evaluation.

Nursing Considerations

• Use clonazepam cautiously in elderly patients (who may be more sensitive to CNS effects) and patients with mixed seizure disorder (because drug can increase the risk of generalized tonic-clonic seizures), renal failure, or respiratory disease and difficult secretions (because clonazepam increases salivation).
• Monitor blood drug level, CBC, and liver function test results during long-term or high-dose therapy, as ordered.
• **WARNING** Don't stop drug abruptly; expect to taper dosage gradually to avoid withdrawal effects and seizures.
PATIENT TEACHING
• Instruct patient to take drug exactly as prescribed. Explain that stopping it abruptly can cause seizures and withdrawal effects.

- Advise patient to avoid alcohol and sleep-inducing drugs during therapy. Instruct him to consult prescriber before taking any OTC drugs.
- Urge patient to carry medical identification indicating his seizure disorder and drug therapy.
- Warn patient that drug may cause drowsiness.
- Instruct patient to report if he experiences difficulty urinating, palpitations, persistent drowsiness, seizure activity, severe dizziness, and other disruptive adverse reactions.
- Suggest that parents monitor child's performance in school because clonazepam can cause drowsiness and inattentiveness.

clorazepate dipotassium

Apo-Clorazepate (CAN), Novo-Clopate (CAN), Tranxene (CAN), Tranxene-SD, Tranxene-SD Half Strength

Class, Category, and Schedule

Chemical class: Benzodiazepine
Therapeutic class: Alcohol withdrawal adjunct, antianxiety drug, anticonvulsant
Pregnancy category: Not rated
Controlled substance schedule: IV

Indications and Dosages

▶ *To relieve anxiety signs and symptoms*
CAPSULES, TABLETS
Adults and adolescents. *Initial:* 15 mg at bedtime or 7.5 to 15 mg b.i.d. Dosage adjusted, as needed, to 15 to 60 mg daily in divided doses b.i.d. to q.i.d. *Maximum:* 90 mg daily.
E.R. TABLETS
Adults and adolescents. 11.25 mg daily as substitute for capsules or tablets in patients taking 3.75 mg t.i.d. of those forms; 22.5 mg daily as substitute for capsules or tablets in patients taking 7.5 mg t.i.d. of those forms.

▶ *To relieve signs and symptoms of acute alcohol withdrawal*
CAPSULES, TABLETS
Adults. *Initial:* 30 mg followed by 15 mg b.i.d. to q.i.d. on day 1 of therapy; 15 mg three to six times on day 2; 7.5 to 15 mg t.i.d. on day 3; 7.5 mg b.i.d. to q.i.d. on day 4; and 3.75 mg b.i.d. to q.i.d. thereafter. *Maximum:* 90 mg daily.

▶ *As adjunct to treat partial seizure disorder*
CAPSULES, TABLETS
Adults and adolescents. *Initial:* Up to 7.5 mg t.i.d. Increased, if

needed, by up to 7.5 mg/wk. *Maximum:* 90 mg daily.
Children ages 9 to 12. *Initial:* 7.5 mg b.i.d. Increased, if needed,
by up to 7.5 mg/wk. *Maximum:* 60 mg daily.
E.R. TABLETS
Adults and adolescents. 11.25 mg daily as substitute for capsules or tablets in patients taking 3.75 mg t.i.d. of those forms;
22.5 mg daily as substitute for capsules or tablets in patients taking 7.5 mg t.i.d. of those forms.
DOSAGE ADJUSTMENT Initial dosage reduced to 3.75 to
15 mg daily to treat anxiety in elderly patients.

Route	Onset	Steady State	Peak	Half-Life	Duration
P.O.	Unknown	5 to 14 days	Unknown	40 to 50 hr	Unknown

Mechanism of Action
Potentiates the action of gamma-aminobutyric acid (GABA) and other inhibitory neurotransmitters by binding to specific benzodiazepine receptor
sites in the limbic and cortical areas of the CNS. GABA inhibits excitatory
stimulation, which helps control emotional behavior and suppresses the
spread of seizure activity caused by seizure-producing foci in the cortex,
thalamus, and limbic structures. The drug also helps relieve signs and symptoms of alcohol withdrawal by depressing the CNS.

Contraindications
Angle-closure glaucoma, hypersensitivity to chlorazepate dipotas-
sium or its components

Interactions
DRUGS
*barbiturates, MAO inhibitors, opioids, other antidepressants, phenothi-
azines:* Potentiated effects of clorazepate
*cimetidine, disulfiram, fluoxetine, isoniazid, ketoconazole, metoprolol, oral
contraceptives, propoxyphene, propranolol, valproic acid:* Increased
blood clorazepate level
clozapine: Possibly increased risk of shock
ACTIVITIES
alcohol use: Potentiated effects of clorazepate

Adverse Reactions
CNS: Anxiety, ataxia, confusion, depression, dizziness, drowsiness, fatigue, headache, insomnia, irritability, nervousness, psychosis, slurred speech, tremor

CV: Hypotension
EENT: Blurred vision, diplopia, dry mouth
GI: Anorexia, constipation, diarrhea, elevated liver function test results, nausea, vomiting
GU: Elevated serum BUN and creatinine levels, incontinence, libido changes, menstrual irregularities, urine retention
HEME: Decreased hematocrit
SKIN: Rash
Other: Drug dependence

Overdose

Monitor patient for signs and symptoms of overdose, including bradycardia, coma, confusion, dyspnea, hyporeflexia, seizures, severe drowsiness, shakiness, slurred speech, staggering, and weakness.

Maintain an open airway, institute continuous cardiac monitoring and seizure precautions, and administer continuous I.V. fluids, as prescribed, to maintain blood pressure and promote diuresis. If patient is conscious and isn't at risk for coma or seizures, be prepared to induce vomiting or perform gastric lavage to decrease drug absorption. Expect that oral activated charcoal may also be prescribed.

For an unconscious patient, anticipate assisting with insertion of an endotracheal tube and then performing gastric lavage. The tube's inflated cuff will help prevent aspiration of gastric contents into the lungs. Anticipate giving a benzodiazepine receptor antagonist such as flumazenil to reverse sedative effects. Be aware that flumazenil may induce seizures, especially in a patient who has been undergoing long-term benzodiazepine therapy or has ingested a cyclic antidepressant.

If excitation occurs, be aware that a barbiturate shouldn't be used because it may increase excitement and prolong CNS depression. Dialysis is ineffective for treating benzodiazepine overdose. Institute suicide precautions according to facility policy, and anticipate psychiatric re-evaluation.

Nursing Considerations

- **WARNING** Be aware that prolonged use of even a therapeutic dosage can lead to dependence.
- Monitor liver function test results during therapy.
- **WARNING** Don't stop drug abruptly. Expect to taper dosage gradually to prevent withdrawal symptoms and seizures.

PATIENT TEACHING
- Tell patient to take clorazepate with food if GI distress occurs.

- Advise patient to avoid alcohol and other CNS depressants while taking drug.
- Because drug may cause drowsiness, advise patient to avoid hazardous activities until he knows how the drug affects him.
- Instruct patient to keep tablets in their original container. Advise him to protect drug from heat, light, and moisture because drug is sensitive to these conditions.
- Instruct patient to swallow E.R. tablets whole.

clozapine
Clozaril, Fazaclo

Class and Category
Chemical class: Dibenzodiazepine derivative
Therapeutic class: Antipsychotic drug
Pregnancy category: B

Indications and Dosages
▶ *To treat severe schizophrenia that fails to respond to standard drug treatment; to reduce risk of recurrent suicidal behavior in schizophrenia or schizoaffective disorders*
ORALLY DISINTEGRATING TABLETS, TABLETS
Adults. *Initial:* 12.5 mg once or twice daily. Increased by 25 to 50 mg daily to 300 to 450 mg daily by the end of 2 wk. Subsequent dosage adjustments shouldn't exceed 100 mg once or twice per wk. *Maximum:* 900 mg daily.

Route	Onset	Steady State	Peak	Half-Life	Duration
P.O.	1 to 6 hr	8 to 10 days	Unknown	4 to 12 hr	4 to 12 hr

Mechanism of Action
May produce antipsychotic effects by interfering with dopamine binding to dopamine—especially D_4—receptors in the limbic region of the brain and by antagonizing adrenergic, cholinergic, histaminic, and serotoninergic receptors.

Contraindications
Angle-closure glaucoma, coma, history of clozapine-induced agranulocytosis or severe granulocytopenia, hypersensitivity to clozapine or its components, myeloproliferative disorders, paralytic ileus, severe CNS depression, uncontrolled epilepsy, WBC count below 3,500/mm^3

Interactions
DRUGS

anticholinergics: Potentiated anticholinergic effects
benzodiazepines, psychotropic drugs: Additive hypotensive effects, increased risk of cardiopulmonary collapse
bone marrow depressants: Potentiated myelosuppressive effects
carbamazepine, phenytoin: Decreased blood clozapine level
cimetidine, ciprofloxacin, erythromycin: Increased blood clozapine level
CNS depressants: Increased CNS depression
digoxin, warfarin: Increased serum levels of digoxin and warfarin, displacement of clozapine from its binding site
lithium: Increased risk of confusion, dyskinesia, neuroleptic malignant syndrome, and seizures
selective serotonin reuptake inhibitors: Markedly increased blood clozapine level, increased risk of adverse effects and leukocytosis

ACTIVITIES

alcohol use: Increased CNS depression
caffeine: Increased blood clozapine level

Adverse Reactions
CNS: Agitation, akinesia, anxiety, ataxia, confusion, depression, dizziness, drowsiness, fatigue, fever, headache, hyperkinesia, hypokinesia, insomnia, lethargy, myoclonic jerks, neuroleptic malignant syndrome, nightmares, restlessness, rigidity, sedation, seizures, sleep disturbance, slurred speech, syncope, tardive dyskinesia, tremor, vertigo, weakness
CV: Cardiac arrest, cardiomyopathy, chest pain, deep vein thrombosis, ECG changes, hypertension, hypotension, orthostatic hypotension, tachycardia
EENT: Blurred vision, dry mouth, increased nasal congestion, increased salivation, pharyngitis, tongue numbness or soreness
ENDO: Ketoacidosis, severe hyperglycemia
GI: Abdominal discomfort, anorexia, constipation, diarrhea, elevated liver function test results, heartburn, nausea, vomiting
GU: Abnormal ejaculation, darkened urine, urinary frequency and urgency, urinary incontinence, urine retention
HEME: Agranulocytosis, eosinophilia, leukopenia, neutropenia
MS: Back or leg pain, muscle spasm or weakness, myalgia
RESP: Dyspnea, respiratory arrest
SKIN: Jaundice, rash
Other: Weight gain

Overdose

Clozapine overdose has no specific antidote. Monitor patient for signs and symptoms of overdose, including arrhythmias, coma, drowsiness, excitement, hallucinations, hypotension, increased salivation, nervousness, respiratory depression, restlessness, seizures, and tachycardia.

Maintain an open airway, institute continuous cardiac monitoring and seizure precautions, and monitor vital signs. Expect to induce vomiting or perform gastric lavage. Administer activated charcoal and sorbitol, as prescribed, to decrease drug absorption. Anticipate the use of angiotensin, dihydroergotamine, norepinephrine, or physostigmine to counteract the anticholinergic effects of clozapine. Be aware that epinephrine shouldn't be used to treat hypotension because of the risk of reversed epinephrine effect. Also, procainamide and quinidine shouldn't be used to treat arrhythmias because of the risk of additive anticholinergic effects. Clozapine is highly protein bound, so dialysis, forced diuresis, exchange transfusions, and hemoperfusion are ineffective for treating overdose. Expect to continue cardiac monitoring for several days because clozapine may have delayed effects. Institute suicide precautions according to facility policy, and anticipate psychiatric re-evaluation.

Nursing Considerations

• Use clozapine cautiously in elderly patients with dementia-related psychosis because they're at increased risk for serious or fatal adverse reactions.
• Monitor patients with known cardiovascular disease for hypotension and arrhythmias. Be aware that those who have hepatic or renal dysfunction may have altered drug metabolism or excretion. Expect to adjust dosage more slowly with these patients.
• Be aware that, although rare, clozapine can cause severe or life-threatening adverse reactions, such as agranulocytosis, cardiac or respiratory arrest, deep vein thrombosis, neuroleptic malignant syndrome, and severe hyperglycemia that leads to ketoacidosis in nondiabetic patients. It also rarely may produce seizures and tardive dyskinesia. Monitor patient closely throughout drug therapy, and take safety and infection-control precautions.
• **WARNING** Make sure patient has a baseline WBC count and an absolute neutrophil count (ANC) before starting therapy and then every week for the first 6 months of therapy. If WBC count remains at 3,500/mm^3 or greater and ANC re-

mains at 2,000/mm^3 or greater during the first 6 months of continuous clozapine therapy, expect to monitor WBC count and ANC every 2 weeks for the next 6 months. If counts continue to be stable, expect to monitor WBC count and ANC every 4 weeks thereafter. Be aware that when clozapine is discontinued, WBC count and ANC must be checked weekly for at least 4 weeks from the day the drug was discontinued or until WBC count is 3,500/mm^3 or greater and ANC is 2,000/mm^3 or greater.

• If mild leukopenia (WBC count of 3,000 to 3,500/mm^3) or mild granulocytopenia (ANC of 1,500 to 2,000/mm^3) occurs, expect to monitor patient's WBC count and ANC twice weekly until values return to normal; then resume regular monitoring schedule.

• If moderate leukopenia (WBC count of 2,000 to 3,000/mm^3) or moderate granulocytopenia (ANC of 1,000 to 1,500/mm^3) occurs, expect to withhold clozapine temporarily and begin daily monitoring of patient's WBC count and ANC, as ordered, until improvement occurs. Then follow manufacturer guidelines for resuming drug and revised monitoring schedule.

• If severe leukopenia (WBC count less than 2,000/mm^3) and severe granulocytopenia (ANC less than 1,000/mm^3) occur, expect clozapine to be discontinued permanently, and begin daily monitoring of patient's WBC count and ANC, as ordered, until improvement occurs. Then follow manufacturer guidelines for revised monitoring schedule for length of time recommended.

• If patient develops any degree of leukopenia and granulocytopenia, assess the patient for flulike symptoms or other evidence of infection. Be prepared to provide supportive care, as ordered.

• Monitor temperature. A transient temperature elevation above 100.4° F (38° C) may occur, usually within the first 3 weeks of therapy.

PATIENT TEACHING

• Tell patient that he'll receive only a 1-week supply at a time.

• If patient takes orally disintegrating tablets (Fazaclo), tell him to leave tablet in unopened blister pack until he's ready to take it. Instruct him to remove tablet by peeling foil back, not by pushing tablet through foil, and then to immediately place tablet in mouth and let it dissolve before swallowing. Explain that no water is needed.

• Inform patient that he'll need weekly blood tests to check for blood dyscrasias. Teach him how to recognize their signs and symptoms (including fatigue, fever, sore throat, and weakness) and urge him to report them to his prescriber if they occur.

• Instruct patient to take safety precautions and avoid potentially hazardous activities until he knows how the drug affects him.

• Advise patient to get up slowly from a lying or sitting position to minimize effects of orthostatic hypotension.

• Stress to the patient the importance of notifying prescriber if he stops taking clozapine for more than 2 days. Tell him not to re-start drug on his own because dosage will need to be changed.

• Tell patient to consult prescriber before using alcohol or taking an OTC drug.

• Advise women of childbearing age to notify prescriber as soon as pregnancy occurs or is suspected.

desipramine hydrochloride
Norpramin, Pertofrane (CAN)

Class and Category
Chemical class: Dibenzazepine derivative
Therapeutic class: Antidepressant
Pregnancy category: C

Indications and Dosages
▶ *To treat depression*
TABLETS
Adults. *Initial:* 100 to 200 mg daily as a single dose or in divided doses. Increased gradually to 300 mg daily, if needed. *Maximum:* 300 mg daily.
Adolescents. *Initial:* 25 to 50 mg daily in divided doses. Increased gradually, if needed. *Maximum:* 100 mg daily.
Children ages 6 to 12. *Initial:* 10 to 30 mg daily, or 1 to 5 mg/kg, in divided doses.
DOSAGE ADJUSTMENT Initial dosage decreased to 25 to 50 mg daily in divided doses for elderly patients, then increased gradually, if needed, to maximum of 150 mg daily.

Route	Onset	Steady State	Peak	Half-Life	Duration
P.O.	2 to 3 wk	2 to 11 days	Unknown	12 to 27 hr	Unknown

Mechanism of Action
Blocks serotonin and norepinephrine reuptake by adrenergic nerves, which normally release these neurotransmitters from their storage sites when activated by a nerve impulse. By blocking reuptake, this tricyclic antidepressant increases serotonin and norepinephrine levels at nerve synapses, which may elevate mood and reduce depression.

Contraindications
Acute recovery phase of an MI; hypersensitivity to desipramine, other tricyclic antidepressants, or their components; MAO inhibitor therapy within 14 days

Interactions
DRUGS

activated charcoal: Prevention of desipramine absorption, causing reduced therapeutic effects of desipramine

barbiturates: Decreased blood desipramine level, increased CNS depression

bupropion, haloperidol, H₂-receptor antagonists, valproic acid: Increased blood level and adverse effects of desipramine

carbamazepine: Increased blood carbamazepine level, decreased blood desipramine level

cimetidine: Increased blood desipramine level and anticholinergic effects, including blurred vision, dry mouth, and urine retention

clonidine: Increased risk of hypertensive crisis

dicumarol: Increased anticoagulant effect

grepafloxacin, quinolones, sparfloxacin: Increased risk of arrhythmias, including torsades de pointes

guanethidine: Antagonized antihypertensive effect of guanethidine

levodopa: Delayed levodopa absorption, increased risk of hypotension

MAO inhibitors: Increased risk of life-threatening adverse effects, such as hyperpyretic or hypertensive crisis and severe seizures

phenothiazines: Increased blood desipramine level, possibly inhibited phenothiazine metabolism, increased risk of neuroleptic malignant syndrome

quinidine: Increased blood quinidine level

rifamycins: Decreased desipramine effects

selective serotonin reuptake inhibitors: Increased desipramine effects

sympathomimetics: Possibly arrhythmias, possibly increased or decreased vasopressor effects of sympathomimetics

ACTIVITIES

alcohol use: Possibly increased CNS depression, respiratory depression, hypotension, and effects of alcohol

Adverse Reactions
CNS: Agitation, akathisia, anxiety, ataxia, confusion, CVA, delusions, disorientation, dizziness, drowsiness, exacerbation of psychosis, extrapyramidal reactions, fatigue, headache, hypomania, insomnia, lack of coordination, nervousness, nightmares, paresthesia, peripheral neuropathy, restlessness, seizures, sleep disturbance, suicidal ideation, tremor, weakness

CV: Arrhythmias, including heart block; hypertension; hypotension; palpitations

EENT: Black tongue, blurred vision, dry mouth, mydriasis, stomatitis, taste perversion, tinnitus

ENDO: Breast enlargement and galactorrhea (in women), gynecomastia (in men), hyperglycemia, hypoglycemia, syndrome of inappropriate ADH secretion

GI: Abdominal cramps, anorexia, constipation, diarrhea, elevated liver function test results, elevated pancreatic enzyme levels, epigastric distress, hepatitis, ileus, increased appetite, nausea, vomiting

GU: Acute renal failure, impotence, libido changes, nocturia, painful ejaculation, testicular swelling, urinary frequency and hesitancy, urine retention

HEME: Agranulocytosis, eosinophilia, thrombocytopenia

SKIN: Acne, alopecia, dermatitis, diaphoresis, dry skin, flushing, petechiae, photosensitivity, pruritus, purpura, rash, urticaria

Other: Angioedema, drug fever, weight gain

Overdose

Monitor patient for signs and symptoms of overdose, including agitation, arrhythmias, confusion, disturbed concentration, drowsiness, dyspnea, fever, hallucinations, irregular heartbeat, mydriasis, restlessness, seizures, unusual fatigue, vomiting, and weakness.

Maintain an open airway, institute continuous ECG monitoring (for at least 5 days), and closely observe patient's blood pressure, respiratory rate, and temperature. Be prepared to treat arrhythmias with lidocaine and sodium bicarbonate, as prescribed. Anticipate possible digitalization to prevent heart failure. Institute seizure precautions according to facility protocol, and administer anticonvulsant therapy, as prescribed.

Be prepared to perform gastric lavage to decrease drug absorption. Expect to administer activated charcoal followed by a bowel stimulant to increase drug elimination. Tricyclic antidepressants are highly protein bound, making dialysis, exchange transfusions, and forced diuresis ineffective for treating overdose.

Be aware that I.V. physostigmine isn't routinely recommended, but it may be prescribed for a patient in a coma with respiratory depression, serious arrhythmias, severe hypertension, or uncontrollable seizures to reverse desipramine's anticholinergic effects.

Institute suicide precautions according to facility policy, and anticipate psychiatric re-evaluation.

Nursing Considerations

• Use desipramine with extreme caution in patients with cardiovascular disease, glaucoma, seizure disorder, thyroid disease, or urine retention.

- **WARNING** Expect drug to produce sedation and, possibly, lower seizure threshold. Take safety and seizure precautions, according to facility protocol.
- **WARNING** Monitor children and adolescents closely for suicidal thinking and behavior because desipramine increases the risk of suicidal ideation in these age groups.
- Monitor patient's blood glucose level often.
- Be prepared to obtain a blood sample for leukocyte and differential counts if patient develops a fever during therapy.
- Expect to discontinue drug as soon as possible before elective surgery because of its possible adverse cardiovascular effects.

PATIENT TEACHING

- **WARNING** Alert parents to watch their child or adolescent closely for abnormal thinking or behavior or an increase in aggression or hostility. If unusual changes occur, stress importance of notifying prescriber.
- Advise patient to use sunscreen when outdoors and to avoid sunlamps and tanning beds.
- Instruct patient to notify prescriber immediately if she experiences fainting, a fast and pounding heartbeat, severe agitation or restlessness, or strange behavior or thoughts.
- Caution patient not to stop drug abruptly; doing so may cause dizziness, headache, hyperthermia, irritability, malaise, nausea, sleep disturbances, and vomiting.
- Advise patient not to drink alcoholic beverages because doing so increases risk of adverse CNS reactions.
- Advise patient to avoid potentially hazardous activities until she knows how the drug affects her.
- If patient has diabetes, advise her to frequently monitor her blood glucose level.

desvenlafaxine succinate

Pristiq

Class and Category

Chemical class: Phenylethylamine derivative
Therapeutic class: Antidepressant
Pregnancy category: C

Indications and Dosages

▶ *To treat major depressive disorder*
E.R. TABLETS
Adults. 50 mg once daily.

DOSAGE ADJUSTMENT For patients with end-stage renal disease, dosage decreased to 50 mg every other day.

Route	Onset	Peak	Duration
P.O.	4 to 5 days	Unknown	Unknown

Mechanism of Action

Inhibits neuronal reuptake of serotonin and norepinephrine, raising serotonin and norepinephrine levels at nerve synapses. This action elevates mood and reduces depression.

Contraindications

Hypersensitivity to desvenlafaxine or its components, use of an MAO inhibitor within 14 days

Interactions

DRUGS

amitriptyline, clomipramine, desipramine, doxepin, haloperidol, imipramine, linezolid, lithium, nortriptyline, protriptyline, St. John's wort, tramadol, trazodone, triptans: Possibly serotonin syndrome

aspirin, NSAIDs: Increased risk of bleeding

CYP3A4 inhibitors, such as ketoconazole: Increased plasma desvenlafaxine level

Drugs metabolized by CYP2D6: Possibly increased plasma level of these drugs

Drugs metabolized by CYP3A4: Possibly decreased plasma level of these drugs

MAO inhibitors: Increased risk of hypertension; hyperthermia; mental status changes, including coma and delirium; muscle rigidity; and severe myoclonus

warfarin: Possibly increased PT, partial thromboplastin time, and INR

Adverse Reactions

CNS: Abnormal dreams, anxiety, asthenia, attention disturbance, chills, depression, dizziness, drowsiness, extrapyramidal disorder, fatigue, headache, hypomania, insomnia, irritability, jitters, mania, mood changes, nervousness, paresthesia, seizures, serotonin syndrome, somnolence, suicidal ideation, syncope, tremor

CV: Elevated serum lipid levels, hypertension, palpitations, sinus tachycardia

EENT: Angle-closure glaucoma, blurred vision, dry mouth, epi-

staxis, mydriasis, tinnitus
GI: Anorexia, constipation, diarrhea, nausea, vomiting
GU: Anorgasmia (women), decreased libido, ejaculation disorders, impotence, urinary hesitatancy
HEME: Life-threatening hemorrhages
SKIN: Diaphoresis, ecchymosis, hematoma, petechiae
Other: Hyponatremia, weight loss

Overdose

Monitor patient for signs and symptoms of overdose, including agitation, change in level of consciousness ranging from somnolence to coma, ECG changes (especially prolonged QT interval, bundle branch block, QRS prolongation), liver necrosis, rhabdomyolysis, seizures, serotonin syndrome, tachycardia, and tremor.

Maintain an open airway, and institute continuous ECG monitoring and seizure precautions according to facility protocol.

To decrease drug absorption, be prepared to perform gastric lavage and administer activated charcoal, as prescribed. Hemodialysis is ineffective because desvenlafaxine has a large distribution volume.

Institute suicide precautions according to facility policy, and anticipate psychiatric re-evaluation.

Nursing Considerations

• Use desvenlafaxine cautiously in patients with seizure disorders, mania, or hypomania because drug may worsen these conditions.
• **WARNING** Monitor patient closely for life-threatening serotonin syndrome, which may cause mental status changes such as agitation, hallucinations, and coma; autonomic instability such as tachycardia, labile blood pressure; hyperthemia; neuromuscular changes such as hyperrreflexia and incoordination; and GI problems such as nausea, vomiting and diarrhea.
• Monitor blood pressure often during desvenlafaxine therapy because drug may cause dose-related increase in supine diastolic pressure. Expect to reduce or stop drug, as prescribed, if increase develops.
• If patient takes desvenlafaxine for depression, watch for suicidal tendencies, especially when therapy starts or dosage changes.
• Monitor patient's serum sodium level, as ordered, and watch for evidence of hyponatremia, such as headache, difficulty concentrating, memory impairment, confusion, weakness, and unsteadiness. Report any abnormality immediately to prescriber.

- **WARNING** Avoid stopping desvenlafaxine abruptly because doing so may cause asthenia, dizziness, headache, insomnia, and nervousness.

PATIENT TEACHING
- Instruct patient not to crush or chew E.R. tablets.
- Advise patient to avoid alcohol during desvenlafaxine therapy.
- Caution patient not to stop taking desvenlafaxine abruptly.
- Urge patient to notify prescriber if she becomes pregnant during therapy because she'll need a different antidepressant. Taking desvenlafaxine during the third trimester increases the risk of complications in the infant after birth.
- Advise patient to tell prescriber about other prescribed drugs or OTC products she takes because of the risk of drug interactions.

dexmedetomidine hydrochloride

Precedex

Class and Category

Chemical class: Imidazole derivative
Therapeutic class: Sedative-hypnotic
Pregnancy category: C

Indications and Dosages

▶ *To sedate intubated and mechanically ventilated patients in an ICU setting*

I.V. INFUSION

Adults. *Initial:* 1 mcg/kg as a loading dose infused over 10 min. *Maintenance:* 0.2 to 0.7 mcg/kg/hr, individualized and titrated to desired level of sedation. *Maximum:* 0.7 mcg/kg/hr for up to 24 hr.

DOSAGE ADJUSTMENT Dosage possibly reduced in patients with hepatic or renal impairment and in elderly and debilitated patients.

Route	Onset	Steady State	Peak	Half-Life	Duration
I.V.	Unknown	Unknown	Unknown	2 hr	Unknown

Contraindications

Hypersensitivity to dexmedetomidine or its components

Interactions

DRUGS

anesthetics, hypnotics, opiate agonists, sedatives: Additive therapeutic effects of all drugs

Mechanism of Action

Selectively stimulates alpha$_2$-adrenergic receptors to produce analgesia, relief of anxiety, and sedation, without producing respiratory depression. Alpha$_2$-adrenergic receptors are found in the CNS, vascular smooth muscle, and other organs and tissues, such as the intestine, pancreas, salivary glands, and fat cells. In the CNS, dexmedetomidine activates the presynaptic alpha$_2$-adrenergic receptors, which inhibits the release of norepinephrine, and activates the postsynaptic alpha$_2$-adrenergic receptors. Dexmedetomidine also binds to the alpha$_2$-adrenergic receptors in the spinal cord, which inhibits sympathetic activity, causing a decrease in blood pressure and heart rate, and thus analgesia, relief of anxiety, and sedation.

Adverse Reactions

CNS: Dizziness, light-headedness, syncope, tiredness
CV: Atrial fibrillation, AV block, cardiac arrest, heart block, hypertension, hypotension, sinus bradycardia
GI: Nausea
GU: Oliguria
HEME: Anemia, leukocytosis
RESP: Hypoxia, pleural effusion, pulmonary edema
Other: Pain

Overdose

Monitor patient for signs and symptoms of overdose, including bradycardia, cardiac arrest, first- and second-degree AV block, and hypotension. Expect to decrease or stop infusion and institute supportive measures—such as increasing the flow rate of I.V. fluids, elevating lower extremities, and administering vasopressors—as prescribed. Anticipate the use of atropine or glycopyrrolate, as prescribed, to treat bradycardia.

Nursing Considerations

- Dilute drug by adding 2 ml of dexmedetomidine injection concentrate to 48 ml of sodium chloride for injection to produce a concentration of 4 mcg/ml.
- Administer drug only in ICU setting, and expect to monitor heart rate and blood pressure continuously because drug may cause bradycardia or hypotension.
- Infuse drug slowly through a mechanical infusion pump for proper control of infusion rate. Rapid infusion may result in a loss of alpha$_2$-adrenergic receptor selectivity.
- Monitor patient for transient hypertension during initial loading

dose (first 10 minutes) because drug may cause peripheral vaso-constriction. Expect to decrease infusion rate if this occurs.
- Be aware that drug should only be administered for 24 hours or less.
- Expect to use a reduced dosage in elderly and debilitated patients, who may be more sensitive to the drug's hypotensive and bradycardic effects.
- If dexmedetomidine is administered with an anesthetic, a hypnotic, an opiate agonist, or a sedative, expect to give a reduced dosage of both drugs because of the additive effects.
- If patient has a history of heart block or heart failure, monitor her for bradycardia.
- Be aware that the patient will be rousable, alert, and able to respond when stimulated and then quickly return to a sleeplike state.

PATIENT TEACHING
- Advise patient to notify prescriber of other drugs she's taking, including nonprescription drugs, because they may interact with dexmedetomidine.
- Alert patient that vital signs will be frequently monitored.

dexmethylphenidate hydrochloride
Focalin, Focalin XR

Class, Category, and Schedule
Chemical class: d-threo-enantiomer of methylphenidate
Therapeutic class: CNS stimulant
Pregnancy category: C
Controlled substance schedule: II

Indications and Dosages
▶ *To treat attention deficit hyperactivity disorder (ADHD)*
TABLETS
Adults and children age 6 and over who are new to methylphenidate. 2.5 mg b.i.d. at least 4 hr apart, increased in weekly increments of 2.5 to 5 mg. *Maximum:* 10 mg b.i.d.
Adults and children age 6 and over who are currently taking methylphenidate. One-half of racemic methylphenidate dosage. *Maximum:* 10 mg b.i.d. at least 4 hr apart.
DOSAGE ADJUSTMENT Drug stopped if no improvement within 1 month after appropriate dosage adjustments. Dosage decreased or drug stopped for paradoxical aggravation of symptoms or adverse reactions.

E.R. CAPSULES, E.R. TABLETS
Adults who are new to methylphenidate. 10 mg daily, increased after 1 wk as needed to 20 mg daily.
Children age 6 and over who are new to methylphenidate.
5 mg daily, increased as needed in weekly intervals by 5-mg increments. *Maximum:* 20 mg daily.
Adults and children age 6 and over who are currently taking methylphenidate. One-half of racemic methylphenidate dosage. *Maximum:* 20 mg daily.

Mechanism of Action
May block the reuptake of norepinephrine and dopamine into presynaptic neurons in the cerebral cortex, which increases the availability of norepinephrine and dopamine in the extraneuronal space.

Contraindications
Diagnosis or family history of Tourette's syndrome; glaucoma; hypersensitivity to dexmethylphenidate, methylphenidate, or their components; marked anxiety, tension, and agitation; motor tics; pre-existing structural cardiac abnormalities; use within 14 days of MAO inhibitor therapy

Interactions
DRUGS
anticoagulants (oral), anticonvulsants, antidepressants (tricyclic and selective serotonin reuptake inhibitors): Possibly decreased metabolism of these drugs
antihypertensives: Decreased therapeutic effect of these drugs
dopamine and other vasopressors: Increased therapeutic effect of these drugs
MAO inhibitors: Increased adverse effects and risk of hypertensive crisis

Adverse Reactions
CNS: Cerebral arteritis or occlusion, dizziness, drowsiness, dyskinesia, fever, headache, insomnia, motor or vocal tics, nervousness, seizures, Tourette's syndrome, toxic psychosis
CV: Angina, arrhythmias, hypertension, hypotension, increased or decreased pulse rate, palpitations, tachycardia
EENT: Accommodation abnormality, blurred vision
GI: Abdominal pain, anorexia, nausea
HEME: Thrombocytopenic purpura

MS: Arthralgia
SKIN: Erythema multiforme, exfoliative
dermatitis, necrotizing vasculitis, rash, urticaria
Other: Weight loss with prolonged dexmethylphenidate therapy

Overdose

Dexmethylphenidate overdose has no specific antidote. Monitor patient for evidence of overdose, including agitation, cardiac arrhythmias, seizures followed by coma, confusion, diaphoresis, delirium, dry mouth, euphoria, flushing, hallucinations, headache, hyperpyrexia, hyperreflexia, hypertension, muscle twitching, mydriasis, palpitations, tachycardia, tremor, and vomiting.

Maintain an open airway, and provide supportive and symptomatic care to ensure adequate circulatory function. Institute seizure precautions according to facility policy. Plan to treat hyperpyrexia with cooling blankets, as prescribed. If overdose is severe, expect to administer a short-acting barbiturate to manage the signs and symptoms of overdose and then perform gastric lavage. After the lavage, expect to administer oral activated charcoal and then a laxative to decrease drug absorption. The effectiveness of dialysis for dexmethylphenidate overdose is unknown.

Institute suicide precautions according to facility policy, and anticipate psychiatric re-evaluation.

Nursing Considerations

• **WARNING** Be aware that dexmethylphenidate may induce CNS stimulation and psychosis and may worsen behavior and thought disorders. Use drug cautiously in children who have psychosis. Keep in mind that, when signs and symptoms of ADHD occur with acute stress reactions or with pre-existing structural cardiac abnormalities, treatment with dexmethylphenidate usually isn't indicated because it may worsen the reaction or lead to sudden death. Also be aware that withdrawal symptoms may occur with long-term use.
• Monitor pulse rate and blood pressure in patients with hypertension, even mild hypertension, because drug may increase blood pressure and cause arrhythmias, including tachycardia. Report abnormal findings, including exertional chest pain, unexplained syncope or other symptoms of cardiac disease.
• Be aware that dexmethylphenidate shouldn't be used to treat severe depression or to prevent or treat normal fatigue.
• **WARNING** Monitor patient for signs of physical or psychological dependence. Use drug cautiously in patients with a history of drug abuse, including alcoholism.

- Monitor CBC and differential and platelet counts, as ordered, during prolonged therapy.
- Expect to stop drug if seizures occur. Drug may lower seizure threshold, especially in patients with a history of seizures or EEG abnormalities.
- Monitor children on long-term therapy for signs of growth suppression, which has occurred during long-term use of stimulants.
- Note that dosages of drugs affected by dexmethylphenidate, such as anticoagulants and antihypertensives, may need adjustment.
- Assess patient with a history of motor or vocal tics or psychological disorders for worsening of these conditions during dexmethylphenidate therapy.
- Monitor children and adolescents for first-time manifestation of psychotic or manic symptoms. If present, notify prescriber and expect drug to be discontinued.

PATIENT TEACHING
- Tell patient that extended-release capsules should either be taken whole, without being chewed, crushed, or divided, or capsule contents should be sprinkled on a small amount of applesauce.
- Stress importance of taking drug exactly as prescribed because misuse of this drug may cause serious adverse cardiovascular reactions, including sudden death.
- Encourage patient to notify her prescriber if she experiences excessive nervousness, fever, insomnia, nausea, palpitations, or rash while undergoing dexmethylphenidate therapy.
- Caution patient with seizure disorder that drug may cause seizures.
- Advise patient to protect drug from light and moisture.
- Teach patient (or parent) to watch for improvement in signs and symptoms of ADHD, such as decreased impulsiveness and increased attention. Stress the need for continued follow-up care, and suggest participation in an ADHD program.

dextroamphetamine sulfate
Dexedrine, Dexedrine Spansule, Dextrostat, Liquadd

Class, Category, and Schedule
Chemical class: Phenylisopropylamine
Therapeutic class: CNS stimulant
Pregnancy category: C
Controlled substance schedule: II

Indications and Dosages

▶ *To treat attention deficit hyperactivity disorder (ADHD)*
E.R. CAPSULES, ORAL SOLUTION, TABLETS
Children age 6 and over. 5 mg once or twice daily; then increased by 5 mg daily at 1-wk intervals until desired response occurs. *Maximum:* 40 mg daily.
Children ages 3 to 6. 2.5 mg daily; then increased by 2.5 mg daily at 1-wk intervals until desired response occurs. *Maximum:* 40 mg daily.
▶ *To treat narcolepsy*
E.R. CAPSULES, TABLETS
Adults and children age 12 and over. *Initial:* 10 mg daily; then increased by 10 mg daily at 1-wk intervals until desired response occurs. *Maximum:* 60 mg daily for adults.
Children ages 6 to 12. *Initial:* 5 mg daily; then increased by 5 mg daily at 1-wk intervals until desired response occurs. *Maximum:* 40 mg daily.

Route	Onset	Steady State	Peak	Half-Life	Duration
P.O.	Unknown	Unknown	Unknown	10 to 12 hr*	Unknown

Mechanism of Action

May produce CNS stimulant effects by facilitating the release and blocking the reuptake of norepinephrine at the adrenergic nerve terminals and by directly stimulating alpha and beta receptors in the peripheral nervous system. Dextroamphetamine also causes the release and blocks the reuptake of dopamine in limbic regions of the brain. The drug's main action appears to be in the cerebral cortex and, possibly, the reticular activating system. Drug also may stimulate inhibitory autoreceptors in the brain. These actions cause decreased motor restlessness, increased mental alertness, and diminished drowsiness and fatigue. The peripheral actions include increased blood pressure and mild bronchodilation and respiratory stimulation.

Contraindications

Advanced arteriosclerosis, agitation, glaucoma, history of drug abuse, hypersensitivity to dextroamphetamine or its components, hyperthyroidism, MAO inhibitor therapy within 14 days, moderate to severe hypertension, structural cardiac abnormalities, symptomatic cardiovascular disease

* For adults. Half-life is 6 to 8 hr for children.

Interactions
DRUGS
anesthetics (inhaled): Increased risk of severe ventricular arrhythmias
antacids (calcium- and magnesium-containing), carbonic anhydrase inhibitors, citrates, sodium bicarbonate: Increased effects of dextroamphetamine
antihypertensives, diuretics used as antihypertensives: Possibly decreased hypotensive effects
ascorbic acid: Decreased absorption and effects of dextroamphetamine
beta blockers: Increased risk of hypertension or excessive bradycardia, possibly heart block
CNS stimulants: Additive CNS stimulation
digoxin, levodopa: Possibly arrhythmias
ethosuximide, phenobarbital, phenytoin: Delayed intestinal absorption of these drugs
glutamic acid hydrochloride, urinary acidifiers (including ammonium chloride, sodium acid phosphate): Increased excretion of dextroamphetamine, leading to decreased blood dextroamphetamine level and effects
haloperidol, loxapine, molindone, phenothiazines, pimozide, thioxanthenes: Reduced antipsychotic effectiveness of these drugs; inhibited CNS stimulant effects of dextroamphetamine
MAO inhibitors: Potentiated effects of dextroamphetamine; possibly hypertensive crisis
meperidine: Increased analgesia
metrizamide: Increased risk of seizures
norepinephrine: Possibly increased adrenergic effect of norepinephrine
propoxyphene: Increased CNS stimulation effects; risk of fatal convulsions
sympathomimetics: Increased cardiovascular effects of both drugs
thyroid hormones: Enhanced effects of both drugs
tricyclic antidepressants: Possibly increased cardiovascular effects
FOODS
acidic juices: Decreased absorption and effects of dextroamphetamine

Adverse Reactions
CNS: Agitation, anxiety, CVA, depression, dizziness, drowsiness, emotional lability, fatigue, fever, headache, insomnia, irritability, light-headedness, mania, motor tics, nervousness, psychoses, seizures, tremor

CV: Arrhythmias, hypertension, MI, sudden death, tachycardia
EENT: Accommodation abnormality, blurred vision, dry mouth, taste perversion
GI: Abdominal pain, anorexia, constipation, diarrhea, nausea, vomiting
GU: Decreased libido
RESP: Dyspnea
SKIN: Diaphoresis
Other: Weight loss

Overdose

Dextroamphetamine overdose has no specific antidote. Monitor patient for signs and symptoms of overdose, including abdominal cramps, arrhythmias, chest pain, confusion, delirium, diaphoresis, diarrhea, dizziness, dyspnea, flushing, hallucinations, hyperpyrexia, hypertension or hypotension, irregular heartbeat, nausea, pallor, palpitations, panic reaction, paranoia, photosensitive mydriasis, polypnea, psychotic reactions, rhabdomyolysis, shock, syncope, tachypnea, toxic psychosis, tremor, unusual fatigue, vomiting, and weakness. Monitor patient for cardiac and respiratory changes. If possible, isolate her to limit external stimuli.

Expect to provide symptomatic and supportive treatment, including maintenance of respiratory and cardiovascular function. Anticipate performing gastric lavage or inducing vomiting to decrease drug absorption. Also anticipate using I.V. fluids to manage hypotension, as needed. Expect to administer drugs and fluids, as prescribed, to enhance diuresis. Be aware that drug treatment to acidify urine may also be prescribed to increase drug excretion, except in patients with hemoglobinemia, myoglobinuria, or rhabdomyolysis because of increased risk of renal failure. Be prepared to administer a barbiturate or chlorpromazine to control CNS stimulation and phentolamine to manage hypertension. If patient ingested the extended-release form of dextroamphetamine, expect to continue treating the signs and symptoms of overdose until they have resolved because the pellets are coated for gradual release.

Institute suicide precautions according to facility policy, and anticipate psychiatric re-evaluation.

Nursing Considerations

- Be aware that extended-release capsules shouldn't be used to start therapy and shouldn't be given when the daily dosage is less than the amount provided in the extended-release form.

• Administer first dose of the regular tablet form when patient awakens and additional doses at 4- to 6-hour intervals.

• Expect to use extended-release capsules when once-a-day dosing is possible and to administer the dose 10 to 14 hours before bedtime to prevent insomnia.

• Keep in mind that, when signs and symptoms of ADHD occur with acute stress reactions or with pre-existing structural cardiac abnormalities, treatment with dextroamphetamines usually isn't indicated because it may worsen the reaction or lead to sudden death.

• Monitor pulse rate and blood pressure in patients who have hypertension, including even mild hypertension, because drug may increase blood pressure and cause arrhythmias, including tachycardia. Report abnormal findings, including exertional chest pain, unexplained syncope or other symptoms suggestive of cardiac disease, to prescriber.

• Monitor children and adolescents for first-time manifestation of psychotic or manic symptoms. If present, notify prescriber and expect drug to be discontinued.

• If the patient is a child, monitor growth and development because drug may adversely affect growth.

• Assess patient for potential drug tolerance, dependence, or drug-seeking behavior. Be alert for signs and symptoms of long-term dextroamphetamine abuse, including hyperactivity, irritability, marked insomnia, personality changes, and severe dermatoses.

• If patient has a history of Tourette's syndrome, motor or vocal tics, or psychological disorders, assess her for worsening of the condition during dextroamphetamine therapy.

• **WARNING** If drug therapy is stopped, assess patient for withdrawal signs and symptoms, such as abdominal pain, depression, nausea, tremor, unusual fatigue, vomiting, and weakness. Anticipate restarting drug therapy and gradually tapering dosage, as prescribed.

PATIENT TEACHING

• Advise patient to take dextroamphetamine with food or after a meal because anorexia may occur.

• Advise patient not to take drug with acidic juice because it may decrease drug's absorption and effects.

• Instruct patient or caregiver that extended-release capsules should be swallowed whole.

• Stress importance of taking drug exactly as prescribed because misuse of this drug may cause serious adverse cardiovascular reactions, including sudden death.

- Urge patient to avoid potentially hazardous activities until she knows how the drug affects her.
- Inform patient of drug's abuse potential and stress importance of not altering dosage unless prescribed.
- Inform parents or caregivers that child may be placed on drug-free weekend and holiday schedule, as prescribed, if signs and symptoms of ADHD are controlled.

diazepam

Apo-Diazepam (CAN), Diastat, Diazepam Intensol, Dizac, Novo-Dipam (CAN), Valium, Vivol (CAN)

Class, Category, and Schedule

Chemical class: Benzodiazepine
Therapeutic class: Anticonvulsant, antianxiety drug, sedative-hypnotic, skeletal muscle relaxant
Pregnancy category: D
Controlled substance schedule: IV

Indications and Dosages

▶ *To relieve anxiety*
ORAL SOLUTION, TABLETS
Adults. 2 to 10 mg b.i.d. to q.i.d.
DOSAGE ADJUSTMENT Dosage reduced to 2 to 2.5 mg once or twice daily and increased gradually as needed and tolerated for elderly or debilitated patients.
Children age 6 months and over. *Initial:* 1 to 2.5 mg t.i.d. or q.i.d. Increased gradually as needed and tolerated.
I.V. OR I.M. INJECTION
Adults. 2 to 5 mg every 3 to 4 hr, p.r.n., for moderate anxiety; 5 to 10 mg every 3 to 4 hr, p.r.n., for severe anxiety.
Children. Individualized dosage. *Maximum:* 0.25 mg/kg given over 3 min and repeated after 15 to 30 min if needed and after another 15 to 30 min if needed.
▶ *To treat signs and symptoms of acute alcohol withdrawal*
ORAL SOLUTION, TABLETS
Adults. 10 mg t.i.d. or q.i.d. during first 24 hr; then 5 mg t.i.d. or q.i.d., if needed.
I.V. OR I.M. INJECTION
Adults. 10 mg and then 5 to 10 mg in 3 to 4 hr, if needed.
▶ *To provide muscle relaxation, sedation*

ORAL SOLUTION, TABLETS

Adults. 2 to 10 mg t.i.d. or q.i.d.

DOSAGE ADJUSTMENT Dosage reduced to 2 to 2.5 mg once or twice daily and increased gradually as needed and tolerated for elderly or debilitated patients.

Children age 6 months and over. *Initial:* 1 to 2.5 mg t.i.d. or q.i.d. Increased gradually as needed and tolerated.

I.V. OR I.M. INJECTION

Adults. 5 to 10 mg and then 5 to 10 mg in 3 to 4 hr, if needed.

DOSAGE ADJUSTMENT Dosage reduced to 2 to 5 mg/dose and increased as needed and tolerated for debilitated patients.

▶ *To treat seizures*

ORAL SOLUTION, TABLETS

Adults. 2 to 10 mg b.i.d. to q.i.d.

DOSAGE ADJUSTMENT Dosage reduced to 2 to 2.5 mg once or twice daily and increased gradually as needed and tolerated for elderly or debilitated patients.

Children age 6 months and over. *Initial:* 1 to 2.5 mg t.i.d. or q.i.d. Increased gradually as needed and tolerated.

▶ *To treat status epilepticus and severe recurrent seizures*

I.V. INJECTION

Adults. 5 to 10 mg repeated every 10 to 15 min, as needed, up to a cumulative dose of 30 mg. Regimen repeated, if needed, in 2 to 4 hr. (Use I.M. route if I.V. access is impossible.)

Children age 5 and over. 1 mg repeated every 2 to 5 min, as needed, up to a cumulative dose of 10 mg. Regimen repeated, if needed, in 2 to 4 hr.

Children ages 1 month to 5 years. 0.2 to 0.5 mg repeated every 2 to 5 min, as needed, up to a cumulative dose of 5 mg. Regimen repeated, if needed, in 2 to 4 hr.

RECTAL GEL

Adults and adolescents. 0.2 mg/kg rounded up to next available unit dose (or rounded down for elderly or debilitated patient). Repeated in 4 to 12 hr, if needed.

Children ages 6 to 12. 0.3 mg/kg rounded up to next available unit dose. Repeated in 4 to 12 hr, if needed.

Children ages 2 to 6. 0.5 mg/kg rounded up to next available unit dose. Repeated in 4 to 12 hr, if needed.

Route	Onset	Steady State	Peak	Half-Life	Duration
P.O.	Unknown	5 to 14 days	Unknown	20 to 80 hr	Unknown
P.R.	Unknown	Unknown	Unknown	46 hr	Unknown

Mechanism of Action

May potentiate the effects of gamma-aminobutyric acid (GABA) and other in-hibitory neurotransmitters by binding to specific benzodiazepine receptors in the limbic and cortical areas of the CNS. GABA inhibits excitatory stimula-tion, which helps control emotional behavior. The limbic system contains a highly dense area of benzodiazepine receptors, which may explain the drug's antianxiety effects. Diazepam suppresses the spread of seizure activity caused by seizure-producing foci in the cortex, thalamus, and limbic structures.

Incompatibilities

Don't mix diazepam emulsion for I.M. injection with glycopyrro-late or morphine or administer emulsion through an infusion set that contains polyvinyl chloride. Don't mix diazepam injection with aqueous solutions.

Contraindications

Acute angle-closure glaucoma, hypersensitivity to diazepam or its components, untreated open-angle glaucoma

Interactions

DRUGS

antacids: Altered rate of diazepam absorption

cimetidine, disulfiram, fluoxetine, fluvoxamine, isoniazid, itraconazole, ketoconazole, metoprolol, oral contraceptives, propoxyphene, propranolol, valproic acid: Decreased diazepam metabolism, increased blood level and risk of adverse effects of diazepam

CNS depressants: Increased CNS depression

digoxin: Increased serum digoxin level and risk of digitalis toxicity

levodopa: Decreased antidyskinetic effect of levodopa

probenecid: Faster onset or more prolonged effects of diazepam

ranitidine: Delayed elimination and increased blood level of di-azepam

rifampin: Decreased blood diazepam level

theophyllines: Antagonized sedative effect of diazepam

ACTIVITIES

alcohol use: Increased CNS depression

Adverse Reactions

CNS: Anterograde amnesia, anxiety, ataxia, confusion, depression, dizziness, drowsiness, fatigue, headache, insomnia, lethargy, light-headedness, sedation, sleepiness, slurred speech, tremor, vertigo

CV: Hypotension, palpitations, tachycardia

EENT: Blurred vision, diplopia, increased salivation
GI: Anorexia, constipation, diarrhea, nausea, vomiting
GU: Libido changes, urinary incontinence, urine retention
RESP: Respiratory depression
SKIN: Dermatitis
Other: Physical and psychological dependence

Overdose

Monitor patient for evidence of overdose including bradycardia, coma, confusion, dyspnea, hyporeflexia, seizures, severe drowsiness, shakiness, slurred speech, staggering, and weakness.

Maintain an open airway, institute continuous cardiac monitoring, and administer continuous I.V. fluids, as prescribed, to maintain blood pressure and promote diuresis. Institute seizure precautions according to facility protocol.

If patient is conscious and not at risk for coma or seizures, be prepared to induce vomiting or perform gastric lavage to decrease drug absorption. Expect that oral activated charcoal may also be prescribed.

If patient is unconscious, anticipate assisting with insertion of an endotracheal tube and then performing gastric lavage. The inflated cuff of the endotracheal tube will help prevent aspiration of gastric contents into the lungs.

Anticipate giving a benzodiazepine receptor antagonist, such as flumazenil, to reverse the sedative effects. Be aware that flumazenil may induce seizures, especially if patient has been undergoing long-term benzodiazepine therapy or has ingested a cyclic antidepressant. If excitation occurs, be aware that a barbiturate shouldn't be used because it may increase excitement and prolong CNS depression. Dialysis is ineffective for treating benzodiazepine overdose.

Institute suicide precautions according to facility policy, and anticipate psychiatric re-evaluation.

Nursing Considerations

* Expect to monitor patients with pulmonary disease because diazepam may cause respiratory depression and increased salivation and bronchial secretions.
* Mix concentrated oral solution (Intensol) with liquid or semi-solid food for administration. Use supplied calibrated dropper for accurate dosing.
* Protect diazepam injection from light. Don't use solution that's more than slightly yellow or that contains precipitate.

- Administer I.M. injection into deltoid muscle for rapid and complete absorption. Administration into other sites may cause slow, erratic absorption.
- Before administering emulsion form, ask if patient is allergic to soybeans because this form contains soybean oil.
- For an infant or a child, administer I.V. injection slowly over 3 minutes in a dose not to exceed 0.25 mg/kg.
- Administer emulsion form within 6 hours of opening ampule because this form contains no preservatives and allows rapid microbial growth. Use polyethylene-lined or glass infusion sets and polyethylene or polypropylene plastic syringes for administration. Don't use a filter with a pore size of less than 5 microns because it may break down the emulsion.
- Don't mix emulsion form with anything other than its emulsion base, otherwise it may become unstable and increase the risk of serious adverse reactions.
- Monitor patient for adverse reactions, especially if she has hypoalbuminemia, which increases the risk of sedation.
- **WARNING** Observe patient for indications of physical and psychological dependence, such as a strong desire or need to continue taking diazepam, a need to increase the dose to maintain drug effects, and post-therapy withdrawal signs and symptoms, such as abdominal cramps, insomnia, irritability, nervousness, and tremor.

PATIENT TEACHING
- Instruct patient not to take more drug than prescribed, more often, or for a longer time. Warn her that physical and psychological dependence can occur, and teach her to recognize the signs and symptoms.
- Advise patient not to take drug to relieve everyday stress.
- Advise patient to avoid potentially hazardous activities until she knows how the drug affects her.
- Advise patient to avoid CNS depressants and alcohol during therapy.
- Instruct patient not to abruptly stop taking drug without prescriber supervision. If patient has a history of seizures, warn her that abrupt withdrawal may trigger them.
- Instruct patient to mix Diazepam Intensol with water, soda, or a similar beverage; applesauce; or pudding just before taking it. Caution her not to save the mixture for later. Also, tell patient to use calibrated dropper that's provided to measure each dose.
- If the rectal form is prescribed, teach patient to administer it.

Other Therapeutic Uses
Diazepam is also indicated for the following:
• To provide preoperative sedation
• To reduce anxiety before cardioversion
• To reduce anxiety before endoscopic procedures
• To treat tetanus

diethylpropion hydrochloride
Tenuate, Tenuate Dospan, Tepanil Ten-Tab

Class, Category, and Schedule
Chemical class: Phenylalkylamine
Therapeutic class: Appetite suppressant
Pregnancy category: B
Controlled substance schedule: IV

Indications and Dosages
▶ *As adjunct to treat exogenous obesity with caloric restriction, exercise, and behavior modification*
E. R. TABLETS
Adults and children age 16 and over. 75 mg daily at mid-morning.
TABLETS
Adults and children age 16 and over. 25 mg t.i.d. 1 hr before meals.

Route	Onset	Steady State	Peak	Half-Life	Duration
P.O.	Unknown	Unknown	Unknown	4 to 6 hr	6 to 8 hr
P.O. (E.R.)	Unknown	Unknown	Unknown	4 to 6 hr	12 hr

Mechanism of Action
Stimulates the release of norepinephrine and dopamine from adrenergic nerve terminals in the lateral hypothalamic feeding center of the cerebral cortex and reticular activating system, which reduces appetite. By stimulating the CNS, other effects may also occur, including reduced gastric acid production and increased metabolism, which may be effective in treating obesity.

Contraindications
Advanced arteriosclerosis; agitation; cerebral ischemia; glaucoma; history of alcohol or drug abuse; hypersensitivity to diethylpropion, other sympathomimetic amines, or their components; hy-

perthyroidism; MAO inhibitor therapy within 14 days; moderate to severe hypertension; symptomatic cardiovascular disease

Interactions
DRUGS

antacids (calcium- and magnesium-containing), carbonic anhydrase inhibitors, citrates, sodium bicarbonate: Increased blood diethylpropion level

amphetamines, other appetite suppressants, selective serotonin reuptake inhibitors: Possibly increased risk of cardiac valve dysfunction

anesthetics (inhaled): Increased risk of arrhythmias

antihypertensives (especially clonidine, guanadrel, guanethidine, methyldopa, rauwolfia alkaloids): Decreased hypotensive effect of these drugs

ascorbic acid: Increased excretion of diethylpropion, causing decreased blood diethylpropion level

CNS stimulants, thyroid hormones: Additive CNS stimulation

insulin, oral antidiabetic drugs: Altered blood glucose level

MAO inhibitors: Potentiated effects of diethylpropion; possibly hypertensive crisis

phenothiazines: Reduced anorexic effect of diethylpropion

tricyclic antidepressants: Possibly potentiated adverse cardiovascular effects

urinary acidifiers (including ammonium chloride, potassium or sodium phosphates): Decreased blood diethylpropion level

vasopressors (especially catecholamines): Possibly potentiated vasopressor effect of these drugs

ACTIVITIES

alcohol use: Increased adverse CNS effects

Adverse Reactions

CNS: Blurred vision, CNS stimulation, depression, dizziness, euphoria, headache, hyperactivity, insomnia, irritability, lightheadedness, nervousness, numbness on one side of the face or body, mania, psychosis, severe headache, syncope, tremor
CV: Chest pain, hypertension, palpitations, peripheral edema
EENT: Dry mouth, taste perversion
GI: Constipation, epigastric pain, nausea, vomiting
GU: Dysuria, impotence, libido changes, polyuria
HEME: Agranulocytosis, leukopenia
RESP: Dyspnea
SKIN: Dermatoses, hives, rash
Other: Diaphoresis, exercise intolerance

Overdose

Diethylpropion overdose has no specific antidote. Monitor patient for signs and symptoms of overdose, including abdominal cramps, arrhythmias, coma, confusion, diarrhea, dyspnea, hallucinations, hostility, hyperreflexia, hyperthermia, labile blood pressure, nausea, panic reaction, restlessness, seizures, shock, tachypnea, tremor, and vomiting. Expect fatigue and depression to follow CNS excitement.

Maintain an open airway, monitor vital signs, and protect patient from self-injury. Be prepared to administer a drug—such as a barbiturate, diazepam, or phenytoin—to control CNS stimulation and seizures. Institute seizure precautions according to facility protocol. Anticipate administering a drug such as lidocaine to control arrhythmias, phentolamine or a nitrate to manage hypertension, and a beta blocker to control tachycardia.

Perform gastric lavage or induce vomiting, and then give activated charcoal, as prescribed, to decrease absorption. Expect to begin drug therapy to promote urine acidification and I.V. fluids, as prescribed, to increase drug excretion. Be aware that the effectiveness of hemodialysis or peritoneal dialysis is unknown.

Institute suicide precautions according to facility policy, and anticipate psychiatric re-evaluation.

Nursing Considerations

- Be aware that drug may cause physical and psychological dependence. Monitor patient for signs and symptoms of drug abuse, which may include hyperactivity, insomnia, personality changes, psychosis, severe dermatoses, and severe irritability.
- Monitor patient for chest pain, dyspnea, exercise intolerance, peripheral edema, and syncope, which may indicate cardiac valve dysfunction or pulmonary hypertension.
- Monitor patients with a history of epilepsy because diethylpropion may increase seizure activity. Follow seizure precautions according to facility protocol.
- Assess patient for evidence of infection and delayed healing because diethylpropion can cause agranulocytosis and leukopenia.
- To overcome night hunger, administer the third dose of the day midevening, as prescribed.
- **WARNING** Expect to taper diethylpropion gradually before discontinuing to prevent withdrawal and increased rebound appetite. Watch for withdrawal signs and symptoms, which may include abdominal cramps, depression, insomnia, nau-

sea, nightmares, severe fever, and tremor. Notify prescriber immediately if signs and symptoms persist or worsen.

PATIENT TEACHING

- Advise patient to notify prescriber immediately of chest pain, dyspnea, exercise intolerance, peripheral edema, or syncope.
- Instruct patient to swallow the extended-release tablets whole and to not break, crush, or chew them.
- Instruct patient to take last dose at least 4 to 6 hours before bedtime to prevent insomnia.
- Instruct patient to take drug exactly as prescribed because of the risk of addiction. Caution patient that tolerance to drug's effects may develop in a few weeks and that long-term drug use may cause psychological or physical dependence. Teach the patient that the drug will be gradually reduced to avoid withdrawal signs and symptoms.
- Explain that changes in eating and activity behaviors are necessary for long-term weight loss. Stress the importance of maintaining a reduced caloric intake and routine exercise program.
- Instruct patient to avoid alcohol because it increases the risk of developing confusion, dizziness, light-headedness, and syncope.
- Advise patient to avoid potentially hazardous activities until she knows how the drug affects her.
- Instruct patient to report evidence of infection, such as sore throat and fever, or delayed healing or unusual bleeding to her prescriber; drug may cause agranulocytosis or leukopenia.
- Urge patient to schedule regular dental checkups because drug may decrease salivary flow, which may increase the risk of gingival disorders. Suggest that patient suck on ice chips or use sugarless candy or gum to prevent dry mouth.
- Caution patient that drug may cause a false-positive result in urine drug screen for amphetamines.
- Advise patient to notify prescriber immediately of known or suspected pregnancy.
- Advise patient against breast-feeding while taking diethylpropion.

dihydroergotamine mesylate

D.H.E. 45, Dihydroergotamine-Sandoz (CAN), Migranal

Class and Category

Chemical class: Semisynthetic ergot alkaloid
Therapeutic class: Antimigraine drug
Pregnancy category: X

Indications and Dosages

▶ *To treat acute migraine*

I.V. INJECTION

Adults. 1 mg, repeated in 1 hr, if needed. *Maximum:* 2 mg/24 hr, 6 mg/wk.

I.M. INJECTION

Adults. 1 mg at first sign of headache, repeated every hr up to 3 mg, if needed. *Maximum:* 3 mg/24 hr, 6 mg/wk.

NASAL SPRAY

Adults. 1 spray (0.5 mg) in each nostril, repeated in 15 min for a total dose of 2 sprays in each nostril or 2 mg. *Maximum:* 3 mg/24 hr, 4 mg/wk.

Route	Onset	Steady State	Peak	Half-Life	Duration
I.V.	In 5 min	Unknown	15 min to 2 hr	15 hr	About 8 hr
I.M.	15 to 30 min	Unknown	15 min to 2 hr	Unknown	3 to 4 hr
Nasal	In 30 min	Unknown	30 to 60 min	About 10 hr	Unknown

Mechanism of Action

Produces intracranial and peripheral vasoconstriction by binding to all known 5-hydroxytryptamine$_1$ (5-HT$_1$) receptors, alpha$_1$- and alpha$_2$-adrenergic receptors, and dopaminergic receptors. Activation of 5-HT$_1$ receptors on intracranial blood vessels probably constricts large intracranial arteries and closes arteriovenous anastomoses to relieve migraine headache. Activation of 5-HT$_1$ receptors on sensory nerves in the trigeminal system also may inhibit the release of proinflammatory neuropeptides.

Peripherally, dihydroergotamine causes vasoconstriction by stimulating alpha-adrenergic receptors. At therapeutic doses, the drug inhibits norepinephrine reuptake, increasing vasoconstriction. Dihydroergotamine constricts veins more than arteries, increasing venous return while decreasing venous stasis and pooling.

Contraindications

Coronary artery disease (including vasospasm); hemiplegic or basilar migraine; hypersensitivity to dihydroergotamine or other ergot alkaloids; hypertension; malnutrition; peripheral vascular disease or previous vascular surgery; pregnancy; sepsis; severe hepatic or renal impairment; severe pruritus; uncontrolled hypertension; use of macrolide antibiotics or protease inhibitors; use within 24 hours of 5-HT$_1$ agonist, ergotamine-containing or ergot-type drug, or methysergide

Interactions

DRUGS

beta blockers: Possibly peripheral vasoconstriction and peripheral ischemia, increased risk of gangrene

macrolides, protease inhibitors: Possibly increased risk of vasospasm, acute ergotism with peripheral ischemia

nitrates: Decreased antianginal effects of nitrates

other ergot drugs, including ergoloid mesylates, ergonovine, methylergonovine, methysergide, and sumatriptan: Increased risk of serious adverse effects from nasal dihydroergotamine

systemic vasoconstrictors: Risk of severe hypertension

ACTIVITIES

smoking: Possibly increased ischemic response to ergot therapy

Adverse Reactions

CNS: Anxiety, confusion, dizziness, fatigue, headache, paresthesia, somnolence, weakness

CV: Bradycardia, chest pain, peripheral vasospasm (calf or heel pain with exertion, cool and cyanotic hands and feet, leg weakness, weak or absent pulses), tachycardia

EENT: Abnormal vision; dry mouth; epistaxis, nasal congestion or rhinitis, and sore nose (nasal spray); miosis; pharyngitis; sinusitis; taste perversion

GI: Diarrhea, nausea, vomiting

MS: Muscle stiffness

SKIN: Localized edema of face, feet, fingers, and lower legs; sensation of heat or warmth; sudden diaphoresis

Overdose

Monitor patient for signs and symptoms of overdose, including diarrhea, dizziness, drowsiness, epigastric pain or bloating, hypertension followed by hypotension, loss of consciousness, hemiparesis, respiratory depression, seizures, severe confusion, shock, tachycardia, vomiting, and weakness.

Maintain an open airway, and be prepared for endotracheal intubation in case patient develops respiratory depression. Monitor vital signs, institute continuous ECG monitoring, and assess capillary refill, peripheral pulses, skin sensation, and warmth. Institute seizure precautions according to facility protocol.

Administer I.V. fluids to increase elimination of dihydroergotamine. Expect to treat seizures with a benzodiazepine, such as diazepam or lorazepam, as prescribed. Monitor patient for hypotension, and be prepared to put patient in Trendelenburg's position and administer I.V. fluids or volume expanders. Be aware that vasopressors may add to the vasoconstricting effects of dihydroergotamine.

After an overdose, signs and symptoms of cerebral ischemia or peripheral ischemia may occur 24 hours later. Assess patient for anxiety; confusion; cyanosis of hands or feet; itching of skin; leg weakness; pain in arms, legs, and lower back; paresthesia; red or violet blisters on the hands and feet; and weak or absent pulses. If patient develops peripheral ischemia, apply warmth, such as with warm blankets, to her extremities, and handle the extremities carefully to prevent tissue damage. If she develops severe coronary ischemia, administer a vasodilator, such as nitroglycerin or nitroprusside, as prescribed. Be aware that low-dose heparin may also be prescribed to treat vasospasm.

Nursing Considerations

• Assess peripheral pulses, skin sensation, warmth, and capillary refill. After giving nasal dihydroergotamine, monitor patient for signs and symptoms of widespread blood vessel constriction and adverse reactions caused by decreased circulation to many body areas.

PATIENT TEACHING

• Instruct patient to use nasal spray when headache pain—not aura—begins.

• Teach her to prime spray pump by squeezing it four times.

• Advise patient to wait 15 minutes between each set of nasal sprays.

• Remind patient to take drug only as needed, not daily.

• Urge patient to lie down in a quiet, dark room after using drug.

• Instruct patient to use more drug if headache returns or worsens but not to exceed maximum prescribed amount or dosing schedule.

• Instruct patient to discard residual nasal spray in an open ampule after 8 hours.

• If patient experiences a headache different from her usual migraines, caution her not to use dihydroergotamine and to notify prescriber.

• Inform patient that nasal form of drug won't relieve pain other than throbbing headaches and to avoid smoking which may cause an ischemic response.

• Advise patient to avoid alcohol, which can cause or worsen headaches, and smoking, which can cause an ischemic response.

- Warn patient about possible dizziness during or after a migraine for which she took dihydroergotamine.

diphenhydramine hydrochloride

Allerdryl (CAN), Banophen, Benadryl, Benadryl Allergy, Diphenhist Captabs, Genahist, Hyrexin, Nytol QuickCaps, Siladryl, Sleep-Eze D Extra Strength, Unisom SleepGels Maximum Strength

Class and Category

Chemical class: Ethanolamine derivative
Therapeutic class: Antidyskinetic, sedative-hypnotic
Pregnancy category: B

Indications and Dosages

▶ *To treat sleep disorders*
CAPSULES, TABLETS
Adults and adolescents. 50 mg 20 to 30 min before bedtime.
▶ *To treat signs and symptoms of Parkinson's disease and drug-induced extrapyramidal reactions in elderly patients who can't tolerate more potent antidyskinetics*
CAPSULES, ELIXIR, TABLETS
Adults. 25 mg t.i.d. increased gradually to 50 mg q.i.d., if needed. *Maximum:* 300 mg daily.
I.V. OR I.M. INJECTION
Adults and adolescents. 10 to 50 mg q.i.d., as needed. *Maximum:* 100 mg/dose, 400 mg daily.

Route	Onset	Steady State	Peak	Half-Life	Duration
P.O.	15 to 60 min	Unknown	1 to 3 hr	1 to 4 hr	6 to 8 hr
I.V.	Immediate	Unknown	1 to 3 hr	1 to 4 hr	6 to 8 hr
I.M.	30 min	Unknown	1 to 3 hr	1 to 4 hr	6 to 8 hr

Mechanism of Action

Parkinsonism is characterized by an imbalance in some of the neurotransmitters in the CNS, such as acetylcholine and dopamine. People who have Parkinson's disease have an excess of acetylcholine, which causes a characteristic tremor. The antidyskinetic effect of diphenhydramine relieves the tremor, possibly by inhibiting the actions of acetylcholine in the CNS, which are mediated by muscarinic receptors. The sedative effect of diphenhydramine occurs because the drug crosses the blood-brain barrier and blocks histamine receptors in the CNS and possibly antagonizes serotonin, acetylcholine, and alpha-adrenergic receptor sites.

Contraindications

Bladder neck obstruction, hypersensitivity to diphenhydramine or its components, lower respiratory tract signs and symptoms (including asthma), MAO inhibitor therapy, angle-closure glaucoma, pyloroduodenal obstruction, stenosing peptic ulcer, symptomatic prostatic hyperplasia

Interactions

DRUGS

apomorphine: Possibly decreased emetic response to apomorphine in treatment of poisoning

barbiturates, other CNS depressants: Possibly increased CNS depression

MAO inhibitors: Increased anticholinergic and CNS depressant effects of diphenhydramine

ACTIVITIES

alcohol use: Possibly increased CNS depression

Adverse Reactions

CNS: Confusion, dizziness, drowsiness
CV: Arrhythmias, palpitations, tachycardia
EENT: Blurred vision, diplopia
GI: Epigastric distress, nausea
HEME: Agranulocytosis, hemolytic anemia, thrombocytopenia
RESP: Thickened bronchial secretions
SKIN: Photosensitivity

Overdose

Diphenhydramine overdose has no specific antidote. Monitor patient for signs and symptoms, including arrhythmias, clumsiness, dyspnea, facial flushing, hallucinations, hypotension, insomnia, seizures, severe drowsiness, and severe dryness of mouth, nose, or throat.

Maintain an open airway, and be prepared to administer oxygen, institute continuous ECG monitoring, and administer I.V. fluids, as prescribed, to maintain blood pressure. Institute seizure precautions according to facility protocol.

Be prepared to induce vomiting with ipecac syrup, as prescribed, taking precautions to prevent aspiration, especially in infants and children. Perform gastric lavage with isotonic or 0.45NS, as prescribed, if patient is unable to vomit. Expect to administer a saline cathartic such as milk of magnesia, as prescribed, to increase drug elimination.

Administer vasopressors, as needed, to treat hypotension;

however, be aware that epinephrine shouldn't be used because it may further lower blood pressure. Stimulants also shouldn't be used because they may cause seizures.

   Institute suicide precautions according to facility policy, and anticipate psychiatric re-evaluation.

Nursing Considerations
- Expect to give parenteral form of diphenhydramine only when oral ingestion isn't possible.
- Keep elixir container tightly closed. Protect elixir and parenteral forms from light.
- Expect to discontinue drug at least 72 hours before skin tests for allergies because drug may inhibit cutaneous histamine response, thus producing false-negative results.

PATIENT TEACHING
- Advise patient to take drug with food to minimize GI distress.
- Because drug may cause drowsiness, advise patient to avoid hazardous activities until she knows how the drug affects her.
- Urge patient to avoid alcohol while taking diphenhydramine.
- Instruct her to use sunscreen to avoid photosensitivity reactions.
- Advise patient to avoid taking other OTC drugs that contain diphenhydramine to prevent additive effects

Other Therapeutic Uses
Diphenhydramine is also indicated for the following:
- To treat hypersensitivity reactions, such as allergic conjunctivitis, perennial and seasonal allergic rhinitis, transfusion reactions, uncomplicated allergic skin eruptions, and vasomotor rhinitis
- To provide antitussive effects
- To prevent motion sickness or treat vertigo

disulfiram
Antabuse

Class and Category
Chemical class: Thiuram derivative
Therapeutic class: Alcohol abuse deterrent
Pregnancy category: Not rated

Indications and Dosages
▶ *As adjunct to maintain sobriety in treatment of chronic alcoholism*
TABLETS
Adults. *Initial:* Up to 500 mg daily for 1 to 2 wk. *Maintenance:* 125 to 500 mg daily. *Maximum:* 500 mg daily.

Route	Onset	Steady State	Peak	Half-Life	Duration
P.O.	In 1 to 2 hr	Unknown	Unknown	Unknown	Up to 14 days

Mechanism of Action

In the liver, alcohol is oxidized by the enzyme alcohol dehydrogenase to acetaldehyde. Acetaldehyde is oxidized to acetate by the enzyme acetaldehyde dehydrogenase, which enters the hepatic circulation, as shown above right. Disulfiram inhibits acetaldehyde dehydrogenase, preventing breakdown of acetaldehyde to acetate. Ingesting even a small amount of alcohol after taking disulfiram raises the blood acetaldehyde level to 5 to 10 times normal, as shown below right, and causes alcohol hypersensitivity. Also, disulfiram's major metabolite, diethyldithiocarbamate, inhibits norepinephrine synthesis and may cause the drug's hypotensive effect. Disulfiram doesn't alter the rate at which alcohol is eliminated.

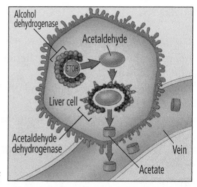

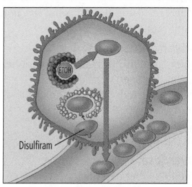

Contraindications

Alcohol intoxication; coronary artery occlusion; hypersensitivity to disulfiram or its components or fungicides, pesticides, or rubber; psychosis; recent use of alcohol, alcohol-containing preparations, metronidazole, or paraldehyde; severe myocardial disease

Interactions

DRUGS

alfentanil: Decreased plasma clearance and prolonged duration of action of alfentanil

amoxicillin-clavulanate, bacampicillin: Possibly disulfiram-alcohol reaction

ascorbic acid: Possibly interference with disulfiram-alcohol reaction
CNS depressants: Possibly increased CNS depressant effects of either drug
isoniazid: Increased risk of additive neurotoxic effect of disulfiram; possibly increased adverse CNS effects
metronidazole: Risk of CNS toxicity, resulting in confusion and psychosis
oral anticoagulants: Possibly increased anticoagulant effects
paraldehyde: Decreased paraldehyde metabolism, increased blood paraldehyde level
phenytoin: Possibly increased blood phenytoin level and risk of phenytoin toxicity
tricyclic antidepressants: Possibly temporary delirium
FOODS
caffeine: Possibly increased cardiovascular and CNS effects of caffeine
ACTIVITIES
alcohol use: Disulfiram-alcohol reaction (if used within 14 days of disulfiram therapy)

Adverse Reactions

CNS: Drowsiness, headache, peripheral neuropathy, psychotic reaction, tiredness
EENT: Blurred vision, garlic or metallic taste, optic atrophy, optic neuritis
GU: Impotence
SKIN: Rash

Overdose

The following describes treatment of a severe disulfiram reaction after alcohol consumption.

Be aware that mild reactions are usually self-limiting and followed by complete recovery, but signs and symptoms may progress to include arrhythmias, heart failure, MI, respiratory depression, seizures, shock, and unconsciousness. The reaction may be fatal, usually if the disulfiram dosage exceeds 500 mg daily and the patient ingested two alcoholic drinks, but deaths have occurred with lower doses and the ingestion of one alcoholic drink.

Maintain an open airway, institute continuous ECG monitoring, and be prepared to administer oxygen or a mixture of 95% oxygen with 5% carbon dioxide. Monitor serum potassium level, especially in patients taking digoxin, and treat hypokalemia, as needed and prescribed. Institute seizure precautions according to facility protocol.

Expect to treat hypotension with I.V. fluids or plasma and to administer ephedrine sulfate, as prescribed. Be aware that a phenothiazine shouldn't be administered because it may worsen hypotension. Anticipate possible use of large amounts of I.V. ascorbic acid (1 g) or antihistamines.

Nursing Considerations

• Know that disulfiram is given only to patients who are highly motivated to stop drinking and who are receiving psychotherapy or substance abuse counseling.

• Be aware that alcohol content of patient's other drugs should be checked before starting therapy.

• **WARNING** Never give drug to patient who is intoxicated; also, never give drug without patient's knowledge.

• If needed, crush tablet and mix with fluids before administration.

• Don't give drug within 14 days of patient's ingestion of a substance that contains alcohol.

• Expect alcohol ingestion during disulfiram therapy to produce a severe reaction that lasts from 30 minutes to several hours. Signs and symptoms may include angina, anxiety, blurred vision, confusion, diaphoresis, dyspnea, heart failure, hypotension, nausea, palpitations, sinus tachycardia, syncope, thirst, throbbing headache, throbbing in neck, vertigo, vomiting, and weakness. A deep sleep usually follows.

• **WARNING** Be aware that ingestion of two or more alcoholic beverages with a disulfiram dose greater than 500 mg daily may cause respiratory depression, arrhythmias, and cardiac arrest.

• If patient takes phenytoin, monitor blood phenytoin level before and during disulfiram therapy, and adjust dosage of either drug as prescribed. Drug interactions may not occur if disulfiram therapy starts before phenytoin therapy. Be aware that a subtherapeutic phenytoin level may result if disulfiram therapy stops.

• If patient takes an oral anticoagulant, monitor PT before and during disulfiram therapy, and adjust anticoagulant dosage as prescribed. Drug interactions may not occur if disulfiram therapy starts before warfarin therapy. If disulfiram therapy stops, be prepared to adjust warfarin dosage to avoid loss of hypoprothrombinemic effects.

• Expect some adverse reactions—such as drowsiness, headache, and impotence—to subside over time or with a brief dosage reduction.

- Because one-fifth of a disulfiram dose may stay in the body for 1 week or longer, know that alcohol ingestion may continue to produce unpleasant signs and symptoms for up to 2 weeks after therapy stops.
- Expect therapy to last months to years, depending on patient's ability to abstain from alcohol.

PATIENT TEACHING

- Teach patient's household and family members about precautions needed and risks associated with disulfiram therapy.
- Inform patient that drug doesn't cure alcoholism but does help deter alcohol consumption.
- If patient reports daytime drowsiness, advise her to take drug in the evening.
- Warn patient to avoid alcohol-containing substances—such as cough syrup, sauces, and vinegar—during therapy because a disulfiram-alcohol reaction may occur after ingesting as little as 15 ml of 100-proof alcohol. Encourage patient to avoid alcohol-containing liniments and lotions as well.
- Teach patient what to expect if a disulfiram-alcohol reaction occurs. Inform her that a deep sleep usually follows the reaction.
- Advise patient that a reaction can occur up to 14 days after therapy stops and that a severe reaction may cause arrhythmias, cardiac arrest, and respiratory depression.
- Instruct patient to carry medical identification that indicates drug, describes possible reactions, and lists someone to notify in case of emergency.

donepezil hydrochloride

Aricept

Class and Category

Chemical class: Piperidine derivative
Therapeutic class: Antidementia drug
Pregnancy category: C

Indications and Dosages

▶ *To treat dementia of the Alzheimer's type*

ORAL SOLUTION, ORALLY DISINTEGRATING TABLETS, TABLETS

Adults. *Initial:* 5 mg at bedtime. After 4 to 6 wk, dosage increased to 10 mg at bedtime, as indicated. *Maximum:* 10 mg daily.

Route	Onset	Steady State	Peak	Half-Life	Duration
P.O.	Unknown	15 days	Unknown	70 hr	Unknown

Mechanism of Action

Reversibly inhibits acetylcholinesterase and improves acetylcholine level at cholinergic synapses. Raising the acetylcholine level in the cerebral cortex may improve cognition. Donepezil becomes less effective as Alzheimer's disease progresses and the number of intact cholinergic neurons declines.

Contraindications

Hypersensitivity to donepezil, piperidine derivatives, or their components

Interactions

DRUGS

anticholinergics: Possibly interference with activity of these drugs
carbamazepine, dexamethasone, phenobarbital, phenytoin, rifampin: Increased donepezil elimination rate
cholinergic agonists, neuromuscular blockers: Possibly synergistic effects of these drugs
ketoconazole, quinidine: Inhibited donepezil metabolism
NSAIDs: Possibly increased gastric acid secretion and increased risk of GI bleeding

Adverse Reactions

CNS: Depression, dizziness, dream disturbances, fatigue, headache, insomnia, seizures, somnolence, syncope
CV: Abnormal ECG, bradycardia, chest pain, edema, heart failure, hypertension, hypotension
GI: Anorexia, constipation, diarrhea, nausea, vomiting
GU: Urinary frequency
MS: Arthralgia, muscle spasms
SKIN: Ecchymosis
Other: Angioedema

Overdose

Monitor patient for evidence of cholinergic crisis, including bradycardia, hypotension, increasing muscle weakness (which may affect respiratory muscles), nausea, respiratory depression, salivation, seizures, sweating, and vomiting. Maintain an open airway, monitor vital signs, and be prepared to assist with artificial respiration, if needed. Use seizure precautions according to facility protocol. Expect to give a tertiary anticholinergic, such as atropine, as an antidote. Expect to give 1 to 2 mg I.V. initially, and adjust additional doses based on patient's response.

Be aware that the effectiveness of hemodialysis, hemoperfusion, or peritoneal dialysis in removing donepezil or its metabolites is unknown. Institute suicide precautions according to facility policy, and anticipate psychiatric re-evaluation.

Nursing Considerations

• Use donepezil cautiously in patients with bladder obstruction because drug's weak peripheral cholinergic effect could obstruct outflow.

• Use drug cautiously in patients with asthma, emphysema, chronic bronchitis, or other pulmonary disorders because drug has a weak affinity for peripheral cholinesterase, which may increase bronchoconstriction and bronchial secretions.

• If patient has cardiac disease, monitor her for bradycardia, which may result from increased vagal tone caused by drug's inhibition of peripheral cholinesterase. Reduced heart rate may be especially significant if patient has bradycardia, sick sinus syndrome, or other supraventricular arrhythmia.

• Take safety precautions if patient experiences dizziness or other adverse CNS reactions.

PATIENT TEACHING

• Advise patient to take donepezil just before going to bed.

• Inform her that drug may be taken with or without food.

• If patient takes orally disintegrating tablets, intruct her to place the tablet on her tongue, let it dissolve, and then drink water.

• Instruct patient to avoid potentially hazardous activities, such as driving, until she knows how the drug affects her. Encourage her to take safety precautions to prevent falling if she experiences adverse reactions, such as dizziness.

• If patient has a history of peptic ulcer disease or gastric irritation, explain that drug may aggravate these conditions by increasing gastric acid secretion.

• Caution patient to avoid NSAIDs during therapy because of risk of GI bleeding. Urge her to notify prescriber immediately if she notices black, tarry stools.

doxepin hydrochloride

Novo-Doxepin (CAN), Sinequan, Triadapin (CAN)

Class and Category

Chemical class: Dibenzoxepin derivative
Therapeutic class: Antidepressant
Pregnancy category: Not rated

Indications and Dosages

▶ *To treat mild to moderate depression or anxiety*
CAPSULES, ORAL SOLUTION
Adults and adolescents. 75 to 150 mg daily at bedtime. *Maximum:* 150 mg daily.
▶ *To treat mild to moderate depression or anxiety with organic disease*
CAPSULES, ORAL SOLUTION
Adults and adolescents. 25 to 50 mg daily.
▶ *To treat severe depression or anxiety*
CAPSULES, ORAL SOLUTION
Adults and adolescents. 50 mg t.i.d., gradually increased to 300 mg daily, as indicated.

Route	Onset	Steady State	Peak	Half-Life	Duration
P.O.	2 to 3 wk	Unknown	Unknown	6 to 8 hr	Unknown

Mechanism of Action

May block serotonin and norepinephrine reuptake by adrenergic nerves. In this way, the tricyclic antidepressant raises serotonin and norepinephrine levels at nerve synapses, which may elevate mood and reduce depression.

Incompatibilities

Don't mix doxepin solution with carbonated beverages or grape juice.

Contraindications

Acute recovery phase of an MI; concurrent use of MAO inhibitor; glaucoma; hypersensitivity to doxepin, other tricyclic antidepressants, or their components; urine retention

Interactions

DRUGS
amantadine, anticholinergics, antidyskinetics, antihistamines: Possibly intensified anticholinergic effects, causing confusion, hallucinations, and nightmares
anticonvulsants: Possibly lowered seizure threshold and decreased effects of these drugs
antithyroid drugs: Possibly increased risk of agranulocytosis
barbiturates, carbamazepine: Increased doxepin metabolism, decreased blood doxepin level, possibly lowered seizure threshold
bupropion, clozapine, cyclobenzaprine, haloperidol, loxapine, maprotiline, molindone, phenothiazines, thioxanthenes: Possibly prolonged and in-

tensified sedative and anticholinergic effects of either drug, possibly increased risk of seizures

cimetidine, flecainide, quinidine, phenothiazines, propaferone, SSRIs, tricyclic antidepressants: Increased blood doxepin level from inhibited systemic clearance, resulting in increased risk of toxicity

clonidine, guanadrel, guanethidine: Increased risk of hypertension, especially during second week of doxepin therapy

CNS depressants: Possibly potentiated CNS depression, hypotension, and respiratory depression

corticosteroids: Possibly worsened depression

direct-acting sympathomimetics, such as epinephrine and norepinephrine: Potentiated effects of these drugs

disulfiram: Possibly transient delirium

fluoxetine: Possibly increased blood doxepin level

MAO inhibitors: Possibly hyperpyrexia, hypertension, seizures, and death

oral anticoagulants: Possibly increased anticoagulant effects of these drugs

pimozide: Increased risk of arrhythmias

probucol: Possibly prolonged QT interval and increased risk of ventricular tachycardia

thyroid hormones: Possibly increased therapeutic and toxic effects of both drugs

tolazamide: Possibly severe hypoglycemia

ACTIVITIES

alcohol use: Possibly enhanced CNS depression, hypotension, and respiratory depression

Adverse Reactions

CNS: Confusion, delirium, dream disturbances, drowsiness, fatigue, hallucinations, headache, nervousness, parkinsonism, restlessness, sedation, seizures, suicidal ideation, tremor
CV: ECG changes, orthostatic hypotension, palpitations
EENT: Blurred vision, dry mouth, taste perversion
GI: Constipation, diarrhea, heartburn, ileus, increased appetite, nausea, vomiting,
GU: Decreased libido, ejaculation disorders
SKIN: Diaphoresis, jaundice
Other: Weight gain

Overdose

Monitor patient for evidence of overdose, including agitation, arrhythmias, confusion, disturbed concentration, drowsiness, dyspnea, fever, hallucinations, irregular heartbeat, mydriasis, restlessness, seizures, unusual fatigue, vomiting, and weakness.

Maintain an open airway, institute continuous ECG monitoring (for at least 5 days), and closely monitor patient's blood pressure, respiratory rate, and temperature. Be prepared to treat arrhythmias with lidocaine and sodium bicarbonate, as prescribed. Anticipate possible digitalization to prevent heart failure. Institute seizure precautions according to facility protocol, and administer an anticonvulsant, as prescribed.

Be prepared to perform gastric lavage to decrease drug absorption. Expect to administer activated charcoal and then a bowel stimulant to enhance drug elimination. Tricyclic antidepressants are highly protein bound, making dialysis, exchange transfusions, and forced diuresis ineffective for treating overdose.

Be aware that I.V. physostigmine isn't routinely recommended, but it may be prescribed for comatose patients with respiratory depression, serious arrhythmias, severe hypertension, or uncontrollable seizures to reverse the anticholinergic effects of doxepin.

Institute suicide precautions according to facility policy, and anticipate psychiatric re-evaluation.

Nursing Considerations
- If desired, mix oral solution in 120 ml of grapefruit, orange, pineapple, or tomato juice; milk; or water.
- Expect to observe adverse reactions within a few hours after giving drug.
- Evaluate patient for therapeutic response: decreased anxiety, apprehension, depression, fear, guilt, somatic signs and symptoms, and worry; increased energy; and more restful sleep.
- Keep in mind that abrupt withdrawal of doxepin after prolonged therapy can cause cholinergic rebound effects, including diarrhea, nausea, and vomiting.
- Plan to discontinue drug, as prescribed, several days before elective surgery to avoid hypertension.
- Monitor patient (particularly a child or an adolescent) closely for suicidal thinking and behavior; drug increases risk of suicidal ideation, especially when therapy starts or dosage changes.
- Monitor elderly patients for signs and symptoms of parkinsonism, especially with high-dose therapy.
- Be alert for seizures. Patients with a seizure disorder may need an increased anticonvulsant dosage to maintain seizure control.
- Know that, for patients with asthma or sulfite sensitivity, doxepin tablets may aggravate asthma or cause allergic reactions because they contain sulfites.

- Monitor diabetic patient's blood glucose level closely; drug may alter glucose metabolism.
- If patient takes a thyroid hormone, be alert for increased responses to both drugs and, possibly, exaggerated drug-induced effects, such as arrhythmias and CNS stimulation. Untreated hypothyroidism prevents adequate response to therapy.

PATIENT TEACHING
- Urge parents to watch their child or adolescent closely for abnormal thinking or behavior or an increase in aggression or hostility. If such changes occur, stress need to notify prescriber.
- Instruct patient to avoid alcohol during doxepin therapy because mental alertness may decrease.
- Advise diabetic patient to measure her blood glucose level more often than usual.

duloxetine hydrochloride
Cymbalta

Class and Category
Chemical class: Selective serotonin and norepinephrine reuptake inhibitor
Therapeutic class: Antidepressant, neuropathic pain reliever
Pregnancy category: C

Indications and Dosages
▶ *To treat major depressive disorder*
E.R. CAPSULES
Adults. 20 mg b.i.d. Or, 60 mg daily or 30 mg b.i.d.
▶ *To relieve neuropathic pain in diabetic peripheral neuropathy*
E.R. CAPSULES
Adults. 60 mg daily.
▶ *To treat generalized anxiety disorder*
E.R. CAPSULES
Adults. *Initial:* 30 to 60 mg once daily, increased in 30-mg increments weekly, as needed. *Maximum:* 120 mg once daily.

Route	Onset	Peak	Duration
P.O.	Unknown	6 hr	Unknown

Contraindications
Hepatic insufficiency, hypersensitivity to duloxetine or its components, uncontrolled angle-closure glaucoma, tryptophan therapy, use within 14 days of an MAO inhibitor

Mechanism of Action

Inhibits neuronal serotonin, norepinephrine, and dopamine reuptake to potentiate serotonergic and noradrenergic activity in the CNS. These activities may elevate mood and inhibit pain signals stemming from peripheral nerves adversely affected by chronically elevated serum glucose levels.

Interactions

DRUGS

amiodarone, celecoxib, cimetidine, erythromycin, fluoxetine, fluvoxamine, haloperidol, ketoconazole, methadone, paroxetine, quinidine, quinolones, ritonavir: Increased blood duloxetine level

amiodarone, amitriptyline, desipramine, flecainide, haloperidol, imipramine, methadone, nortriptyline, phenothiazines, propafenone, ritonavir, thioridazine: Increased blood levels of these drugs

aspirin, NSAIDs, warfarin: Increased risk of bleeding

CNS drugs: Increased effect of duloxetine

MAO inhibitors, serotonergic drugs, triptans: Serious, sometimes fatal, autonomic instability, hyperthermia, myoclonus, rigidity

plasma protein binders (warfarin, phenytoin): Increased free concentration of these drugs and increased risk of adverse reactions

serotonergic drugs: Increased risk of serotonin syndrome

ACTIVITIES

alcohol use: Increased risk of hepatotoxicity

Adverse Reactions

CNS: Anxiety, asthenia, dizziness, fatigue, fever, headache, insomnia, serotonin syndrome, somnolence, suicidal ideation, tremor

CV: Hypertension, palpitations, peripheral edema

EENT: Blurred vision, dry mouth, naso-pharyngitis, pharyngitis

ENDO: Hot flashes

GI: Anorexia, constipation, diarrhea, indigestion, hepatotoxicity, nausea, upper abdominal pain, vomiting

GU: Abnormal orgasm, decreased libido, erectile or ejaculatory dysfunction, urinary frequency

HEME: Abnormal bleeding events, leukopenia, thrombocytopenia

MS: Arthralgia, back pain, extremity pain, muscle cramp, myalgia

RESP: Cough, upper respiratory tract infection

SKIN: Diaphoresis, pruritus, Stevens-Johnson syndrome

Other: Angioedema, hyponatremia, weight loss

Overdose

Duloxetine overdose has no specific antidote. Monitor patient for signs and symptoms of overdose, including seizures, serotonin syndrome (agitation, confusion, diaphoresis, diarrhea, fever, hyperactive reflexes, hyperthermia, labile blood pressure, nausea, poor coordination, restlessness, shaking, tachycardia, talking or acting with uncontrolled excitement, tremor, twitching, and vomiting), somnolence, and vomiting.

Maintain an open airway. Monitor vital signs, institute continuous ECG monitoring and assess capillary refill, peripheral pulses, skin sensation, and warmth. Institute seizure precautions according to facility protocol and expect to treat seizures with a barbiturate, a benzodiazepine or other type of anticonvulsant agent, as prescribed. If serotonin syndrome occurs, be prepared to administer cyproheptadine and use cooling blanket for temperature regulation as needed, and prescribed. Provide additional symptomatic and supportive therapy as indicated.

To decrease drug absorption, be prepared to give activated charcoal, as prescribed. Don't induce emesis. Be aware that forced diuresis, dialysis, hemoperfusion, and exchange transfusion aren't likely to be effective because of duloxetine's large volume of distribution. Institute suicide precautions according to facility policy, and anticipate psychiatric re-evaluation.

Nursing Considerations

- Avoid giving duloxetine to patients with severe renal impairment or end-stage renal disease that requires hemodialysis because blood drug levels increase significantly in these patients. Also avoid duloxetine in patients with hepatic insufficiency because drug is metabolized by the liver.
- Use duloxetine cautiously in patients with delayed gastric emptying because drug has an enteric coating that resists dissolution until it reaches an area where pH exceeds 5.5.
- Give duloxetine cautiously to patients with a history of mania (which it may activate) and patients with a seizure disorder (because drug effects aren't known in these patients).
- **WARNING** Monitor patient closely during duloxetine therapy for evidence of serotonin syndrome, such as agitation, hallucinations, coma tachycardia, labile blood pressure, hyperthermia, hyperreflexia incoordination, nausea, vomiting, or diarrhea. If present, notify prescriber and expect to stop drug and provide supportive therapy, as ordered. Concurrent therapy with serotonergic drugs or MAO inhibitors increases risk.

- Obtain baseline blood pressure before duloxetine therapy starts, and assess it periodically thereafter for changes. If orthostatic hypotension occurs during duloxetine therapy, notify prescriber; drug may need to be discontinued.
- Monitor serum sodium level, especially in patients who are elderly, who take diuretics, or who have volume depletion, because drug may lower serum sodium level.
- Monitor patient's hepatic function, as ordered, because drug may increase the risk of hepatotoxicity.
- If patient (particularly a child or an adolescent) takes duloxetine for depression, watch closely for suicidal tendencies, especially when therapy starts or dosage changes.
- **WARNING** Assess patient for bleeding that may range from ecchymoses, hematomas, epistaxis and petechiae to life-threatening hemorrhages. Notify prescriber if bleeding occurs, and anticipate stopping duloxetine.
- Discontinue duloxetine gradually, when possible, to avoid sudden onset of such adverse effects as irritability, dizziness, sensory disturbances, and seizures.

PATIENT TEACHING
- Tell patient to take capsule whole and not to chew it, crush it, or sprinkle contents on food or liquids because doing so alters enteric coating and may affect drug absorption.
- Inform patient that full effect of drug may take weeks; stress the importance of continuing to take drug as directed.
- Advise against excessive alcohol consumption while taking duloxetine because it may increase risk of hepatic dysfunction.
- Explain that duloxetine therapy must be stopped gradually, not abruptly, to avoid adverse reactions.
- Instruct patient to notify prescriber of any serious or troublesome adverse effects.
- Advise patient to avoid hazardous activities until drug's CNS effects are known.
- If patient (particularly a child or an adolescent) takes duloxetine for depression, urge caregivers to watch closely for suicidal tendencies, particularly when therapy starts or dosage changes.
- Instruct patient to rise slowly from a lying or sitting position to minimize the effects of lowered blood pressure.
- Instruct female patients of childbearing potential to notify prescriber if they are, could be, or wish to become pregnant during therapy; duloxetine may cause adverse reactions in neonates exposed to it during the third trimester.

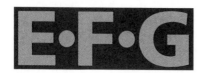

eletriptan hydrobromide
Relpax

Class and Category
Chemical class: Serotonin 5-HT$_{1D}$–receptor agonist
Therapeutic class: Antimigraine agent
Pregnancy category: C

Indications and Dosages
▶ *To relieve acute migraine attacks with or without aura*
TABLETS
Adults. *Initial:* 20 or 40 mg as a single dose. Repeated in 2 hr, as needed and ordered. *Maximum:* 40 mg as single dose, 80 mg daily.

Mechanism of Action
May stimulate 5-hydroxytryptamine$_1$ (5-HT$_1$) receptors, causing selective vasoconstriction of inflamed and dilated cranial blood vessels in carotid circulation, which decreases carotid arterial blood flow and relieves acute migraines.

Contraindications
Bibasilar or hemiplegic migraine, cardiovascular disease (significant), cerebrovascular syndromes (CVA, transient ischemic attack), hepatic impairment (severe), hypersensitivity to eletriptan or components, ischemic bowel disease, ischemic or vasospastic coronary artery disease (CAD), peripheral vascular disease, uncontrolled hypertension, use within 24 hours of another serotonin 5-HT$_1$–receptor agonist or ergot-type drug, use within 72 hours of a potent CYP3A4 inhibitor

Interactions
DRUGS
clarithromycin, ketoconazole, itraconazole, nefazodone, nelfinavir, ritonavir, troleandomycin and other potent CYP3A4 inhibitors: Increased metabolism of eletriptan and decreased blood eletriptan level

ergot-containing drugs, 5-HT₁-receptor agonists: Possibly additive or prolonged vasoconstrictive effects

fluoxetine, fluvoxamine, paroxetine, sertraline: Increased risk of weakness, hyperreflexia, and incoordination

Adverse Reactions

CNS: Asthenia, dizziness, headache, paresthesia, somnolence, tiredness, weakness

CV: Chest tightness, pain, or pressure; coronary artery vasospasm; hypertension, MI or myocardial ischemia (transient); ventricular fibrillation or tachycardia

EENT: Dry mouth, throat tightness

GI: Abdominal pain, cramps, discomfort, or pressure; dysphagia; indigestion; nausea

SKIN: Flushing

Other: Feeling of warmth, pain, or pressure

Overdose

Eletriptan overdose has no specific antidote. Montior patient for signs and symptoms of overdose, including hypertension, arrhythmias, and chest pain. Monitoring should continue for at least 20 hours or longer if signs and symptoms persist because eletriptan's half-life is 4 hours.

Maintain an open airway, and be prepared to assist with endotracheal intubation if patient develops respiratory depression. Monitor vital signs and cardiac monitor for arrhythmias, especially ventricular fibrillation and tachycardia. Expect to give symptomatic and supportive care, as needed. The effect of hemodialysis or peritoneal dialysis is unknown.

Institute suicide precautions according to facility policy, and anticipate psychiatric re-evaluation.

Nursing Considerations

- Ensure that patients who are at risk for CAD undergo a satisfactory CV evaluation before you administer the first dose of eletriptan and that they have a periodic re-evaluation of their cardiac status during intermittent long-term therapy.
- Obtain an ECG immediately after first dose in patients with CV risk factors but who have had a satisfactory CV evaluation because of the drug's potential to cause coronary vasospasm.
- Evaluate patient for CV signs and symptoms after giving eletriptan, and notify prescriber if they occur. Expect drug to be with-

held, as ordered, while patient undergoes an extensive CV workup, and discontinued if abnormalities are detected.
• Monitor patient's blood pressure during therapy because of drug's potential to increase blood pressure.

PATIENT TEACHING
• Advise patient to take eletriptan as soon as possible after onset of migraine symptoms.
• Urge patient to contact prescriber and avoid taking drug if headache symptoms aren't typical.
• Remind patient not to exceed prescribed daily dose.
• Instruct patient to seek emergency care for chest, jaw, or neck tightness after taking eletriptan because these may indicate adverse CV reactions; subsequent doses may require ECG monitoring.
• Urge patient to report palpitations to prescriber.
• Advise patient to avoid potentially hazardous activities until drug's CNS effects are known.
• Encourage yearly ophthalmic examinations for patients who require prolonged eletriptan therapy.
• Instruct patient to inform prescriber of all drugs he's taking, including OTC products and herbal remedies.

entacapone
Comtan

Class and Category
Chemical class: Catechol-O-methyltransferase (COMT) inhibitor
Therapeutic class: Antidyskinetic
Pregnancy category: C

Indications and Dosages
▶ *As adjunct to manage signs and symptoms of Parkinson's disease*
TABLETS
Adults. 200 mg with each dose of carbidopa and levodopa. *Maximum:* 1,600 mg daily.

Route	Onset	Steady State	Peak	Half-Life	Duration
P.O.	Unknown	Unknown	Unknown	1.5 to 3.5 hr	Unknown

Contraindications
Hypersensitivity to entacapone or its components, use within 14 days of nonselective MAO inhibitor therapy

Mechanism of Action

Entacapone is a selective and reversible inhibitor of catechol-*O*-methyltransferase (COMT), the major metabolizing enzyme for levodopa. Normally, levodopa is metabolized by COMT in the peripheral circulation to 3-methoxy-4-hydroxy-L-phenylalanine (3-OMD). An inactive metabolite, 3-OMD enters the bloodstream and competes with levodopa for transport across the blood-brain barrier to the CNS, as shown above right.

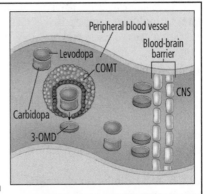

Entacapone inhibits COMT by binding to an active site on the COMT enzyme, which causes a decrease in the blood level of 3-OMD and makes more levodopa available for diffusion into the CNS. After levodopa crosses the blood-brain barrier, it's converted to dopa-

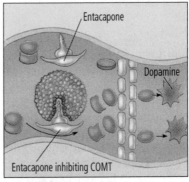

mine, as shown below right. Depleted dopamine stores are thought to cause Parkinson's disease. By replenishing dopamine stores, entacapone increases dopaminergic stimulation in the brain and reduces the symptoms of Parkinson's disease.

Entacapone has no antidyskinetic properties of its own, so it's prescribed as adjunctive therapy with carbidopa-levodopa to treat the signs and symptoms of Parkinson's disease. Carbidopa is given with levodopa because it inhibits the peripheral distribution of levodopa, making more levodopa available for transport to the brain. Carbidopa doesn't cross the blood-brain barrier.

Interactions
DRUGS

ampicillin, chloramphenicol, cholestyramine, erythromycin, probenecid, rifampin: Decreased biliary excretion of entacapone

apomorphine, bitolterol, dobutamine, dopamine, epinephrine, isoetharine,

isoproterenol, methyldopa, norepinephrine: Possibly increased heart rate, arrhythmias, and excessive changes in blood pressure
MAO inhibitors (nonselective): Possibly inhibited entacapone metabolism

Adverse Reactions

CNS: Agitation, anxiety, asthenia, chills, dizziness, dyskinesia, fatigue, fever, hallucinations, hyperkinesia, hypokinesia, somnolence
EENT: Dry mouth
GI: Abdominal pain, constipation, diarrhea, indigestion, gastritis, nausea
GU: Brown-orange urine, dysuria
MS: Back pain
RESP: Cough, dyspnea
SKIN: Diaphoresis, purpura

Overdose

Information about the signs and symptoms of entacapone overdose isn't available; however, assess patient for dyspnea or worsening dyskinesia, which may indicate serious adverse reactions and possibly overdose.

Anticipate performing gastric lavage to decrease absorption of entacapone. Administer repeated doses of charcoal, as prescribed, to enhance elimination. Be aware that entacapone is highly protein bound, so hemodialysis and hemoperfusion are ineffective for treating entacapone overdose.

Institute suicide precautions according to facility policy, and anticipate psychiatric re-evaluation.

Nursing Considerations

- **WARNING** Be aware that entacapone shouldn't be discontinued abruptly because doing so may cause signs and symptoms like those of neuroleptic malignant syndrome, such as altered level of consciousness, confusion, elevated creatine kinase level, fever, and muscle rigidity. Patients also may have a rapid re-emergence of parkinsonian signs and symptoms.
- Monitor patient for drug-induced diarrhea during first 4 to 12 weeks of entacapone therapy.
- Assist patient with activities as necessary because drug may increase occurrence of orthostatic hypotension or syncope if he's susceptible to either one.
- Monitor patient for worsening dyskinesia because entacapone potentiates dopaminergic adverse effects of levodopa and may

exacerbate pre-existing dyskinesia.
- Be aware that drug may be taken with a selective MAO inhibitor, such as selegiline.

PATIENT TEACHING
- Instruct patient to always take entacapone with carbidopa-levodopa because drug has no antidyskinetic effect of its own.
- Inform patient that dizziness and sleepiness are more common at beginning of treatment, especially in those with hypotension.
- Advise patient not to participate in potentially hazardous activities until he knows how the drug affects him, especially if he's also taking a CNS depressant.
- If patient is scheduled for surgery, tell him to inform surgeon and anesthesiologist about entacapone use beforehand because COMT inhibitors may interact with drugs used during surgery.
- Caution patient that entacapone may increase adverse effects of carbidopa and levodopa, such as nausea and uncontrolled movements. If these adverse effects do increase, advise him to contact prescriber immediately because carbidopa and levodopa dosage may need to be lowered.
- Inform patient that urine may turn brown-orange while he's taking entacapone but that this is a harmless effect.

ergoloid mesylates
(dihydrogenated ergot alkaloids)
Gerimal, Hydergine, Hydergine LC

Class and Category
Chemical class: Dihydrogenated ergot alkaloid derivative
Therapeutic class: Antidementia adjunct, cerebral metabolic enhancer
Pregnancy category: Not rated

Indications and Dosages
▶ *To treat age-related decline in mental capacity*
CAPSULES, ORAL SOLUTION, S.L. TABLETS, TABLETS
Adults. 1 to 2 mg t.i.d.

Route	Onset	Steady State	Peak	Half-Life	Duration
P.O.	3 wk or more	Unknown	Unknown	2 to 5 hr	Unknown

Contraindications
Acute or chronic psychosis, hypersensitivity to ergoloid mesylates or their components

Mechanism of Action

May increase cerebral metabolism, blood flow, and oxygen uptake. These actions may elevate neurotransmitter levels.

Interactions

DRUGS

delavirdine, efavirenz, indinavir, nelfinavir, saquinavir: Increased risk of ergotism (blurred vision, dizziness, and headache)
dopamine: Increased risk of gangrene

Adverse Reactions

CNS: Dizziness, headache, light-headedness, syncope
CV: Bradycardia, orthostatic hypotension
EENT: Blurred vision, nasal congestion, tongue soreness (with S.L. tablets)
GI: Abdominal cramps, anorexia, nausea, vomiting
SKIN: Flushing, rash

Overdose

Information about the signs and symptoms of ergoloid mesylates overdose isn't available; however, assess patient for anorexia, blurred vision, dizziness, epigastric pain, flushing, headache, nasal congestion, nausea, syncope, and vomiting, which may indicate serious adverse reactions and possibly overdose. Expect to give symptomatic and supportive care, as needed.

Nursing Considerations

• Expect ergoloid mesylates to be prescribed only after a pathophysiologic cause for mental decline has been ruled out.
• Measure blood pressure and pulse rate and rhythm before therapy begins, and monitor them frequently during therapy.
• If bradycardia or hypotension develops, expect to discontinue drug permanently.

PATIENT TEACHING

• Stress the importance of adhering to prescribed dosage and schedule.
• Teach caregiver to place S.L. ergoloid tablet under patient's tongue and withhold food, fluids, and cigarettes until tablet dissolves.
• Instruct patient not to swallow S.L. tablets.
• Advise caregiver to skip a missed dose and resume the regular dosing schedule. Warn against doubling the dose, and urge

caregiver to notify prescriber if patient misses two or more doses in a row.
- Instruct caregiver to store drug in a tightly closed, light-resistant container.
- Inform caregiver and family that drug may take 3 to 4 weeks to produce effects.
- Stress the importance of follow-up care.

ergotamine tartrate

Ergomar (CAN), Ergostat, Gynergen (CAN), Medihaler Ergotamine (CAN)

Class and Category

Chemical class: Ergot alkaloid
Therapeutic class: Vascular headache suppressant
Pregnancy category: X

Indications and Dosages

▶ *To relieve vascular headaches, such as migraine and migraine variants*

S.L. TABLETS

Adults. *Initial:* 2 mg at first sign of attack and repeated every 30 min, p.r.n. *Maximum:* 6 mg daily and no more than twice weekly, at least 5 days apart.

TABLETS

Adults. *Initial:* 1 to 2 mg at first sign of attack and repeated every 30 min, p.r.n. Dosage increased to 3 mg for subsequent attacks if needed and if lower dose was well tolerated. *Maximum:* 6 mg daily.

ORAL INHALATION AEROSOL

Adults. 1 (360-mcg) inhalation at first sign of attack and repeated every 5 min, p.r.n. *Maximum:* 2.16 mg daily and no more than twice weekly, at least 5 days apart.

Route	Onset	Steady State	Peak	Half-Life	Duration
P.O., S.L.	Unknown	Unknown	1 to 5 hr	21 hr	Unknown

Contraindications

Coronary artery disease, hypersensitivity to ergot alkaloids, hypertension, impaired hepatic or renal function, malnutrition, peripheral vascular disease (Raynaud's disease, severe arteriosclerosis, syphilitic arteritis, thromboangiitis obliterans, thrombophlebitis), pregnancy or risk of pregnancy, sepsis, severe pruritus

Mechanism of Action

Directly stimulates vascular smooth muscles, constricting arteries and veins and depressing vasomotor centers in the brain. Ergotamine decreases the firing of serotonergic (5-hydroxytryptaminergic, 5-HT) neurons, possibly resulting in headache suppression. The drug also interacts with alpha-adrenergic receptors, which may cause constriction of cerebral blood vessels.

Interactions

DRUGS

beta blockers: Increased risk of vasoconstriction and, possibly, peripheral gangrene

erythromycin, troleandomycin: Increased risk of peripheral vasospasm and ischemia

nitrates: Increased ergotamine effects, decreased antianginal effects of nitrates, increased risk of hypertension

sumatriptan: Possibly additive vasoconstriction

vasoconstrictors: Increased risk of dangerous hypertension

ACTIVITIES

smoking: Possibly increased risk of peripheral vasoconstriction and ischemia

Adverse Reactions

CNS: Anxiety, confusion, dizziness, drowsiness, paresthesia, severe headache

CV: Chest pain, fast or slow heart rate, heart valve fibrosis, increased or decreased blood pressure, MI, weak pulse

EENT: Dry mouth, miosis, vision changes

GI: Nausea, vomiting

MS: Arm, back, or leg pain; muscle weakness in legs

SKIN: Cold, cyanotic, or pale feet or hands; pruritus

Other: Edema of face, feet, fingers, or lower legs; physical dependence

Overdose

Monitor patient for signs and symptoms of overdose, including bloating or epigastric pain, diarrhea, dizziness, drowsiness, hemiparesis, hypertension followed by hypotension, loss of consciousness, respiratory depression, seizures, severe confusion, shock, tachycardia, vomiting, and weakness.

Maintain an open airway, and be prepared to perform endotracheal intubation if patient develops respiratory depression. Monitor vital signs, institute continuous ECG monitoring, and assess capillary refill, peripheral pulses, skin sensation, and warmth. Institute seizure precautions according to facility protocol.

To decrease drug absorption in a conscious patient, be prepared to induce vomiting with syrup of ipecac or perform gastric lavage. Also be prepared to give activated charcoal or a saline cathartic, such as sodium or magnesium sulfate, as prescribed.

For an unconscious patient, anticipate assisting with the insertion of an endotracheal tube and then performing gastric lavage. The inflated cuff of the endotracheal tube will help prevent aspiration of gastric contents into the lungs.

Administer I.V. fluids to enhance elimination of ergotamine. Expect to treat seizures with a benzodiazepine, such as diazepam or lorazepam, as prescribed. Monitor patient for hypotension, and be prepared to put him in Trendelenburg's position and administer I.V. fluids or volume expanders. Be aware that a vasopressor may add to the vasoconstricting effects of ergotamine.

About 24 hours after an acute overdose, signs and symptoms of cerebral ischemia or peripheral ischemia may occur. Assess patient for anxiety; confusion; cyanosis of hands or feet; itching of skin; leg weakness; pain in arms, legs, and lower back; paresthesia; red or violet blisters on the hands and feet; and weak or absent pulses. If patient develops peripheral ischemia, expect to apply warmth, such as with warm blankets to his extremities, and handle the extremities carefully to prevent tissue damage. If he develops coronary ischemia and it's severe, expect to administer a vasodilator, such as nitroglycerin or nitroprusside. Be aware that low-dose heparin may also be prescribed to treat vasospasm.

Nursing Considerations

- Use ergotamine cautiously in elderly patients.
- If patient receives long-term therapy, monitor him for pain control; he may need increasingly higher doses to obtain relief.
- Notify prescriber at the first sign of vasospasm, and expect to discontinue drug.

PATIENT TEACHING

- Teach patient to take a tablet at the first sign of headache and to lie down in a quiet, dark room.
- Instruct patient not to swallow S.L. tablet but to let it dissolve under his tongue. Advise him not to drink, eat, or smoke until tablet has dissolved.
- Stress the importance of adhering to prescribed dosage and schedule because of drug's potential for dependence.
- Warn patient not to smoke while taking ergotamine because

the combination of drug and nicotine, which also constricts vessels, may increase the risk of peripheral vascular ischemia.
- Advise patient to notify prescriber if usual doses fail to relieve headaches or if headache frequency or severity increases.
- Urge patient to avoid alcohol because it worsens headaches. Also, suggest that patient avoid excessive cold, which may increase peripheral vasoconstriction.
- Instruct patient to notify prescriber if an infection develops because severe infection may increase sensitivity to drug.
- Advise patient to notify prescriber if he experiences chest pain; numbness, pain, or tingling in fingers or toes; pulse rate changes; swelling of face, feet, fingers, or lower legs; or vision changes.

Other Therapeutic Uses
Ergotamine tartrate is also indicated for the following:
- To treat cluster headaches

escitalopram oxalate
Lexapro

Class and Category
Chemical class: Pure S1 enantiomer of racemic bicyclic phthalane derivative citalopram
Therapeutic class: Antidepressant
Pregnancy category: C

Indications and Dosages
▶ *To treat generalized anxiety disorder or major depression*
ORAL SOLUTION, TABLETS
Adults. *Initial:* 10 mg daily in morning or evening, increased to 20 mg daily after 1 wk or more, as needed.
DOSAGE ADJUSTMENT Dosage shouldn't exceed 10 mg daily for elderly patients and those with hepatic impairment.

Mechanism of Action
Inhibits reuptake of the neurotransmitter serotonin by CNS neurons, thereby increasing the amount of serotonin available in nerve synapses. An elevated serotonin level may result in elevated mood and reduced depression.

Contraindications
Hypersensitivity to escitalopram, citalopram, or its components; use within 14 days of an MAO inhibitor

Interactions

DRUGS

aspirin, NSAIDs, warfarin: Possibly increased risk of bleeding
carbamazepine: Possibly increased escitalopram clearance
cimetidine: Possibly increased plasma escitalopram level
CNS drugs: Additive CNS effects
lithium: Possible enhancement of the serotonergic effects of escitalopram
MAO inhibitors: Possibly hyperpyretic episodes, hypertensive crisis, serotonin syndrome, and severe seizures
metoprolol: Increased plasma metoprolol level with decreased cardioselectivity of metoprolol
naratriptan, sumatriptan, zolmitriptan: Possibly weakness, hyperreflexia, and incoordination
St. John's wort: Increased risk of serotonin syndrome
sibutramine: Increased risk of serotonin syndrome

ACTIVITIES

alcohol use: Possibly increased cognitive and motor effects of alcohol

Adverse Reactions

CNS: Abnormal gait, aggression, akathisia, delirium, dizziness, dyskinesia, dystonia, extrapyramidal effects, fatigue, headache, hypomania, insomnia, lethargy, mania, myoclonus syndrome, neuroleptic malignant syndrome, paresthesia, seizures, serotonin syndrome, somnolence, suicidal ideation
CV: Atrial fibrillation, hypotension, MI, prolonged QT interval, thrombosis, torsades de pointes, ventricular arrhythmias
EENT: Diplopia, dry mouth, nystagmus, rhinitis, sinusitis, toothache, visual hallucinations
ENDO: Syndrome of inappropriate ADH secretion
GI: Abdominal pain, constipation, decreased appetite, diarrhea, flatulence, GI bleeding or hemorrhage, hepatic necrosis, hepatitis, indigestion, nausea, pancreatitis, vomiting
GU: Acute renal failure, anorgasmia, decreased libido, ejaculation disorders, impotence, priapism
HEME: Bleeding, decreased prothrombin time, hemolytic anemia, thrombocytopenia
MS: Neck or shoulder pain, rhabdomyolysis
RESP: Pulmonary embolism
SKIN: Ecchymosis, erythema multiforme, increased sweating, toxic epidermal necrolysis
Other: Anaphylaxis, angioedema, flulike symptoms

Overdose

Escitalopram overdose has no specific antidote. Monitor patient for signs and symptoms of overdose, including seizures, coma, dizziness, hypotension, insomnia, nausea and vomiting, tachycardia, somnolence, ECG changes (prolonged QT interval, torsades de pointes), and acute renal failure.

Maintain an open airway, and provide oxygen therapy, as needed and prescribed. Monitor vital signs, institute continuous ECG monitoring, and assess capillary refill, peripheral pulses, skin sensation, and warmth. Institute seizure precautions according to facility protocol, and expect to treat seizures with a barbiturate, a benzodiazepine, or other anticonvulsant, as prescribed. Administer I.V. fluids and a vasopressor, as prescribed, to combat hypotension. Provide additional symptomatic and supportive therapy as indicated.

To decrease drug absorption, be prepared to perform gastric lavage followed by administration of oral activated charcoal, as prescribed. Be aware that forced diuresis, dialysis, hemoperfusion, and exchange transfusion are not likely to be effective because of escitalopram's large volume of distribution.

Institute suicide precautions according to facility policy, and anticipate psychiatric re-evaluation.

Nursing Considerations

- Use escitalopram cautiously in patients with a history of mania or seizures, patients with severe renal impairment, or those with diseases or conditions that produce altered metabolism or hemodynamic responses.
- Monitor patient for hypo-osmolarity of serum and urine and for hyponatremia, which may indicate escitalopram-induced syndrome of inappropriate ADH secretion.
- Observe patient for signs of misuse or abuse, such as development of tolerance, increasing dosage without approval, and drug-seeking behavior, because escitalopram's potential for physical and psychological dependence is unknown.
- Expect prescriber to reassess patient periodically to determine continued need for therapy and confirm appropriate dosage.
- If patient takes escitalopram for depression (particularly a child or an adolescent), watch closely for suicidal tendencies, especially when therapy starts or dosage changes; depression may worsen temporarily at these times.
- If drug will be stopped, expect to taper dosage to avoid serious adverse reactions.

PATIENT TEACHING
• Inform patient that alcohol use isn't recommended during escitalopram therapy because it may decrease his ability to think clearly and perform motor skills.
• Advise patient to avoid potentially hazardous activities until drug's CNS effects are known.
• Instruct patient that drug shouldn't be taken with citalopram hydrobromide because of potentially additive effects.
• Tell patient that improvement may not be noticed for 1 to 4 weeks after therapy begins. Emphasize the importance of continuing therapy as prescribed.
• Warn patient not to stop taking escitalopram abruptly. Explain that tapering the dosage gradually helps to avoid withdrawal symptoms.
• Urge patient to inform prescriber of any OTC drugs he takes because of potential for interactions.
• Particularly if patient is a child or an adolescent and is taking escitalopram for depression, urge caregivers to watch closely for evidence of suicidal tendencies, especially when therapy starts or dosage changes.

estazolam

Class, Category, and Schedule
Chemical class: Benzodiazepine
Therapeutic class: Sedative-hypnotic
Pregnancy category: X
Controlled substance schedule: IV

Indications and Dosages
▶ *To treat insomnia*
TABLETS
Adults. 1 to 2 mg at bedtime.
DOSAGE ADJUSTMENT Starting dose reduced to 0.5 mg for small or debilitated elderly patients.

Mechanism of Action
May potentiate the effects of gamma-aminobutyric acid (GABA) and other inhibitory neurotransmitters by binding to specific benzodiazepine receptors in the limbic and cortical areas of the CNS. By binding to these receptors, estazolam increases GABA's inhibitory effects and blocks cortical and limbic arousal.

Route	Onset	Steady State	Peak	Half-Life	Duration
P.O.	Unknown	2 to 3 days	Unknown	8 to 28 hr	6 to 8 hr

Contraindications

Acute angle-closure glaucoma; hypersensitivity to estazolam, other benzodiazepines, or their components; pregnancy; psychosis

Interactions

DRUGS

barbiturates, carbamazepine, phenytoin, rifampin: Possibly decreased blood estazolam level

carbamazepine: Possibly increased blood carbamazepine level

cimetidine, diltiazem, disulfiram, erythromycin, fluoxetine, fluvoxamine, isoniazide, itraconazole, ketoconazole, nefazodone, oral contraceptives, propoxyphene, ranitidine, verapamil: Possibly increased blood level and impaired hepatic metabolism of estazolam

clozapine: Possibly cardiac arrest or respiratory depression

CNS depressants: Possibly potentiated CNS depression

levodopa: Possibly decreased therapeutic effects of levodopa

FOODS

grapefruit juice: Possibly increased blood level and impaired hepatic metabolism of estazolam

ACTIVITIES

alcohol use: Possibly potentiated CNS depression

Adverse Reactions

CNS: Amnesia, anxiety, ataxia, confusion, delusions, depression, dizziness, drowsiness, euphoria, headache, hypokinesia, irritability, malaise, nervousness, slurred speech, tremor

CV: Chest pain, palpitations, tachycardia

EENT: Blurred vision, dry mouth, increased salivation, photophobia

GI: Abdominal pain, constipation, diarrhea, nausea, thirst, vomiting

GU: Libido changes

RESP: Respiratory depression

SKIN: Diaphoresis

Other: Physical or psychological dependence

Overdose

Monitor patient for evidence of overdose, including bradycardia, coma, confusion, dyspnea, hyperreflexia, seizures, severe drowsiness, shakiness, slurred speech, staggering, and weakness.

Maintain open airway, institute continuous cardiac monitoring, and administer continuous I.V. fluids, as prescribed, to maintain blood pressure and promote diuresis. Institute seizure precautions according to facility protocol.

To decrease absorption of drug in a conscious patient who isn't at risk for coma or seizures, be prepared to induce vomiting or perform gastric lavage. Expect that oral activated charcoal may also be prescribed.

For an unconscious patient, anticipate assisting with the insertion of an endotracheal tube and then performing gastric lavage. The inflated cuff of the endotracheal tube will help prevent aspiration of gastric contents into the lungs.

Anticipate the use of a benzodiazepine receptor antagonist, such as flumazenil, to reverse sedative effects. Be aware that flumazenil may induce seizures, especially in a patient who has taken benzodiazepines long-term or ingested a cyclic antidepressant. If excitation occurs, be aware that a barbiturate shouldn't be used because it may increase excitement and prolong CNS depression. Dialysis is ineffective for benzodiazepine overdose.

Institute suicide precautionary measures according to facility policy, and anticipate psychiatric re-evaluation.

Nursing Considerations

- Use estazolam with extreme caution in patients with a history of drug or alcohol abuse because of the risk of addiction. Expect to give drug for no more than 12 weeks for the same reason.
- Use drug cautiously in elderly or debilitated patients and those with depression or impaired hepatic, renal, or respiratory function.
- Expect to stop estazolam gradually to prevent withdrawal signs and symptoms, especially if patient has a history of seizures.

PATIENT TEACHING
- Warn patient not to exceed prescribed dosage or to take estazolam longer than prescribed because of the risk of addiction.
- Because estazolam can reduce alertness, advise patient to avoid potentially hazardous activities until he knows how the drug affects him.
- Advise patient not to drink alcohol or take another CNS depressant during estazolam therapy because of the risk of additive effects.
- Warn elderly or debilitated patients and those with impaired renal or hepatic function about the risk of excessive sedation or mental impairment. Urge patient to notify prescriber if these problems occur.

• Caution patient who takes 2-mg dosage for a prolonged time against stopping drug abruptly; withdrawal signs and symptoms may develop.

eszopiclone
Lunesta

Class, Category, and Schedule
Chemical class: Pyrrolopyrazine derivative of cyclopyrrolone class
Therapeutic class: Sedative-hypnotic
Pregnancy category: C
Controlled substance schedule: IV

Indications and Dosages
▶ *To treat insomnia*
TABLETS
Adults. *Initial:* 2 mg immediately before bedtime. May be increased to 3 mg at bedtime, as needed. *Maintenance:* 3 mg at bedtime.
DOSAGE ADJUSTMENT For elderly patients who have trouble falling asleep or patients with severe hepatic impairment, dosage decreased to 1 mg immediately before bedtime. For elderly patients who have trouble staying asleep, dosage may be increased to 2 mg at bedtime.

Route	Onset	Peak	Duration
P.O.	Unknown	1 hr	Unknown

Mechanism of Action
May potentiate the effects of the inhibitory neurotransmitter gamma-aminobutyric acid (GABA) by binding close to or with benzodiazepine receptors in the limbic and cortical areas of the CNS. By binding to these receptor sites and areas, eszopiclone increases GABA's inhibitory effects and blocks cortical and limbic arousal, thereby inducing and maintaining sleep.

Contraindications
Hypersensitivity to eszopiclone or its components

Interactions
DRUGS
clarithromycin, itraconazole, ketoconazole, nefazodone, nelfinavir, ritonavir, troleandomycin: Increased blood level of eszopiclone

rifampin: Decreased blood level of eszopiclone
ACTIVITIES
alcohol use: Additive effect on psychomotor performance

Adverse Reactions

CNS: Anxiety, confusion, depression, dizziness, hallucinations, headache (including migraine), nervousness, neuralgia, sleep-driving, somnolence, unusual dreams
CV: Chest pain, peripheral edema
EENT: Dry mouth, taste perversion
ENDO: Gynecomastia
GI: Diarrhea, hepatitis, indigestion, nausea, vomiting
GU: Decreased libido, dysmenorrhea, UTI
RESP: Asthma, respiratory tract infection
SKIN: Pruritus, rash
Other: Anaphylaxis, angioedema, generalized pain, heatstroke, viral infection

Overdose

Monitor patient for signs and symptoms of eszopiclone overdose, including hypotension and an exaggeration of the drug's effects, especially somnolence, impaired consciousness, and coma.

Maintain an open airway, and monitor vital signs. Flumazenil, a benzodiazepine antidote, may be useful in treating eszopiclone overdose. Administer dosage prescribed, and expect to repeat at 60-second intervals, as needed. Accumulated dosage should not exceed 3 mg in 1-hour interval. Be aware that flumazenil may induce seizures, especially in a patient who has been taking benzodiazepines long-term or has ingested a cyclic antidepressant. If excitation occurs, be aware that a barbiturate shouldn't be used because it may increase excitement and prolong CNS depression.

Give I.V. fluids or volume expanders as needed and prescribed to treat hypotension. Provide additional symptomatic and supportive therapy as indicated. Usefulness of dialysis is unknown.

Institute suicide precautions according to facility policy, and anticipate psychiatric re-evaluation.

Nursing Considerations

• Use eszopiclone cautiously in patients with severe mental depression or reduced respiratory function; drug may intensify depression and lead to respiratory depression.
• **WARNING** Monitor patient closely for allergic reactions that, although rare, may be severe. If patient experiences dyspnea, throat closing, or nausea and vomiting, notify prescriber im-

mediately and be prepared to provide airway management and other emergency care and to discontinue eszopiclone.

• Monitor patient for worsening insomnia and emergence of abnormal thinking or behavior because eszopiclone may unmask them; patient will need a more extensive work-up.

PATIENT TEACHING

• Instruct patient not to exceed prescribed eszopiclone dosage and not to abruptly stop taking the drug because withdrawal symptoms may occur.

• Because eszopiclone can reduce alertness, advise patient to take drug immediately before bedtime and to avoid hazardous activities until drug's CNS effects are known.

• Caution patient to avoid alcohol and CNS depressants during therapy because of additive effects.

• Advise female patient of childbearing age to notify prescriber if she becomes or intends to become pregnant during therapy.

• Inform patient that sleep may be disturbed for the first few nights after he stops taking drug.

• Urge patient to notify prescriber about insomnia that lasts longer than 7 days despite eszopiclone therapy.

• Instruct family to report any episodes of sleep-driving, in which patient drives while not fully awake and usually has no recall of the event.

• Advise patient to stop drug and seek emergency care immediately if he has trouble breathing, throat closing, or nausea and vomiting.

ethchlorvynol

Placidyl

Class, Category, and Schedule

Chemical class: Chlorinated tertiary acetylenic carbinol
Therapeutic class: Sedative-hypnotic
Pregnancy category: C
Controlled substance schedule: IV

Indications and Dosages

▶ *To provide short-term relief from insomnia*

CAPSULES

Adults. 0.5 to 1 g at bedtime for no longer than 1 wk.

Route	Onset	Steady State	Peak	Half-Life	Duration
P.O.	15 to 60 min	Unknown	Unknown	10 to 20 hr	5 hr

Mechanism of Action
Exerts sedative-hypnotic, muscle relaxant, and anticonvulsant effects possibly by depressing the reticular activating system.

Contraindications
Hypersensitivity to ethchlorvynol or its components, porphyria

Interactions
DRUGS
CNS depressants, tricyclic antidepressants: Increased CNS depression
oral anticoagulants: Decreased anticoagulant effects
ACTIVITIES
alcohol use: Increased CNS depression

Adverse Reactions
CNS: Ataxia, dizziness, facial numbness, fatigue, lightheadedness, syncope, unsteadiness, weakness
CV: Hypotension
EENT: Blurred vision, unpleasant aftertaste
GI: Epigastric pain, indigestion, nausea, vomiting
HEME: Thrombocytopenia
SKIN: Jaundice, rash, urticaria
Other: Physical and psychological dependence

Overdose
Monitor patient for signs and symptoms of overdose, including bradycardia, chills, coma, easy bleeding or bruising, fever, hypothermia, nystagmus, pale skin, pancytopenia, respiratory depression, sore throat, and weakness.

Maintain open airway and monitor pulmonary function; obtain blood gases, as needed. Be prepared to assist with endotracheal intubation if patient experiences respiratory depression. Monitor patient's temperature because of the risk of hypothermia.

To decrease absorption of drug in a conscious patient who isn't at risk for coma, be prepared to perform gastric lavage. For an unconscious patient, anticipate assisting with the insertion of an endotracheal tube and then performing gastric lavage. The inflated cuff of the endotracheal tube will help prevent aspiration of gastric contents into the lungs.

Be aware that hemoperfusion, using the Amberlite column technique, is an effective treatment for ethchlorvynol overdose. Hemodialysis and peritoneal dialysis with the use of aqueous and oil dialysates may also be effective.

Institute suicide precautionary measures according to facility policy, and anticipate psychiatric re-evaluation.

Nursing Considerations
- If patient awakens too early after taking 0.5 or 0.75 g of ethchlorvynol at bedtime, ask prescriber if he may take a single supplemental dose of 200 mg.
- Assess patient for signs and symptoms of addiction if he has taken drug for 2 weeks or longer.
- Be aware that ethchlorvynol shouldn't be given for longer than 1 week. If patient has received prolonged therapy, expect to discontinue drug gradually to prevent withdrawal. Notify prescriber if you detect diaphoresis, hallucinations, irritability, muscle twitching, nausea, nervousness, restlessness, seizures, sleep disturbance, tremor, vomiting, and weakness.

PATIENT TEACHING
- Caution patient not to exceed prescribed dosage or dosing frequency because of ethchlorvynol's habit-forming potential. Instruct him not to use drug for more than 1 week.
- Advise patient to take drug with food or milk to minimize adverse GI reactions.
- If patient has taken ethchlorvynol for a prolonged period, warn against stopping drug abruptly; advise him to contact prescriber for guidelines to reduce dosage.
- Direct patient to avoid alcohol and other CNS depressants during therapy because they increase the risk of adverse reactions.
- Advise patient to avoid potentially hazardous activities until he knows how the drug affects him.

ethosuximide
Zarontin

Class and Category
Chemical class: Succinimide derivative
Therapeutic class: Anticonvulsant
Pregnancy category: Not rated

Indications and Dosages
▶ *To manage absence seizures in a patient who also has generalized tonic-clonic seizures*
CAPSULES, SYRUP
Adults and children age 6 and over. *Initial:* 500 mg daily.

Maintenance: Increased by 250 mg every 4 to 7 days until control is achieved with minimal adverse reactions.
Children ages 3 to 6. *Initial:* 250 mg daily. *Maintenance:* Increased by 250 mg every 4 to 7 days until control is achieved with minimal adverse reactions.

Route	Onset	Steady State	Peak	Half-Life	Duration
P.O.	Unknown	4 to 7 day	Unknown	56 to 60 hr*	Unknown

Mechanism of Action
Elevates the seizure threshold and reduces the frequency of attacks by depressing the motor cortex and elevating the threshold of CNS response to convulsive stimuli.

Contraindications
Hypersensitivity to ethosuximide, succinimides, or their components

Interactions
DRUGS
carbamazepine, phenobarbital, phenytoin, primidone: Possibly decreased blood ethosuximide level
CNS depressants: Possibly increased CNS depression
haloperidol: Possibly decreased blood haloperidol level
loxapine, MAO inhibitors, maprotiline, molindone, phenothiazines, pimozide, tricyclic antidepressants: Possibly lowered seizure threshold and reduced therapeutic effect of ethosuximide
valproic acid: Increased or decreased blood ethosuximide level
ACTIVITIES
alcohol use: Possibly increased CNS depression

Adverse Reactions
CNS: Aggressiveness, ataxia, decreased concentration, dizziness, drowsiness, euphoria, fatigue, headache, hyperactivity, irritability, lethargy, nightmares, sleep disturbance
EENT: Gingival hypertrophy, myopia, tongue swelling
GI: Abdominal and epigastric pain, abdominal cramps, anorexia, diarrhea, hiccups, indigestion, nausea, vomiting
GU: Increased libido, microscopic hematuria, vaginal bleeding

---

* For adults. Half-life is 30 to 36 hr for children.

HEME: Agranulocytosis, aplastic anemia, eosinophilia, leukopenia, pancytopenia
SKIN: Erythematous and pruritic rash, hirsutism, Stevens-Johnson syndrome, systemic lupus erythematosus, urticaria
Other: Hypersensitivity reactions, weight loss

Overdose

Monitor patient for signs and symptoms of overdose, including CNS depression, nausea, respiratory depression, and vomiting. Maintain open airway, and be prepared to assist with endotracheal intubation if patient experiences respiratory depression.

To decrease absorption of drug in a conscious patient who isn't at risk for coma, be prepared to induce vomiting. For an unconscious patient, anticipate assisting with the insertion of an endotracheal tube and then performing gastric lavage. The inflated cuff of the endotracheal tube will help prevent aspiration of gastric contents into the lungs. Expect that activated charcoal or cathartics may also be prescribed. Hemodialysis may be effective for treating ethosuximide overdose.

Institute suicide precautions according to facility policy, and anticipate psychiatric re-evaluation.

Nursing Considerations

- Use ethosuximide with extreme caution in patients with hepatic or renal disease.
- Give other anticonvulsants concurrently, as prescribed, to control generalized tonic-clonic seizures.
- Monitor CBC and platelet count and assess for signs of infection, such as cough, fever, and pharyngitis. Also, routinely evaluate liver and renal function test results.
- Take safety precautions because drug may cause adverse CNS reactions, such as dizziness and drowsiness.

PATIENT TEACHING
- Stress the importance of complying with ethosuximide regimen.
- Advise patient to take a missed dose as soon as he remembers unless it's nearly time for the next dose. Warn him not to double the dose.
- Instruct patient not to engage in potentially hazardous activities until he knows how the drug affects him.
- Caution patient not to stop taking drug abruptly; doing so increases the risk of absence seizures.
- Advise patient to notify prescriber if she is, is planning to become, or could be pregnant. Drug may cause fetal defects.

ethotoin
Peganone

Class and Category
Chemical class: Hydantoin derivative
Therapeutic class: Anticonvulsant
Pregnancy category: D

Indications and Dosages
▶ *To treat tonic-clonic and simple or complex partial seizures as initial or adjunct therapy, or when other drugs are ineffective*
TABLETS
Adults and adolescents. *Initial:* 500 mg to 1 g on the first day in 4 to 6 divided doses, increased over several days until desired response is reached. *Maintenance:* 2 to 3 g daily in 4 to 6 divided doses. *Maximum:* 3 g daily.
Children. *Initial:* Up to 750 mg daily, based on weight and age, in 4 to 6 divided doses, adjusted as needed and tolerated. *Maintenance:* 500 mg to 1 g daily in 4 to 6 divided doses. *Maximum:* 3 g daily.
DOSAGE ADJUSTMENT For debilitated patients, initial dosage lowered to reduce the risk of adverse reactions.

Route	Onset	Steady State	Peak	Half-Life	Duration
P.O.	Unknown	Unknown	Unknown	3 to 9 hr	Unknown

Mechanism of Action
Limits the spread of seizure activity and the start of new seizures by regulating voltage-dependent sodium and calcium channels in neurons, inhibiting calcium movement across neuronal membranes, and enhancing sodium-potassium adenosine triphosphatase activity in neurons and glial cells. These actions may result from ethotoin's ability to slow the recovery rate of inactivated sodium channels.

Contraindications
Hematologic disorders; hepatic dysfunction; hypersensitivity to ethotoin, phenytoin, other hydantoins, or their components

Interactions
DRUGS
acetaminophen: Increased risk of hepatotoxicity with long-term acetaminophen use

amiodarone: Possibly increased blood ethotoin level and risk of toxicity

antacids: Possibly decreased ethotoin effectiveness

bupropion, clozapine, loxapine, MAO inhibitors, maprotiline, phenothiazines, pimozide, thioxanthenes: Possibly lowered seizure threshold and decreased therapeutic effects of ethotoin; possibly intensified CNS depressant effects of these drugs

chloramphenicol, cimetidine, disulfiram, fluconazole, isoniazid, methylphenidate, metronidazole, omeprazole, phenylbutazone, ranitidine, salicylates, sulfonamides, trimethoprim: Possibly impaired metabolism of these drugs and increased risk of ethotoin toxicity

corticosteroids, cyclosporine, digoxin, disopyramide, doxycycline, furosemide, levodopa, mexiletine, quinidine: Decreased therapeutic effects of these drugs

diazoxide: Possibly decreased therapeutic effects of both drugs

estrogens, progestins: Decreased therapeutic effects of these drugs, increased blood ethotoin level

folic acid, leucovorin: Increased ethotoin metabolism, decreased seizure control

haloperidol: Possibly lowered seizure threshold and decreased ethotoin effects; possibly decreased blood haloperidol level

insulin, oral antidiabetic drugs: Possibly increased blood glucose level and decreased therapeutic effects of these drugs

lidocaine: Increased metabolism of lidocaine, leading to reduced concentration

methadone: Possibly increased methadone metabolism, leading to withdrawal signs and symptoms

molindone: Possibly lowered seizure threshold, impaired absorption, and decreased therapeutic effects of ethotoin

oral anticoagulants: Possibly impaired metabolism of these drugs and increased risk of ethotoin toxicity; possibly increased anticoagulant effect initially, but decreased effect with prolonged therapy

oral contraceptives containing estrogen and progestin: Possibly breakthrough bleeding and decreased contraceptive effectiveness

rifampin: Possibly decreased therapeutic effects of ethotoin

streptozocin: Possibly decreased therapeutic effects of streptozocin

sucralfate: Possibly decreased ethotoin absorption

tricyclic antidepressants: Possibly lowered seizure threshold and decreased therapeutic effects of ethotoin; possibly decreased blood level of tricyclic antidepressants

valproic acid: Possibly decreased blood ethotoin level, increased blood valproic acid level

vitamin D analogues: Decreased vitamin D analogue activity; risk of anticonvulsant-induced rickets and osteomalacia
xanthines: Possibly inhibited ethotoin absorption and increased clearance of xanthines
ACTIVITIES
alcohol use: Possibly decreased ethotoin effectiveness, enhanced CNS depressant effects

Adverse Reactions

CNS: Clumsiness, confusion, drowsiness, excitement, peripheral neuropathy, sedation, slurred speech, stuttering, tremor
EENT: Nystagmus
GI: Constipation, diarrhea, nausea, vomiting
HEME: Agranulocytosis, leukopenia, thrombocytopenia
SKIN: Rash, Stevens-Johnson syndrome, toxic epidermal necrolysis
Other: Lymphadenopathy, systemic lupus erythematosus

Overdose

Hydantoin overdose has no specific antidote. Monitor patient for signs and symptoms of overdose, including ataxia, blurred vision, confusion, dizziness, drowsiness, dysarthria, hyperreflexia, nausea, nystagmus, seizures, slurred speech, staggering, tiredness, tremor, and vomiting.

Maintain an open airway, and expect to give oxygen and a vasopressor, as prescribed, for cardiovascular, CNS, and respiratory depression. Take seizure precautions according to facility protocol.

Be prepared to induce vomiting or perform gastric lavage, and administer activated charcoal and cathartic, as prescribed, to decrease absorption. Be aware that dialysis, diuresis, exchange transfusions, and plasmapheresis are ineffective for treating hydantoin overdose because these drugs aren't eliminated by the kidneys.

Monitor patient's hematologic status following recovery because hydantoins may cause agranulocytosis, leukopenia, and thrombocytopenia. Institute suicide precautions according to facility policy, and anticipate psychiatric re-evaluation.

Nursing Considerations

• Obtain CBC and differential before treatment and at monthly intervals for the first few months of ethotoin therapy, as ordered.
• **WARNING** Be aware that ethotoin shouldn't be abruptly dis-

continued because doing so could cause status epilepticus. Plan to reduce dosage gradually or substitute another drug, as prescribed, when discontinuing ethotoin.

- Monitor patient for signs and symptoms of infection or unusual bleeding because ethotoin may cause hematologic toxicity.
- Because of ethotoin's potential for hepatotoxicity, monitor liver function test results, and expect drug to be discontinued if test results are abnormal.
- Notify prescriber immediately and expect ethotoin to be discontinued and substituted with another drug if depressed blood counts, enlarged lymph nodes, or rash develops.
- Be aware that ethotoin may be substituted for phenytoin without loss of seizure control if patient develops severe gum hyperplasia or other adverse effects. Expect ethotoin dosage to be four to six times greater than phenytoin dosage.
- Institute and maintain seizure precautions according to facility protocol.

PATIENT TEACHING

- Instruct patient to take ethotoin exactly as prescribed and not to abruptly discontinue it.
- Advise patient to take drug with food to enhance absorption and reduce adverse GI effects.
- Advise patient to report easy bruising, epistaxis, fever, malaise, petechiae, or sore throat to prescriber immediately.
- Instruct patient to keep medical appointments to monitor drug effectiveness and check for adverse reactions. Explain the need for periodic laboratory tests.
- Urge patient to avoid alcohol during therapy.
- Caution patient to avoid potentially hazardous activities until he knows how the drug affects him.
- Encourage patient to obtain medical identification indicating his diagnosis and drug therapy.

felbamate

Felbatol

Class and Category

Chemical class: Dicarbamate
Therapeutic class: Anticonvulsant
Pregnancy category: C

Indications and Dosages

▶ *To treat partial seizures in patients who don't respond to other drugs*

ORAL SUSPENSION, TABLETS

Adults and adolescents over age 14. *Initial:* 1,200 mg daily in divided doses t.i.d. or q.i.d. Dosage increased over several weeks based on patient response. *Maximum:* 3,600 mg daily.

Children ages 2 to 14. *Initial:* 15 mg/kg daily in divided doses t.i.d. or q.i.d. Dosage increased over several wk based on patient response. *Maximum:* 3,600 mg daily or 45 mg/kg daily.

▶ *As adjunct to treat generalized or partial seizures associated with Lennox-Gastaut syndrome in children*

ORAL SUSPENSION, TABLETS

Children ages 2 to 14. *Initial:* 15 mg/kg daily in divided doses t.i.d. or q.i.d. while decreasing other anticonvulsants by 20% to control blood levels. Felbamate dosage increased by 15 mg/kg daily every wk. *Maximum:* 3,600 mg daily or 45 mg/kg daily.

DOSAGE ADJUSTMENT Dosage reduced by 50% in patients with renal impairment.

Route	Onset	Steady State	Peak	Half-Life	Duration
P.O.	Unknown	Unknown	Unknown	13 to 23 hr	Unknown

Mechanism of Action

May exert anticonvulsant effects by antagonizing the amino acid glycine. When glycine binds to *N*-methyl-D-aspartate (NMDA) receptors in the CNS, receptor-gated calcium ion channels open more often—an important factor in initiating seizures. Felbamate may raise the seizure threshold by blocking NMDA receptors so that glycine can't bind to them.

Contraindications

Hepatic dysfunction; history of blood dyscrasias; hypersensitivity to felbamate, other carbamates, or their components

Interactions

DRUGS

carbamazepine: Decreased blood carbamazepine level and increased felbamate clearance, resulting in decreased blood felbamate level

fosphenytoin, phenytoin: Increased blood phenytoin level and increased felbamate clearance, resulting in decreased blood felbamate level

methsuximide: Increased adverse effects of methsuximide

oral contraceptives: Possibly decreased effectiveness of oral contraceptives

phenobarbital: Decreased blood felbamate level, increased blood phenobarbital level and risk of adverse effects

valproic acid: Increased blood valproic acid level and increased risk of adverse effects

Adverse Reactions

CNS: Abnormal gait, aggressiveness, agitation, anxiety, dizziness, drowsiness, fever, headache, insomnia, mood changes, tremor

EENT: Altered taste, diplopia, rhinitis

GI: Abdominal pain, anorexia, constipation, diarrhea, elevated liver function test results, hepatic failure, indigestion, nausea, vomiting

HEME: Aplastic anemia, leukopenia, pancytopenia, thrombocytopenia

RESP: Upper respiratory tract infection

SKIN: Photosensitivity, purpura, rash

Other: Anaphylaxis, lymphadenopathy, weight loss

Overdose

Information about felbamate overdose is limited, and the only signs and symptoms that have been reported include mild gastric distress and a resting heart rate of 100 beats/min.

Expect to give symptomatic and supportive care, as needed. To decrease absorption of the drug, be prepared to induce vomiting or perform gastric lavage. The effects of hemodialysis on felbamate overdose are unknown.

Institute suicide precautions according to facility policy, and anticipate psychiatric re-evaluation.

Nursing Considerations

- Check liver function test results before starting felbamate therapy, and expect to monitor test results every 1 to 2 weeks during treatment. Notify prescriber immediately and expect to discontinue drug if test results become abnormal.
- Plan to taper dosage by one-third every 4 to 5 days as prescribed. If patient receives adequate amounts of other anticonvulsant drugs, felbamate may be discontinued without tapering, if needed.
- **WARNING** Assess patient for signs and symptoms of aplastic anemia and bone marrow depression, which may occur with felbamate use. Signs and symptoms may not appear until several months after therapy begins. Expect to stop felbamate therapy if bone marrow depression develops.
- If patient receives adjunctive therapy, expect adverse reactions to resolve as other anticonvulsant dosages decrease.

PATIENT TEACHING
• Direct patient to shake suspension before using and to use a calibrated spoon or container to measure each dose.
• Instruct patient to store felbamate oral suspension and tablets at room temperature.
• Because drug may cause photosensitivity, urge patient to protect his skin from sun and to avoid sunlamps and tanning booths.
• Inform patient that dizziness and drowsiness may occur. Advise him to avoid potentially hazardous activities until he knows how the drug affects him.
• Warn patient not to stop taking felbamate abruptly.
• Advise patient to return for ordered liver function tests and to report yellow skin or eyes and dark urine to prescriber.
• Instruct patient to tell prescriber if he experiences bleeding, infection, or fatigue.
• Advise patient to carry medical identification that indicates his condition and drug therapy.
• Because felbamate decreases oral contraceptive effectiveness, discuss alternate contraceptive methods with female patient.

flumazenil

Anexate (CAN), Romazicon

Class and Category

Chemical class: Imidazobenzodiazepine derivative
Therapeutic class: Benzodiazepine antidote
Pregnancy category: C

Indications and Dosages

▶ *To reverse sedation from benzodiazepine therapy*
I.V. INJECTION
Adults. 0.2 mg, repeated after 45 to 60 sec if response is inadequate and then repeated every 1 min, if needed. If sedation recurs, regimen is repeated every 20 min or more. *Maximum:* 1 mg over 5 min or 3 mg in 1-hr period.
▶ *To reverse benzodiazepine toxicity or suspected overdose*
I.V. INJECTION
Adults. 0.2 mg followed by 0.3 mg 30 to 60 sec later if response is inadequate and then 0.5 mg repeated every 1 min. If sedation recurs, regimen is repeated every 20 min. *Maximum:* 3 mg in 1-hr period.

Route	Onset	Steady State	Peak	Half-Life	Duration
I.V.	1 to 2 min	Unknown	6 to 10 min	41 to 79 min	Variable

Mechanism of Action
Antagonizes the CNS effects of benzodiazepines by competing for their binding sites.

Contraindications
Evidence of tricyclic antidepressant overdose; hypersensitivity to flumazenil, benzodiazepines, or their components; use of benzodiazepine to control intracranial pressure, a potentially life-threatening condition, or status epilepticus

Interactions
DRUGS
benzodiazepines: Benzodiazepine withdrawal signs and symptoms, including seizures
tetracyclic or tricyclic antidepressant overdose: High risk of seizures
nonbenzodiazepine agonists: Loss of effectiveness of nonbenzodiazepine agonists
FOODS
all foods: Increased flumazenil clearance (by half) with food ingestion during I.V. injection

Adverse Reactions
CNS: Agitation, anxiety, ataxia, confusion, dizziness, drowsiness, emotional lability, fatigue, headache, hypoesthesia, insomnia, paresthesia, resedation, seizures, tremor, vertigo
CV: Hot flashes, hypertension, palpitations
EENT: Blurred vision, diplopia, dry mouth
GI: Nausea, vomiting
RESP: Dyspnea, hyperventilation, hypoventilation
SKIN: Diaphoresis, flushing, rash
Other: Injection site pain and thrombophlebitis

Overdose
Giving excessively high doses of flumazenil to reverse the effects of benzodiazepines may cause agitation, anxiety, hyperesthesia (increased sensitivity to sensory stimuli), increased muscle tone, and seizures. Expect to treat seizures with a barbiturate, a benzodiazepine, and phenytoin, as prescribed, and to institute seizure precautions according to facility protocol.

Be aware that no serious adverse reactions have been reported when high doses of flumazenil have been administered to patients who haven't taken a benzodiazepine.

Nursing Considerations

• Use flumazenil cautiously in patients with cardiac disease. Assess patient for increased stress or anxiety from benzodiazepine withdrawal because cardiac patient's blood pressure may rise.

• Give flumazenil undiluted or diluted in a syringe with D_5W, normal saline solution, or lactated Ringer's solution. Give over 15 to 30 seconds directly into tubing of a free-flowing compatible I.V. solution. Use a large vein, if possible, to minimize pain at site. Avoid extravasation because drug may irritate tissue.

• Be aware that drug may cause signs and symptoms of benzodiazepine withdrawal in drug-dependent patient. Also, abrupt awakening from benzodiazepine overdose can cause agitation, dysphoria, and increased adverse reactions.

• Be aware that benzodiazepine reversal may cause an anxiety or a panic attack for patient with a history of these episodes. Expect to adjust dosage carefully.

• Monitor patient for signs and symptoms of resedation and hypoventilation for at least 2 hours after giving flumazenil because drug has a short half-life. Be aware that patient shouldn't be discharged until the risk of resedation is gone.

PATIENT TEACHING

• Caution patient to avoid alcohol and OTC drugs for 10 to 24 hours after flumazenil administration.

• Advise patient to avoid potentially hazardous activities for 18 to 24 hours after discharge.

• Inform patient and family that agitation, emotional lability, fear, and panic attack (if patient has a history of them) may occur. Tell them to seek medical care for depression, trouble breathing, flushing, hyperventilation, insomnia, palpitations, and tremor.

• Because drug doesn't always reverse amnesia quickly, provide written instructions or instruct caregiver even if patient is alert.

fluoxetine hydrochloride

Prozac, Prozac Weekly, Sarafem

Class and Category

Chemical class: Phenylpropylamine derivative
Therapeutic class: Antibulimic drug, antidepressant, antiobsessional
Pregnancy category: C

Indications and Dosages

▶ *To treat depression*
CAPSULES, ORAL SOLUTION, TABLETS (PROZAC)
Adults. *Initial:* 20 mg daily in the morning. Dosage increased every 4 to 8 wk as needed. Dosage greater than 20 mg daily given b.i.d. morning and noon. *Maximum:* 80 mg daily.
Children age 8 and over and adolescents. *Initial:* 10 mg daily. Dosage increased after 1 wk to 20 mg daily.
DOSAGE ADJUSTMENT For lower-weight children, dosage increased to 20 mg daily only if improvement insufficient after several wk.
DELAYED-RELEASE CAPSULES (PROZAC WEEKLY)
Adults. 90 mg weekly, starting 7 days after last 20-mg daily dose.
▶ *To treat obsessive-compulsive disorder*
CAPSULES, ORAL SOLUTION, TABLETS (PROZAC)
Adults. *Initial:* 20 mg daily in the morning. Dosage increased every 4 to 8 wk as needed. Dosage greater than 20 mg daily given b.i.d. morning and noon. *Maximum:* 80 mg daily.
Children age 7 and over and adolescents. *Initial:* 10 mg daily. Dosage increased after 2 wk to 20 mg daily. Subsequent dosage increased, as needed, at intervals of at least several wk. *Maintenance:* 20 to 60 mg daily.
DOSAGE ADJUSTMENT For lower-weight children, dosage increased above 10 mg daily only if clinical improvement remains insufficient after several wk. Maintenance dosage for such patients should not exceed 30 mg daily.
▶ *To treat moderate to severe bulimia nervosa (Prozac)*
CAPSULES, ORAL SOLUTION, TABLETS
Adults. 60 mg daily in the morning. Some patients may be prescribed a lower dose, which is adjusted to 60 mg daily as tolerated.
▶ *To treat panic disorder with or without agoraphobia*
CAPSULES, ORAL SOLUTION, TABLETS (PROZAC)
Adults. *Initial:* 10 mg daily. Dosage increased in 1 wk to 20 mg daily, as needed. *Maximum:* 60 mg daily.
▶ *To treat premenstrual dysmorphic diosorder*
CAPSULES, (SARAFEM)
Adult women. 20 mg daily. Dosage increased as needed. *Maximum:* 80 mg daily.
DOSAGE ADJUSTMENT Dose or frequency reduced for patients with hepatic impairment or concurrent illness, those who take multiple medications, and for elderly patients.

Route	Onset	Steady State	Peak	Half-Life	Duration
P.O.*	1 to 6 wk†	4 wk	Unknown	4 to 6 days‡	Unknown

Mechanism of Action
Selectively inhibits reuptake of the neurotransmitter serotonin by CNS neurons and increases the amount of serotonin that's available in nerve synapses. An elevated serotonin level may result in elevated mood and, consequently, reduced depression.

Contraindications
Hypersensitivity to selective serotonin reuptake inhibitors or their components, pimozide therapy, use within 14 days of MAO inhibitor therapy

Interactions
DRUGS

alprazolam, diazepam: Possibly prolonged half-life of these drugs
aspirin, NSAIDs, warfarin: Increased anticoagulant activity and risk of bleeding
buspirone: Decreased buspirone effects
clozapine, fluphenazine, haloperidol, maprotiline, trazodone: Increased risk of adverse effects
CYP2D6-metabolized drugs, such as antiarrhythmics (especially flecainide, propafenone), selected antidepressants (tricyclics), antipyschotics (phenothiazines and most atypicals), thioridazine, and vinblastine: Increased plasma levels of these drugs and increased risk of serious adverse reactions
linezolid, lithium, serotonergics (such as amphetamines and other psychostimulants, antidepressants, and dopamine agonists), St. John's wort, tramadol, triptans: Increased risk of serotonin syndrome
MAO inhibitors: Possibly severe and life-threatening adverse effects
phenytoin: Increased blood phenytoin level and risk of toxicity
pimozide: Possibly bradycardia or prolonged QT interval
tricyclic antidepressants: Increased risk of adverse effects, including seizures
tryptophan: Increased risk of central and peripheral toxicity

Adverse Reactions
CNS: Anxiety, chills, dream disturbances, drowsiness, fatigue,

---

* Capsules, oral solution, and tablets.
† For depression and bulimia; 5 wk for obsessive-compulsive disorder.
‡ For long-term administration; 1 to 3 days for single dose.

fever, headache, hypomania, insomnia, mania, nervousness, restlessness, seizures, somnolence, suicidal ideation, tremor, vertigo, weakness, yawning

CV: Hypotension, palpitations

EENT: Abnormal vision, dry mouth, pharyngitis, sinusitis

ENDO: Galactorrhea, gynecomastia, hypoglycemia

GI: Anorexia, diarrhea, indigestion, nausea

GU: Decreased libido, ejaculation disorders, impotence

HEME: Altered platelet function, unusual bleeding

MS: Arthralgia, myalgia

RESP: Dyspnea

SKIN: Diaphoresis, erythema multiforme, pruritus, rash, urticaria

Other: Flulike signs and symptoms, hyponatremia, weight loss

Overdose

Fluoxetine overdose has no specific antidote. Monitor patient for signs and symptoms of overdose, including agitation, drowsiness, hypomania (talking or acting with uncontrolled excitement), nausea, restlessness, seizures, tachycardia, tremor, and vomiting.

Maintain an open airway, institute continuous ECG monitoring, and maintain patient's temperature. Expect to treat seizures with an anticonvulsant, such as diazepam, as prescribed, and institute seizure precautions according to facility protocol.

To decrease absorption of drug, be prepared to perform gastric lavage with appropriate airway protection. Expect that activated charcoal with sorbitol may be prescribed. Induced vomiting isn't recommended. Be aware that dialysis, forced diuresis, exchange transfusions, and hemoperfusion are ineffective for treating fluoxetine overdose because the drug is highly protein bound and has a large volume of distribution in the body.

If the patient has also ingested a tricyclic antidepressant, monitor him for signs and symptoms of tricyclic antidepressant toxicity, including constipation, dry mouth, light-headedness, memory loss, slowed thinking and acting, and sedation. Fluoxetine inhibits the metabolism of the tricyclic antidepressant, so these effects may be observed for 3 weeks or more.

Institute suicide precautions according to facility policy, and anticipate psychiatric re-evaluation.

Nursing Considerations

• Use fluoxetine cautiously in patients with a history of seizures.

• **WARNING** Avoid giving fluoxetine within 14 days of an MAO inhibitor or starting MAO inhibitor therapy within

5 weeks of discontinuing fluoxetine.

- **WARNING** If patient takes another drug that raises serotonin level (such as an amphetamine or other psychostimulant, a dopamine agonist, a triptan, another antidepressant, or tryptophan), assess him for serotonin syndrome, a rare but serious adverse effect of selective serotonin reuptake inhibitors. Signs and symptoms include agitation, autonomic instability (such as tachycardia, labile blood pressure, hyperthemia), confusion, diaphoresis, diarrhea, fever, hyperactive reflexes, poor coordination, restlessness, shaking, talking or acting with uncontrolled excitement, tremor, twitching, and vomiting.

- If patient takes fluoxetine for depression (particularly a child or an adolescent), monitor him closely for suicidal tendencies, especially when therapy starts and dosage changes, because depression may temporarily worsen during these times.

- Monitor patient closely for evidence of GI bleeding, especially if he takes a drug known to cause it, such as aspirin, an NSAID, or warfarin.

- Monitor patients with diabetes mellitus for altered blood glucose levels because drug may cause hypoglycemia during therapy and hyperglycemia when therapy stops. Expect to adjust dosage of antidiabetic drug, as prescribed.

- Check patient's serum sodium level, as ordered, because fluoxetine may lower it, especially in elderly patients or those who take diuretics or have volume depletion. If hyponatremia develops, notify prescriber and expect to provide supportive care, which may include discontinuation of fluoxetine.

- Expect patient taking drug for PMDD to be re-evaluated in 6 months to determine whether fluoxetine therapy should be continued.

- When drug is no longer needed, expect to taper dosage, as ordered, to minimize adverse reactions.

PATIENT TEACHING

- Instruct family or caregiver to observe patient closely for suicidal tendencies, especially when therapy starts or dosage changes, and particularly if patient is a child or teenager.

- Warn patient not to abruptly stop taking fluoxetine because serious adverse effects can occur.

- **WARNING** Inform patient that fluoxetine increases the risk of serotonin syndrome, a rare but serious complication. Teach patient to recognize its signs and symptoms, including diaphoresis, diarrhea, fever, hyperactive reflexes, mood changes,

rapid heart rate, restlessness, and shivering or shaking, and advise him to notify prescriber immediately if they occur.
- Caution patient to avoid potentially hazardous activities until he knows how the drug affects him.
- Advise patient to consult prescriber if he intends to take an OTC or prescription drug, if he develops a rash or hives or, for female patient, if she becomes or intends to become pregnant during therapy.
- Explain that drug may take several weeks to reach full effect.
- Instruct patient to schedule and maintain follow-up appointments for re-evaluation of signs and symptoms.
- Urge patient to notify prescriber if he develops a rash or hives.

fluphenazine decanoate
Modecate (CAN), Modecate Concentrate (CAN), Prolixin Decanoate
fluphenazine enanthate
Moditen Enanthate (CAN), Prolixin Enanthate
fluphenazine hydrochloride
Apo-Fluphenazine (CAN), Moditen HCl (CAN), Permitil, Permitil Concentrate, PMS Fluphenazine (CAN), Prolixin, Prolixin Concentrate

Class and Category
Chemical class: Phenothiazine, propylpiperazine derivative
Therapeutic class: Antipsychotic drug
Pregnancy category: Not rated

Indications and Dosages
▶ *To control psychotic disorders*
ELIXIR, ORAL SOLUTION, TABLETS (FLUPHENAZINE HYDROCHLORIDE)
Adults and adolescents. *Initial:* 2.5 to 10 mg daily in divided doses every 6 to 8 hr. When signs and symptoms are controlled, dosage reduced to 1 to 5 mg daily. *Maximum:* 20 mg/dose with caution.
Children. 250 to 750 mcg once daily to q.i.d.
I.M. INJECTION (FLUPHENAZINE HYDROCHLORIDE)
Adults and adolescents. *Initial:* 1.25 mg, increased based on patient response up to 2.5 to 10 mg daily in divided doses every 6 to 8 hr. *Maximum:* 10 mg daily.
DOSAGE ADJUSTMENT For elderly or debilitated patients, dosage reduced to 1 to 2.5 mg daily in divided doses every 6 to 8 hr.

I.M. OR SUBCUTANEOUS INJECTION (FLUPHENAZINE DECANOATE OR ENANTHATE)
Adults. *Initial:* 12.5 to 25 mg every 1 to 4 wk, as needed (decanoate). For doses over 50 mg, next dose increased cautiously by 12.5 mg. Or 25 mg every 2 wk, with dose and dosing interval adjusted based on patient response (enanthate). *Maximum:* 100 mg/dose.
Adolescents and children over age 12. *Initial:* 6.25 to 18.75 mg/wk (decanoate), increased to 12.5 to 25 mg every 1 to 3 wk, based on patient response.
Children ages 5 to 12. 3.125 to 12.5 mg every 1 to 3 wk (decanoate), based on patient response.

Route	Onset	Steady State	Peak	Half-Life	Duration
P.O.	In 1 hr	4 to 7 days	Variable	14 to 15 hr	6 to 8 hr
I.M.*	In 1 hr	Unknown	Variable	14 to 15 hr	6 to 8 hr
I.M., SubQ†	In 24 to 72 hr	4 to 6 wk	Variable	6 to 10 days‡	1 to 6 wk§

Mechanism of Action
May block postsynaptic dopamine$_2$ (D$_2$) receptor sites in the CNS. This action may depress areas of the brain that control activity and aggression, including the cerebral cortex, hypothalamus, and limbic system.

Incompatibilities
Don't mix fluphenazine hydrochloride oral solution with caffeine-containing beverages, such as coffee and cola; pectins, such as apple juice; or tannins, such as tea. They're physically incompatible.

Contraindications
Blood dyscrasias, bone marrow depression, cerebral arteriosclerosis, coma, concomitant use of large amounts of another CNS depressant, coronary artery disease, hepatic dysfunction, hypersensitivity to phenothiazines, myeloproliferative disorders, severe CNS depression, severe hypertension or hypotension, subcortical brain damage

---

* For hydrochloride.
† For decanoate and enanthate.
‡ For decanoate; 3.6 days for enanthate.
§ For decanoate; 2 wk for enanthate.

Interactions
DRUGS
adsorbent antidiarrheals, antacids (aluminum- and magnesium-containing): Possibly inhibited absorption of fluphenazine
amantadine, anticholinergics: Possibly intensified adverse effects of both drugs
amphetamines: Possibly decreased therapeutic effects of both drugs
antihypertensives: Possibly severe hypotension
antithyroid drugs: Increased risk of agranulocytosis
beta blockers: Possibly increased blood levels and risk of adverse effects of both drugs
bromocriptine: Decreased bromocriptine effects
CNS depressants: Possibly prolonged and intensified CNS depression
erythromycin: Possibly inhibited fluphenazine metabolism
guanethidine: Decreased hypotensive effect of guanethidine
levodopa: Possibly decreased antidyskinetic effect of levodopa
lithium: Possibly neurotoxicity (disorientation, extrapyramidal reactions, unconsciousness)
meperidine: Excessive sedation and hypotension
metrizamide: Increased risk of seizures when injected in subarachnoid area during fluphenazine therapy
oral anticoagulants: Possibly decreased anticoagulant effects
pimozide, other drugs that prolong QT interval: Prolonged QT interval and risk of arrhythmias
thiazide diuretics: Increased risk of hyponatremia, hypotension, and water intoxication
tricyclic antidepressants: Possibly prolonged and intensified sedation
ACTIVITIES
alcohol use: Possibly increased CNS depression and increased risk of heatstroke

Adverse Reactions
CNS: Ataxia, cerebral edema, dizziness, drowsiness, headache, insomnia, lightheadedness, nervousness, seizures, slurred speech, syncope, worsening psychotic signs and symptoms
CV: AV conduction disorders, bradycardia, cardiac arrest, hypercholesterolemia, hypertension, orthostatic hypotension, prolonged QT interval, shock, ST-segment depression, tachycardia
EENT: Blurred vision, dry mouth, glaucoma, increased salivation, laryngeal edema, laryngospasm, miosis, mydriasis, nasal congestion, papillary hypertrophy of the tongue, parotid gland enlargement, photophobia, pigmentary retinopathy, ptosis
ENDO: Breast engorgement (females), galactorrhea, hyper-

glycemia, hypoglycemia, mastalgia, syndrome of inappropriate ADH secretion

GI: Anorexia, constipation, diarrhea, fecal impaction, ileus, increased appetite, nausea, vomiting

GU: Amenorrhea, bladder paralysis, decreased libido, enuresis, menstrual irregularities, polyuria, urinary frequency, urinary incontinence, urine retention

HEME: Anemia, aplastic anemia, eosinophilia, leukopenia, thrombocytopenia, thrombocytopenic or nonthrombocytopenic purpura

RESP: Bronchospasm, dyspnea, increased respiratory depth

SKIN: Contact dermatitis, dry skin, eczema, erythema, jaundice, photosensitivity, pruritus, seborrhea

Other: Heatstroke, hyponatremia, lupuslike signs and symptoms, weight gain

Overdose

Monitor patient for signs and symptoms of overdose, including agitation, areflexia or hyperreflexia, arrhythmias, blurred vision, cardiac arrest, CNS toxicity, coma, confusion, disorientation, drowsiness, dry mouth, dyspnea, heart failure, hyperpyrexia, hypotension, hypothermia, mydriasis, pulmonary edema, QRS complex changes, respiratory depression, seizures, shock, stupor, tachycardia, ventricular fibrillation, and vomiting.

Maintain an open airway, monitor patient for arrhythmias, and maintain temperature. Institute seizure precautions according to facility protocol. Expect to administer phenytoin to control arrhythmias and norepinephrine or phenylephrine and I.V. fluids to treat hypotension, as prescribed. Epinephrine shouldn't be used because of risk of paradoxical hypotension. Anticipate digitalizing patient for heart failure, as prescribed. To manage seizures, expect to administer diazepam, followed by phenytoin. Avoid barbiturates because they may potentiate respiratory and CNS depression.

Perform gastric lavage, and administer activated charcoal, as prescribed. Be aware that vomiting shouldn't be induced because of the potential for impaired consciousness or dystonic reactions of the head and neck. Anticipate administering benztropine or diphenhydramine, as prescribed, to manage acute parkinsonian effects. Dialysis is ineffective for treating phenothiazine overdose. Expect to continue ECG monitoring for at least 5 days. Be aware that phenothiazine tablets are visible on X-ray.

Institute suicide precautions according to facility policy, and anticipate psychiatric re-evaluation.

Nursing Considerations
• Use fluphenazine cautiously in patients with a history of glaucoma or renal impairment.
• For I.M. and subcutaneous injection, use at least a 21G needle.
• Monitor temperature; a significant, unexplained rise can indicate intolerance and a need to discontinue drug. Notify prescriber immediately if this occurs.
• Assess patient for signs of hepatic failure, such as jaundice.
• Notify prescriber about worsening psychotic signs and symptoms: agitation, catatonic state, confusion, depression, hallucinations, lethargy, paranoid reactions.

PATIENT TEACHING
• If patient takes elixir form , instruct him to keep it in an amber or opaque bottle because drug is sensitive to light.
• Tell patient not to mix oral solution with beverages that contain caffeine (coffee, cola), pectins (apple juice), or tannins (tea).
• Warn patient that he may become dizzy or lightheaded.
• Teach patient how to prevent heatstroke, orthostatic hypotension, and photosensitivity reactions.
• Warn patient not to stop taking fluphenazine abruptly.

flurazepam hydrochloride
Apo-Flurazepam (CAN), Dalmane, Novo-Flupam (CAN), Somnol (CAN)

Class, Category, and Schedule
Chemical class: Benzodiazepine
Therapeutic class: Sedative-hypnotic
Pregnancy category: Not rated
Controlled substance schedule: IV

Indications and Dosages
▶ *To treat insomnia characterized by difficulty falling asleep, frequent nocturnal awakenings, or early-morning awakening*
CAPSULES
Adults. 15 to 30 mg at bedtime.
DOSAGE ADJUSTMENT Initial dose reduced to 15 mg for elderly or debilitated patients until individual response is known.

Route	Onset	Steady State	Peak	Half-Life	Duration
P.O.	15 to 45 min	7 to 10 days	Unknown	2 to 3 hr*	7 to 8 hr

Mechanism of Action

May potentiate the effects of gamma-aminobutyric acid (GABA) and other inhibitory neurotransmitters by binding to specific benzodiazepine receptor sites in the limbic and cortical areas of the CNS. By binding to these receptor sites, flurazepam increases GABA's inhibitory effects and blocks cortical and limbic arousal.

Contraindications

Acute angle-closure glaucoma, breast-feeding, hypersensitivity to other benzodiazepines, itraconazole or ketoconazole therapy, psychosis

Interactions

DRUGS

cimetidine, diltiazem, disulfiram, erythromycin, fluoxetine, fluvoxamine, itraconazole, nefazodone, estrogen-containing oral contraceptives, propoxyphene, ranitidine, verapamil: Possibly increased blood level and impaired hepatic metabolism of flurazepam

clozapine: Possibly cardiac arrest or respiratory depression

CNS depressants: Possibly potentiated CNS depression

levodopa: Possibly decreased therapeutic effects of levodopa

FOODS

grapefruit juice: Possibly increased blood level and impaired hepatic metabolism of flurazepam

ACTIVITIES

alcohol use: Possibly potentiated CNS and respiratory depression

Adverse Reactions

CNS: Amnesia, anxiety, ataxia, confusion, delusions, depression, dizziness, drowsiness, euphoria, headache, hypokinesia, irritability, malaise, nervousness, sleep-driving, slurred speech, tremor

CV: Chest pain, palpitations, tachycardia

EENT: Blurred vision, dry mouth, increased salivation, photophobia

GI: Abdominal pain, constipation, diarrhea, nausea, thirst, vomiting

GU: Libido changes

SKIN: Diaphoresis

Other: Anaphylaxis, angioedema, physical or psychological dependence

---

* 47 to 100 hr for active metabolite, N-desalkylflurazepam.

Overdose

Monitor patient for signs and symptoms of overdose, including bradycardia, coma, confusion, dyspnea, hyporeflexia, seizures, severe drowsiness, shakiness, slurred speech, staggering, and weakness.

Maintain an open airway, institute continuous cardiac monitoring, and administer continuous I.V. fluids, as prescribed, to maintain blood pressure and promote diuresis. Institute seizure precautions according to facility protocol.

To decrease absorption of drug in a conscious patient who isn't at risk for coma or seizures, be prepared to induce vomiting or perform gastric lavage. Expect that oral activated charcoal may also be prescribed.

For an unconscious patient, anticipate assisting with the insertion of an endotracheal tube and then performing gastric lavage. The inflated cuff of the endotracheal tube will help prevent aspiration of gastric contents into the lungs.

Anticipate the use of a benzodiazepine receptor antagonist, such as flumazenil, to reverse the sedative effects. Be aware that flumazenil may induce seizures, especially in a patient who has been using benzodiazepines long-term or one who has also ingested a cyclic antidepressant. If excitation occurs, be aware that a barbiturate shouldn't be used because it may increase excitement and prolong CNS depression. Dialysis is ineffective for treating benzodiazepine overdose.

Institute suicide precautions according to facility policy, and anticipate psychiatric re-evaluation.

Nursing Considerations

• Use flurazepam cautiously in patients with severe mental depression or reduced respiratory function; drug may intensify depression and lead to respiratory depression.
• Expect to use lowest effective dose in elderly or debilitated patients to minimize the risk of ataxia, confusion, dizziness, and oversedation.
• Monitor liver function test results, as appropriate.
• **WARNING** Monitor patient closely for allergic reactions that, although rare, may be severe. If patient develops dyspnea, throat closing, or nausea and vomiting, notify prescriber immediately and be prepared to stop flurazepam and provide airway management and other emergency care as needed.
• Monitor patient for worsening of insomnia or the emergence of thinking or behavior abnormalities because flurazepam may unmask their existence requiring a more extensive work up.

PATIENT TEACHING
• Instruct patient not to exceed prescribed flurazepam dosage and not to stop drug abruptly.
• Warn patient that drug may cause morning dizziness or drowsiness.
• Because flurazepam can reduce alertness, advise patient to avoid potentially hazardous activities until he knows how the drug affects him.
• Caution patient to avoid alcohol and CNS depressants during therapy.
• Advise female patient to notify prescriber if she becomes or intends to become pregnant during therapy.
• Inform patient that flurazepam becomes increasingly effective on the second or third consecutive night of use.
• Inform patient that his sleep may be disturbed for the first few nights after stopping drug.
• Advise patient to notify prescriber if insomnia lasts longer than 7 days despite flurazepam therapy.
• Tell family to report sleep-driving, in which patient drives while not fully awake, usually with no recall of the event.
• Advise patient to stop drug and seek emergency care immediately if he experiences difficulty breathing, throat closing, or nausea and vomiting.

fluvoxamine maleate
Luvox, Luvox CR

Class and Category
Chemical class: Aralkylketone derivative
Therapeutic class: Antiobsessional drug, antianxiety drug
Pregnancy category: C

Indications and Dosages
▶ *To treat social anxiety disorder*
E.R. CAPSULES
Adults. 100 mg at bedtime, increased in 50-mg increments once weekly, as needed. *Maximum:* 300 mg daily.
▶ *To treat obsessive-compulsive disorder*
TABLETS
Adults. *Initial:* 50 mg at bedtime, increased by 50 mg every 4 to 7 days, if needed. *Maximum:* 300 mg daily.
Children ages 8 to 17. *Initial:* 25 mg at bedtime, increased by 25 mg every 4 to 7 days, if needed. *Maximum:* 200 mg daily.

E R. CAPSULES

Adults. 100 mg at bedtime, increased in 50-mg increments once weekly, as needed. *Maximum:* 300 mg daily.

DOSAGE ADJUSTMENT Doses divided for adults taking more than 100 mg daily of tablet form and children taking more than 50 mg daily; given in 2 equal doses b.i.d. or 2 unequal doses with larger dose at bedtime.

Route	Onset	Steady State	Peak	Half-Life	Duration
P.O.	3 to 10 wk	10 days	Unknown	15 to 20 hr	Unknown

Mechanism of Action

May potentiate serotonin's action by blocking its reuptake at neuronal membranes. An elevated serotonin level may result in elevated mood and, consequently, reduced depression and anxiety, which commonly accompany obsessive-compulsive disorder.

Contraindications

Alosetron, astemizole, cisapride, pimozide, terfenadine, thioridazine, or tizanidine therapy; hypersensitivity to fluvoxamine maleate or its components; use within 14 days of MAO inhibitor therapy

Interactions

DRUGS

alosetron: Increased plasma alosetron level

alprazolam: Increased plasma alprazolam level

antihistamines: Increased risk of impaired mental and motor skills

astemizole, cisapride, terfenadine: Possibly fatal prolonged QT interval

benzodiazepines: Decreased benzodiazepine clearance, possibly impaired memory and motor skills

buspirone: Decreased buspirone effects, increased blood fluvoxamine level, paradoxical worsening of obsessive-compulsive disorder

carbamazepine: Increased risk of carbamazepine toxicity

clozapine: Increased blood clozapine level

diltiazem: Increased risk of bradycardia

haloperidol: Increased blood haloperidol level, possibly delayed recall and reduced memory and attention span

lithium: Possibly increased serotonin reuptake action of fluvoxamine

MAO inhibitors: Possibly serious or fatal reactions (such as agitation, autonomic instability, coma, delirium, fluctuating vital signs, hyperthermia, myoclonus, and rigidity)

methadone: Possibly significantly increased blood methadone level, increased risk of methadone toxicity

metoprolol, propranolol: Increased blood levels of these drugs, possibly reduced diastolic blood pressure and heart rate induced by these drugs

serotonergics (such as amphetamines and other psychostimulants, antidepressants, and dopamine agonists): Serotonin syndrome

sympathomimetics: Possibly increased effects of sympathomimetics and increased risk of serotonin syndrome

tacrine: Increased blood level and therapeutic and adverse effects of tacrine

theophylline: Decreased theophylline clearance, increased risk of theophylline toxicity

tricyclic antidepressants: Increased blood levels of antidepressants

warfarin: Increased blood warfarin level, prolonged PT

FOODS

caffeine: Possibly decreased hepatic clearance of caffeine

ACTIVITIES

smoking: Increased fluvoxamine metabolism

Adverse Reactions

CNS: Agitation, anxiety, apathy, chills, confusion, depression, dizziness, drowsiness, fatigue, headache, hypomania, insomnia, malaise, mania, nervousness, sedation, tremor, vertigo, yawning

CV: Palpitations, tachycardia

EENT: Altered taste, blurred vision, dry mouth

GI: Anorexia, constipation, diarrhea, flatulence, indigestion, nausea, vomiting

GU: Decreased libido, ejaculation disorders, impotence, urinary frequency, urine retention

MS: Muscle twitching

RESP: Dyspnea, upper respiratory tract infection

SKIN: Diaphoresis, rash

Other: Flulike signs and symptoms, weight gain

Overdose

Fluvoxamine overdose has no specific antidote. Monitor patient for signs and symptoms of overdose, including abnormal liver function test results, bradycardia, coma, diarrhea, dizziness, dry mouth, ECG changes, hypotension, mydriasis, myoclonus, seizures, tachycardia, tremor, and urine retention.

Maintain an open airway, and institute continuous ECG monitoring. Expect to continue monitoring patient for 48 hours because absorption of drug may be delayed. Be alert to the possibility that the patient also may have ingested other drugs. Institute seizure precautions according to facility protocol.

To decrease absorption of drug, be prepared to induce vomiting or perform gastric lavage. Expect that activated charcoal may be prescribed for up to 24 hours after overdose because drug absorption may be delayed. Be aware that dialysis and forced diuresis are ineffective for treating the overdose because fluvoxamine is extensively distributed in the tissues.

Institute suicide precautions according to facility policy, and anticipate psychiatric re-evaluation.

Nursing Considerations
- Use fluvoxamine cautiously in patients with cardiovascular disease, impaired hepatic or renal function, mania, seizures, or suicidal tendencies.
- **WARNING** Be aware that fluvoxamine shouldn't be given within 14 days of an MAO inhibitor.
- **WARNING** If patient receives another drug that raises the serotonin level by a different mechanism, assess him for serotonin syndrome, a rare but serious complication of certain selective serotonin reuptake inhibitors. Signs and symptoms include agitation, confusion, diaphoresis, diarrhea, fever, hyperactive reflexes, lack of coordination, muscle twitching, restlessness, shivering, talking or acting with uncontrolled excitement, and tremor. Drugs that raise the serotonin level include amphetamines and other psychostimulants, antidepressants (buspirone, lithium), dopamine agonists, MAO inhibitors, and tryptophan.

PATIENT TEACHING
- Caution patient not to drink alcohol during therapy.
- Advise patient to avoid potentially hazardous activities until he knows how the drug affects him.
- **WARNING** Inform patient that fluvoxamine increases the risk of the rare but serious serotonin syndrome. Encourage him to notify the prescriber immediately if signs and symptoms develop.
- Caution patient not to stop taking fluvoxamine abruptly. Explain that gradual tapering helps avoid withdrawal signs and symptoms.
- If patient takes extended-release capsules, instruct him to swallow them whole and not to crush or chew them.

fosphenytoin sodium

Cerebyx

Class and Category

Chemical class: Hydantoin derivative
Therapeutic class: Anticonvulsant
Pregnancy category: D

Indications and Dosages

▶ *To treat status epilepticus*

I.V. INFUSION, I.M. INJECTION

Adults and adolescents. *Initial:* 15 to 20 mg of phenytoin equivalent (PE)/kg I.V. at 100 to 150 PE/min. *Maintenance:* 4 to 6 mg PE/kg daily I.V. or I.M. in divided doses b.i.d. to q.i.d. *Maximum:* 30 mg PE/kg as total loading dose.

Children. *Initial:* 15 to 20 mg PE/kg I.V. given at up to 3 mg PE/kg/min. *Maintenance:* 4 to 6 mg PE/kg daily I.V. or I.M. in divided doses b.i.d. to q.i.d.

▶ *To prevent or treat seizures during and after neurosurgery*

I.V. INFUSION, I.M. INJECTION

Adults and adolescents. *Initial:* 10 to 20 mg PE/kg I.V., not to exceed 150 mg PE/min. *Maintenance:* 4 to 6 mg PE/kg daily I.V. or I.M. in divided doses b.i.d. to q.i.d. *Maximum:* 30 mg PE/kg as total loading dose.

Route	Onset	Steady State	Peak	Half-Life	Duration
I.V.	Unknown	Unknown	Unknown	8 to 15 min*	Unknown

Mechanism of Action

Is converted from fosphenytoin (a prodrug) to phenytoin, which limits the spread of seizure activity and the start of new seizures by regulating voltage-dependent sodium and calcium channels in neurons, inhibiting calcium movement across neuronal membranes, and enhancing the sodium-potassium adenosine triphosphatase activity in neurons and glial cells. These actions may stem from phenytoin's ability to slow the recovery rate of inactivated sodium channels.

Contraindications

Hypersensitivity to fosphenytoin, phenytoin, other hydantoins, or their components

---

* Conversion half-life of fosphenytoin to phenytoin.

Interactions

DRUGS

acetaminophen (long-term use): Increased risk of hepatotoxicity
acyclovir: Decreased blood phenytoin level, loss of seizure control
alfentanil: Increased clearance and decreased effectiveness of alfentanil
amiodarone, fluoxetine: Possibly increased blood phenytoin level and risk of toxicity
antacids: Possibly decreased phenytoin effectiveness
antineoplastics: Increased phenytoin metabolism
beta blockers: Increased myocardial depression
bupropion, clozapine, loxapine, MAO inhibitors, maprotiline, phenothiazines, pimozide, thioxanthenes: Possibly lowered seizure threshold and decreased therapeutic effects of phenytoin, possibly intensified CNS depressant effects of these drugs
calcium: Possibly impaired phenytoin absorption
calcium channel blockers: Possibly increased blood phenytoin level
carbamazepine: Decreased blood carbamazepine level, possibly increased blood phenytoin level and risk of toxicity
chloramphenicol, cimetidine, disulfiram, isoniazid, methylphenidate, metronidazole, phenylbutazone, ranitidine, salicylates, sulfonamides, trimethoprim: Possibly impaired metabolism of these drugs, increased risk of phenytoin toxicity
CNS depressants: Possibly increased CNS depression
contraceptives (estrogen- and progestin-containing): Possibly breakthrough bleeding and decreased contraceptive effectiveness
corticosteroids, cyclosporine, digoxin, disopyramide, doxycycline, furosemide, levodopa, mexiletine, quinidine: Decreased therapeutic effects of these drugs
diazoxide: Possibly decreased therapeutic effects of both drugs
dopamine: Possibly sudden hypotension or cardiac arrest after I.V. fosphenytoin administration
estrogens, progestins: Decreased therapeutic effects, increased blood phenytoin level
felbamate: Possibly impaired metabolism and increased blood level of phenytoin
fluconazole, itraconazole, ketoconazole, miconazole: Increased blood phenytoin level
folic acid: Increased phenytoin metabolism, decreased seizure control
haloperidol: Possibly lowered seizure threshold and decreased phenytoin effects; possibly decreased blood haloperidol level

insulin, oral antidiabetic drugs: Possibly increased blood glucose level and decreased therapeutic effects of these drugs

lamotrigine: Possibly decreased therapeutic effects of lamotrigine

lidocaine: Possibly decreased blood lidocaine level, increased myocardial depression

lithium: Increased risk of lithium toxicity

methadone: Possibly increased methadone metabolism, leading to withdrawal signs and symptoms

molindone: Possibly lowered seizure threshold, impaired absorption, and decreased therapeutic effects of phenytoin

omeprazole: Possibly increased blood phenytoin level

oral anticoagulants: Possibly impaired metabolism of these drugs and increased risk of phenytoin toxicity; possibly increased anticoagulant effects initially and then decreased effects with prolonged therapy

rifampin: Possibly decreased therapeutic effects of phenytoin

streptozocin: Possibly decreased therapeutic effects of streptozocin

sucralfate: Possibly decreased phenytoin absorption

tricyclic antidepressants: Possibly lowered seizure threshold and decreased therapeutic effects of phenytoin; possibly decreased blood antidepressant level

valproic acid: Decreased blood phenytoin level, increased blood valproic acid level

vitamin D analogues: Decreased vitamin D analogue activity

xanthines: Possibly inhibited phenytoin absorption and increased clearance of xanthines

zaleplon: Increased clearance and decreased effectiveness of zaleplon

ACTIVITIES

alcohol use: Possibly decreased phenytoin effectiveness

Adverse Reactions

CNS: Agitation, amnesia, asthenia, ataxia, cerebral edema, chills, coma, confusion, CVA, delusions, depression, dizziness, emotional lability, encephalitis, encephalopathy, extrapyramidal reactions, fever, headache, hemiplegia, hostility, hypoesthesia, lack of coordination, malaise, meningitis, nervousness, neurosis, paralysis, personality disorder, positive Babinski's sign, seizures, somnolence, speech disorders, stupor, subdural hematoma, syncope, transient paresthesia, tremor, vertigo

CV: Atrial flutter, bradycardia, bundle-branch block, cardiac arrest, cardiomegaly, edema, heart failure, hypertension, hypotension, orthostatic hypotension, palpitations, PVCs, shock, tachycardia, thrombophlebitis

EENT: Amblyopia, conjunctivitis, diplopia, dry mouth, earache, epistaxis, eye pain, gingival hyperplasia, hearing loss, hyperacusis, increased salivation, loss of taste, mydriasis, nystagmus, pharyngitis, photophobia, rhinitis, sinusitis, taste perversion, tinnitus, tongue swelling, visual field defects
ENDO: Diabetes insipidus, hyperglycemia, ketosis
GI: Anorexia, constipation, diarrhea, dysphagia, elevated liver function test results, flatulence, gastritis, GI bleeding, hepatic necrosis, hepatitis, ileus, indigestion, nausea, vomiting
GU: Albuminuria, dysuria, incontinence, oliguria, polyuria, renal failure, urine retention, vaginal candidiasis
HEME: Anemia, easy bruising, leukopenia, thrombocytopenia
MS: Arthralgia, back pain, leg cramps, muscle twitching, myalgia, myasthenia, myoclonus, myopathy
RESP: Apnea, asthma, atelectasis, bronchitis, dyspnea, hemoptysis, hyperventilation, hypoxia, increased cough, increased sputum production, pneumonia, pneumothorax
SKIN: Contact dermatitis, diaphoresis, maculopapular or pustular rash, photosensitivity, skin discoloration, skin nodule, Stevens-Johnson syndrome, transient pruritus, urticaria
Other: Cachexia, cryptococcosis, dehydration, facial edema, flulike signs and symptoms, hyperkalemia, hypokalemia, hypophosphatemia, infection, injection site reaction, lymphadenopathy, sepsis

Overdose
Fosphenytoin overdose has no specific antidote. Monitor patient for signs and symptoms of overdose, including ataxia, blurred vision, confusion, dizziness, drowsiness, dysarthria, hyperreflexia, nausea, nystagmus, seizures, slurred speech, staggering, tiredness, tremor, and vomiting.

Maintain an open airway, and expect to give oxygen and a vasopressor, as prescribed, for cardiovascular, CNS, and respiratory depression. Take seizure precautions according to facility protocol.

Be prepared to induce vomiting or perform gastric lavage and administer activated charcoal and a cathartic, as prescribed, to decrease absorption. Be aware that dialysis, diuresis, exchange transfusions, and plasmapheresis are ineffective for treating fosphenytoin overdose because the drug isn't eliminated by the kidneys.

The metabolites of fosphenytoin may contribute to toxicity, causing metabolic acidosis and an elevated serum phosphate level. Because phosphate toxicity can lead to hypocalcemia, monitor patient's ionized calcium level, and assess him for signs and symptoms of hypocalcemia, including muscle spasms, paresthesia, and seizures. Monitor patient's hematologic status following recovery because fosphenytoin may cause agranulocytosis, leukopenia, and thrombocytopenia.

Institute suicide precautions according to facility policy, and anticipate psychiatric re-evaluation.

Nursing Considerations

- Express the dosage, concentration, and infusion rate of fosphenytoin in PE units. Misreading an order or a label could result in massive overdose.
- Refrigerate unopened fosphenytoin at 2° to 8° C (36° to 46° F), but don't freeze.
- Dilute drug in D_5W or normal saline solution to 1.5 to 25 mg PE/ml.
- Inspect parenteral solution before administration. Discard solution that contains particles or is discolored.
- Be aware that drug shouldn't be given I.M. for status epilepticus because I.V. route allows faster onset and peak.
- Keep in mind that I.V. fosphenytoin administration doesn't require use of a filter, as does phenytoin administration.
- Don't give fosphenytoin solution faster than 150 mg PE/minute because of the risk of hypotension. For a 50-kg (110-lb) patient, infusion typically takes 5 to 7 minutes. Fosphenytoin can be given more rapidly than I.V. phenytoin.
- Follow loading dose with maintenance dosage of oral or parenteral phenytoin or parenteral fosphenytoin, as prescribed.
- As prescribed, give I.V. benzodiazepine (such as lorazepam or diazepam) with fosphenytoin; otherwise, drug's full antiepileptic effect won't be immediate.
- Monitor ECG, blood pressure, and respiratory function for 10 to 20 minutes after infusion ends.
- Expect to obtain blood fosphenytoin (phenytoin) level 2 hours after I.V. infusion or 4 hours after I.M. injection. Therapeutic level generally ranges from 10 to 20 mcg/ml; steady-state may take several days to several weeks to reach.
- Be aware that I.V. or I.M. fosphenytoin may be substituted for oral phenytoin sodium at same total daily dose and frequency. If prescribed, give daily amount in two or more divided doses to maintain seizure control.
- When switching between phenytoin and fosphenytoin, remember that small differences in phenytoin bioavailability can lead to significant changes in blood phenytoin level and an increased risk of toxicity.

- If drug causes transient, infusion-related paresthesia and pruritus, decrease or discontinue infusion, as ordered.
- Monitor CBC for thrombocytopenia or leukopenia—signs of hematologic toxicity. Also monitor serum albumin level and results of renal and liver function tests.
- Anticipate increased frequency and severity of adverse reactions after I.V. administration in patients with hepatic or renal impairment or hypoalbuminemia.
- Stop drug, as ordered, if signs of hypersensitivity develop: acute hepatotoxicity (hepatic necrosis and hepatitis), fever, lymphadenopathy, and skin reactions during first 2 months of therapy.
- Monitor blood phenytoin level to detect early signs and symptoms of toxicity, such as diplopia, nausea, severe confusion, slurred speech, and vomiting. Expect to reduce or stop drug if such signs or symptoms develop.
- **WARNING** Monitor patient for seizures; at toxic levels, phenytoin is excitatory.
- **WARNING** If patient has bradycardia or heart block rhythm, notify prescriber and expect to withhold drug because severe cardiovascular reactions and death could occur.
- Expect to give vitamin D supplement if patient has inadequate dietary intake and is on long-term anticonvulsant treatment.
- Document type, onset, and characteristics of seizures, as well as response to treatment.

PATIENT TEACHING
- Inform patient that fosphenytoin typically is used short-term.
- Instruct patient to notify prescriber immediately about bothersome signs and symptoms, especially rash and swollen glands.
- Because gingival hyperplasia may develop during long-term therapy, stress need for good oral hygiene and gum massage.
- Urge patient to consume adequate amounts of vitamin D.

gabapentin
Neurontin

Class and Category
Chemical class: Cyclohexane-acetic acid derivative
Therapeutic class: Anticonvulsant
Pregnancy category: C

Indications and Dosages
▶ *As adjunct to treat partial seizures*

CAPSULES, ORAL SOLUTION, TABLETS
Adults and adolescents. *Initial:* 300 mg t.i.d., increased gradually based on patient response. *Maintenance:* 900 to 1,800 mg daily. *Maximum:* 3,600 mg daily.
DOSAGE ADJUSTMENT Dosage reduced to 300 mg b.i.d. if creatinine clearance is 30 to 60 ml/min/1.73 m^2; to 300 mg daily if creatinine clearance is 15 to 29 ml/min/1.73 m^2; and to 300 mg every other day if creatinine clearance is less than 15 ml/min/1.73 m^2.

Route	Onset	Steady State	Peak	Half-Life	Duration
P.O.	Unknown	Unknown	Unknown	5 to 7 hr*	Unknown

Mechanism of Action
Is structurally similar to endogenous gamma-aminobutyric acid (GABA), the most common inhibitory neurotransmitter in the brain. Although gababentin's exact mechanism of action is unknown, GABA is known to inhibit the rapid firing of neurons, which is associated with seizures.

Contraindications
Hypersensitivity to gabapentin or its components

Interactions
DRUGS
antacids (aluminum- and magnesium-containing): Decreased gabapentin bioavailability
CNS depressants: Increased CNS depression
ACTIVITIES
alcohol use: Increased CNS depression

Adverse Reactions
CNS: Agitation, altered proprioception, amnesia, anxiety, apathy, aphasia, asthenia, ataxia, cerebellar dysfunction, chills, CNS tumors, confusion, CVA, decreased or absent reflexes, delusions, depersonalization, depression, disappearance of aura, dizziness, dream disturbances, dysesthesia, dystonia, emotional lability, euphoria, facial paralysis, fatigue, fever, hallucinations, headache, hemiplegia, hostility, hyperkinesia, hyperreflexia, hypoesthesia, hypotonia, intracranial hemorrhage, lack of coordination, malaise,

---

* For normal renal function; 52 hr for impaired renal function; 132 hr for anuric patients on nondialysis days.

migraine headache, nervousness, occipital neuralgia, paranoia, paresis, paresthesia, positive Babinski's sign, psychosis, sedation, seizures, somnolence, stupor, subdural hematoma, suicidal tendencies, syncope, tremor, vertigo

CV: Angina, hypertension, hypotension, murmur, palpitations, peripheral edema, peripheral vascular insufficiency, tachycardia, vasodilation

EENT: Abnormal vision, amblyopia, blepharospasm, cataracts, conjunctivitis, diplopia, dry eyes and mouth, earache, epistaxis, eye hemorrhage, eye pain, gingival bleeding, gingivitis, glossitis, hearing loss, increased salivation, inner ear infection, loss of taste, nystagmus, pharyngitis, photophobia, ptosis (bilateral or unilateral), rhinitis, sensation of fullness in ears, stomatitis, taste perversion, tinnitus, tooth discoloration, visual field defects

ENDO: Blood glucose fluctuations

GI: Abdominal pain, anorexia, constipation, diarrhea, elevated liver enzymes, fecal incontinence, flatulence, gastroenteritis, hemorrhoids, hepatitis, hepatomegaly, increased appetite, indigestion, jaundice, melena, nausea, thirst, vomiting

GU: Acute renal failure, decreased libido, impotence

HEME: Anemia, coagulation defect, leukopenia, thrombocytopenia

MS: Arthralgia, arthritis, back pain, bone fractures, dysarthria, joint stiffness or swelling, muscle twitching, myalgia, positive Romberg test result, tendinitis

RESP: Apnea, cough, dyspnea, pneumonia, pseudocroup

SKIN: Abrasion, acne, alopecia, cyst, diaphoresis, dry skin, eczema, erythema multiforme, hirsutism, pruritus, purpura, rash, seborrhea, Stevens-Johnson syndrome, urticaria

Other: Angioedema, dehydration, facial edema, hyponatremia, lymphadenopathy, viral infection, weight gain or loss

Overdose

Gabapentin overdose has no specific antidote. Monitor patient for evidence of overdose, including diarrhea, diplopia, dysarthria, lethargy, and somnolence.

Maintain an open airway, and give symptomatic and supportive care, as needed. Be aware that gabapentin isn't metabolized and is eliminated by the kidneys as unchanged drug; hemodialysis is an effective treatment for gabapentin overdose.

Take suicide precautions according to facility policy, and anticipate psychiatric re-evaluation.

Nursing Considerations

• As needed, open gabapentin capsules, and mix contents with

fruit juice or water or a semisolid food, such as applesauce or pudding, before administration.
- Administer initial dose at bedtime to minimize adverse reactions, especially ataxia, dizziness, fatigue, and somnolence.
- Give drug at least 2 hours after giving an antacid.
- Don't exceed 12 hours between doses on a three-times-a-day schedule.
- Be aware that routine monitoring of blood gabapentin level is unnecessary.
- **WARNING** To discontinue drug or switch to an alternate anticonvulsant, expect to change gradually over at least 1 week, as prescribed, to avoid loss of seizure control.
- Monitor renal function test results, and expect to adjust dosage, if necessary.

PATIENT TEACHING
- If patient has trouble swallowing gabapentin capsules, advise him to open them and sprinkle contents in juice or water or on soft food immediately before use.
- Tell patient not to take drug within 2 hours after an antacid.
- Advise patient to take a missed dose as soon as he remembers. If the next scheduled dose is less than 2 hours away, tell him to wait 1 to 2 hours before taking it and then resume his regular dosing schedule. Caution against doubling the dose.
- Caution patient not to stop taking drug abruptly.
- Inform patient that he may develop ataxia, dizziness, drowsiness, and nystagmus. Advise him to avoid potentially hazardous activities until he knows how the drug affects him.
- To prevent complications from adverse oral reactions (such as gingivitis), encourage patient to use good oral hygiene and to seek routine dental care.
- Inform patient that drug's adverse effects usually are mild to moderate and decline with continued use.
- Urge patient to keep follow-up appointments with prescriber to check progress.

galantamine hydrobromide
Razadyne, Razadyne ER

Class and Category
Chemical class: Tertiary alkaloid
Therapeutic class: Antidementia drug
Pregnancy category: B

Indications and Dosages

▶ *To treat mild to moderate dementia of Alzheimer's type*

TABLETS

Adults. *Initial:* 4 mg b.i.d. Dosage increased by 8 mg daily every 4 wk, if tolerated. *Maximum:* 12 mg b.i.d.

E.R. CAPSULES

Adults. *Initial:* 8 mg daily. Dosage increased by 8 mg daily every 4 wk, if tolerated. *Maximum:* 24 mg daily.

DOSAGE ADJUSTMENT For patients with moderately impaired hepatic or renal function, maximum dosage shouldn't exceed 16 mg daily.

Route	Onset	Steady State	Peak	Half-Life	Duration
P.O.	Unknown	Unknown	About 1 hr	7 hr	Unknown

Mechanism of Action

Reduces acetylcholine metabolism by competitively and reversibly inhibiting the brain enzyme acetylcholinesterase. Acetylcholine-producing neurons degenerate in the brains of patients with Alzheimer's disease. Inhibition of acetylcholinesterase increases the amount of acetylcholine, which is necessary for nerve impulse transmission.

Contraindications

Hypersensitivity to galantamine hydrobromide or its components, severe hepatic or renal impairment (creatinine clearance less than 9 ml/min/1.73 m²)

Interactions

DRUGS

amitriptyline, fluoxetine, fluvoxamine, quinidine: Possibly decreased galantamine clearance

anticholinergics: Possibly interference with cholinesterase activity

cholinergic agonists, cholinesterase inhibitors, neuromuscular blockers: Possibly exaggerated effects of these drugs and galantamine

cimetidine: Possibly increased galantamine bioavailability

ketoconazole, paroxetine: Increased galantamine bioavailability

Adverse Reactions

CNS: Aggression, asthenia, CVA, depression, dizziness, fatigue, fever, headache, insomnia, malaise, somnolence, suicidal ideation, suicide, syncope, transient ischemic attacks, tremor

CV: Atrial arrhythmias, AV block, bradycardia, cardiac failure, chest pain, dependent edema, hypotension, myocardial infarction or ischemia, ventricular tachycardia

EENT: Rhinitis

GI: Abdominal pain, anorexia, diarrhea, esophageal perforation, flatulence, GI bleeding, indigestion, nausea, vomiting

GU: Hematuria, incontinence, renal insufficiency or failure, UTI

HEME: Anemia, thrombocytopenia

Other: Dehydration, hypokalemia, weight loss

Overdose

Tertiary anticholinergics, such as atropine sulfate, may be used as an antidote for galantamine overdose. Monitor patient for signs and symptoms of galantamine overdose, including abdominal cramps, bradycardia, defecation, diaphoresis, dyspnea, hypotension, increased salivation, lacrimation, muscle weakness (which may affect the respiratory muscles), nausea, seizures, urination, and vomiting.

Maintain an open airway, and be prepared to assist with endotracheal intubation, as needed. Monitor patient for cardiovascular effects, such as bradycardia and hypotension. Institute seizure precautions according to facility protocol. Be aware that the effect of hemodialysis on galantamine overdose is unknown.

Institute suicide precautions according to facility policy, and anticipate psychiatric re-evaluation.

Nursing Considerations

- Give galantamine twice daily with morning and evening meals, and ensure adequate fluid intake to prevent GI signs and symptoms.
- If therapy is interrupted for several days, expect to restart drug at lowest dose because drug's benefits are lost when it is discontinued.
- Monitor patient's heart rate closely because drug can have vagotonic effects on heart's sinoatrial and atrioventricular nodes, which can lead to bradycardia.
- If patient is at risk for ulcer disease or is using an NSAID, monitor him for signs and symptoms of active or occult GI bleeding because gastric acid secretion may increase as a result of increased cholinergic activity.
- If patient has severe asthma or obstructive pulmonary disease, watch for worsening signs and symptoms; galantamine has cholinergic-like effects that may precipitate bronchospasm.
- Continue to assess patient for progressive deterioration of men-

tal status because drug becomes less effective as Alzheimer's disease progresses and the number of intact cholinergic neurons declines.

PATIENT TEACHING

• To minimize adverse reactions, instruct patient or caregiver to administer regular-strength form with morning and evening meals and extended-release form once in the morning with food.

• Explain to patient and caregiver the importance of maintaining adequate fluid intake during therapy.

• Advise patient or caregiver to notify prescriber immediately if therapy is stopped for several days. Prescriber may restart drug at lowest dose.

• Advise patient not to drive or perform activities requiring high levels of alertness, especially during first weeks of treatment, because drug may cause dizziness and drowsiness.

• Inform patient and family members that drug isn't a cure for Alzheimer's disease.

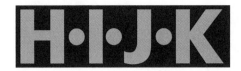

halazepam
Paxipam

Class, Category, and Schedule
Chemical class: Benzodiazepine
Therapeutic class: Antianxiety drug
Pregnancy category: D
Controlled substance schedule: IV

Indications and Dosages
▶ *To manage anxiety*
TABLETS
Adults. 20 to 40 mg t.i.d. or q.i.d. *Optimal:* 80 to 160 mg daily.
DOSAGE ADJUSTMENT Dosage reduced to 20 mg once or twice daily if needed for elderly and debilitated patients.

Route	Onset	Steady State	Peak	Half-Life	Duration
P.O.	Slow	5 to 14 days	Unknown	14 hr	6 to 8 hr

Mechanism of Action
May potentiate the effects of gamma-aminobutyric acid (GABA) and other inhibitory neurotransmitters by binding to specific benzodiazepine receptor sites in the limbic and cortical areas of the CNS. By binding to these receptor sites, halazepam increases the inhibitory effects of GABA and blocks cortical and limbic arousal.

Contraindications
Acute angle-closure glaucoma, hypersensitivity to halazepam or its components, itraconazole or ketoconazole therapy, psychosis

Interactions
DRUGS
antacids: Possibly altered rate of halazepam absorption
barbiturates, CNS depressants, opioids: Increased CNS depression, possibly sedation and impaired motor function
cimetidine, diltiazem, disulfiram, erythromycin, fluoxetine, fluvoxamine,

isoniazid, itraconazole, ketoconazole, metoprolol, nefazodone, oral contraceptives, propoxyphene, propranolol, ranitidine, valproic acid, verapamil: Decreased clearance, increased blood level, and increased risk of adverse effects of halazepam

clozapine: Possibly respiratory depression

digoxin: Increased blood digoxin level and risk of digitalis toxicity

levodopa: Decreased antidyskinetic effect

neuromuscular blockers: Increased or blocked neuromuscular blockade

theophyllines: Decreased sedative effect of halazepam

ACTIVITIES

alcohol use: Increased CNS depression, possibly sedation and impaired motor function

smoking: Decreased halazepam effectiveness

Adverse Reactions

CNS: Agitation, anxiety, ataxia, confusion, depression, dizziness, drowsiness, euphoria, headache, irritability, nervousness, slurred speech, tremor, weakness

CV: Angina, palpitations, sinus tachycardia

EENT: Diplopia, dry mouth, tinnitus

GI: Abdominal cramps or pain, constipation, diarrhea, increased salivation, nausea, vomiting

GU: Decreased libido, dysuria

MS: Arthralgia

SKIN: Pruritus, rash

Overdose

Monitor patient for evidence of overdose, including bradycardia, coma, confusion, dyspnea, hyporeflexia, seizures, severe drowsiness, shakiness, slurred speech, staggering, and weakness.

Maintain open airway, institute continuous cardiac monitoring, and administer I.V. fluids, as prescribed, to maintain blood pressure and promote diuresis. Institute seizure precautions according to facility protocol.

To decrease drug absorption in a conscious patient who isn't at risk for coma or seizures, be prepared to induce vomiting or perform gastric lavage. Expect that oral activated charcoal may also be prescribed. For an unconscious patient, anticipate assisting with the insertion of an endotracheal tube and then performing gastric lavage. The inflated cuff of the endotracheal tube will help prevent aspiration of gastric contents into the lungs.

Anticipate the use of a benzodiazepine receptor antagonist, such as flumazenil, to reverse the sedative effects. Be aware that flumazenil may induce seizures, especially if the patient has been undergoing long-term benzodiazepine treatment or has also ingested a cyclic antidepressant. If excitation occurs, be aware that a barbiturate shouldn't be used because it may increase excitement and prolong CNS depression. Dialysis is ineffective for treating benzodiazepine overdose.

Institute suicide precautionary measures according to facility policy, and anticipate psychiatric re-evaluation.

Nursing Considerations

- Use halazepam cautiously in patients with impaired hepatic or renal function, seizure disorders, or suicidal tendencies.
- Be aware that risk of halazepam addiction and abuse is high.
- Monitor renal and liver function test results, as appropriate, during long-term treatment.
- Expect to withdraw drug gradually over 2 weeks to avoid withdrawal signs and symptoms, which include anxiety, confusion, insomnia, psychosis, and seizures.

PATIENT TEACHING

- Instruct patient to take halazepam exactly as prescribed and not to stop taking it abruptly because withdrawal signs and symptoms may occur.
- Caution patient to avoid alcohol and other CNS depressants during therapy. Advise her to avoid OTC drugs, such as cough and cold remedies, because they may contain CNS depressants.
- Advise patient to avoid potentially hazardous activities until she knows how the drug affects her.
- Instruct patient to report depression, difficulty voiding, double vision, persistent drowsiness, and rash.
- Explain that drug's full effects may not occur for 6 weeks.

haloperidol

Apo-Haloperidol (CAN), Haldol, Novo-Peridol (CAN), Peridol (CAN)

haloperidol decanoate

Haldol Decanoate, Haldol LA (CAN)

haloperidol lactate

Haldol, Haldol Concentrate

Class and Category

Chemical class: Butyrophenone derivative
Therapeutic class: Antidyskinetic, antipsychotic drug
Pregnancy category: Not rated (haloperidol, haloperidol lactate), C (haloperidol decanoate)

Indications and Dosages

▶ *To treat psychotic disorders*
ORAL SOLUTION, TABLETS
Adults and adolescents. 0.5 to 5 mg b.i.d. or t.i.d. *Maximum:* Usually 100 mg daily.
Children ages 3 to 12. 0.05 mg/kg daily in divided doses b.i.d. or t.i.d. Increased by 0.5 mg every 5 to 7 days, if needed. *Maximum:* 0.15 mg/kg daily.

▶ *To treat nonpsychotic behavior disorders and Tourette's syndrome*
ORAL SOLUTION, TABLETS
Adults and adolescents. 0.5 to 5 mg b.i.d. or t.i.d. *Maximum:* Usually 100 mg daily.
Children ages 3 to 12. 0.05 to 0.075 mg/kg daily in divided doses b.i.d. or t.i.d. Increased by 0.5 mg every 5 to 7 days, if needed. *Maximum:* 0.075 mg/kg daily.
DOSAGE ADJUSTMENT Initial dosage reduced to 0.5 to 2 mg b.i.d. or t.i.d., if needed, for elderly or debilitated patients.

▶ *To treat acute psychotic episodes*
I.M. INJECTION
Adults and adolescents. *Initial:* 2 to 5 mg followed by subsequent doses as often as every 60 min. Alternatively, if signs and symptoms are controlled, dose may be repeated every 4 to 8 hr. *Maximum:* Usually 100 mg daily. First oral dose may be given 12 to 24 hr after last parenteral dose.

▶ *To provide long-term antipsychotic therapy for patients who require parenteral therapy*
LONG-ACTING I.M. (DECANOATE) INJECTION
Adults. *Initial:* 10 to 15 times the daily oral dose up to 100 mg. Repeated every 4 wk, if needed. *Maximum:* 300 mg/mo.

Route	Onset	Steady State	Peak	Half-Life	Duration
P.O.	Unknown	Unknown	Unknown	12 to 37 hr	Unknown
I.M.*	Unknown	3 mo[†]	3 to 4 days[‡]	3 wk[§]	Unknown

Mechanism of Action
May block postsynaptic dopamine receptors in the limbic system and increase brain turnover of dopamine, producing an antipsychotic effect.

---

* For haloperidol decanoate and lactate.
[†] For haloperidol decanoate.
[‡] For haloperidol decanoate only; 30 to 45 min for haloperidol lactate.
[§] For haloperidol decanoate; 17 to 25 hr for haloperidol lactate.

Contraindications

Blood dyscrasias, bone marrow depression, cerebral arteriosclerosis, coma, concomitant use of large amounts of another CNS depressant, coronary artery disease, epilepsy, hepatic dysfunction, hypersensitivity to haloperidol or its components, Parkinson's disease, severe hypertension or hypotension, severe CNS depression, subcortical brain damage

Interactions

DRUGS

amphetamines: Possibly decreased stimulant effects of amphetamines and decreased antipsychotic effect of haloperidol

anticholinergics, antidyskinetics, antihistamines: Increased anticholinergic effect and risk of decreased antipsychotic effect of haloperidol

anticonvulsants: Possibly decreased effectiveness of anticonvulsants and decreased blood haloperidol level

bromocriptine: Possibly decreased effectiveness of bromocriptine

bupropion: Lowered seizure threshold, increased risk of major motor seizure

CNS depressants: Increased CNS depression and risk of respiratory depression and hypotension

diazoxide: Possibly hypoglycemia

dopamine (high-dose therapy): Possibly decreased vasoconstriction

ephedrine: Possibly decreased vasopressor effect of ephedrine

epinephrine: Possibly severe hypotension and tachycardia

fluoxetine: Increased risk of severe and frequent extrapyramidal effects

guanadrel, guanethidine: Decreased hypotensive effects of these drugs

levodopa, pergolide: Possibly decreased therapeutic effects of these drugs

lithium: Increased risk of neurotoxicity

MAO inhibitors, maprotiline, tricyclic antidepressants: Increased sedative and anticholinergic effects of these drugs

metaraminol: Possibly decreased vasopressor effect of metaraminol

methoxamine: Decreased vasopressor effect, shortened duration of action of methoxamine

methyldopa: Possibly disorientation, slowed or difficult thought processes

phenylephrine: Decreased vasopressor response to phenylephrine

ACTIVITIES

alcohol use: Increased CNS depression and risk of respiratory depression and hypotension

Adverse Reactions

CNS: Agitation, anxiety, confusion, drowsiness, euphoria, extrapyramidal reactions that may be irreversible (akathisia, pseudoparkinsonism, tardive dyskinesia), hallucinations, headache, insomnia, neuroleptic malignant syndrome, restlessness, slurred speech, tremor, vertigo
CV: Cardiac arrest, hypertension, orthostatic hypotension, prolonged QT interval, ventricular arrhythmias
EENT: Blurred vision, dry mouth, increased salivation (all drug forms); stomatitis (oral solution)
ENDO: Breast engorgement, galactorrhea
GI: Constipation, nausea, vomiting
GU: Decreased libido, difficult ejaculation, impotence, menstrual irregularities, urine retention
HEME: Anemia, leukocytosis, leukopenia
SKIN: Diaphoresis, photosensitivity, rash
Other: Heatstroke, weight gain

Overdose

Monitor patient for signs and symptoms of overdose, including coma, dizziness, dyspnea, hypotension, jerking, muscle tremors, respiratory depression, stiffness, tiredness, uncontrolled movements, and weakness.

Maintain an open airway, institute continuous ECG monitoring, and assess patient for prolonged QT interval and torsades de pointes. Be prepared to treat arrhythmias, as needed and prescribed.

Give albumin, I.V. fluids, or plasma to treat hypotension and circulatory collapse. Expect that a vasopressor, such as norepinephrine, may also be prescribed. Be aware that epinephrine shouldn't be used because it may cause paradoxical hypotension. Expect to manage severe extrapyramidal reactions with benztropine or diphenhydramine, as prescribed.

To decrease drug absorption in a conscious patient who isn't at risk for coma, be prepared to induce vomiting or perform gastric lavage. Expect that activated charcoal may also be prescribed. For an unconscious patient, anticipate assisting with the insertion of an endotracheal tube and then performing gastric lavage. The inflated cuff of the endotracheal tube will help prevent aspiration of gastric contents into the lungs. Know that dialysis is ineffective for treating haloperidol overdose.

Institute suicide precautionary measures according to facility policy, and anticipate psychiatric re-evaluation.

Nursing Considerations
- Use haloperidol cautiously in patients with a history of prolonged QT interval, patients with uncorrected electrolyte disorders, and patients taking class IA or III antiarrhythmics because of a heightened risk for prolonged QT interval. Monitor elderly patients closely because they may be more susceptible to prolonged QT interval.
- Before giving oral solution, dilute it using a beverage with a pH less than 4, such as cola or apple, orange, or tomato juice.
- Administer haloperidol decanoate (long-acting form prepared in sesame oil to produce slow, sustained release) by deep I.M. injection into gluteal muscle using Z-track technique and 21G needle. Don't give more than 3 ml at one site. Expect to reach a stable blood level after third or fourth dose.
- Be aware that injection solution may develop a slight yellow discoloration but that this change doesn't affect drug potency.
- **WARNING** Parenteral haloperidol should never be given intravenously; doing so could cause such life-threatening adverse effects as sudden death, prolonged QT interval, and torsades de pointes.
- If patient is receiving long-term therapy, especially if she's elderly and taking a large dose, monitor her for tardive dyskinesia (potentially irreversible involuntary movements).
- If extrapyramidal reactions occur during the first few days of treatment, reduce dosage, as prescribed.
- Don't stop haloperidol abruptly unless severe adverse reactions occur.
- Watch for evidence of neuroleptic malignant syndrome (altered mental status, arrhythmias, fever, muscle rigidity), a rare but possibly fatal disorder linked to antipsychotic drugs.

PATIENT TEACHING
- Advise patient to take haloperidol exactly as prescribed and not to stop taking it abruptly because withdrawal signs and symptoms may occur.
- Instruct patient to dilute liquid form with juice or cola before taking it to prevent oral mucosal irritation.
- Caution patient to avoid skin contact with oral solution because it may cause a rash.
- Advise patient to take tablets with food or a full glass of milk or water to reduce GI distress.
- Instruct patient to maintain adequate fluid intake and to take precautions against heatstroke.

- Urge patient not to drink alcohol during therapy.
- Caution patient to avoid driving and other potentially hazardous activities if sedation occurs.
- Instruct patient to report repetitive movements, tremor, and vision changes to prescriber.

hydroxyzine hydrochloride
Apo-Hydroxyzine (CAN), Atarax, Multipax (CAN), Novo-Hydroxyzin (CAN), Vistaril

hydroxyzine pamoate
Vistaril

Class and Category
Chemical class: Piperazine derivative
Therapeutic class: Antianxiety drug, sedative-hypnotic
Pregnancy category: C

Indications and Dosages
▶ *To relieve anxiety and induce sedation and hypnosis*
CAPSULES, ORAL SUSPENSION, SYRUP, TABLETS
Adults and adolescents. 50 to 100 mg as a single dose.
Children. 600 mcg/kg as a single dose.
I.M. INJECTION
Adults and adolescents. 50 to 100 mg every 4 to 6 hr., p.r.n. (for antianxiety effects); 50 mg as a single dose (for sedative-hypnotic effects).

Route	Onset	Steady State	Peak	Half-Life	Duration
P.O.	15 to 60 min	Unknown	Unknown	20 to 25 hr	4 to 6 hr
I.M.	20 to 30 min	Unknown	Unknown	20 to 25 hr	4 to 6 hr

Mechanism of Action
Suppresses activity at subcortical level of the CNS, producing a calming effect without CNS depression. Hydroxyzine crosses the blood-brain barrier and inhibits histamine action. It also blocks central histaminergic receptors and may antagonize other CNS receptor sites, such as those for serotonin, acetylcholine, and alpha-adrenergic stimulation, producing sedative-hypnotic effects.

Contraindications
Breast-feeding; early pregnancy; hypersensitivity to cetirizine, hydroxyzine, or their components

Interactions
DRUGS
anticholinergics: Possibly increased anticholinergic effects; risk of paralytic ileus
apomorphine: Possibly decreased emetic response to apomorphine in treatment of poisoning
CNS depressants: Increased CNS depression
MAO inhibitors: Increased anticholinergic and CNS depressant effects of hydroxyzine
ACTIVITIES
alcohol use: Increased CNS depression

Adverse Reactions
CNS: Drowsiness, hallucinations, headache, involuntary motor activity, seizures, tremor
EENT: Dry mouth
SKIN: Pruritus, rash, urticaria
Other: Allergic reaction, injection site pain

Overdose
Hydroxyzine overdose has no specific antidote. Monitor patient for evidence of overdose, including arrhythmias; clumsiness; dyspnea; facial flushing; hallucinations; hypotension; insomnia; seizures; severe drowsiness; and severe dryness of mouth, nose, and throat.

Maintain an open airway and be prepared to give oxygen, institute continuous ECG monitoring, and give I.V. fluids, as prescribed, to maintain blood pressure. Institute seizure precautions according to facility protocol. Give a vasopressor, as needed, to treat hypotension; however, be aware that epinephrine shouldn't be used because it may further lower blood pressure. A stimulant also shouldn't be used because it may cause seizures.

Be prepared to induce vomiting with ipecac syrup, as prescribed, taking precautions to prevent aspiration, especially in infants and children. If patient is unable to vomit, perform gastric lavage with isotonic or 0.45NS, as prescribed. Expect to administer a saline cathartic such as milk of magnesia, as prescribed, to enhance drug elimination.

Institute suicide precautionary measures according to facility policy, and anticipate psychiatric re-evaluation.

Nursing Considerations
• Don't give hydroxyzine by subcutaneous or I.V. route because tissue necrosis may occur.

• Inject I.M. form deep into a large muscle using Z-track method.
• If patient takes another CNS depressant, watch for oversedation.
PATIENT TEACHING
• Urge patient to avoid alcohol.
• Caution patient about drowsiness, and tell her to avoid potentially hazardous activities until she knows how the drug affects her.
• Instruct female patient to alert prescriber if she is or could be pregnant because drug will need to be discontinued during early pregnancy.

Other Therapeutic Uses
Hydroxyzine hydrochloride is also indicated for the following:
• To treat pruritus
• To provide antiemetic effects
• As adjunct to permit reduction in preoperative and postoperative opioid dosage

imipramine hydrochloride
Apo-Imipramine (CAN), Impril (CAN), Norfranil, Novo-Pramine (CAN), Tipramine, Tofranil
imipramine pamoate
Tofranil-PM
Class and Category
Chemical class: Dibenzazepine derivative
Therapeutic class: Antidepressant
Pregnancy category: Not rated
Indications and Dosages
▶ *To treat depression*
CAPSULES
Adults. *Initial:* 75 mg daily at bedtime, gradually increased as needed and tolerated. *Maximum:* 300 mg daily (hospitalized patients), 200 mg daily (outpatients).
TABLETS
Adults. *Initial:* 25 to 50 mg t.i.d. or q.i.d., gradually increased as needed and tolerated. *Maximum:* 300 mg daily (hospitalized patients), 200 mg daily (outpatients).
DOSAGE ADJUSTMENT Initial dosage reduced to 25 mg at bedtime for depressed elderly patients and then adjusted as needed and tolerated up to 100 mg daily in divided doses.
Adolescents. *Initial:* 25 to 50 mg daily in divided doses, adjusted

as needed and tolerated. *Maximum:* 100 mg daily.
Children ages 6 to 12. 10 to 30 mg daily in divided doses b.i.d.

Route	Onset	Steady State	Peak	Half-Life	Duration
P.O.	2 to 3 wk	2 to 5 days	Unknown	11 to 25 hr	Unknown

Mechanism of Action

May interfere with reuptake of serotonin (and possibly other neurotransmitters) at presynaptic neurons, thus enhancing serotonin's effects at postsynaptic receptors. By restoring normal levels of neurotransmitters at nerve synapses, this tricyclic antidepressant may elevate mood and reduce depression.

Contraindications

Acute recovery period after an MI; hypersensitivity to imipramine, other tricyclic antidepressants, or their components; use within 2 weeks of MAO inhibitor therapy

Interactions

DRUGS

amantadine, anticholinergics, antidyskinetics, antihistamines: Risk of increased anticholinergic effects, including confusion, hallucinations, and nightmares
anticonvulsants: Risk of increased CNS depression, increased risk of seizures, decreased effectiveness of imipramine
antithyroid drugs: Possibly agranulocytosis
barbiturates, carbamazepine: Possibly decreased blood level and effectiveness of imipramine
cimetidine, fluoxetine: Possibly increased blood imipramine level
clonidine, guanadrel, guanethidine: Possibly decreased antihypertensive effects of these drugs, increased CNS depressant effects of clonidine
CNS depressants: Increased CNS depression, respiratory depression, and hypotension
disulfiram, ethchlorvynol: Risk of delirium, increased CNS depressant effects of ethchlorvynol
estramustine, estrogens, oral contraceptives (estrogen-containing): Risk of increased bioavailability of imipramine, increased depression
MAO inhibitors: Increased risk of hypertensive crisis, severe seizures, and death
oral anticoagulants: Possibly increased anticoagulant activity
pimozide, probucol: Risk of arrhythmias

sympathomimetics (including ophthalmic epinephrine and vasoconstrictive local anesthetics): Increased risk of arrhythmias, hyperpyrexia, hypertension, tachycardia

thyroid hormones: Risk of increased therapeutic and adverse effects of both drugs

ACTIVITIES

alcohol use: Increased CNS depression, increased alcohol effects

Adverse Reactions

CNS: Anxiety, ataxia, chills, confusion, CVA, delirium, dizziness, drowsiness, excitation, extrapyramidal reactions, fever, hallucinations, headache, insomnia, nervousness, nightmares, parkinsonism, seizures, suicidal thinking, tremor

CV: Arrhythmias, orthostatic hypotension, palpitations

EENT: Blurred vision, dry mouth, increased intraocular pressure, pharyngitis, taste perversion, tinnitus, tongue swelling

ENDO: Gynecomastia, syndrome of inappropriate ADH secretion

GI: Constipation, diarrhea, heartburn, ileus, increased appetite, nausea, vomiting

GU: Impotence, libido changes, testicular swelling, urine retention

HEME: Agranulocytosis, bone marrow depression

RESP: Wheezing

SKIN: Alopecia, diaphoresis, jaundice, photosensitivity, pruritus, rash, urticaria

Other: Allergic reaction, facial edema, weight gain

Overdose

Monitor patient for signs and symptoms of overdose, including agitation, arrhythmias, confusion, disturbed concentration, drowsiness, dyspnea, fever, hallucinations, irregular heartbeat, mydriasis, restlessness, seizures, unusual fatigue, vomiting, and weakness.

Maintain open airway, institute continuous ECG monitoring (for at least 5 days), and closely observe patient's blood pressure, respiratory rate, and temperature. Be prepared to treat arrhythmias with lidocaine and sodium bicarbonate, as prescribed. Anticipate possible digitalization to prevent heart failure. Institute seizure precautions according to facility protocol, and administer anticonvulsant therapy, as prescribed.

Be prepared to perform gastric lavage to decrease drug absorption. Expect to administer activated charcoal followed by a bowel stimulant to enhance drug elimination. Because tricyclic antidepressants are highly protein bound, dialysis, exchange transfusions, and forced diuresis are ineffective for treating overdose.

Be aware I.V. physostigmine isn't routinely recommended, but it may be prescribed to reverse the anticholinergic effects of imipramine in comatose patients with respiratory depression, serious arrhythmias, severe hypertension, or uncontrollable seizures.

Institute suicide precautionary measures according to facility policy, and anticipate psychiatric re-evaluation.

Nursing Considerations

- Use imipramine cautiously in patients with a history of urine retention or angle-closure glaucoma because anticholinergic effects may cause urine retention and increased intraocular pressure.
- **WARNING** Don't administer an MAO inhibitor within 2 weeks of imipramine. Otherwise, the patient may experience hypertensive crisis, seizures, and death.
- Assess patient for adverse reactions; often, they occur during first 2 hours of therapy.
- Monitor blood pressure for orthostatic hypotension, with patient in supine and standing positions, before and during imipramine therapy and before dosage increases.
- Anticipate increased risk of arrhythmias in patients with a history of cardiac disease.
- Monitor patients, especially children and adolescents, closely for suicidal tendencies, especially when therapy starts and dosage changes.
- Expect mood to improve after 2 to 3 weeks of therapy.
- Avoid abrupt withdrawal of drug in patients who receive long-term therapy. Such withdrawal may cause headache, malaise, nausea, sleep disturbance, and vomiting.
- Taper drug gradually, as ordered, a few days before surgery to avoid the risk of hypertension during surgery.
- If patient experiences signs and symptoms of infection, such as fever or pharyngitis, obtain CBC, as ordered.
- Limit drug access for potentially suicidal patient.

PATIENT TEACHING
- Advise patient to take imipramine exactly as prescribed. Warn her that stopping drug abruptly may cause headache, malaise, nausea, trouble sleeping, and vomiting.
- Urge parents to monitor child or adolescent closely for suicidal tendencies, especially when therapy starts and dosage changes.
- Advise patient to report chills, difficulty urinating, dizziness, excessive sedation, fever, palpitations, signs and symptoms of an allergic reaction, and sore throat.

- Caution patient to avoid potentially hazardous activities until she knows how the drug affects her.
- Urge patient to avoid alcohol during imipramine therapy because of the risk of increased CNS depression and alcohol effects.
- Suggest eating small, frequent meals to help relieve nausea.
- Instruct patient to avoid prolonged exposure to sunlight because of the risk of photosensitivity.
- Inform men about possible impotence and altered libido.
- If patient reports dry mouth, suggest sugarless candy or gum to relieve it. Tell her to check with prescriber if dry mouth persists after 2 weeks.

Other Therapeutic Uses

Imipramine hydrochloride is also indicated for the following:
- As adjunct to treat childhood enuresis

ipecac syrup

Ipecac Syrup

Class and Category

Chemical class: Cephaelis acuminata or Cephaelis ipecacuanha derivative
Therapeutic class: Emetic
Pregnancy category: C

Indications and Dosages

▶ *To induce vomiting after drug overdose and certain types of poisoning*
SYRUP

Adults and children older than age 12. 15 to 30 ml followed by 8 oz (240 ml) of water. Dose repeated if vomiting doesn't start within 20 to 30 min.

Children ages 1 to 12. 15 ml preceded or followed by 4 to 8 oz (120 to 240 ml) of water. Dose repeated if vomiting doesn't begin within 20 to 30 min.

Infants ages 6 months to 1 year. 5 to 10 ml preceded or followed by 4 to 8 oz (120 to 240 ml) of water.

Route	Onset	Steady State	Peak	Half-Life	Duration
P.O.	20 to 30 min	Unknown	Unknown	Unknown	20 to 25 min

Contraindications

Loss of gag reflex, poisoning with strychnine or corrosives (such as alkaloid substances, petroleum distillates, and strong acids), seizures, semiconsciousness or unconsciousness, severe inebriation, shock

> **Mechanism of Action**
> Induces vomiting by irritating the gastric mucosa and stimulating the medullary chemoreceptor trigger zone in the CNS.

Interactions
DRUGS
activated charcoal: Neutralization of emetic effect

Adverse Reactions
CNS: Depression, drowsiness
EENT: Aspiration of vomitus, coughing
GI: Diarrhea, indigestion

Overdose
If patient takes an excessive dose of ipecac or fails to vomit after it's administered, overdose may occur. Severe toxicity has also occurred from the inadvertent administration of ipecac fluidextract (which is 14 times more concentrated than ipecac syrup) in a dosage appropriate for ipecac syrup. Monitor patient for signs and symptoms of overdose, including abdominal cramps, atrial fibrillation, coma, decreased myocardial contractility, dyspnea, GI bleeding, heart failure, hypotension, myocarditis, nausea, seizures, shock, tachycardia, and T-wave depression.

Maintain open airway, begin continuous ECG monitoring, and institute seizure precautions according to facility protocol.

Expect to administer activated charcoal, as prescribed, to adsorb the ipecac, and perform gastric lavage. Anticipate the use of a cardiac glycoside, as prescribed, or the insertion of a pacemaker to treat the cardiotoxic effects of ipecac overdose.

Nursing Considerations
- Give ipecac syrup, followed by plenty of water, only to conscious patients. Give young or frightened children water before or after ipecac.
- Expect vomiting to begin 20 to 30 minutes after patient takes drug.
- If vomiting doesn't occur within 30 minutes of second dose, prepare to perform gastric lavage.
- Don't give ipecac after ingestion of petroleum distillates, such as

gasoline, or caustic substances because doing so could cause further injury to esophagus.

• If activated charcoal also will be given to treat overdose or poisoning, expect to give it after patient vomits or 30 minutes after second dose if no vomiting occurs because activated charcoal will adsorb ipecac and inhibit its action.

• Be alert for possibility of abuse by anorexic and bulimic patients, who use ipecac to purge after binging. Long-term ipecac use can cause cardiotoxicity and toxic myopathy.

PATIENT TEACHING

• Inform patient of ipecac's effects.

• Instruct adult patient to drink 8 oz (240 ml) of water after taking drug. Instruct a child to drink 4 to 8 oz (120 to 240 ml) of water before or after taking drug.

• Inform patient or parents of child that diarrhea may occur after taking drug.

• Urge parents to keep ipecac syrup at home (along with the telephone number of a poison control center), and teach them how to administer it in case of poisoning.

• **WARNING** Advise parents that ipecac syrup has replaced ipecac fluidextract and ipecac tincture and that they should check their home supply and update it, if needed. Inform them that ipecac fluidextract is 14 times more concentrated than ipecac syrup and can cause serious, possibly toxic effects if administered incorrectly.

isocarboxazid

Marplan

Class and Category

Chemical class: Hydrazine derivative
Therapeutic class: Antidepressant
Pregnancy category: C

Indications and Dosages

▶ *To treat major depression*
TABLETS
Adults and adolescents over age 16. *Initial:* 10 mg b.i.d., increased by 10 mg daily every 2 to 4 days, as needed and tolerated. *Maximum:* 60 mg daily.

Route	Onset	Steady State	Peak	Half-Life	Duration
P.O.	7 to 10 days	Unknown	Unknown	Unknown	10 days

Mechanism of Action

Irreversibly binds to MAO, reducing its activity and resulting in increased levels of neurotransmitters, including serotonin and the catecholamine neurotransmitters dopamine, epinephrine, and norepinephrine. This regulation of CNS neurotransmitters helps ease depression. After 2 to 4 weeks of continuous therapy, alpha$_2$- or beta-adrenergic and serotonin receptors become desensitized, which also produces an antidepressant effect.

Contraindications

Cardiovascular disease; cerebrovascular disease; heart failure; hepatic disease; history of headaches; hypersensitivity to isocarboxazid or its components; hypertension; pheochromocytoma; severe renal impairment; use of an anesthetic, an antihypertensive, bupropion, buspirone, carbamazepine, a CNS depressant, cyclobenzaprine, dextromethorphan, meperidine, a selective serotonin reuptake inhibitor, a sympathomimetic, or a tricyclic antidepressant; use within 14 days of other MAO inhibitor

Interactions

DRUGS

anticholinergics, antidyskinetics, antihistamines: Increased anticholinergic effect; prolonged CNS depressant effect of antihistamines
anticonvulsants: Increased CNS depression, possibly altered pattern of seizures
antihypertensives, diuretics: Increased hypotensive effect
bromocriptine: Possibly interference with bromocriptine effects
bupropion: Increased risk of bupropion toxicity
buspirone: Increased risk of hypertension
caffeine-containing drugs: Increased risk of dangerous arrhythmias and severe hypertension
carbamazepine, cyclobenzaprine, maprotiline, other MAO inhibitors: Increased risk of hyperpyretic crisis, hypertensive crisis, severe seizures, and death; altered pattern of seizures with carbamazepine
CNS depressants: Increased CNS depression
dextromethorphan: Increased risk of excitation, hypertension, and hyperpyrexia
doxapram: Increased vasopressor effects of either drug
fluoxetine, paroxetine, sertraline, trazodone, tricyclic antidepressants: Increased risk of potentially fatal serotonin syndrome
guanadrel, guanethidine: Increased risk of hypertension
haloperidol, loxapine, molindone, phenothiazines, pimozide, thioxan-

thenes: Prolonged and intensified anticholinergic, hypotensive, and sedative effects of these drugs or isocarboxazid

insulin, oral antidiabetic drugs: Increased hypoglycemic effects

levodopa: Increased risk of sudden or moderate to severe hypertension

local anesthetics (with epinephrine or levonordefrin): Possibly severe hypertension

meperidine, other opioid analgesics: Increased risk of coma, hyperpyrexia, hypotension, immediate excitation, rigidity, seizures, severe hypertension, severe respiratory depression, shock, sweating, and death

methyldopa: Increased risk of hallucinations, headache, hyperexcitability, and severe hypertension

methylphenidate: Increased CNS stimulant effect

metrizamide: Decreased seizure threshold, increased risk of seizures

oral anticoagulants: Increased anticoagulant activity

phenylephrine (nasal or ophthalmic): Potentiated vasopressor effect of phenylephrine

rauwolfia alkaloids: Increased risk of moderate to severe hypertension, CNS depression (when isocarboxazid is added to rauwolfia alkaloid therapy), CNS excitation and hypertension (when rauwolfia alkaloid is added to isocarboxazid therapy)

spinal anesthetics: Increased risk of hypotension

sympathomimetics: Prolonged and intensified cardiac stimulant and vasopressor effects

tryptophan: Increased risk of confusion, disorientation, hyperreflexia, hyperthermia, hyperventilation, mania or hypomania, and shivering

FOODS

aged cheese; avocados; bananas; fava or broad beans; cured meat or sausage; overripe fruit; pickled fish, meats or poultry; protein extract; smoked fish, meats, or poultry; soy sauce; yeast extract; and other foods high in tyramine or other pressor amines: Increased risk of dangerous arrhythmias and severe hypertensive crisis

ACTIVITIES

use of alcohol-containing products that also may contain tyramine, such as beer (including reduced-alcohol and alcohol-free beer), hard liquor, liqueurs, sherry, and wine: Increased risk of hypertensive crisis

Adverse Reactions

CNS: Agitation, dizziness, drowsiness, fever, headache, insomnia, intracranial bleeding, overstimulation, restlessness, sedation, suicidal thinking, tremor, weakness

CV: Bradycardia, chest pain, edema, hypertensive crisis, orthostatic hypotension, palpitations, tachycardia
EENT: Blurred vision, dry mouth, mydriasis, photophobia, yellowing of sclera
GI: Abdominal pain, anorexia, constipation, diarrhea, elevated liver function test results, increased appetite, nausea
GU: Darkened urine, oliguria, sexual dysfunction
HEME: Leukopenia
MS: Muscle spasms, myoclonus, neck stiffness
SKIN: Clammy skin, diaphoresis, jaundice, rash
Other: Unusual weight gain

Overdose

Monitor patient for signs and symptoms of overdose, including anxiety, confusion, cool and clammy skin, diaphoresis, dizziness, drowsiness, dyspnea, fever, hallucinations, headache, hyperreflexia or hyporeflexia, hypertension or hypotension, insomnia, irritability, muscle stiffness, respiratory depression, seizures, and tachycardia. Signs and symptoms may be minimal for the first 12 hours and reach a maximum by 24 to 48 hours, so frequently monitor patient during this time period.

Maintain open airway, administer oxygen, as ordered, and be prepared to assist with endotracheal intubation if patient develops respiratory failure. Monitor temperature, and expect to treat hyperpyrexia with an antipyretic and a cooling blanket, as prescribed. Anticipate using I.V. fluids and a vasopressor, such as norepinephrine, to treat hypotension and an alpha-adrenergic blocker, such as phentolamine or phenoxybenzamine, to treat hypertension. Expect to treat seizures with diazepam, and be aware that a phenothiazine shouldn't be used because of possible hypotensive effects. Institute seizure precautions according to facility protocol.

Be prepared to induce vomiting or perform gastric lavage, followed by the administration of activated charcoal, as prescribed, to decrease absorption of isocarboxazid. Take precautions to protect patient's airway against aspiration. Hemodialysis, hemoperfusion, and peritoneal dialysis may be effective for treating isocarboxazid overdose.

Expect to administer dantrolene, 2.5 mg/kg daily in divided doses, as prescribed to treat signs and symptoms of a hypermetabolic state, including coma, hyperpyrexia, hyperreflexia, muscle rigidity, respiratory failure, tachycardia, and tremor. Monitor patient for hepatotoxicity and pleural and pericardial effusion.

Institute suicide precautionary measures according to facility policy, and anticipate psychiatric re-evaluation.

Nursing Considerations

• Monitor patient's blood pressure during isocarboxazid therapy to detect hypertensive crisis and to decrease the risk of orthostatic hypotension.

• **WARNING** Notify prescriber immediately if patient experiences signs and symptoms of hypertensive crisis (drug's most serious adverse effect), such as chest pain, headache, neck stiffness, and palpitations. Expect to stop drug immediately if these occur.

• Keep phentolamine readily available to treat hypertensive crisis. Give 5 mg by slow I.V. infusion, as prescribed, to reduce blood pressure without causing excessive hypotension. Use external cooling measures, as prescribed, to manage fever.

• Expect to wait 10 to 14 days, as prescribed, when switching patient from one MAO inhibitor to another or when switching from a dibenzazepine-related drug, such as amitriptyline or perphenazine, to avoid hypertensive crisis.

• Monitor patient with a history of epilepsy for seizures because isocarboxazid may alter seizure threshold. Institute seizure precautions according to facility protocol.

• Monitor liver function test results and assess patient for abdominal pain, darkened urine, and jaundice because isocarboxazid may cause hepatic dysfunction.

• Expect to observe some therapeutic effect within 7 to 10 days, but keep in mind that full effect may not occur for 4 to 8 weeks.

• Be aware that, for maintenance therapy, the smallest dose possible should be used. Once clinical effect has been achieved, expect to decrease the dosage slowly over several weeks.

• Keep dietary restrictions in place for at least 2 weeks after stopping isocarboxazid because of the slow recovery from drug's enzyme-inhibiting effects.

• Ideally, expect to stop drug 10 days before elective surgery, as prescribed, to avoid hypotension.

• Anticipate that coadministration with a selective serotonin reuptake inhibitor may cause confusion, diaphoresis, diarrhea, seizures, and other less severe signs and symptoms.

• Monitor patient for suicidal tendencies, especially when therapy starts and dosage changes. Institute suicide precautions according to facility policy, and notify prescriber immediately.

- Monitor patient for sudden insomnia. If it develops, notify prescriber and be prepared to administer isocarboxazid early in the day.

PATIENT TEACHING
- Inform patient and family members that therapeutic effects of isocarboxazid may take several weeks to become evident and that she should continue taking drug as prescribed.
- Caution patient to rise slowly from a lying or sitting position to minimize effects of orthostatic hypotension.
- **WARNING** Instruct patient to avoid the following foods, beverages, and drugs during isocarboxazid therapy and for 2 weeks afterward: alcohol-free and reduced-alcohol beer and wine; appetite suppressants; beer; broad beans; cheese (except cottage and cream cheese); chocolate and caffeine in large quantities; dry sausage (including Genoa salami, hard salami, Lebanon bologna, and pepperoni); hay fever drugs; inhaled asthma drugs; liver; meat extract; OTC cold and cough preparations (including those containing dextromethorphan), nasal decongestants (tablets, drops, or sprays); pickled herring; products that contain tryptophan; protein-rich foods that may have undergone protein changes by aging, fermenting, pickling, or smoking; sauerkraut; sinus drugs; weight-loss preparations; yeast extracts (including brewer's yeast in large quantities); yogurt; and wine.
- Urge parents to monitor child or adolescent closely for suicidal tendencies, especially when therapy starts and dosage changes.
- Advise patient to notify prescriber immediately about chest pain, dizziness, headache, nausea, neck stiffness, palpitations, rapid heart rate, sweating, and vomiting.
- Advise patient to inform all health care providers (including dentists) that she takes an MAO inhibitor because certain drugs are contraindicated within 2 weeks of therapy.
- Urge patient to avoid potentially hazardous activities until she knows how the drug affects her.
- Suggest that patient change position slowly to minimize effects of orthostatic hypotension.
- Urge patient with diabetes mellitus who's taking insulin or an oral antidiabetic drug to monitor blood glucose level frequently during therapy because isocarboxazid may affect glucose control.
- Caution patient not to stop taking drug abruptly to avoid recurrence of original signs and symptoms.

isometheptene mucate, dichloralphenazone, and acetaminophen

Amidrine, I.D.A., Iso-Acetozone, Isocom, Midchlor, Midrin, Migquin, Migragap, Migratine, Migrazone, Migrend, Migrex, Mitride (all contain 325 mg of acetaminophen, 100 mg of dichloralphenazone, and 65 mg of isometheptene mucate)

Class and Category

Chemical class: Sympathomimetic amine
Therapeutic class: Analgesic
Pregnancy category: Not rated

Indications and Dosages

▶ *To relieve migraine headache*
CAPSULES
Adults. 2 capsules followed by 1 capsule every hr until relief occurs. *Maximum:* 5 capsules/12 hr.

Route	Onset	Steady State	Peak	Half-Life	Duration
P.O.	30 to 60 min	Unknown	1 to 3 hr	1 to 4 hr	3 to 4 hr

Mechanism of Action

Isometheptene mucate constricts dilated cranial and cerebral arterioles by sympathomimetic action, which reduces stimuli that lead to vascular headaches. Dichloralphenazone reduces the patient's emotional reaction to pain through its mild sedative effect. Acetaminophen raises the pain threshold by acting on the hypothalamus.

Contraindications

Heart disease; hepatic disease; hypersensitivity to acetaminophen, dichloralphenazone, or isometheptene; MAO inhibitor therapy within 14 days; severe renal disease; uncontrolled glaucoma; uncontrolled hypertension

Interactions

DRUGS
CNS depressants: Additive sedative effects
hepatic enzyme inducers, other hepatotoxic drugs: Increased risk of hepatotoxicity
MAO inhibitors: Increased risk of severe hypertension and hyperpyrexia

ACTIVITIES
alcohol use: Additive sedative effects, increased risk of hepatotoxicity

Adverse Reactions

CNS: Dizziness, drowsiness
CV: Irregular heartbeat
HEME: Anemia, methemoglobinemia
SKIN: Rash

Overdose

Treatment for overdose should account for the potential toxic effects of isometheptene mucate, dichloralphenazone, and acetaminophen. Monitor patient for signs and symptoms of overdose, including abdominal distress, anorexia, diaphoresis, diarrhea, nausea, and vomiting. These signs and symptoms are typical of acetaminophen overdose, but they don't always occur. The first indication of an overdose may be elevated liver function test results, occurring 2 to 4 days after overdose.

Maintain open airway, and monitor temperature and fluid and electrolyte levels. Institute continuous ECG monitoring, and assess patient for an irregular heartbeat, which may be caused by the excessive sympathetic stimulation or vasoconstrictive effects of isometheptene mucate.

Be prepared to administer acetylcysteine, the antidote for acetaminophen overdose. Expect to adjust acetylcysteine dosage based on periodic blood acetaminophen levels. Start to monitor blood acetaminophen levels 4 hours after ingestion because blood levels drawn before this time may not be an accurate assessment of hepatotoxicity. Also, monitor liver function tests results, PT, and bilirubin at 24-hour intervals for at least 3 days. Expect to correct hypoglycemia and administer vitamin K, fresh frozen plasma, or clotting factor concentrate, as prescribed, for elevated PT.

Be prepared to perform gastric lavage or induce vomiting to decrease absorption of all three components of the drug. Be aware that activated charcoal shouldn't be used because it may interfere with acetylcysteine. Hemodialysis or hemoperfusion may help remove acetaminophen and trichloroethanol (the active metabolite of dichloralphenazone) from the circulation.

Be alert for signs and symptoms of hepatic and renal dysfunction, which may not occur for 2 to 6 days after ingestion of drug. Observe patient for abdominal pain or swelling, agitation, arrhythmias, cerebral edema, cloudy urine, coagulation abnormalities, coma, confusion, decreased urine output, disseminated intravascular coagulation, GI bleeding, hematuria, hypoglycemia, mental changes, metabolic acidosis, seizures, shock, and stupor.

Institute suicide precautionary measures according to facility policy, and anticipate psychiatric re-evaluation.

Nursing Considerations
• Expect to monitor patients with peripheral vascular disease, recent angina attack, or an MI for arrhythmias and vasoconstriction because isometheptene mucate has sympathomimetic and vasoconstrictive effects.
• Take safety precautions to prevent injury from falls.

PATIENT TEACHING
• **WARNING** Caution patient not to take isometheptene mucate, dichloralphenazone, and acetaminophen if she has taken an MAO inhibitor within the past 14 days; doing so can cause severe hypertension or hyperpyrexia.
• Advise patient to take drug only after a migraine warning sign occurs. Overuse may make drug less effective and headaches worse.
• Instruct patient to lie down in a quiet, dark room after taking drug.
• Drug can cause dizziness or drowsiness, so advise patient to avoid potentially hazardous activities until she knows how the drug affects her.
• Caution patient to avoid alcohol and CNS depressants during therapy because they increase dizziness, drowsiness, and the risk of hepatotoxicity.
• Advise patient to notify prescriber if drug becomes less effective or headaches occur more frequently.
• Teach patient how to read drug labels to avoid taking too much acetaminophen, which can cause hepatic or renal damage.
• Inform patient that decreasing the dose may prevent transient dizziness or rash.
• Instruct patient to store drug away from heat, moisture, and direct light.

Other Therapeutic Uses
Isometheptene mucate, dichloralphenazone, and acetaminophen is also indicated for the following:
• To relieve tension headache

lamotrigine

Lamictal

Class and Category

Chemical class: Phenyltriazine
Therapeutic class: Anticonvulsant
Pregnancy category: C

Indications and Dosages

▶ *As adjunct to treat partial seizures; to treat generalized seizures of Lennox-Gastaut syndrome; and to treat primary generalized tonic-clonic seizures*

CHEWABLE TABLETS, TABLETS

Adults and children age 12 and over taking valproate.
25 mg every other day for 2 wk, followed by 25 mg daily for 2 wk. Increased by 25 to 50 mg every 1 to 2 wk, if needed. *Maintenance:* 100 to 400 mg daily.

Children ages 2 to 12 taking valproate. 0.15 mg/kg daily as a single dose or in divided doses b.i.d. for 2 wk and then 0.3 mg/kg daily as a single dose or in divided doses b.i.d. for next 2 wk. Increased by 0.3 mg/kg every 1 to 2 wk, if needed to reach maintenance dosage. *Maintenance:* 1 to 5 mg/kg daily as a single dose or in divided doses b.i.d. *Maximum:* 200 mg daily.

Adults and children age 12 and over also taking an antiepileptic drug other than carbamazepine, phenytoin, phenobarbital, primidone, or valproate. 25 mg daily for 2 wk, followed by 50 mg daily for 2 wk. Increased by 50 mg every 1 to 2 wk, if needed. *Maintenance:* 225 to 375 mg daily in 2 divided doses b.i.d. *Maximum:* 400 mg daily.

Children ages 2 to 12 also taking an antiepileptic drug other than carbamazepine, phenytoin, phenobarbital, primidone, or valproate. 0.3 mg/kg daily in 1 or 2 divided doses for 2 wk, followed by 0.6 mg/kg daily in 2 divided doses for 2 wk. Increased by 0.6 mg/kg daily every 1 to 2 wk, if needed. *Maintenance:* 4.5 to 7.5 mg/kg daily in 2 divided doses. *Maximum:* 300 mg daily.

Adults and children age 12 and over taking carbamazepine, phenytoin, phenobarbital, primidone but not taking valproate. 50 mg daily for 2 wk and then 100 mg daily in divided doses b.i.d. for 2 wk. Increased by 100 mg every 1 to 2 wk, if needed. *Maintenance:* 300 to 500 mg daily in divided doses b.i.d. *Maximum:* 700 mg daily in divided doses b.i.d.

Children ages 2 to 12 also taking carbamazepine, phenytoin, phenobarbital, primidone but not taking valproate. 0.6 mg/kg daily in divided doses b.i.d. for 2 wk and then 1.2 mg/kg daily in divided doses b.i.d. for 2 wk. Increased by 1.2 mg/kg every 1 to 2 wk, if needed to reach maintenance dosage. *Maintenance:* 5 to 15 mg/kg daily in divided doses b.i.d. *Maximum:* 400 mg daily.

▶ *To treat partial seizures after conversion from carbamazepine, phenytoin, phenobarbital, primidone, or valproate therapy*
CHEWABLE TABLETS, TABLETS

Adults and adolescents age 16 and over converting from carbamazepine, phenytoin, phenobarbital, or primidone. 50 mg daily for 2 wk, followed by 100 mg daily for next 2 wk. Increased by 100 mg daily every 1 to 2 wk (while continuing to take carbamazepine, phenytoin, phenobarbital, or primidone), until usual maintenance dosage—500 mg daily in divided doses b.i.d.—is achieved. Then, carbamazepine, phenytoin, phenobarbital, or primidone dosage tapered in 20% increments weekly over 4 wk and then discontinued.

Adults and adolescents age 16 and over converting from valproate. 25 mg every other day for 2 wk followed by 25 mg daily for 2 wk. Then increased by 25 to 50 mg daily every 1 to 2 wk until reaching 200 mg daily. Then, valproate dosage decreased to 500 mg daily by decrements no greater than 500 mg daily/wk and then maintained at 500 mg daily for 1 wk. After completion of week, lamotrigine dosage increased to 300 mg daily and maintained for 1 wk while valproate dosage simultaneously decreased to 250 mg daily and maintained for 1 wk. Then, lamotrigne dosage increased by 100 mg daily every wk to maintenance dose of 500 mg daily. Once achieved, valproate therapy is discontinued.

▶ *To delay occurrence of mood episodes (depression, mania, hypomania, mixed episodes) as maintenance therapy for bipolar 1 disorder*
CHEWABLE TABLETS, TABLETS

Adults not taking carbamazepine, phenytoin, phenobarbital, primidone, rifampin, or valproate. 25 mg daily for 2 wk, followed by 50 mg daily for 2 wk, followed by 100 mg daily for 1 wk and then increased to 200 mg daily as maintenance dose. *Maximum:* 200 mg daily.

Adults taking valproate. 25 mg every other day for 2 wk, followed by 25 mg daily for 2 wk, followed by 50 mg daily for 1 wk, and then increased to 100 mg daily as maintenance dose.

Adults taking carbamazepine, phenytoin, phenobarbital, primidone, or rifampin but not taking valproate. 50 mg daily for 2 wk, followed by 100 mg daily in divided doses for 2 wk, followed by 200 mg daily in divided doses for 1 wk. Then increased to 300 mg daily in divided doses for 1 wk. Then increased to 400 mg daily in divided doses as maintenance dose.

DOSAGE ADJUSTMENT For patient starting or stopping estrogen-containing oral contraceptives, lamotrigine dosage may need to be adjusted on individual basis. For patients with moderate to severe liver impairment without ascites, dosage reduced by 25%; for patients with severe liver impairment with ascites, dosage reduced by 50%

Route	Onset	Steady State	Peak	Half-Life	Duration
P.O.	Days to wks	Unknown	Unknown	15 to 35 hr*	Unknown

Mechanism of Action

May stabilize neuron membranes by blocking sodium channels in the membranes. This action inhibits the release of excitatory neurotransmitters, such as glutamate and aspartate, through these channels. By blocking the release of neurotransmitters, lamotrigine inhibits the spread of seizure activity in the brain and reduces seizure frequency.

Contraindications

Hypersensitivity to lamotrigine or its components

Interactions

DRUGS

acetaminophen (long-term use) olanzapine, rifampin: Possibly decreased blood lamotrigine level

carbamazepine: Decreased blood lamotrigine level; possibly increased incidence of dizziness, diplopia, ataxia, and blurred vision

---

* For lamotrigine taken alone. Half-life is 8 to 20 hr when taken with an enzyme-inducing anticonvulsant; 59 hr when taken with valproic acid only; and 28 hr when taken with an enzyme-inducing anticonvulsant and valproic acid.

folate inhibitors, such as co-trimoxazole and methotrexate: Increased blood lamotrigine level

oral contraceptives: Decreased blood lamotrigine level during 3-week hormone-active therapy and increased blood lamotrigine level during 1-wk hormone-inactive period; possibly reduced effectiveness of oral contraceptives

oxcarbazepine: Possibly increased incidence of headache, dizziness, nausea, and somnolence

phenobarbital, phenytoin, primidone: Decreased blood lamotrigine level, possibly increased CNS depression

topiramate: Increased blood topiramate level

valproic acid: Increased blood lamotrigine level, decreased lamotrigine clearance, decreased blood valproic acid level

ACTIVITIES

alcohol use: Possibly increased CNS depression

Adverse Reactions

CNS: Amnesia, anxiety, ataxia, confusion, depression, dizziness, drowsiness, emotional lability, fever, headache, increased seizure activity, lack of coordination, suicidal thoughts

CV: Chest pain

EENT: Blurred vision, diplopia, dry mouth, nystagmus

GI: Abdominal pain, anorexia, constipation, diarrhea, hepatic failure, vomiting

HEME: Anemia, aplastic anemia, disseminated intravascular coagulation, eosinophilia, leukopenia, neutropenia, pancytopenia, pure red cell aplasia, thrombocytopenia

SKIN: Petechiae, photosensitivity, pruritus, rash, Stevens-Johnson syndrome, toxic epidermal necrolysis

Other: Acute multiorgan failure, angioedema, flulike signs and symptoms, lymphadenopathy

Overdose

Monitor patient for signs and symptoms of overdose, including ataxia, coma, decreased salivation, dizziness, drowsiness, dysarthria, headache, nystagmus, seizures, tachycardia, and widened QRS complex.

Maintain an open airway and begin continuous ECG monitoring. Monitor ECG for changes, especially widened QRS complex. Institute seizure precautions according to facility protocol.

To decrease absorption of drug in a conscious patient who isn't at risk for coma or seizures, be prepared to induce vomiting or perform gastric lavage. Expect that oral activated charcoal may also be prescribed. For an unconscious patient, anticipate assisting with the insertion of an endotracheal tube and then performing gastric lavage. The inflated cuff of the endotracheal tube will help prevent aspiration of gastric contents into the lungs. The effectiveness of hemodialysis on the elimination of lamotrigine is unknown.

Institute suicide precautions according to facility policy, and anticipate psychiatric re-evaluation.

Nursing Considerations

- Use cautiously in patients with illnesses that could affect metabolism or elimination of lamotrigine, such as renal, hepatic, or cardiac impairment.
- Monitor patient for adverse reactions, especially suicidal thoughts, at start of therapy and with each dosage increase.
- If patient is taking the chewable tablet, give him a small amount of juice or water to help him swallow the drug.
- Be aware that the chewable tablet may be dissolved in a teaspoonful of water or juice for about 1 minute, then the solution swirled and taken immediately, to make drug easier to swallow.
- **WARNING** Lamotrigine may cause severe, potentially life-threatening rashes. Notify prescriber at first sign of rash and expect to discontinue drug. Be aware that patient shouldn't be restarted on lamotrigine after rash subsides.
- Monitor patient for seizure activity during therapy.
- Be aware that abrupt discontinuation of lamotrigine may cause increased seizure activity. Expect to taper dosage over at least 2 weeks, even for the treatment of bipolar disorder.

PATIENT TEACHING

- Advise patient to take lamotrigine exactly as prescribed and not to discontinue drug abruptly because doing so may increase seizure activity.
- Instruct patient taking the chewable tablet that it may be swallowed whole, chewed, or dissolved in a small amount of liquid (about 1 teaspoonful) for 1 minute, then swirled and swallowed immediately.
- Advise patient to notify prescriber immediately if fever, flulike signs or symptoms, lymphadenopathy, or rash occurs.
- Caution patient or caregiver about possibility of suicidal thoughts, especially when therapy begins or dosage changes.
- Instruct patient to report increased seizure activity, vision changes, and vomiting.
- Caution patient to avoid potentially hazardous activities until he knows how the drug affects him.

- Advise patient to avoid direct sunlight and to wear protective clothing to minimize the risk of photosensitivity.
- Instruct patient to wear medical identification stating that he takes an anticonvulsant.
- Tell female patient to notify prescriber if she starts or stops an oral contracepticve or other source of female hormones or if she is, could be, or intends to become pregnant.

levetiracetam

Keppra

Class and Category

Chemical class: Pyrrolidine derivative
Therapeutic class: Anticonvulsant
Pregnancy category: C

Indications and Dosages

▶ *As adjunct to treat partial seizures*
ORAL SOLUTION, TABLETS

Adults and adolescents over age 16. *Initial:* 500 mg b.i.d., increased by 1,000 mg daily every 2 wk if needed. *Maximum:* 3,000 mg daily.

Children ages 4 to 16. *Initial:* 10 mg/kg b.i.d., increased by 20 mg/kg daily every 2 wk until reaching recommended dose of 60 mg/kg daily.

I.V. INFUSION

Adults and adolescents over age 16. *Initial:* 500 mg infused over 15 minutes b.i.d., increased by 1,000 mg daily every 2 wk, if needed. *Maximum:* 3,000 mg daily.

▶ *As adjunct to treat myoclonic seizures in patients with juvenile myoclonic epilepsy*
ORAL SOLUTION, TABLETS

Adults and children age 12 and over. *Initial:* 500 mg b.i.d., increased by 1,000 mg daily every 2 wk, if needed. *Maximum:* 3,000 mg daily.

▶ *As adjunct to treat primary generalized tonic-clonic seizures in patients with idiopathic generalized epilepsy*
ORAL SOLUTION, TABLETS

Adults and children age 6 and over. *Initial:* 500 mg b.i.d., increased by 1,000 mg daily every 2 wk, as needed. *Maximum:* 3,000 mg daily.

DOSAGE ADJUSTMENT Maximum dosage reduced to

2,000 mg daily for patients with creatinine clearance of 50 to 80 ml/min/1.73 m^2; to 1,500 mg daily for creatinine clearance of 30 to 49 ml/min/1.73 m^2; and to 1,000 mg daily for creatinine clearance of less than 30 ml/min/1.73 m^2. For patients with end-stage renal disease who are receiving dialysis, expect to give an additional 250 to 500 mg, as prescribed, after each dialysis session. For children unable to tolerate 60 mg/kg daily, dosage reduced to point of tolerance.

Route	Onset	Steady State	Peak	Half-Life	Duration
P.O.	Unknown	2 days	Unknown	7 hr	Unknown

Mechanism of Action

May protect against secondary generalized seizure activity by selectively preventing the coordination of epileptiform burst firing. Levetiracetam doesn't appear to involve inhibitory and excitatory neurotransmission.

Contraindications

Hypersensitivity to levetiracetam or its components

Adverse Reactions

CNS: Abnormal gait, aggression, agitation, anger, anxiety, apathy, asthenia, ataxia, confusion, coordination difficulties, depersonalization, depression, dizziness, emotional lability, fatigue, hallucinations, headache, hostility, hyperkinesias, increased reflexes, insomnia, irritability, mental or mood changes, nervousness, neurosis, paresthesia, personality disorder, psychosis, seizures, somnolence, suicidal thinking, vertigo
EENT: Amblyopia, conjunctivitis, diplopia, ear pain, pharyngitis, rhinitis, sinusitis
GI: Anorexia, constipation, diarrhea, elevated liver enzymes, gastroenteritis, hepatic failure, hepatitis, pancreatitis, vomiting
GU: Albuminuria
HEME: Decreased hemtatocrit, hemoglobin, and total mean RBC count; leukopenia; neutropenia; pancytopenia; thrombocytopenia
MS: Neck pain
RESP: Asthma, cough
SKIN: Alopecia, ecchymosis, pruritus, rash, skin discoloration, vesiculobullous rash
Other: Dehydration, facial edema, infection, influenza, weight loss

Overdose

Be aware that information about levetiracetam overdose is limited; the only symptom reported has been drowsiness.

Maintain an open airway, and monitor vital signs and clinical status. To decrease drug absorption, be prepared to induce vomiting or perform gastric lavage. Hemodialysis is an effective treatment for levetiracetam overdose and may remove 50% of the drug in a 4-hour treatment.

Institute suicide precautions according to facility policy, and anticipate psychiatric re-evaluation.

Nursing Considerations

• Know that children who weigh 20 kg or less should only be given oral solution form.
• For intravenous use, dilute parenteral levetiracetam in 100 ml of a compatible diluent such as sodium chloride injection, lactated Ringer's injection, or 5% dextrose injection. Use within 24 hours.
• Monitor patient for drug compliance during first 4 weeks of levetiracetam therapy, when adverse reactions are most common.
• Monitor patient for seizure activity during levetiracetam therapy. As appropriate, implement seizure precautions according to facility policy.
• Be aware that certain adverse effects, such as somnolence, fatigue, coordination difficulties, and behavioral abnormalities, may occur more often in patients taking levetiracetam for partial seizure disorders.
• Be aware that stopping levetiracetam abruptly may increase seizure activity. Expect to taper dosage gradually.

PATIENT TEACHING

• Caution patient that levetiracetam may cause dizziness and drowsiness, especially during first 4 weeks of therapy.
• Advise patient to avoid activities that require a high level of alertness until he knows how the drug affects him.
• Caution patient not to stop taking levetiracetam abruptly; inform him that drug dosage should be tapered under prescriber's direction to avoid breakthrough seizures.
• If patient is already taking an anticonvulsant, tell him to continue taking it, as prescribed, along with levetiracetam.
• Encourage patient to avoid alcohol during levetiracetam therapy because alcohol can increase drowsiness and dizziness.
• Instruct patient to see prescriber regularly so that his progress can be monitored.

- Inform patient that levetiracetam may cause changes in behavior, such as aggression, depression, irritability, and, rarely, psychotic symptoms or thoughts of suicide. If any negative behavior occurs, urge him to notify prescriber.

levodopa

Larodopa

Class and Category

Chemical class: Dihydroxyphenylalanine isomer, metabolic precursor of dopamine
Therapeutic class: Antidyskinetic
Pregnancy category: Not rated

Indications and Dosages

▶ *To manage signs and symptoms of primary Parkinson's disease, postencephalitic parkinsonism, and parkinsonism caused by CNS injury from carbon monoxide or manganese intoxication*

CAPSULES, TABLETS

Adults and children age 12 and over. *Initial:* 250 mg daily in divided doses b.i.d. to q.i.d. Increased by 100 to 750 mg every 3 to 7 days, as indicated. *Maximum:* 8 g daily.

Route	Onset	Steady State	Peak	Half-Life	Duration
P.O.	14 to 21 days*	Unknown	Unknown	45 to 90 min	5 hr

Contraindications

Angle-closure glaucoma, history of melanoma, hypersensitivity to levodopa or its components, suspicious undiagnosed skin lesions, use within 14 days of MAO inhibitor therapy

Interactions

DRUGS

antacids: Increased blood levodopa level
antihypertensives: Risk of orthostatic hypotension
benzodiazepines: Possibly decreased therapeutic effects of levodopa
bromocriptine: Possibly additive effects of levodopa
furazolidone, MAO inhibitors, procarbazine: Risk of severe hypertension
haloperidol, loxapine, molindone, papaverine, phenothiazines, phenytoin, rauwolfia alkaloids: Decreased effects of levodopa
inhaled anesthetics, sympathomimetics: Increased risk of arrhythmias

* With multiple doses.

Mechanism of Action

By supplementing a low level of endogenous dopamine, levodopa helps control alterations in voluntary muscle movement (such as tremors and rigidity) associated with Parkinson's disease. Dopamine, a neurotransmitter that's synthesized and released by neurons leading from substantia nigra to basal ganglia, is essential for normal motor function. By stimulating peripheral and central dopaminergic$_2$ (D_2) receptors on postsynaptic cells, dopamine inhibits the firing of striatal neurons (such as cholinergic neurons). In Parkinson's disease, progressive degeneration of these neurons substantially reduces the supply of intrasynaptic dopamine. Levodopa, a dopamine precursor, increases the dopamine supply in neurons, making more available to stimulate dopaminergic receptors.

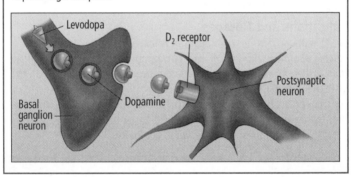

iron salts: Possibly decreased blood level and effectiveness of levodopa

methyldopa: Possibly toxic CNS effects

metoclopramide: Possibly worsening of Parkinson's disease and decreased therapeutic effects of metoclopramide

pyridoxine (vitamin B$_6$): Decreased antidyskinetic effect of levodopa

FOODS

high-protein food: Decreased levodopa absorption

ACTIVITIES

cocaine use: Increased risk of arrhythmias

Adverse Reactions

CNS: Aggressiveness, anxiety, ataxia, confusion, delusions, dizziness, dream disturbances, dyskinesia, dystonia, euphoria, hallucinations, headache, increased tremor, insomnia, malaise, mood changes, severe depression, suicidal tendencies, syncope, weakness

CV: Arrhythmias, hot flashes, orthostatic hypotension, palpitations

EENT: Bitter aftertaste, blurred vision, darkened saliva, diplopia, dry mouth, increased salivation, mydriasis, tooth clenching and grinding
GI: Abdominal pain, anorexia, constipation, diarrhea, flatulence, GI bleeding, hepatotoxicity, hiccups, indigestion, nausea, vomiting
GU: Darkened urine, priapism, urine retention
SKIN: Darkened sweat, diaphoresis, rash

Overdose

An early indication of overdose is blepharospasm, or eyelid spasm, so monitor patient for increased blinking or spasms of the eyelids. Acute overdose of levodopa has no specific antidote.

Maintain an open airway, institute ECG monitoring, and assess patient for arrhythmias. Expect to perform gastric lavage to decrease drug absorption. Administer I.V. fluids and an antiarrhythmic, as prescribed. The effectiveness of hemodialysis is unknown.

Institute suicide precautions according to facility policy, and anticipate psychiatric re-evaluation.

Nursing Considerations

- Expect to discontinue levodopa 6 to 8 hours before surgery to avoid interactions with anesthetics.
- Observe patient for mental or behavioral changes and suicidal tendencies. Notify prescriber immediately if they occur.
- Monitor patient for muscle twitching and blepharospasm, and report them immediately; they're early indications of overdose.
- Expect patient to be tested for acromegaly and diabetes during long-term levodopa therapy. Also expect to monitor hematopoietic, hepatic, and renal function.

PATIENT TEACHING

- Advise patient to take levodopa with meals if he experiences adverse GI reactions.
- Because protein impairs drug absorption, instruct patient to avoid high-protein meals during levodopa therapy and to distribute protein intake equally throughout the day.
- Caution patient to avoid excessive use of vitamins and fortified cereals that contain vitamin B_6 or iron, which can reduce levodopa's effects.
- Instruct patient to report fainting, increased muscle tremor, difficult urination, and severe or persistent nausea and vomiting.
- Urge patient to continue taking drug even if results of therapy aren't evident immediately.
- Inform patient that saliva, sweat, and urine may darken but that the change is harmless.

- Direct patient to protect drug from heat, light, and moisture and to discard darkened pills because they have lost their potency.
- Advise patient to change position slowly to minimize effects of orthostatic hypotension.
- Caution male patient about risk of priapism (persistent, painful erection that lasts longer than 4 hours), and urge him to seek medical treatment immediately if it occurs.

lisdexamfetamine dimesylate
Vyvanse

Class and Category
Chemical class: Sympathomimetic amine
Therapeutic class: CNS stimulant
Pregnancy category: C

Indications and Dosages
▶ *To treat attention deficit hyperactivity disorder (ADHD)*
CAPSULES
Children ages 6 to 12. *Initial:* 30 mg once daily in the morning, increased as needed in increments of 20 mg daily every wk. *Maximum:* 70 mg daily.

Route	Onset	Peak	Duration
P.O.	Unknown	1 hr	Unknown

Mechanism of Action
Produces CNS stimulation, probably by facilitating release and blocking reuptake of norepinephrine at adrenergic nerve terminals, by stimulating alpha and beta receptors in the peripheral nervous system, and by releasing and blocking reuptake of dopamine in the limbic region of the brain. By these actions, lisdexamfetamine decreases restlessness and increases alertness.

Contraindications
Advanced arteriosclerosis; agitation; glaucoma; history of drug abuse, hypersensitivity, or idiosyncratic reaction to lisdexamfetamine, other sympathomimetic amines, or their components; hyperthyroidism; MAO inhibitor therapy within 14 days; moderate to severe hypertension; symptomatic cardiovascular disease; history of seizures

Interactions
DRUGS
acetazolamide, alkalinizers (such as sodium bicarbonate), some thiazides: Increased blood level and effects of lisdexamfetamine
adrenergic blockers: Inhibited adrenergic blockade
antihistamines: Possibly reduced sedation from antihistamine
antihypertensives: Possibly decreased antihypertensive effects
chlorpromazine: Inhibited CNS-stimulant effects of lisdexamfetamine
ethosuximide: Possibly delayed ethosuximide absorption
GI acidifiers (such as ascorbic acid), reserpine: Decreased lisdexamfetamine absorption
guanethidine: Decreased antihypertensive effect and decreased lisdexamfetamine absorption
haloperidol: Decreased CNS stimulation
lithium carbonate: Possibly decreased anorectic and stimulant effects of lisdexamfetamine
MAO inhibitors: Potentiated effects of lisdexamfetamine; possibly hypertensive crisis
meperidine: Increased analgesia
methenamine: Increased urine excretion and decreased effects of lisdexamfetamine
norepinephrine: Possibly increased adrenergic effect of norepinephrine
phenobarbital, phenytoin: Synergistic anticonvulsant action
propoxyphene: Increased CNS stimulation and potentially fatal seizures
sympathomimetic drugs: Increased stimulant effect
tricyclic antidepressants: Possibly increased antidepressant effects and decreased lisdexamfetamine effects
urinary acidifiers (such as ammonium chloride and sodium acid phosphate): Increased amphetamine excretion and decreased amphetamine blood level and effects
veratrum alkaloids: Decreased hypotensive effect

Adverse Reactions
CNS: Affect lability, anxiety, dizziness, fever, headache, insomnia, irritability, psychomotor hyperactivity, seizures, somnolence, tic
CV: Ventricular hypertrophy
EENT: Dry mouth
GI: Anorexia, nausea, vomiting, upper abdominal pain
SKIN: Rash
Other: Weight loss

Overdose

Lisdexamfetamine overdose has no specific antidote. Monitor patient for signs and symptoms of overdose, including abdominal cramps, arrhythmias, chest pain, confusion, delirium, diaphoresis, diarrhea, dizziness, dyspnea, faintness, flushing, hallucinations, hyperpyrexia, hypertension or hypotension, irregular heartbeat, nausea, pallor, palpitations, panic reaction, paranoia, photosensitive mydriasis, polypnea, psychotic reactions, rhabdomyolysis, shock, syncope, tachypnea, toxic psychosis, tremor, unusual fatigue, vomiting, and weakness. Monitor patient for cardiac and respiratory changes. If possible, isolate patient to limit external stimuli.

Expect to provide symptomatic and supportive treatment, including performing gastric lavage or inducing vomiting. Anticipate use of I.V. fluids to manage hypotension, as needed. Expect to administer drugs and fluids to enhance diuresis, as prescribed. Be aware that drug treatment to induce urine acidification may also be prescribed to increase drug excretion, except for patients with hemoglobinemia, myoglobinuria, or rhabdomyolysis because of increased risk of renal failure. Be prepared to administer drugs such as a barbiturate or chlorpromazine to control CNS stimulation and phentolamine to manage hypertension.

Institute emergency supportive measures, and protect patient from self-injury. Implement suicide precautions according to facility policy, and anticipate psychiatric re-evaluation.

Nursing Considerations

- **WARNING** If patient has symptoms such as chest pain or fainting, notify prescriber immediately.
- **WARNING** Be aware that lisdexamfetamine shouldn't be given to children with structural cardiac abnormalities, cardiomyopathy, or other serious heart problems or rhythm abnormalities because even usual CNS-stimulant dosages increase the risk of sudden death in these children.
- Use lisdexamfetamine cautiously in children with hypertension, heart failure, recent MI, or ventricular arrhythmia because drug may increase blood pressure and worsen these conditions.
- Monitor patient's blood pressure closely; stimulant drugs such as lisdexamfetamine may increase it.
- Monitor patients with psychosis, bipolar illness, or a history of aggression or hostility; CNS stimulation may worsen symptoms.
- Assess growth pattern in pediatric patients because stimulants such as lisdexamfetamine may suppress growth. If this occurs,

notify prescriber and expect therapy to be halted.
- If patient has a history of seizures or EEG abnormality, watch for seizure activity because stimulants may lower the seizure threshold. Rarely, lisdexamfetamine may cause seizures in a child with no history of them. Take seizure precautions in all patients, and notify prescriber if a seizure occurs. Expect to discontinue lisdexamfetamine, as prescribed.
- Take safety precautions because stimulants may alter accommodation and cause blurred vision. Although these effects haven't been reported with lisdexamfetamine, the drug is a known stimlulant.
- Be aware that therapy may be stopped temporarily to assess the continued need for it, as evidenced by a return of hyperactivity and attention deficit.

PATIENT TEACHING
- **WARNING** Tell patient to contact his prescriber immediately if he develops such symptoms as chest pain or fainting.
- Instruct child and parents that capsule may be opened and contents dissolved in a glass of water; it should be drunk immediately.
- Tell child and parents that drug should only be taken in the morning because taking it later in the day may cause insomnia.
- Advise child and parents to report any signs or symptoms that suggest heart disease, such as exertional chest pain or unexplained syncope.
- Urge parents and child to avoid hazardous activities until drug effects are known.

lithium carbonate
Carbolith (CAN), Duralith (CAN), Eskalith, Eskalith CR, Lithane, Lithizine (CAN), Lithobid, Lithonate, Lithotabs

lithium citrate
Cibalith-S

Class and Category
Chemical class: Alkaline metal, monovalent cation
Therapeutic class: Antidepressant, antimanic drug
Pregnancy category: D

Indications and Dosage
▶ *To treat recurrent bipolar affective disorder; to prevent bipolar disorder depression*

CAPSULES, TABLETS
Adults and children age 12 and over. *Initial:* 300 to 600 mg t.i.d. *Maintenance:* 300 mg t.i.d. or q.i.d. *Maximum:* 2,400 g daily.
Children up to age 12. 15 to 20 mg/kg daily in divided doses b.i.d. or t.i.d.
E.R. TABLETS
Adults and children age 12 and over. *Initial:* 900 to 1,800 mg daily in divided doses b.i.d. or t.i.d. *Maintenance:* 450 mg b.i.d. or 300 mg t.i.d. *Maximum:* 2,400 g daily.
SLOW-RELEASE CAPSULES
Adults and children age 12 and over. 600 to 900 mg on day 1, increased to 1,200 to 1,800 mg daily in divided doses t.i.d. *Maintenance:* 900 to 1,200 mg daily in divided doses t.i.d. *Maximum:* 2,400 g daily.
SYRUP (LITHIUM CITRATE)
Adults and children age 12 and over. 8 to 16 mEq (equivalent of 300 to 600 mg of lithium carbonate) t.i.d. *Maintenance:* Equivalent of 300 mg of lithium carbonate t.i.d. or q.i.d. *Maximum:* Equivalent of 2,400 g daily of lithium carbonate.
Children up to age 12. 0.4 to 0.5 mEq (equivalent of 15 to 20 mg of lithium carbonate)/kg daily in divided doses b.i.d. or t.i.d.

Route	Onset	Steady State	Peak	Half-Life	Duration
P.O.	1 to 3 wk	12 hr	Unknown	24 hr*	Unknown

Mechanism of Action
May increase presynaptic degradation of the catecholamine neurotransmitters serotonin, dopamine, and norepinephrine; inhibit their release at neuronal synapses; and decrease postsynaptic receptor sensitivity. These actions may correct the overactive catecholamine systems in patients with mania.

Lithium's antidepressant action may result from enhanced serotonergic activity. The neurotransmitter serotonin produces feelings of well-being.

Contraindications
Blood dyscrasias, bone marrow depression, brain damage, cerebrovascular disease, coma, coronary artery disease, excessive intake of another CNS depressant, hypersensitivity to lithium or its components, impaired hepatic function, myeloproliferative disorders, severe depression, severe hypertension or hypotension

---

* For adults. Half-life is 18 hr for adolescents; 36 hr for elderly patients.

Interactions
DRUGS

ACE inhibitors, NSAIDs, piroxicam: Possibly increased blood lithium level and increased risk of lithium toxicity

acetazolamide, sodium bicarbonate, urea, xanthines: Decreased blood lithium level

calcium channel blockers, molindone: Increased risk of neurotoxicity from lithium

calcium iodide, iodinated glycerol, potassium iodide: Possibly increased hypothyroid effects of both drugs

carbamazepine: Possibly increased therapeutic effects of carbamazepine and neurotoxic effect of lithium

chlorpromazine, other phenothiazines: Possibly impaired GI absorption and decreased blood levels of these drugs; possibly masking of early signs and symptoms of lithium toxicity

desmopressin, lypressin, vasopressin: Possibly impaired antidiuretic effects of these drugs

diuretics (loop and osmotic): Increased lithium reabsorption by kidneys, possibly leading to lithium toxicity

fluoxetine, methyldopa, metronidazole: Increased risk of lithium toxicity

haloperidol and other antipsychotics: Increased risk of irreversible neurotoxicity and brain damage

neuromuscular blockers: Risk of prolonged paralysis or weakness

norepinephrine: Possibly decreased therapeutic effects of norepinephrine and severe respiratory depression

selective serotinin reuptake inhibitors: Increased risk of adverse reactions, especially agitation, confusion, diarrhea, dizziness, tremor

thyroid hormones: Possibly hypothyroidism

tricyclic antidepressants: Possibly severe mood swings from mania to depression

FOODS

high-sodium foods: Increased excretion and possibly decreased therapeutic effects of lithium

Adverse Reactions

CNS: Ataxia, coma, confusion, depression, dizziness, drowsiness, headache, lethargy, mania, seizures, syncope, tremor (in hands), vertigo

CV: Arrhythmias (including bradycardia and tachycardia), ECG changes, edema

EENT: Dental caries, dry mouth, exophthalmos

ENDO: Diabetes insipidus, euthyroid goiter, hypothyroidism, myxedema

GI: Abdominal distention and pain, anorexia, diarrhea, nausea, thirst
GU: Stress incontinence, urinary frequency
HEME: Leukocytosis
MS: Muscle twitching and weakness
RESP: Dyspnea
SKIN: Acne; alopecia; dry, thin hair; pruritus; rash
Other: Cold sensitivity, weight gain or loss

Overdose

Monitor patient for signs and symptoms of overdose, including anorexia, ataxia, blurred vision, confusion, diarrhea, dizziness, drowsiness, lack of coordination, muscle weakness, nausea, polyuria, slurred speech, seizures, tinnitus, tremor, and vomiting.

Maintain an open airway, monitor fluid and electrolyte levels, and obtain blood lithium level every 3 hours. Institute seizure precautions according to facility protocol.

To decrease drug absorption in a conscious patient who isn't at risk for seizures, be prepared to induce vomiting or perform gastric lavage. For an unconscious patient, anticipate assisting with the insertion of an endotracheal tube and then performing gastric lavage. The inflated cuff of the endotracheal tube will help prevent aspiration of gastric contents into the lungs.

To enhance drug elimination, anticipate the use of acetazolamide, aminophylline, mannitol, or urea, as prescribed. Hemodialysis is effective for treating lithium overdose. Be aware that the patient may need the dialysis treatment repeated because drug levels may rebound after 5 to 8 hours when the drug gets redistributed from the tissues to the blood.

Institute suicide precautions according to facility policy, and anticipate psychiatric re-evaluation.

Nursing Considerations

- Administer lithium after meals to slow absorption from GI tract and reduce adverse reactions. Dilute syrup with juice or other flavored drink before giving it.
- Note that 5 ml of lithium citrate equals 8 mEq of lithium ion or 300 mg of lithium carbonate.
- Expect to monitor blood lithium level two or three times weekly during first month and then weekly to monthly during maintenance therapy and when starting or stopping NSAID therapy. In uncomplicated cases, plan to monitor lithium level every 2 to 3 months.

• Be aware that lithium has a narrow therapeutic range. Even a slightly high blood level is dangerous, and some patients exhibit signs of toxicity at normal levels.

• Expect prescriber to decrease dosage after acute manic episode is controlled.

• **WARNING** Be aware that lithium affects the normal shift of intracellular and extracellular potassium ions, which can cause ECG changes, such as flattened or inverted T waves, and can increase the risk of cardiac arrest.

• Monitor patient's ECG, renal and thyroid function test results, and serum electrolyte levels, as appropriate, during lithium treatment.

• **WARNING** Be aware that lithium can cause reversible leukocytosis, which usually peaks within 7 to 10 days of starting therapy; WBC count typically returns to baseline within 10 days after lithium is discontinued.

• Weigh patient daily to detect sudden weight changes.

• Frequently monitor blood glucose level in diabetic patient because lithium alters glucose tolerance.

• Palpate thyroid gland to detect enlargement because drug may cause goiter.

• Ensure that patient's fluid and sodium intake is adequate during treatment.

PATIENT TEACHING

• Advise patient to take lithium with or after meals to minimize adverse reactions.

• Instruct patient to swallow E.R. or slow-release forms whole.

• Direct patient to mix syrup form with juice or other flavored drink before taking it.

• Inform patient that frequent urination, nausea, and thirst may occur during the first few days of treatment.

• Caution patient not to stop taking lithium or adjust dosage without first consulting prescriber.

• Instruct patient to report signs and symptoms of toxicity, such as diarrhea, drowsiness, muscle weakness, tremor, uncoordinated body movements, and vomiting.

• Urge patient to avoid potentially hazardous activities until he knows how the drug affects him.

• Advise patient to maintain normal fluid and sodium intake during therapy.

• Emphasize the importance of complying with scheduled checkups and laboratory tests.

lorazepam

Apo-Lorazepam (CAN), Ativan, Lorazepam Intensol, Novo-Lorazem (CAN), Nu-Loraz (CAN)

Class, Category, and Schedule

Chemical class: Benzodiazepine
Therapeutic class: Antianxiety drug, anticonvulsant, sedative
Pregnancy category: D (parenteral), Not rated (oral)
Controlled substance schedule: IV

Indications and Dosages

▶ *To treat anxiety*
ORAL CONCENTRATE, TABLETS
Adults and adolescents. 1 to 3 mg b.i.d. or t.i.d. *Maximum:* 10 mg daily.
DOSAGE ADJUSTMENT For elderly or debilitated patients, initial dosage may be reduced to 0.5 to 2 mg daily, divided.
▶ *To treat insomnia caused by anxiety*
ORAL CONCENTRATE, TABLETS
Adults and adolescents. 2 to 4 mg at bedtime.
DOSAGE ADJUSTMENT Dosage may be reduced for elderly or debilitated patients.
▶ *To treat status epilepticus*
I.V. INJECTION
Adults and adolescents. *Initial:* 4 mg at a rate of 2 mg/min. Repeated in 10 to 15 min if seizures continue. *Maximum:* 8 mg/ 24 hr.

Route	Onset	Steady State	Peak	Half-Life	Duration
P.O.	Unknown	2 to 3 days	Unknown	12 hr	Unknown
I.V.	5 min	Unknown	Unknown	10 to 20 hr	12 to 24 hr

Incompatibilities

Don't mix I.V. lorazepam in same syringe as buprenorphine.

Contraindications

Acute angle-closure glaucoma, hypersensitivity to lorazepam, benzodiazepines, or their components; intra-arterial administration; psychosis

Interactions

DRUGS
aminophylline, theophylline: Possibly reduced sedative effects of lorazepam
clozapine: Increased risk of marked sedation, excessive salivation,

Mechanism of Action

Causes hyperpolarization of selected CNS cell membranes, which helps relieve anxiety and reduce the incidence of seizures. Normally, when an impulse reaches a presynaptic nerve ending in the CNS, it releases neurotransmitters that bring about a response in the postsynaptic neuron. Gamma-aminobutyric acid (GABA) is the main inhibitory neurotransmitter. When GABA is released from the presynaptic nerve ending, as shown top right, it interacts with the GABA binding site located on the GABA receptor that's imbedded in the cell membrane of the postsynaptic neuron. This causes the chloride channel in the GABA receptor to open and chloride (Cl^-) ions to flow into the cell, causing hyperpolarization of the cell membrane. The end result is that excitatory stimulation is inhibited.

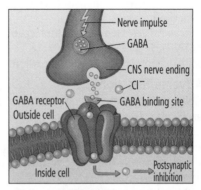

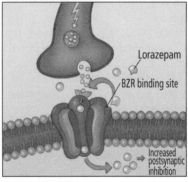

Lorazepam, a benzodiazepine, enhances the actions of GABA. The limbic system and cortical areas of the CNS contain a highly dense area of benzodiazepine receptors (BZRs), which are contained within the GABA receptors. When lorazepam engages with a BZR binding site, as shown immediately above, it increases the opening frequency of the chloride channels. This causes hyperpolarization of the cell membrane, which results in increased inhibition in the CNS and helps to relieve anxiety. The anticonvulsant action of lorazepam also results from hyperpolarization of the cell membrane, which suppresses the spread of seizure activity.

hypotension, ataxia, delirium, and respiratory arrest
CNS depressants: Additive CNS depression, including potentially fatal respiratory depression
digoxin: Possibly increased blood digoxin level and risk of digitalis toxicity

fentanyl: Possibly decreased therapeutic effects of fentanyl
probenecid: Possibly increased therapeutic and adverse effects of
lorazepam
valproate: Increased plasma lorazepam level
ACTIVITIES
alcohol use: Increased CNS depression

Adverse Reactions

CNS: Amnesia, anxiety, ataxia, coma, confusion, delusions, depression, dizziness, drowsiness, euphoria, extrapyramidal symptoms, headache, hypokinesia, irritability, malaise, nervousness, seizures, slurred speech, suicidal ideation, tremor
CV: Bradycardia, cardiac arrest, chest pain, hypotension, palpitations, tachycardia
EENT: Blurred vision, dry mouth, increased salivation, photophobia
ENDO: Syndrome of inappropriate ADH secretion
GI: Abdominal pain, constipation, diarrhea, nausea, thirst, vomiting
GU: Libido changes
HEME: Agranulocytosis, pancytopenia, thrombocytopenia
MS: Muscle weakness
RESP: Apnea, respiratory depression, worsening of sleep apnea or obstructive pulmonary disease
SKIN: Diaphoresis
Other: Phlebitis (I.V.), physical and psychological dependence, withdrawal signs and symptoms

Overdose

Monitor patient for evidence of overdose, including bradycardia, coma, confusion, dyspnea, hyporeflexia, seizures, severe drowsiness, shakiness, slurred speech, staggering, and weakness.

Maintain an open airway, institute continuous cardiac monitoring, and administer I.V. fluids, as prescribed, to maintain blood pressure and promote diuresis. Institute seizure precautions according to facility protocol.

To decrease drug absorption in a conscious patient who isn't at risk for coma or seizures, be prepared to induce vomiting or perform gastric lavage. Expect that oral activated charcoal may also be prescribed. For an unconscious patient, anticipate assisting with the insertion of an endotracheal tube and then performing gastric lavage. The inflated cuff of the endotracheal tube will help prevent aspiration of gastric contents into the lungs.

Anticipate giving a benzodiazepine receptor antagonist, such as flumazenil, to reverse the sedative effects of lorazepam, although flumazenil may induce seizures, especially in a patient who has taken benzodiazepines long-term or has ingested a cyclic antidepressant. If excitation occurs, a barbiturate shouldn't be used because it may increase excitement and prolong CNS depression. Dialysis is ineffective for treating benzodiazepine overdose.

Institute suicide precautions according to facility policy, and anticipate psychiatric re-evaluation.

Nursing Considerations

- In a depressed patient, make sure that antidepressant therapy is already in place before starting lorazepam therapy. Untreated depression increases the risk of suicide.
- Use extreme caution when giving lorazepam to elderly patients because it can cause hypoventilation, sedation, and unsteadiness. Also use caution in patients with compromised respiratory function because drug can cause respiratory depression.
- Use cautiously in patients with a history of alcohol or drug abuse or personality disorder because they have an increased risk of physical and psychological dependence. Also use caution in patients with severe hepatic insufficiency or encephalopathy because drug may worsen hepatic encelphalopathy.
- **WARNING** Monitor patient's respiratory status closely because drug may cause life-threatening respiratory depression.
- Dilute I.V. drug with equal amount of sterile water for injection, sodium chloride for injection, or D₅W. Give diluted drug slowly, at a rate not to exceed 2 mg/min.
- During I.V. use, monitor respirations every 5 to 15 minutes and keep emergency resuscitation equipment readily available.
- Dilute the oral concentrate form of lorazepam with a carbonated beverage, juice, or water, or a semisolid food such as applesauce or pudding. Mix before administering it, and don't save any mixture for later use.
- Abrupt drug discontinuation increases the risk of withdrawal signs and symptoms, including anxiety, confusion, insomnia, psychosis, and seizures. Expect to taper dosage gradually, especially in epileptic patients.

PATIENT TEACHING
- Instruct patient to take lorazepam exactly as prescribed and not to stop drug without consulting prescriber because of the risk of withdrawal signs and symptoms.
- Instruct patient or caregiver to use the calibrated dropper provided with the oral concentrate form to ensure correct dosage.

- Instruct patient taking oral concentrate to dilute the solution with a carbonated beverage, juice, or water, or a semisolid food such as applesauce or pudding just before taking drug. Tell him not to save any of the mixture for later use.
- Tell patient to store oral concentrate form in the refrigerator.
- Advise patient to avoid potentially hazardous activities until he knows how the drug affects him.
- Urge patient to avoid alcohol while taking lorazepam because it increases drug's CNS depressant effects.
- Instruct patient to report excessive drowsiness and nausea.
- Inform pregnant patient that lorazepam therapy will need to be discontinued early in third trimester to avoid possible withdrawal symptoms in the baby after delivery.

Other Therapeutic Uses

Lorazepam is also indicated for the following:
- To provide preoperative sedation

loxapine hydrochloride

Loxapac (CAN), Loxitane C, Loxitane IM

loxapine succinate

Loxapac (CAN), Loxitane

Class and Category

Chemical class: Dibenzoxazepine derivative
Therapeutic class: Antipsychotic drug
Pregnancy category: C

Indications and Dosages

▶ *To treat psychotic disorders and schizophrenia*
CAPSULES, ORAL SOLUTION
Adults. *Initial:* 10 mg b.i.d., increased over 7 days. *Maintenance:* 15 to 25 mg b.i.d. to q.i.d. *Maximum:* 250 mg daily.
DOSAGE ADJUSTMENT For elderly patients, dosage reduced to 3 to 5 mg b.i.d.
▶ *To treat acute exacerbations of psychotic disorders*
I.M. INJECTION
Adults. 12.5 to 50 mg every 4 to 6 hr or longer. *Maximum:* 250 mg daily.

Route	Onset	Steady State	Peak	Half-Life	Duration
P.O.	20 to 30 min	Unknown	½ to 3 hr	3 to 4 hr	12 hr
I.M.	Unknown	Unknown	Unknown	12 hr	Unknown

Mechanism of Action

May treat psychotic disorders by blocking dopamine at postsynaptic receptors in the brain. With prolonged use, loxapine enhances antipsychotic effects by causing depolarization blockade of dopamine tracts, resulting in decreased dopamine neurotransmission.

Contraindications

Blood dyscrasias, bone marrow depression, cerebrovascular disease, coma, coronary artery disease, hypersensitivity to loxapine or its components, impaired hepatic function, myeloproliferative disorders, severe drug-induced CNS depression, severe hypertension or hypotension

Interactions

DRUGS

amphetamines, ephedrine: Decreased effects of these drugs
antacids, antidiarrheals (adsorbent): Possibly decreased absorption of oral loxapine
anticholinergics: Possibly increased anticholinergic effects
anticonvulsants: Lowered seizure threshold, increased risk of seizures
antidyskinetics: Possibly antagonized effects of these drugs
bromocriptine: Possibly decreased therapeutic effects of bromocriptine
CNS depressants: Increased CNS depression
dopamine: Possibly decreased alpha-adrenergic effects of dopamine
epinephrine: Possibly severe hypotension or tachycardia, decreased effects of epinephrine
guanadrel, guanethidine, levodopa: Possibly decreased therapeutic effects of these drugs
MAO inhibitors, tricyclic antidepressants: Possibly increased blood levels of these drugs and increased CNS depressant and anticholinergic effects of these drugs and loxapine
metaraminol: Possibly decreased vasopressor effect of metaraminol
methoxamine: Possibly decreased vasopressor effect and duration of action of methoxamine

ACTIVITIES

alcohol use: Increased CNS depression

Adverse Reactions

CNS: Confusion, drowsiness, dystonia, involuntary motor activity, neuroleptic malignant syndrome, pseudoparkinsonism, sleep disturbance, tardive dyskinesia

CV: Orthostatic hypotension
EENT: Blurred vision, dry mouth
ENDO: Galactorrhea, gynecomastia
GI: Constipation, ileus, nausea, vomiting
GU: Menstrual irregularities, sexual dysfunction, urine retention
SKIN: Photosensitivity (mild), rash
Other: Weight gain

Overdose

Monitor patient for signs and symptoms of overdose, including coma, dizziness, drowsiness, dyspnea, hypotension, muscle tremor or stiffness, respiratory depression, seizures, tiredness, uncontrolled movements, and weakness.

Maintain an open airway, and assess patient for CNS and respiratory depression. Be prepared to assist with artificial respiration, as needed. Expect to treat hypotension with I.V. fluids and norepinephrine or phenylephrine, as prescribed. Be aware that epinephrine shouldn't be used because it may further lower patient's blood pressure. Institute seizure precautions according to facility protocol, and anticipate the use of an anticonvulsant.

Loxapine has an antiemetic effect, so ipecac syrup may not induce vomiting. Expect to treat extrapyramidal reactions with an antidyskinetic or diphenhydramine, as needed and prescribed.

Institute suicide precautions according to facility policy, and anticipate psychiatric re-evaluation.

Nursing Considerations

• Be aware that loxapine's full antipsychotic effect may take weeks before it becomes apparent.
• Be aware that parenteral loxapine is intended for I.M. use only. Although the solution may darken to a light amber color, the discoloration won't alter the effectiveness of the drug.
• Measure oral solution with the dropper that's provided by the manufacturer, and dilute drug with grapefruit or orange juice before administering it.
• After giving loxapine I.M., have patient remain lying down for 30 minutes because drug may cause orthostatic hypotension.
• Assess patient for signs of tardive dyskinesia, including involuntary protrusion of tongue and chewing movements. These signs may appear months or years after loxapine therapy begins and may not disappear with dosage reduction.
• Watch for extrapyramidal reactions or parkinsonian signs and symptoms, such as excessive salivation, masklike facies, rigidity,

and tremor, especially in first few days of treatment. Prescriber may reduce dosage to control these signs and symptoms.

• **WARNING** Monitor patient for neuroleptic malignant syndrome, a rare but possibly fatal adverse reaction. Early signs and symptoms include altered mental status, arrhythmias, fever, and muscle rigidity.

PATIENT TEACHING

• Instruct patient to dilute loxapine oral solution with grapefruit or orange juice just before taking. Advise him to use the calibrated dropper that accompanies the solution to ensure the correct dosage.

• Direct patient to avoid taking an antacid or antidiarrheal 2 hours before or after taking loxapine.

• Caution patient to avoid alcohol while taking loxapine.

• Advise patient to change position slowly to minimize effects of orthostatic hypotension.

• Urge patient to avoid potentially hazardous activities until he knows how the drug affects him.

• Advise patient to avoid prolonged exposure to sun and to use sunscreen to minimize the risk of photosensitivity.

• Encourage patient to have periodic eye examinations during therapy.

magnesium sulfate

*(contains 100 to 500 mg of elemental magnesium per 1 ml of injection
and 1 to 5 g of elemental magnesium per 10 ml of injection)*

Class and Category

Chemical class: Cation, electrolyte
Therapeutic class: Anticonvulsant
Pregnancy category: A

Indications and Dosages

▶ *To prevent and control seizures in preeclampsia or eclampsia as well
as seizures caused by epilepsy, glomerulonephritis, or hypothyroidism*
I.V. INFUSION OR INJECTION (MAGNESIUM SULFATE)
Adults. *Loading:* 4 g diluted in 250 ml of compatible solution
and infused over 30 min. *Maintenance:* 1 to 2 g/hr by continuous
infusion.
I.M. INJECTION (MAGNESIUM SULFATE)
Adults. 4 to 5 g every 4 hr, p.r.n.
Children. 20 to 40 mg/kg, repeated p.r.n.

Route	Onset	Steady State	Peak	Half-Life	Duration
I.V.	Immediate	Unknown	Unknown	Unknown	About 30 min
I.M.	1 hr	Unknown	Unknown	Unknown	3 to 4 hr

Mechanism of Action

Assists all enzymes involved in phosphate transfer reactions that use ATP.
Magnesium is required for normal function of the ATP-dependent sodium-
potassium pump in muscle membranes.

   As an anticonvulsant, magnesium depresses the CNS and blocks peripheral neuromuscular impulse transmission by decreasing the amount of available acetylcholine.

Incompatibilities

Don't combine magnesium sulfate with alkali carbonates, ar-
senates, bicarbonates, calcium, clindamycin phosphate, dobuta-

mine, fat emulsions, heavy metals, hydrocortisone sodium succinate, hydroxides, phosphates, polymyxin B, procaine hydrochloride, salicylates, sodium bicarbonate, strontium, and tartrates.

Contraindications
Heart block, hypersensitivity to magnesium salts or any component of magnesium-containing preparations, MI, preeclampsia
2 hours or less before delivery (I.V. form), renal impairment

Interactions
DRUGS
calcium (I.V. salts): Possibly neutralized effects of magnesium sulfate
CNS depressants: Possibly increased CNS depression
digoxin: Possibly cardiac conduction changes and heart block
neuromuscular blockers: Possibly increased neuromuscular blockade
nifedipine: Possibly increased hypotensive response

Adverse Reactions
CNS: Decreased or absent deep tendon reflexes, headache,
slurred speech, weakness
CV: Asystole, bradycardia, cardiac arrest, heart block, hypoten-
sion, prolonged PQ interval, widened QRS complex
EENT: Diplopia
GI: Nausea, vomiting
RESP: Dyspnea, respiratory paralysis
SKIN: Flushing

Overdose
Monitor patient for evidence of hypermagnesemia, as listed in *Adverse Reactions.* Maintain an open airway, and be prepared to assist
with artificial respiration. Institute continuous ECG monitoring,
and assess for changes, including asystole, bradycardia, heart
block, prolonged PQ interval, and widened QRS complex.

Anticipate using I.V. calcium gluconate, as prescribed, to treat
heart block or respiratory depression. Dialysis may increase drug
elimination because the kidneys excrete magnesium.

Nursing Considerations
• Be aware that magnesium sulfate is the elemental form of
magnesium.
• Dilute 50% magnesium sulfate injection to a concentration of
20% before I.V. infusion.
• Expect to administer I.V. magnesium sulfate at a rate that
doesn't exceed 150 mg/minute, except when using the drug to
treat seizures caused by severe eclampsia.

- Have I.V. calcium gluconate or calcium gluceptate readily available to antagonize the toxic effects of hypermagnesemia.
- **WARNING** Observe patient for early signs and symptoms of hypermagnesemia: bradycardia, depressed deep tendon reflexes, diplopia, dyspnea, flushing, hypotension, nausea, slurred speech, vomiting, and weakness. Notify prescriber immediately if patient experiences any of these signs or symptoms.
- **WARNING** Be aware that magnesium may precipitate myasthenic crisis by decreasing patient's sensitivity to acetylcholine.
- If patient is taking a drug that lowers heart rate, such as a beta blocker, frequently assess cardiac status because magnesium may aggravate signs and symptoms of heart block.
- If patient is experiencing renal insufficiency, monitor serum electrolyte levels because he's at risk for magnesium toxicity.
- Be aware that magnesium salts aren't intended for long-term use.

PATIENT TEACHING
- Explain that you'll measure patient's vital signs frequently and use ECG monitoring to detect cardiac changes and respiratory depression.
- Inform the patient that you'll frequently check her patellar reflex (knee jerk) to assess her for toxicity.

Other Therapeutic Uses

Magnesium sulfate is also indicated for the following:
- To correct magnesium deficiency caused by alcoholism, magnesium-depleting drugs, malnutrition, or restricted diet; to prevent magnesium deficiency based on recommended daily allowances
- To treat mild magnesium deficiency
- To treat severe hypomagnesemia
- To relieve constipation
- To evacuate colon for rectal or bowel examination

maprotiline hydrochloride
Ludiomil

Class and Category
Chemical class: Dibenzobicyclooctadiene derivative
Therapeutic class: Antidepressant
Pregnancy category: B

Indications and Dosages

▶ *To treat mild to moderate depression*
TABLETS
Adults and adolescents. *Initial:* 75 mg daily in divided doses for 2 wk. Increased in 25-mg increments as needed and tolerated. *Maintenance:* 150 to 225 mg daily in divided doses; for prolonged therapy, possibly 75 to 150 mg daily in divided doses.
▶ *To treat severe depression in hospitalized patients*
TABLETS
Adults and adolescents. *Initial:* 100 to 150 mg daily in divided doses, increased as needed and tolerated. *Maintenance:* 150 to 225 mg daily in divided doses; for prolonged therapy, possibly 75 to 150 mg daily in divided doses.
DOSAGE ADJUSTMENT For patients over age 60, initial dosage reduced to 25 mg daily and then increased by 25 mg/wk to maintenance dosage of 50 to 75 mg daily in divided doses.

Route	Onset	Steady State	Peak	Half-Life	Duration
P.O.	1 to 3 wk	7 days	3 to 6 wk	27 to 58 hr*	Unknown

Mechanism of Action

Blocks norepinephrine's reuptake at adrenergic nerve fibers. Normally, when a nerve impulse reaches an adrenergic nerve fiber, norepinephrine is released from its storage sites and metabolized in the nerve or at the synapse. Some norepinephrine reaches receptor sites on target organs and tissues, but most is taken back into the nerve and stored by way of the reuptake mechanism. By blocking norepinephrine reuptake, this tetracyclic antidepressant increases its level at nerve synapses. An elevated norepinephrine level may improve mood and, consequently, decrease depression.

Contraindications

Hypersensitivity to maprotiline, mirtazapine, or their components; use within 14 days of MAO inhibitor therapy

Interactions
DRUGS
anticholinergics, antihistamines: Increased atropine-like adverse effects, such as blurred vision, constipation, dizziness, and dry mouth
anticonvulsants: Increased risk of CNS depression, possibly lower seizure threshhold and increased risk of seizures

* 60 to 90 hr for active metabolite.

bupropion, clozapine, haloperidol, loxapine, molindone, phenothiazines, pimozide, thioxanthenes, trazodone, tricyclic antidepressants: Possibly increased anticholinergic effects, lowered seizure threshhold, and increased risk of seizures

cimetidine: Possibly increased blood maprotiline level

clonidine, guanadrel, guanethidine: Possibly decreased antihypertensive effects of these drugs; possibly increased CNS depression (with clonidine)

CNS depressants: Increased risk of CNS depression

estrogens, oral contraceptives containing estrogen: Possibly decreased therapeutic effects and increased adverse effects of maprotiline

MAO inhibitors: Increased risk of hyperpyrexia, hypertensive crisis, severe seizures, or death

sympathomimetics: Increased risk of arrhythmias, hyperpyrexia, hypertension, or tachycardia

thyroid hormones: Increased risk of arrhythmias

ACTIVITIES

alcohol use: Increased risk of CNS depression

Adverse Reactions

CNS: Agitation, dizziness, drowsiness, fatigue, headache, insomnia, seizures, tremor, weakness

EENT: Blurred vision, dry mouth, increased intraocular pressure

ENDO: Gynecomastia

GI: Constipation, diarrhea, epigastric distress, increased appetite, nausea, vomiting

GU: Impotence, libido changes, testicular swelling, urinary hesitancy, urine retention

HEME: Agranulocytosis

SKIN: Diaphoresis, photosensitivity, pruritus, rash

Other: Weight loss

Overdose

Monitor patient for signs and symptoms of overdose, including agitation, coma, dizziness, drowsiness, dyspnea, fever, irregular heartbeat, muscle stiffness or weakness, restlessness, seizures, tachycardia, and vomiting.

Maintain an open airway, institute continuous ECG monitoring and seizure precautions, and closely observe patient's blood pressure, respiratory rate, and temperature. Expect to treat hyperpyrexia with a cooling blanket, as needed. Be prepared to institute supportive measures such as performing gastric lavage to decrease drug absorption. Expect to administer activated charcoal followed by a bowel stimulant to enhance drug elimination, as prescribed. Maprotiline is highly protein bound, so dialysis is ineffective for treating overdose.

To treat hypotension, be prepared to administer I.V. fluids and corticosteroids, as prescribed. Anticipate that the patient may need digitalization to prevent heart failure. To treat arrhythmias, administer sodium bicarbonate to alkalize the blood and phenytoin or propranolol, as prescribed.

Expect to treat seizures with parenteral administration of a benzodiazepine or a barbiturate. If a barbiturate is given, observe the patient for respiratory depression, and have resuscitative equipment available to provide artificial respiration. Be aware that physostigmine shouldn't be administered because of the increased risk of seizures.

Institute suicide precautions according to facility policy, and anticipate psychiatric re-evaluation.

Nursing Considerations

- Give largest dose of maprotiline at bedtime if daytime drowsiness occurs.
- Obtain CBC, as ordered, if fever, sore throat, or other signs or symptoms of agranulocytosis develop.
- Take seizure precautions according to facility policy.
- Expect to taper drug dosage gradually because abrupt drug discontinuation may produce withdrawal signs and symptoms.

PATIENT TEACHING

- Tell patient to take maprotiline exactly as prescribed. Caution against stopping it abruptly because of risk of withdrawal symptoms, including headache, nausea, nightmares, and vertigo.
- Inform patient that she may not feel drug's effects for several weeks.
- Suggest taking drug with food if adverse GI reactions develop.
- Urge patient to report difficulty urinating, excessive drowsiness, fever, or sore throat.
- Advise patient to avoid potentially hazardous activities until she knows how the drug affects her.
- Urge patient to avoid alcohol and other CNS depressants while taking drug.

mazindol

Mazanor, Sanorex

Class, Category, and Schedule

Chemical class: Isoindole

Therapeutic class: Appetite suppressant
Pregnancy category: Not rated
Controlled substance schedule: IV

Indications and Dosages

▶ *As adjunct to treat exogenous obesity with caloric restriction, exercise, and behavior modification*

TABLETS

Adults and children age 16 and over. *Initial:* 1 mg daily. *Usual:* 1 mg t.i.d., 1 hr before meals, or 2 mg daily, 1 hr before lunch. *Maximum:* 3 mg daily.

Route	Onset	Steady state	Peak	Half-Life	Duration
P.O.	30 to 60 min	Unknown	Unknown	10 to 13 hr	8 to 15 hr

Mechanism of Action

Inhibits the reuptake of norepinephrine from adrenergic nerve terminals in the lateral hypothalamic feeding center of the cerebral cortex and reticular activating system. This action decreases appetite. By stimulating the CNS, mazindol causes other effects, including reduced gastric acid production and increased metabolism, which may be effective in treating obesity.

Contraindications

Advanced arteriosclerosis; agitation; cerebral ischemia; glaucoma; history of drug or alcohol abuse; hypersensitivity to mazindol, other sympathomimetic amines, or any of their components; hyperthyroidism; MAO inhibitor therapy within 14 days; moderate to severe hypertension; symptomatic cardiovascular disease

Interactions

DRUGS

antacids (calcium- and magnesium-containing), carbonic anhydrase inhibitors, citrates, sodium bicarbonate: Increased blood mazindol level
amphetamines, other appetite suppressants, selective serotonin reuptake inhibitors: Possibly increased risk of cardiac valve dysfunction
anesthetics (inhaled): Increased risk of arrhythmias
antihypertensives (especially clonidine, guanadrel, guanethidine, methyldopa, rauwolfia alkaloids): Decreased hypotensive effect of these drugs
ascorbic acid: Increased excretion of mazindol, causing decreased blood mazindol level
CNS stimulants, thyroid hormones: Additive CNS stimulation

insulin, oral antidiabetic drugs: Altered blood glucose level
MAO inhibitors: Potentiated effects of mazindol; possibly hypertensive crisis
phenothiazines: Reduced anorexic effect of mazindol
tricyclic antidepressants: Possibly potentiated adverse cardiovascular effects
urinary acidifiers (including ammonium chloride, potassium or sodium phosphates): Decreased blood mazindol level
vasopressors (especially catecholamines): Possibly potentiated vasopressor effect of these drugs
ACTIVITIES
alcohol use: Increased adverse CNS effects

Adverse Reactions

CNS: Cerebral ischemia, CNS stimulation, depression, dizziness, headache, insomnia, light-headedness, mania, nervousness, psychosis, syncope, tremor
CV: Chest pain, hypertension, palpitations, peripheral edema
EENT: Dry mouth
GI: Abdominal pain, constipation, nausea, vomiting
GU: Dysuria
RESP: Dyspnea
SKIN: Hives, rash
Other: Exercise intolerance

Overdose

Appetite suppressant overdose has no specific antidote. Monitor patient for evidence of overdose, including abdominal cramps, arrhythmias, coma, confusion, diarrhea, dyspnea, hallucinations, hostility, hyperreflexia, hyperthermia, labile blood pressure, nausea, panic reaction, restlessness, seizures, shock, tachypnea, tremor, and vomiting. Anticipate fatigue and depression to follow CNS excitement.

Maintain an open airway, monitor vital signs, and protect patient from self-injury. Institute seizure precautions according to facility policy. Expect to perform gastric lavage or induce vomiting and then to give activated charcoal, as prescribed, to decrease absorption. Expect to give a drug to promote urine acidification and I.V. fluids, as prescribed, to increase drug excretion.

Be prepared to give a drug such as a barbiturate, diazepam, or phenytoin to control CNS stimulation and seizures, a drug such as lidocaine to control arrhythmias, a nitrate or phentolamine to manage hypertension, and a beta blocker to control tachycardia. Effectiveness of hemodialysis and peritoneal dialysis is unknown.

Institute suicide precautions according to facility policy, and anticipate psychiatric re-evaluation.

Nursing Considerations

• Be aware that mazindol may cause physical and psychological dependence. Monitor patient for effects of long-term abuse, which may include hyperactivity, insomnia, personality changes, psychosis, severe dermatoses, and severe irritability.

• Monitor patient for chest pain, dyspnea, exercise intolerance, peripheral edema, and syncope, which may indicate cardiac valve dysfunction or pulmonary hypertension.

• **WARNING** Expect to taper drug gradually before discontinuing it to prevent withdrawal and increased rebound appetite. Monitor patient for withdrawal signs and symptoms, which may include abdominal cramps, depression, insomnia, nausea, nightmares, severe fever, and tremor. Notify prescriber immediately if signs and symptoms persist or worsen.

PATIENT TEACHING

• Advise patient to notify prescriber immediately about chest pain, dyspnea, exercise intolerance, peripheral edema, or syncope.

• Instruct patient to take last dose at least 4 to 6 hours before bedtime to prevent insomnia.

• Suggest that patient take mazindol with meals to prevent stomach upset.

• Instruct patient to take drug exactly as prescribed because of the risk of addiction. Tell her that tolerance to drug effects may develop in a few weeks and that long-term use may cause psychological or physical dependence. Explain that the drug will be reduced gradually to avoid withdrawal effects.

• Explain that behavior changes are needed for long-term weight loss. Stress the importance of maintaining a reduced caloric intake and routine exercise program.

• Instruct patient to avoid alcohol because of the risk of increased confusion, dizziness, light-headedness, and syncope.

• Advise patient to avoid potentially hazardous activities until she knows how the drug affects her.

• Teach patient ways to relieve dry mouth, such as sucking on ice chips or using sugarless candy or gum.

• Caution patient that drug may cause a false-positive result in urine drug screen for amphetamines.

• Advise patient to notify prescriber immediately if she knows or suspects that she's pregnant.

memantine hydrochloride

Namenda

Class and Category

Chemical class: N-methyl-D-aspartate receptor antagonist
Therapeutic class: Antidementia agent
Pregnancy category: B

Indications and Dosages

▶ *To treat moderate to severe dementia of the Alzheimer's type*

TABLETS

Adults. *Initial:* 5 mg daily P.O., increased by 5 mg/wk, as needed, to 10 mg daily in two divided doses; then 15 mg daily with one 5-mg and one 10-mg dose daily; then 20 mg daily in two divided doses. *Maintenance:* 20 mg daily.

DOSAGE ADJUSTMENT Dosage reduction probable for patients with renal impairment.

Mechanism of Action

Blocks the action of the excitatory amino acid glutamate on N-methyl-D-aspartate (NMDA) receptor cells in the CNS. In Alzheimer's disease, glutamate levels are abnormally high when brain cells are both at rest and active. Normally, when certain brain cells are resting, magnesium ions block NMDA receptors and prevent the influx of sodium and calcium ions and the outflow of potassium ions. When learning and memory cells are active, glutamate engages with NMDA receptors, magnesium ions are removed from NMDA receptors, and the cells are depolarized. During depolarization, sodium and calcium ions enter brain cells and potassium ions leave. In Alzheimer's disease, excessive circulating glutamate permanently removes magnesium ions and opens ion channels. The excessive influx of calcium may damage brain cells and play a major role in Alzheimer's disease. What's more, dying brain cells release additional glutamate, worsening the cycle of brain cell destruction.

Memantine replaces magnesium on the NMDA receptors of brain cells, closing ion channels and preventing calcium influx and the resulting damage to brain cells. By preventing excessive brain cell death, memantine slows the progression of Alzheimer's disease.

Contraindications

Hypersensitivity to memantine, amantadine, or their components

Interactions

DRUGS

amantadine, dextromethorphan, ketamine: Possibly additive effects *carbonic anhydrase inhibitors, sodium bicarbonate:* Decreased memantine clearance, leading to increased blood drug levels and risk of adverse effects

cimetidine, hydrochlorothiazide, metformin, nicotinic acid, quinidine, ranitidine, triamterene: Possibly increased blood levels of both agents

Adverse Reactions

CNS: Abnormal gait, agitation, akathisia, anxiety, confusion, CVA, delirium, delusions, depression, dizziness, drowsiness, dyskinesia, fatigue, hallucinations, headache, hyperexcitability, insomnia, malaise, neuroleptic malignant syndrome, psychosis, restlessness, seizures, somnolence, tardive dyskinesia

CV: Atrioventricular block, chest pain, claudication, hyperlipidemia, hypertension, peripheral edema, prolonged QT interval, supraventricular tachycardia, tachycardia

ENDO: Hypoglycemia

GI: Acute pancreatitis, anorexia, colitis, constipation, diarrhea, gastroesophageal reflux, gastritis, hepatic failure, ileus, indigestion, nausea, vomiting

GU: Acute renal failure, impotence, urinary incontinence, UTI

HEME: Thrombocytopenia

MS: Arthralgia, back pain

RESP: Bronchitis, cough, dyspnea, upper respiratory tract infection

SKIN: Stevens-Johnson syndrome

Other: Generalized pain, flulike symptoms

Overdose

Memantine overdose has no specific antidote. Monitor patient for signs and symptoms, including restlessness, psychosis, visual hallucinations, somnolence, stupor, and loss of consciousness.

Maintain an open airway, and monitor patient's vital signs closely. Be prepared to administer a urine-acidifying drug to enhance memantine elimination. Provide symptomatic and supportive treatment, as needed and prescribed.

Institute suicide precautions according to facility policy, and anticipate psychiatric re-evaluation.

Nursing Considerations

• Use memantine with caution in patients with renal tubular acidosis or severe UTI because these conditions cause urine to become alkaline, thereby reducing memantine excretion and increasing the risk of adverse reactions.
• Use cautiously in patients with severe hepatic impairment be-

cause drug undergoes partial hepatic metabolism, which may increase risk of adverse reactions.
• Monitor patient's response to memantine, and notify prescriber if serious or bothersome adverse reactions occur.

PATIENT TEACHING
• Advise patient to avoid a diet excessively high in fruits and vegetables because these foods contribute to alkaline urine, which can alter memantine clearance and increase adverse reactions.
• Caution patient to avoid potentially hazardous activities until drug's CNS effects are known.

mephenytoin
Mesantoin

Class and Category
Chemical class: Hydantoin derivative
Therapeutic class: Anticonvulsant
Pregnancy category: Not rated

Indications and Dosages
▶ *To control generalized tonic-clonic, focal, and jacksonian seizures when other drugs are ineffective*

TABLETS
Adults. *Initial:* 50 to 100 mg daily during first wk. Increased by 50 to 100 mg at 1-wk intervals until desired response is reached. *Maintenance:* 200 to 600 mg daily in equally divided doses. *Maximum:* 1.2 g daily.
Children. *Initial:* 25 to 50 mg daily. Increased by 25 to 50 mg at 1-wk intervals until desired response occurs. *Maintenance:* 100 to 400 mg daily in equally divided doses. *Maximum:* 400 mg daily.
▶ *To replace other anticonvulsants*

TABLETS
Adults. 50 to 100 mg daily during first wk. Dosage is gradually increased while dosage of other drug is decreased over 3 to 6 wk.

Route	Onset	Steady State	Peak	Half-Life	Duration
P.O.	30 min	Unknown	Unknown	7 hr*	24 to 48 hr

Contraindications
Hypersensitivity to mephenytoin, phenytoin, other hydantoins, or their components

* 95 to 144 hr for active metabolite, nirvanol.

Mechanism of Action

Limits the spread of seizure activity and the start of new seizures by regulating voltage-dependent sodium and calcium channels in neurons, inhibiting calcium movement across neuronal membranes, and enhancing sodium-potassium adenosine triphosphatase activity in neurons and glial cells.

These actions may result from mephenytoin's ability to slow the recovery rate of inactivated sodium channels.

Interactions

DRUGS

acetaminophen: Increased risk of hepatotoxicity with long-term acetaminophen use

amiodarone: Possibly increased blood mephenytoin level and risk of toxicity

antacids: Possibly decreased mephenytoin effectiveness

antineoplastics: Increased mephenytoin metabolism

bupropion, clozapine, loxapine, MAO inhibitors, maprotiline, phenothiazines, pimozide, thioxanthenes: Possibly lowered seizure threshold and decreased therapeutic effects of mephenytoin, possibly intensified CNS depressant effects of these drugs

calcium channel blockers, fluconazole, itraconazole, ketoconazole, miconazole, omeprazole: Possibly increased blood phenytoin level

carbamazepine: Decreased blood carbamazepine level, possibly increased blood phenytoin level and risk of toxicity

chloramphenicol, cimetidine, disulfiram, isoniazid, methylphenidate, metronidazole, phenylbutazone, ranitidine, salicylates, sulfonamides, trimethoprim: Possibly impaired metabolism of these drugs and increased risk of mephenytoin toxicity

corticosteroids, cyclosporine, digoxin, disopyramide, doxycycline, furosemide, levodopa, mexiletine, quinidine: Decreased therapeutic effects of these drugs

diazoxide: Possibly decreased therapeutic effects of both drugs

estrogens, progestins: Decreased therapeutic effects of these drugs, increased blood phenytoin level

felbamate: Possibly impaired metabolism and increased blood level of phenytoin

fluoxetine: Possibly increased blood phenytoin level and risk of toxicity

folic acid: Increased mephenytoin metabolism, decreased seizure control

haloperidol: Possibly lowered seizure threshold and decreased therapeutic effects of mephenytoin; possibly decreased blood haloperidol level

insulin, oral antidiabetic drugs: Possibly increased blood glucose level and decreased therapeutic effects of these drugs

lamotrigine: Possibly decreased therapeutic effects of lamotrigine

lithium: Increased risk of lithium toxicity

methadone: Possibly increased methadone metabolism, leading to withdrawal symptoms

molindone: Possibly lowered seizure threshold, impaired absorption, and decreased therapeutic effects of mephenytoin

oral anticoagulants: Possibly impaired metabolism of these drugs and increased risk of mephenytoin toxicity; possibly increased anticoagulant effect initially, but decreased effect with prolonged therapy

oral contraceptives (estrogen- and progestin-containing): Possibly breakthrough bleeding and decreased contraceptive effectiveness

rifampin: Possibly decreased therapeutic effects of mephenytoin

streptozocin: Possibly decreased therapeutic effects of streptozocin

sucralfate: Possibly decreased mephenytoin absorption

tricyclic antidepressants: Possibly lowered seizure threshold and decreased therapeutic effects of mephenytoin; possibly decreased blood level of tricyclic antidepressants

valproic acid: Decreased blood phenytoin level, increased blood valproic acid level

vitamin D analogues: Decreased vitamin D analogue activity, risk of anticonvulsant-induced rickets and osteomalacia

xanthines: Possibly inhibited mephenytoin absorption and increased clearance of xanthines

zaleplon: Increased clearance and decreased effectiveness of zaleplon

ACTIVITIES

alcohol use: Possibly decreased mephenytoin effectiveness

Adverse Reactions

CNS: Ataxia, choreoathetoid movements, confusion, dizziness, drowsiness, excitement, fatigue, fever, headache, peripheral neuropathy, sedation, slurred speech, stuttering, tremor

EENT: Gingival hyperplasia, nystagmus

GI: Constipation, diarrhea, nausea, vomiting

HEME: Agranulocytosis, leukopenia, thrombocytopenia

MS: Muscle twitching

SKIN: Rash, Stevens-Johnson syndrome, toxic epidermal necrolysis

Other: Lymphadenopathy, systemic lupus erythematosus

Overdose

Hydantoin overdose has no specific antidote. Monitor patient for signs and symptoms of overdose, including ataxia, blurred vision, confusion, dizziness, drowsiness, dysarthria, hyperreflexia, nausea, nystagmus, seizures, slurred speech, staggering, tiredness, tremor, and vomiting.

Maintain an open airway, and expect to administer oxygen and a vasopressor, as prescribed, for cardiovascular, CNS, and respiratory depression. Institute seizure precautions according to facility protocol.

Be prepared to induce vomiting or perform gastric lavage and to give activated charcoal and cathartic, as prescribed, to decrease drug absorption. Be aware that dialysis, diuresis, exchange transfusions, and plasmapheresis are ineffective for treating hydantoin overdose because these drugs aren't eliminated by the kidney.

Monitor patient's hematologic status following recovery because hydantoins may cause agranulocytosis, leukopenia, and thrombocytopenia.

Institute suicide precautions according to facility policy, and anticipate psychiatric re-evaluation.

Nursing Considerations

• Because of mephenytoin's potentially dangerous adverse effects, expect to use it only when other drugs are ineffective.

• Keep in mind that mephenytoin doesn't control absence seizures.

• **WARNING** Be aware that drug shouldn't be abruptly discontinued because doing so may cause status epilepticus. Plan to reduce dosage gradually or substitute another drug, as prescribed, when discontinuing mephenytoin.

• Obtain CBC and differential before treatment, after 2 weeks of treatment, and then monthly during first year of treatment, as ordered.

• If patient experiences depressed blood counts, enlarged lymph nodes, or rash, notify prescriber immediately and expect to discontinue mephenytoin and substitute another drug.

PATIENT TEACHING

• Instruct patient to take mephenytoin exactly as prescribed and not to discontinue drug abruptly.

• Advise patient to take drug with food to enhance absorption and reduce adverse GI reactions.

• Caution patient on once-a-day therapy to be especially careful not to miss a dose.

- Advise patient to report impaired coordination, persistent headache, rash, severe GI distress, swollen gums or lymph nodes, or unusual bleeding or bruising.
- Encourage patient to maintain good oral hygiene and to have regular checkups with a dentist to reduce the risk of gum disease.
- Instruct patient to keep medical appointments to monitor drug effectiveness and check for adverse reactions. Explain the need for periodic laboratory tests.
- Advise patient to wear or carry medical identification stating that she has epilepsy and takes mephenytoin to prevent seizures.

mephobarbital
Mebaral

Class, Category, and Schedule
Chemical class: Barbiturate derivative
Therapeutic class: Anticonvulsant, sedative
Pregnancy category: D
Controlled substance schedule: IV

Indications and Dosages
▶ *To treat seizures*
TABLETS
Adults. 400 to 600 mg daily as a single dose or in divided doses, usually beginning with low dose and increasing over 4 to 5 days until optimum dosage is determined.
Children age 5 and over. 32 to 64 mg t.i.d. or q.i.d.
Children younger than age 5. 16 to 32 mg t.i.d. or q.i.d.
▶ *To provide sedation*
TABLETS
Adults. 32 to 100 mg t.i.d. or q.i.d.
Children. 16 to 32 mg t.i.d. or q.i.d.

Route	Onset	Steady State	Peak	Half-Life	Duration
P.O.	30 to 60 min	Unknown	Unknown	11 to 67 hr	10 to 16 hr

Contraindications
Hepatic disease or failure; history of addiction to sedatives or hypnotics; hypersensitivity to mephobarbital, other barbiturates, or their components; nephritis; porphyria; severe respiratory disease with obstruction or dyspnea

Mechanism of Action

May reduce seizure activity by reducing transmission of monosynaptic and polysynaptic nerve impulses, which causes decreased excitability in nerve cells. As a sedative, mephobarbital inhibits upward conduction of nerve impulses to the reticular formation of the brain, which disrupts impulse transmission to the cortex. As a result, mephobarbital depresses the CNS and produces drowsiness, hypnosis, and sedation.

Interactions

DRUGS

acetaminophen: Possibly decreased effects of acetaminophen (with long-term mephobarbital use)

anesthetics (halogenated hydrocarbon): Increased risk of hepatotoxicity (with long-term mephobarbital use)

carbamazepine, chloramphenicol, corticosteroids, cyclosporine, dacarbazine, disopyramide, doxycycline, griseofulvin, metronidazole, oral contraceptives, phenylbutazone, quinidine, theophyllines, vitamin D: Decreased effectiveness of these drugs

CNS depressants: Increased CNS depression

divalproex sodium, valproic acid: Increased risk of CNS depression and neurotoxicity

guanadrel, guanethidine: Increased risk of orthostatic hypotension

haloperidol: Possibly decreased blood haloperidol level and change in seizure pattern

hydantoins: Possibly interference with hydantoin metabolism

leucovorin: Possibly decreased anticonvulsant effect of mephobarbital

maprotiline: Possibly increased CNS depression and decreased therapeutic effects of mephobarbital

mexiletine: Possibly decreased blood mexiletine level

oral anticoagulants: Possibly decreased therapeutic effects of anticoagulants, possibly increased risk of bleeding when mephobarbital is discontinued

tricyclic antidepressants: Possibly decreased therapeutic effects of tricyclic antidepressants

ACTIVITIES

alcohol use: Increased CNS depression

Adverse Reactions

CNS: Agitation, anxiety, ataxia, confusion, delusions, depression, dizziness, drowsiness, fever, hallucinations, headache, insomnia, irritability, nervousness, nightmares, paradoxical stimulation, seizures, syncope, tremor

CV: Orthostatic hypotension
EENT: Vision changes
GI: Anorexia, constipation, hepatic dysfunction, nausea, vomiting
HEME: Agranulocytosis
MS: Arthralgia, bone pain, muscle twitching or weakness
RESP: Respiratory depression
SKIN: Exfoliative dermatitis, rash, Stevens-Johnson syndrome
Other: Physical and psychological dependence, weight loss

Overdose

Monitor patient for signs and symptoms of overdose, including bradycardia, Cheyne-Stokes respiration, coma, confusion, decreased or absent reflexes, dyspnea, fever, hypothermia, miosis or mydriasis, oliguria, severe drowsiness, severe weakness, shock, slurred speech, staggering, tachycardia, and unusual eye movements. If patient has signs and symptoms such as continued irritability, insomnia, poor judgment, and severe confusion, the problem may be chronic overdose.

Maintain an open airway, and carefully monitor blood pressure and temperature. If the patient is conscious, be prepared to give ipecac syrup, as prescribed, to induce vomiting. Expect to administer activated charcoal, 30 to 60 g, with water or sorbitol to prevent further absorption and to enhance drug elimination.

For an unconscious patient, anticipate assisting with the insertion of an endotracheal tube and then performing gastric lavage. The inflated cuff of the endotracheal tube will help prevent aspiration of gastric contents into the lungs.

Be prepared to administer a drug to promote urine alkalization in order to enhance drug elimination. Administer I.V. fluids and a vasopressor, as prescribed. For severe cases, anticipate the need for hemodialysis or hemoperfusion. Be aware that, in cases of extreme barbiturate overdose, the patient may have a flat EEG because all electrical activity in the brain has ceased; however, this effect may be reversible.

Institute suicide precautions according to facility policy, and anticipate psychiatric re-evaluation.

Nursing Considerations

• Observe patient for signs and symptoms of physical and psychological dependence on mephobarbital, especially if she's undergoing long-term, high-dose therapy.
• Observe patient for signs and symptoms of chronic barbiturate intoxication, including confusion, insomnia, poor judgment, slurred speech, and unsteady gait.

- If patient receives a drug for acute or chronic pain, assess her for paradoxical stimulation.
- **WARNING** Expect to taper dosage gradually when discontinuing drug. Be aware that withdrawal signs and symptoms can be severe and may cause death. Mild signs and symptoms—including anxiety, muscle twitching, nausea, orthostatic hypotension, and progressive weakness—appear 8 to 12 hours after last drug dose. More severe signs include delirium and seizures.

PATIENT TEACHING

- Advise patient to take mephobarbital exactly as prescribed. Caution her not to stop taking drug abruptly because of the risk of withdrawal signs and symptoms and, for epileptic patients, seizures.
- Instruct patient to avoid alcohol, sleeping pills, and other sedatives while taking mephobarbital because of the risk of increased CNS depression.
- Advise patient to avoid potentially hazardous activities until she knows how the drug affects her.
- Advise patient to change position slowly to minimize effects of orthostatic hypotension.
- Urge patient to report confusion, fever, rash, or severe dizziness.

meprobamate

Apo-Meprobamate (CAN), Equanil, MB-Tab, Meprospan, Miltown, Neuramate

Class, Category, and Schedule

Chemical class: Carbamate derivative
Therapeutic class: Antianxiety drug
Pregnancy category: Not rated
Controlled substance schedule: IV

Indications and Dosages

▶ *To treat anxiety*

S.R. CAPSULES

Adults and adolescents. 400 to 800 mg every morning and bedtime. *Maximum:* 2,400 mg daily.

Children ages 6 to 12. 200 mg every morning and bedtime.

TABLETS

Adults and adolescents. 1,200 to 1,600 mg daily in divided doses t.i.d. or q.i.d. *Maximum:* 2,400 mg daily.

DOSAGE ADJUSTMENT For patients with creatinine clear-

ance of 10 to 50 ml/min/1.73 m², drug administered every
12 hr; with creatinine clearance of less than 10 ml/min/1.73 m²,
drug administered every 18 hr.
Children ages 6 to 12. 200 to 600 mg daily in divided doses
b.i.d. or t.i.d.

Route	Onset	Steady State	Peak	Half-Life	Duration
P.O.	1 hr	Unknown	Unknown	10 hr	Unknown

Mechanism of Action
May act at multiple sites in the CNS, including the thalamus and limbic system. Meprobamate inhibits spinal reflexes, causing CNS relaxation; its sedative effects may account for its anticonvulsant action. It also has muscle relaxant properties.

Contraindications
Hypersensitivity to meprobromate or related drugs, such as
carisoprodol; porphyria

Interactions
DRUGS
CNS depressants: Increased CNS depression
ACTIVITIES
alcohol use: Increased CNS depression

Adverse Reactions
CNS: Ataxia, dizziness, drowsiness, euphoria, headache, paradoxical stimulation, paresthesia, slurred speech, syncope, vertigo, weakness
CV: Arrhythmias, including tachycardia; hypotension; palpitations
EENT: Impaired visual accommodation
GI: Diarrhea, nausea, vomiting
SKIN: Erythematous maculopapular rash, pruritus, urticaria
Other: Physical dependence

Overdose
Monitor patient for signs and symptoms of overdose, including
bradycardia, confusion, dizziness, drowsiness, dyspnea, slurred
speech, staggering, and weakness.

Maintain an open airway, assess patient for dyspnea, and assist
with artificial respiration, as needed. Monitor vital signs and fluid
intake and output.

To decrease drug absorption, be prepared to induce vomiting or perform gastric lavage. Anticipate the use of I.V. fluids or mannitol to promote diuresis and dialysis to enhance drug elimination.

Institute suicide precautions according to facility policy, and anticipate psychiatric re-evaluation.

Nursing Considerations
- If patient has a history of impaired hepatic or renal function, assess effects of meprobamate because the drug is metabolized in the liver and excreted by the kidneys.
- Be aware that the drug may prompt seizures in a patient who has epilepsy. Institute seizure precautions according to facility policy.
- If patient has a history of drug dependence or abuse, use meprobamate cautiously because its use can lead to physical dependence and abuse.
- Observe patient for signs and symptoms of chronic drug intoxication, such as ataxia, slurred speech, and vertigo.
- **WARNING** Expect to taper meprobamate dosage gradually over 2 weeks when discontinuing the drug because abrupt discontinuation can worsen patient's previous symptoms, such as anxiety, or cause withdrawal signs and symptoms, such as confusion, hallucinations, muscle twitching, tremor, and vomiting.

PATIENT TEACHING
- Instruct patient to take meprobamate exactly as directed and not to stop taking it abruptly.
- Advise patient not to crush or chew S.R. capsules.
- Instruct patient to avoid potentially hazardous activities until she knows how the drug affects her.
- Direct patient to avoid alcohol, sedatives, and other CNS depressants while taking meprobamate.
- Inform patient that drug may become less effective after several months of treatment.
- Instruct patient to report rash.

mesoridazine besylate
Serentil

Class and Category
Chemical class: Alkylpiperidine phenothiazine derivative
Therapeutic class: Antipsychotic drug
Pregnancy category: Not rated

Indications and Dosages

▶ *To treat schizophrenia in patients unresponsive to other antipsychotic drugs*

ORAL SOLUTION, TABLETS

Adults and adolescents. 50 mg t.i.d., increased as needed and tolerated. *Maximum:* 400 mg daily.

I.M. INJECTION

Adults and adolescents. 25 mg, repeated in 30 to 60 min, as needed. *Maximum:* 200 mg daily.

Route	Onset	Steady State	Peak	Half-Life	Duration
P.O., I.M.	Up to several wk	4 to 7 days*	6 wk to 6 mo	Unknown	4 to 8 hr

Mechanism of Action

Depresses brain areas that control activity and aggression—including the cerebral cortex, hypothalamus, and limbic system—by blocking postsynaptic dopmaine$_2$ (D$_2$) receptors. Mesoridazine may relieve anxiety by indirectly reducing arousal and increasing the filtering of internal stimuli to the reticular activating system.

Contraindications

Coma; concurrent use of drugs that cause prolonged QT interval or history of arrhythmias or prolonged QT interval; concurrent use of high doses of a CNS depressant; hypersensitivity to mesoridazine, other phenothiazines, or their components; severe CNS depression

Interactions

DRUGS

antacids (aluminum- and magnesium-containing), antidiarrheals (adsorbent): Decreased mesoridazine absorption

amantadine, anticholinergics: Increased anticholinergic effects, possibly decreased therapeutic effects of mesoridazine

aminoglycosides, ototoxic drugs: Masked symptoms of ototoxicity, such as dizziness, tinnitus, and vertigo

anticonvulsants: Possibly lowered seizure threshold

antithyroid drugs: Increased risk of agranulocytosis

appetite suppressants: Possibly antagonized anorectic effect

beta blockers: Increased blood levels of both drugs, possibly result-

---

* For oral route.

ing in additive hypotension, arrhythmias, retinopathy, and tardive dyskinesia

cisapride, disopyramide, erythromycin, pimozide, probucol, procainamide, quinidine: Increased risk of life-threatening arrhythmias and prolonged QT interval

CNS depressants, general anesthetics: Increased CNS depression

dextroamphetamine: Possibly interference with action of either drug

levodopa: Possibly inhibited effects of levodopa

lithium: Possibly decreased absorption of mesoridazine

opioid analgesics: Possibly decreased mesoridazine effects; increased CNS and respiratory depression and orthostatic hypotension; increased risk of severe constipation

oral anticoagulants: Possibly decreased therapeutic effects of anticoagulants

sympathomimetics: Possibly decreased therapeutic effects of these drugs and increased risk of hypotension

thiazide diuretics: Possibly orthostatic hypotension, hyponatremia, and water intoxication

tricyclic antidepressants: Increased tricyclic antidepressant levels, inhibited mesoridazine metabolism, increased risk of neuroleptic malignant syndrome

ACTIVITIES

alcohol use: Increased CNS depression

Adverse Reactions

CNS: Ataxia, dizziness, drowsiness, extrapyramidal reactions (tardive dyskinesia, pseudoparkinsonism), fever, neuroleptic malignant syndrome, restlessness, seizures, slurred speech, syncope, tremor, weakness

CV: Hypotension, orthostatic hypotension, prolonged QT interval, torsades de pointes

EENT: Blurred vision, dry mouth, hypertrophic papillae of tongue, increased salivation, photophobia

ENDO: Galactorrhea, gynecomastia

GI: Constipation, hepatotoxicity, nausea, vomiting

GU: Dysuria, ejaculation disorders, impotence, menstrual irregularities, priapism

HEME: Agranulocytosis, leukopenia, thrombocytopenia

SKIN: Contact dermatitis, decreased sweating, jaundice, photosensitivity, rash

Other: Injection site pain, weight gain

Overdose

Monitor patient for signs and symptoms of overdose, including agitation, areflexia and hyperreflexia, arrhythmias, blurred vision, cardiac arrest, coma, confusion, disorientation, drowsiness, dry mouth, dyspnea, heart failure, hyperpyrexia, hypotension, hypothermia, mydriasis, pulmonary edema, QRS complex changes, respiratory depression, seizures, shock, stupor, tachycardia, ventricular fibrillation, and vomiting.

Maintain an open airway, monitor patient for arrhythmias, and maintain temperature. Institute seizure precautions according to facility protocol. Perform gastric lavage and administer activated charcoal, as prescribed. Be aware that vomiting shouldn't be induced because of the potential for impaired consciousness or dystonic reactions of the head and neck.

Don't administer a drug that may prolong the QT interval—such as disopyramide, procainamide, or quinidine—to treat arrhythmias because these drugs may have an additive effect with mesoridazine. Expect to give phenytoin to control arrhythmias and norepinephrine or phenylephrine and I.V. fluids to treat hypotension, as prescribed. Epinephrine shouldn't be used because of risk of paradoxical hypotension. Anticipate digitalizing patient for heart failure, as prescribed. Expect to treat electrolyte imbalances and maintain acid-base balance, as prescribed, and to administer diazepam followed by phenytoin to manage seizures. Avoid giving barbiturates because they may potentiate CNS and respiratory depression.

Anticipate giving benztropine or diphenhydramine to manage acute dyskinetic effects. Dialysis is ineffective for phenothiazine overdose. Expect to continue ECG monitoring for at least 5 days. Be aware that phenothiazine tablets are visible on X-ray.

Institute suicide precautions according to facility policy, and anticipate psychiatric re-evaluation.

Nursing Considerations

- **WARNING** Mesoridazine may prolong the QT interval and has been associated with torsades de pointes and sudden death. Expect to use drug only if patient has failed to respond to therapy with at least two other antipsychotic drugs.
- Obtain baseline and serial ECG and serum potassium levels, as prescribed. Notify prescriber if QTc interval is greater than 450 milliseconds or if potassium level is abnormal, and expect to discontinue drug immediately.
- Wear gloves when working with liquid and parenteral forms of mesoridazine, and avoid contact with clothing or skin; drug may cause contact dermatitis.

- Dilute oral concentrate form of drug with acidified water, distilled water, or grape or orange juice immediately before administration. Plan to use 2 teaspoonfuls of diluent for each 25 mg of drug.
- Discard injection solution if it's frankly discolored or contains precipitate; slightly yellow color is acceptable.
- Inject I.M. drug deep into upper outer quadrant of buttocks; massage area afterward to prevent sterile abscess.
- Assess patient for hypotension and orthostatic hypotension, especially if she's receiving I.M. form. Notify prescriber if either develops.
- **WARNING** Monitor patient for signs of neuroleptic malignant syndrome, a potentially fatal reaction to antipsychotic drugs, and notify prescriber if they develop. Early signs include altered mental status, fever, hypertension or hypotension, muscle rigidity, and tachycardia.
- Assess patient for signs of blood dyscrasias, including cellulitis, fever, and pharyngitis. If they develop, stop drug, as directed.
- Monitor patient for signs and symptoms of tardive dyskinesia, even after treatment stops. Notify prescriber if they develop.
- Expect to taper dosage before discontinuing drug to avoid adverse reactions, such as dizziness, nausea, tremor, and vomiting.

PATIENT TEACHING

- Instruct patient to take mesoridazine exactly as prescribed and not to stop taking it abruptly.
- Instruct patient to notify her prescriber immediately if she develops symptoms of torsades de pointes, such as dizziness, palpitations, and syncope.
- Teach patient or caregiver to dilute the oral concentrate form of drug with acidified water, distilled water, or grape or orange juice immediately before administration. Tell her to use 2 teaspoonfuls of diluent for each 25 mg of drug.
- Inform patient that I.M. injection may be painful.
- Caution patient to avoid potentially hazardous activities until she knows how the drug affects her.
- Advise patient to change position slowly to minimize effects of orthostatic hypotension.
- Instruct patient to report fever, involuntary facial movements, sore throat, unusual bleeding or bruising, and yellowing of eyes or skin.
- Urge patient to avoid alcohol and prolonged sun exposure during therapy.

• If patient requires long-term mesoridazine therapy, explain the risk of tardive dyskinesia. Also, advise her to have regular eye examinations.
• Instruct patient to tell other prescribers that she's taking mesoridazine before she takes any new drug.

methadone hydrochloride
Dolophine, Methadose

Class, Category, and Schedule
Chemical class: Phenylheptylamine
Therapeutic class: Synthetic opiate agonist
Pregnancy category: C
Controlled substance schedule: II

Indications and Dosages
▶ *To manage opioid detoxification*
DISPERSIBLE TABLETS, ORAL CONCENTRATE, I.M. OR SUBCUTANEOUS INJECTION
Adults. *Initial:* 15 to 40 mg daily or as needed. *Usual:* Dosage individualized based on response. *Maximum:* 120 mg daily.
Children. Dosage individualized based on age and size. *Maximum:* 120 mg daily.
▶ *To maintain opioid abstinence*
DISPERSIBLE TABLETS, ORAL CONCENTRATE
Adults. Dosage individualized based on response. *Maximum:* 120 mg daily.
Children. Dosage individualized based on age and size. *Maximum:* 120 mg daily.
DOSAGE ADJUSTMENT Elderly patients, debilitated patients, and patients with severe hepatic or renal dysfunction, hypothyroidism, Addison's disease, prostatic hyperplasia, or urethral stricture need individualized dosage reduction.

Route	Onset	Steady State	Peak	Half-Life	Duration
P.O.	30 to 60 min	Unknown	½ to 2 hr	13 to 47 hr	4 to 6 hr
I.M.	10 to 20 min	Unknown	1 to 2 hr	Unknown	4 to 5 hr

Mechanism of Action
Binds with and activates opioid receptors (primarily mu receptors) in the spinal cord and in higher levels of the CNS to produce euphoric effects.

Contraindications

Acute or postoperative pain, acute or severe asthma, chronic respiratory disease, diarrhea associated with pseudomembranous colitis or poisoning, hypersensitivity to methadone or its components, respiratory depression, severe inflammatory bowel disease

Interactions

DRUGS

ammonium chloride, ascorbic acid, potassium or sodium phosphate: May precipitate methadone withdrawal signs and symptoms

amitriptyline, chloripramine, nortriptyline: Increased CNS and respiratory depression

anticholinergics: Possibly severe constipation leading to ileus; urine retention

antiemetics, general anesthetics, hypnotics, phenothiazines, sedatives, tranquilizers: Possibly coma, hypotension, respiratory depression, and severe sedation

antihistamines, choral hydrate, glutethimide, MAO inhibitors, methocarbamol: Increased CNS and respiratory depressant effects of methadone

antihypertensives, hypotension-producing drugs: Increased hypotension, risk of orthostatic hypotension

azole antifungals, macrolide antibiotics: Increased or prolonged opioid effect

buprenorphine: Decreased therapeutic effect of methadone, increased respiratory depression, possibly withdrawal symptoms

calcium channel blockers, class IA and class III antiarrhythmics, diuretics, laxatives, mineralocorticoid hormones, neuroleptics, tricyclic antidepressants: Increased risk of electrolyte disturbances and prolonged QT intervals

carbamazepine, phenobarbital, St. John's wort: Possibly precipitation of withdrawal symptoms

cimetidine: Increased analgesic and CNS and respiratory depressant effects of methadone

desipramine: Increased plasma desipramine level

didanosine, stavudine: Decreased plasma levels of these drugs

diuretics: Decreased diuresis

efavirenz, nevirapine, ritonavir, ritonavir and lopinavir: Decreased blood methadone level

hydroxyzine: Increased analgesic, CNS depressant, and hypotensive effects of methadone

loperamide, paregoric: Increased CNS depression, possibly severe constipation

MAO inhibitors: Possibly increased risk of severe adverse reactions
metoclopramide: Possibly antagonized metoclopramide effects on
GI motility
mixed agonist-antagonist analgesics: Possibly withdrawal signs and
symptoms
naloxone: Antagonized analgesic and CNS and respiratory depressant effects of methadone, possibly withdrawal signs and symptoms
naltrexone: Possibly induction or worsening of withdrawal signs
and symptoms if methadone given within 7 days before naltrexone
neuromuscular blockers: Increased or prolonged respiratory depression
opioid analgesics (such as alfentanil and sufentanil): Increased CNS
and respiratory depression, increased hypotension
phenytoin, rifampin: May precipitate withdrawal signs and symptoms
selective serotonin reuptake inhibitors: Possibly increased blood
methadone level and increased risk of methadone toxicity
zidovudine: Increased blood zidovudine level and risk of toxicty
ACTIVITIES
alcohol use: Increased CNS and respiratory depression, possibly hypotension

Adverse Reactions

CNS: Agitation, amnesia, anxiety, asthenia, coma, confusion, decreased concentration, delirium, delusions, depression, dizziness,
drowsiness, euphoria, fever, hallucinations, headache, insomnia,
lethargy, light-headedness, malaise, psychosis, restlessness, sedation, seizures, syncope, tremor
CV: Bradycardia, cardiac arrest, cardiomyopathy, edema, heart
failure, hypotension, orthostatic hypotension, palpitations,
phlebitis, QT-interval prolongation, shock, tachycardia, T-wave
inversion on ECG, torsades de pointes, ventricular fibrillation or
tachycardia
EENT: Blurred vision, diplopia, dry mouth, glossitis, laryngeal
edema or laryngospasm (allergic), miosis, nystagmus, rhinitis
GI: Abdominal cramps or pain, anorexia, biliary tract spasm, constipation, diarrhea, dysphagia, elevated liver function test results,
gastroesophageal reflux, hiccups, ileus and toxic megacolon (in
patients with inflammatory bowel disease), indigestion, nausea,
vomiting
GU: Amenorrhea, decreased ejaculate potency or libido, difficult
ejaculation, impotence, prolonged labor, urinary hesitancy, urine
retention

HEME: Anemia, leukopenia, thrombocytopenia
MS: Arthralgia
RESP: Apnea, asthma exacerbation, atelectasis, bronchospasm, depressed cough reflex, hypoventilation, pulmonary edema, respiratory arrest and depression, wheezing
SKIN: Diaphoresis, flushing, pallor, pruritus
Other: Allergic reaction; facial edema; hypokalemia; hypomagnesemia; injection site edema, pain, rash, or redness; physical and psychological dependence; weight gain; withdrawal signs and symptoms

Overdose

Monitor patient for signs and symptoms of overdose, including bradycardia, cold and clammy skin, confusion, dizziness, drowsiness, dyspnea, hypotension, nervousness, pinpoint pupils, restlessness, seizures, unconsciousness, and weakness.

Maintain an open airway, and be prepared to provide artificial respiration, as needed. Institute seizure precautions according to facility protocol. Administer I.V. fluids and a vasopressor to treat hypotension, as prescribed. Expect to administer naloxone, an opioid antagonist, to reverse the signs and symptoms of overdose. Plan to administer additional doses of naloxone, as needed and prescribed. Be aware that naloxone may precipitate withdrawal signs and symptoms—such as diaphoresis, irritability, large pupils, nausea, tachycardia, tremor, vomiting, and yawning—in physically dependent patients.

To decrease absorption of oral form of drug in a conscious patient who isn't at risk for coma or seizures, be prepared to induce vomiting or perform gastric lavage. For an unconscious patient, anticipate assisting with the insertion of an endotracheal tube and then performing gastric lavage. The inflated cuff of the endotracheal tube will help prevent aspiration of gastric contents into the lungs.

Institute suicide precautions according to facility policy, and anticipate psychiatric re-evaluation.

Nursing Considerations

• Before giving methadone, make sure opioid antagonist and equipment for administering oxygen and controlling respiration are nearby.
• Before therapy begins, assess patient's current drug use, including all prescription and OTC drugs.
• Before administration, dilute oral concentrate with water or an-

other liquid to a volume of 3 oz (90 ml) or more and dissolve dispersible tablets in water or another liquid.

- **WARNING** Give drug cautiously to patients at risk for prolonged QT interval, such as those with cardiac hypertrophy, hypokalemia, or hypomagnesemia; those with a history of cardiac conduction abnormalities; and those taking diuretics or medications that affect cardiac conduction.

- Monitor patient for expected excessive drowsiness, unsteadiness, or confusion during first 3 to 5 days of therapy, and notify prescriber if effects continue to worsen or persist beyond this time.

- **WARNING** Monitor respiratory and circulatory status carefully and at frequent intervals during methadone therapy because respiratory depression, circulatory depression, respiratory arrest, shock, hypotension, and cardiac arrest are potential hazards of therapy. Monitor children frequently for respiratory depression and paradoxical CNS excitation because of their increased sensitivity to drug. Assess patient for excessive or persistent sedation; dosage may need to be adjusted.

- Monitor patient for drug tolerance, especially if she has a history of long-term drug abuse, because methadone can cause physical and psychological dependence.

- Monitor patients who are pregnant or who have liver or renal impairment for increased adverse effects from methadone because drug may have a prolonged duration and cumulative effect in these patients. Methadone may prolong labor by reducing strength, duration, and frequency of uterine contractions, so expect dosage to be tapered before third trimester of pregnancy. Breast-feeding mothers on maintenance therapy who abruptly stop breast-feeding or discontinue methadone therapy put their infants at risk for withdrawal signs and symptoms. Methadone also accumulates in CNS tissue, increasing the risk of seizures in infants.

- Monitor plasma amylase and lipase levels in patients who develop biliary tract spasms because levels may increase up to 2 to 15 times normal. Notify prescriber immediately of any significant or sustained increase.

- Monitor patients with head injuries or other conditions that may increase intracranial pressure (ICP) because methadone may further increase ICP.

- Monitor patient for withdrawal signs and symptoms and tolerance to therapy because physiologic dependence can occur with long-term methadone use. Avoid abrupt discontinuation because withdrawal signs and symptoms will occur within 3 to 4 days after last dose.

• Monitor patient, especially if she's elderly, for cardiac arrhythmias, hypotension, hypovolemia, orthostatic hypotension, and vasovagal syncope because drug may produce cholinergic adverse reactions in patients with cardiac disease, resulting in bradycardia and peripheral vasodilation; dosage decrease may be indicated.

• If patient has prostatic hyperplasia, urethral stricture, or renal disease, watch for urine retention and oliguria because drug can increase tension of detrusor muscle.

• Be prepared to treat anxiety if it occurs. Be aware that anxiety may be confused with symptoms of opioid abstinence and that methadone doesn't have antianxiety effects.

PATIENT TEACHING

• If patient is taking oral concentrate form of methadone, instruct her to dilute it with water or another liquid to a volume of 3 oz (90 ml) or more before administration.

• Instruct patient to dissolve dispersible tablets in water or other liquid before administration.

• Advise patient to notify prescriber of all other drugs she's currently taking and to avoid alcohol and other depressants, such as sleeping pills and tranquilizers, because they may increase drug's CNS depressant effects.

• Instruct patient to take drug only as prescribed and not to change dosage without prescriber approval. Inform patient that abrupt cessation of methadone therapy can precipitate withdrawal signs and symptoms. Urge her to notify prescriber if she develops any concerns over therapy.

• Urge patient to notify prescriber if she has palpitations, dizziness, lightheadedness, or syncope, which may be caused by methadone-induced arrhythmias.

• Instruct patient to avoid activities that require mental alertness because methadone may cause drowsiness or sleepiness.

• Teach patient to change positions slowly to minimize effects of orthostatic hypotension.

• Inform parents of child on methadone maintenance therapy that child may experience unusual excitement or restlessness; advise them to notify prescriber of any change in child's behavior.

• Instruct female patient to notify prescriber immediately if she

becomes pregnant during methadone therapy because drug may cause physical dependence in fetus and withdrawal in neonate.
• Caution patient who is breast-feeding not to stop doing so abruptly and not to stop taking methadone without prescriber's approval because infant may have withdrawal effects.

Other Therapeutic Uses
Methadone hydrochloride is also indicated for the following:
• To treat severe or chronic pain

methamphetamine hydrochloride
Desoxyn, Desoxyn Gradumet

Class, Category, and Schedule
Chemical class: Phenylisopropylamine
Therapeutic class: CNS stimulant
Pregnancy category: C
Controlled substance schedule: II

Indications and Dosages
▶ *To treat attention-deficit hyperactivity disorder (ADHD)*
E.R. TABLETS
Children age 6 and over. 20 to 25 mg daily.
TABLETS
Children age 6 and over. *Initial:* 5 mg daily or b.i.d. Increased by 5 mg every wk. *Maintenance:* 20 to 25 mg daily in divided doses b.i.d.

Route	Onset	Steady State	Peak	Half-Life	Duration
P.O.	Unknown	Unknown	Unknown	4 to 5 hr	6 to 24 hr

Mechanism of Action
May produce CNS stimulation by facilitating norepinephrine's release and blocking its reuptake at adrenergic nerve terminals and by directly stimulating alpha and beta receptors in the peripheral nervous system. Methamphetamine also promotes dopamine release and blocks its reuptake in the brain's limbic regions. The drug appears to act mainly in the cerebral cortex and, possibly, the reticular activating system. These actions decrease motor restlessness, increase alertness, and diminish drowsiness and fatigue. The drug's peripheral actions include increased blood pressure and mild bronchodilation and respiratory stimulation.

Contraindications

Advanced arteriosclerosis; glaucoma; hypersensitivity to methamphetamine, sympathomimetic amines, or their components; hyperthyroidism; history of drug abuse; moderate to severe hypertension; severe agitation; symptomatic cardiovascular disease; use within 14 days of MAO inhibitor therapy

Interactions

DRUGS

ascorbic acid: Decreased methamphetamine absorption and therapeutic effect

beta blockers: Increased risk of heart block, hypotension, and severe bradycardia

CNS stimulants: Increased CNS stimulation and risk of adverse reactions

digoxin, levodopa: Increased risk of arrhythmias

diuretics, other antihypertensives: Possibly decreased antihypertensive effect

ethosuximide, phenobarbital, phenytoin: Possibly delayed absorption of these drugs

haloperidol, phenothiazines: Possibly interference with the therapeutic effects of these drugs and with methamphetamine's CNS stimulation

inhalation anesthetics: Increased risk of ventricular arrhythmias

insulin: Altered insulin requirements

lithium: Possibly antagonized CNS stimulant effects of methamphetamine

MAO inhibitors: Possibly severe hypertension, risk of hypertensive crisis, increased vasopressor effect of methamphetamine

meperidine: Increased risk of hypotension and life-threatening interactions, such as severe respiratory depression and coma

metrizamide (intrathecal): Increased risk of seizures

thyroid hormones: Enhanced effects of both drugs

tricyclic antidepressants: Increased risk of arrhythmias and severe hypertension

urinary acidifiers: Increased metabolism and shortened pharmacologic effects of methamphetamine

urinary alkalizers: Decreased metabolism and prolonged pharmacologic effects of methamphetamine

FOODS

caffeine: Increased methamphetamine effects

Adverse Reactions

CNS: CVA, dizziness, euphoria, headache, hyperactivity, insom-

nia, irritability, mania, nervousness, psychotic episodes, restlessness, talkativeness, tremor
CV: Arrhythmias, chest pain, hypertension, hypotension, MI, palpitations, tachycardia
EENT: Blurred vision, dry mouth, taste perversion
GI: Abdominal cramps, anorexia, constipation, diarrhea, nausea, vomiting
GU: Impotence, libido changes
SKIN: Diaphoresis, urticaria
Other: Physical and psychological dependence

Overdose

Methamphetamine overdose has no specific antidote. Monitor patient for signs and symptoms of overdose, including abdominal cramps, arrhythmias, chest pain, confusion, delirium, diaphoresis, diarrhea, dizziness, dyspnea, flushing, hallucinations, hyperpyrexia, hypertension and hypotension, irregular heartbeat, nausea, pallor, palpitations, panic reaction, paranoia, photosensitive mydriasis, polypnea, psychotic reactions, rhabdomyolysis, shock, syncope, tachypnea, toxic psychosis, tremor, unusual fatigue, vomiting, and weakness. Monitor patient for cardiac and respiratory changes. If possible, isolate her to limit external stimuli.

Expect to provide symptomatic and supportive treatment, including maintenance of respiratory and cardiovascular function. Be prepared to perform gastric lavage or induce vomiting to decrease drug absorption. Anticipate the use of I.V. fluids to manage hypotension, as needed. Expect to administer drugs and fluids to enhance diuresis, as prescribed. Be aware that drug treatment to induce urine acidification may also be prescribed to increase drug excretion, except in patients with hemoglobinemia, myoglobinuria, or rhabdomyolysis because of increased risk of renal failure. Be prepared to administer a drug such as a barbiturate or chlorpromazine to control CNS stimulation and phentolamine to manage hypertension. If the patient ingested the E.R. form of methamphetamine, expect to continue treating the signs and symptoms of overdose until they've resolved because the pellets are coated for gradual release.

Institute suicide precautions according to facility policy, and anticipate psychiatric re-evaluation.

Nursing Considerations

• Be aware that methamphetamine shouldn't be used in patients, especially children and adolescents, with a structural heart defect, cardiomyopathy, a serious heart rhythm abnormality, or

other serious heart condition.
- Monitor patient for exertional chest pain, unexplained syncope, or other symptoms that suggest heart disease. If present, notify prescriber; a cardiac evaluation will be needed, and methamphetamine may need to be discontinued.
- If patient has a history of psychiatric problems or suicidal or homicidal tendencies, monitor him for worsening of these conditions.
- If patient has a history of seizure disorders, monitor her for seizures because drug may lower seizure threshold.
- Observe patient for signs of drug tolerance and, possibly, extreme dependence, which may develop after a few weeks. Be aware that methamphetamine abuse may occur.
- Expect treatment for ADHD to include psychological, educational, and social measures in conjunction with drug therapy.
- Monitor patient for signs or symptoms of chronic methamphetamine intoxication, including hyperactivity, insomnia, irritability, and personality changes. Notify prescriber if such signs occur.

PATIENT TEACHING
- Instruct parent of patient to give methamphetamine at least 6 hours before bedtime to prevent insomnia.
- Explain the high risk of abuse with this drug. Instruct parent of patient not to increase dosage unless advised to do so by prescriber and not to give drug to prevent fatigue.
- Caution parent that patient should not crush or chew E.R. tablets.
- Advise parent that patient should avoid caffeine, which increases drug effects.
- Instruct parent of patient to report signs or symptoms of overstimulation, such as diarrhea, hyperactivity, insomnia, and irritability.
- **WARNING** Advise patient to take methamphetamine exactly as prescribed because misuse may cause serious adverse cardiac effects and even death.

methsuximide
Celontin

Class and Category
Chemical class: Succinimide derivative
Therapeutic class: Anticonvulsant
Pregnancy category: Not rated

Indications and Dosages

▶ *To treat absence seizures unresponsive to other medications*
CAPSULES
Adults and children. *Initial:* 300 mg daily. Increased by 150 to 300 mg daily every 1 to 2 wk until control is achieved with minimal adverse reactions. *Maximum:* 1.2 g daily in divided doses.

Route	Onset	Steady State	Peak	Half-Life	Duration
P.O.	Unknown	Unknown	Unknown	1 to 3 hr*	Unknown

Mechanism of Action

Elevates the seizure threshold and reduces the frequency of attacks by depressing the motor cortex and elevating the threshold of CNS response to convulsive stimuli. Methsuximide is metabolized to the active metabolite N-desmethylmethsuximide, which may add to drug's anticonvulsant effects.

Contraindications

Hypersensitivity to methsuximide, succinimides, or their components

Interactions

DRUGS
carbamazepine, phenobarbital, phenytoin, primidone: Possibly decreased blood methsuximide level
CNS depressants: Possibly increased CNS depression
haloperidol: Change in seizure pattern; possibly decreased blood haloperidol level
loxapine, MAO inhibitors, maprotiline, molindone, phenothiazines, pimozide, thioxanthenes, tricyclic antidepressants: Possibly lowered seizure threshold and reduced therapeutic effect of methsuximide
ACTIVITIES
alcohol use: Possibly increased CNS depression

Adverse Reactions

CNS: Aggressiveness, ataxia, decreased concentration, dizziness, drowsiness, fatigue, fever, headache, insomnia, irritability, mental depression, nightmares, seizures
EENT: Periorbital edema, pharyngitis
GI: Abdominal or epigastric pain, abdominal cramps, abnormal liver function test results, anorexia, diarrhea, hiccups, nausea, vomiting

---

* 34 to 80 hr for the metabolite N-desmethylmethsuximide.

GU: Microscopic hematuria, proteinuria
HEME: Agranulocytosis, aplastic anemia, eosinophilia, leukopenia, pancytopenia
MS: Muscle pain
SKIN: Erythematous and pruritic rash, Stevens-Johnson syndrome, systemic lupus erythematosus, urticaria
Other: Lymphadenopathy

Overdose

Monitor patient for signs and symptoms of overdose, including CNS depression, nausea, respiratory depression, and vomiting. Maintain open airway and be prepared to assist with endotracheal intubation if patient experiences respiratory depression. Methsuximide's active metabolite, N-desmethylmethsuximide, has a long half-life, so be alert to the possibility that the patient may awaken from an initial comatose state then relapse into a coma within 24 hours. Monitor serum N-desmethylmethsuximide level to assess recovery.

To decrease absorption of drug in a conscious patient who isn't at risk for coma, be prepared to induce vomiting. For an unconscious patient, anticipate assisting with the insertion of an endotracheal tube and then performing gastric lavage. The inflated cuff of the endotracheal tube will help prevent aspiration of gastric contents into the lungs. Expect that activated charcoal or a cathartic may also be prescribed. Charcoal hemoperfusion may be effective for treating methsuximide overdose because it removes the N-desmethylmethsuximide metabolite, but forced diuresis and exchange transfusions are ineffective.

Institute suicide precautionary measures according to facility policy, and anticipate psychiatric re-evaluation.

Nursing Considerations

• Monitor CBC and platelet count and assess patient for signs of infection—such as cough, fever, and pharyngitis—because methsuximide may cause blood dyscrasias.
• If patient has a history of hepatic or renal disease, monitor liver function test results and urinalysis results because methsuximide may cause functional changes in the liver and kidneys.
• When administering drug to patient with a history of mixed type of epilepsy, institute seizure precautions according to facility protocol because drug may increase the frequency of generalized tonic-clonic seizures.
• Expect dosage to be carefully and slowly adjusted according to response and withdrawn slowly to avoid causing seizures.

- Plan to use the 150-mg capsule when making dosage adjustments with small children.
- If patient develops depression or aggressiveness, notify her prescriber. Expect to have drug withdrawn slowly if these behavioral changes occur.

PATIENT TEACHING
- Stress the importance of complying with methsuximide regimen.
- Advise patient to take a missed dose as soon as she remembers unless it's nearly time for the next dose. Warn her not to double the dose.
- Instruct patient not to take capsules that are melted or not full because the effectiveness of the drug will be reduced.
- Instruct patient to take the drug with milk or food to reduce gastric irritation.
- Advise patient to notify prescriber if she develops cough, fever, or pharyngitis.
- Urge patient to avoid alcohol because of the increased risk of CNS depression.
- Instruct patient not to engage in potentially hazardous activities until she knows how the drug affects her.
- Caution patient not to stop taking drug abruptly; doing so increases the risk of absence seizures.
- Instruct patient to avoid excessive heat when storing or transporting the drug, such as near an oven or in a closed car, because the capsules can melt easily.

methylphenidate hydrochloride
Concerta, Daytrana, Metadate, Metadate CD, Metadate ER, Methylin, Methylin ER, PMS-Methylphenidate (CAN), Riphenidate (CAN), Ritalin, Ritalin LA, Ritalin SR (CAN), Ritalin-SR

Class, Category, and Schedule
Chemical class: Piperidine derivative
Therapeutic class: CNS stimulant
Pregnancy category: C
Controlled substance schedule: II

Indications and Dosages
▶ *To treat attention-deficit hyperactivity disorder (ADHD)*
E.R. TABLETS, ORAL SOLUTION, S.R. TABLETS, TABLETS
Adults and adolescents. 5 to 20 mg b.i.d. or t.i.d. *Maximum:* 90 mg daily.
Children ages 6 to 12. 5 mg b.i.d. before breakfast and lunch;

increased as ordered by 5 to 10 mg daily at 1-wk intervals. *Maximum:* 60 mg daily.

E.R. ONCE-DAILY TABLETS (CONCERTA)

Adults and adolescents. 18 mg daily; increased in 18-mg increments at 1-wk intervals. *Maximum:* 72 mg daily with dosage not exceeding 2 mg/kg daily.

Children ages 6 to 12. 18 mg daily. *Maximum:* 54 mg daily.

E.R. ONCE-DAILY CAPSULES (METADATE CD)

Children age 6 and over. 20 mg daily, increased to 40 or 60 mg daily based on individual response. *Maximum:* 60 mg daily.

DOSAGE ADJUSTMENT Dosage reduced or drug discontinued if no improvement in signs or symptoms achieved within 1 mo. When maintenance dosage is achieved with tablets, regimen may be switched to E.R. or S.R. tablets.

TRANSDERMAL PATCH

Children ages 6 to 12. *Initial:* 10 mg (12.5-cm patch worn for 9 hours) daily. After 1 wk, increased to 15 mg (18.75-cm patch worn for 9 hours) daily. Then, after 1 wk, increased to 20 mg (25-cm patch worn for 9 hours) daily. Then, after 1 wk, increased to 30 mg (37.5-mg patch worn for 9 hours) daily. *Maintenance:* 30 mg (37.5-mg patch worn for 9 hours) daily.

▶ *To treat narcolepsy*

ORAL SOLUTION, TABLETS

Adults and adolescents. 5 to 20 mg b.i.d. or t.i.d. *Maximum:* 90 mg daily.

Route	Onset	Steady State	Peak	Half-Life	Duration
P.O. (tablets)	Unknown	Unknown	Unknown	1 to 3 hr	3 to 6 hr
P.O. (solution)	Unknown	Unknown	Unknown	1 to 3 hr	3 to 6 hr
P.O. (E.R., S.R.)	Unknown	Unknown	Unknown	1 to 3 hr	About 8 hr
P.O. (E.R. once-daily)	Unknown	Unknown	Unknown	1 to 3 hr	About 12 hr
Transdermal	Unknown	Unknown	Unknown	1 to 3 hr	12 hr

Mechanism of Action

Blocks the reuptake mechanism of dopaminergic neurons in the cerebral cortex and subcortical structures of the brain, including the thalamus. This activity decreases motor restlessness and improves concentration in children with attention deficit hyperactivity disorder.

Methylphenidate also may trigger sympathomimetic activity. This action produces increased motor activity, alertness, mild euphoria, and decreased fatigue in patients with narcolepsy.

Contraindications

Anxiety, depression, glaucoma, hypersensitivity to methylphenidate or its components, motor tics, severe agitation, tension, Tourette's syndrome or family history of it, use within 14 days of MAO inhibitor therapy

Interactions

DRUGS

anticholinergics: Possibly increased anticholinergic effects of both drugs

anticonvulsants, oral anticoagulants, phenylbutazone, tricyclic antidepressants: Inhibited metabolism and increased blood levels of these drugs

diuretics, antihypertensives: Decreased therapeutic effects of these drugs

MAO inhibitors: Possibly increased adverse effects of methylphenidate, possibly severe hypertension

FOODS

caffeine: Increased methylphenidate effects

Adverse Reactions

CNS: Agitation, anxiety, CVA, dizziness, emotional lability, fever, headache, hyperactivity, insomnia, mania, motor tics, nervousness, psychosis, seizures, Tourette's syndrome

CV: Angina, arrhythmias, bradycardia, hypertension, hypotension, MI, palpitations, structural cardiac abnormalities, sudden death, tachycardia

EENT: Accommodation abnormality, blurred vision, dry throat, pharyngitis, rhinitis, sinusitis, vision changes

ENDO: Growth suppression in children (with long-term use)

GI: Abdominal pain, anorexia, diarrhea, elevated liver enzymes, hepatotoxicity, nausea, vomiting

GU: Dysmenorrhea

HEME: Anemia, leukopenia, thrombocytopenia, thrombocytopenic purpura

MS: Arthralgia

RESP: Increased cough, upper respiratory infection

SKIN: Application site irritation (transdermal patch), erythema multiforme, exfoliative dermatitis, rash, urticaria

Other: Angioedema, anaphylaxis, physical and psychological dependence, weight loss

Overdose

Monitor patient for signs and symptoms of overdose, including agitation, coma, confusion, diaphoresis, delirium, dry mouth, euphoria, hallucinations, headache, hyperpyrexia, hyperreflexia, hypertension, muscle twitching, mydriasis, palpitations, seizures, tachycardia, tremor, and vomiting.

Maintain an open airway, and provide supportive and symptomatic care to ensure adequate circulatory function. Institute seizure precautions according to facility policy. Plan to treat hyperpyrexia with cooling blankets, as prescribed. If overdose is severe, expect to administer a short-acting barbiturate to manage the signs and symptoms of overdose and then perform gastric lavage to decrease drug absorption. The effectiveness of dialysis for methylphenidate overdose is unknown.

Institute suicide precautions according to facility policy, and anticipate psychiatric re-evaluation.

Nursing Considerations

- Keep in mind that, when signs and symptoms of ADHD occur with acute stress reactions or with pre-existing structural cardiac abnormalities, treatment with methylphenidate usually isn't indicated because the reaction may worsen or sudden death may occur.
- **WARNING** Be aware that methylphenidate may induce CNS stimulation and psychosis and may worsen behavior disturbances and thought disorders. Use drug cautiously in children with psychosis.
- Monitor children and adolescents for first-time evidence of psychosis or mania. If present, notify prescriber and expect drug to be discontinued.
- Monitor pulse rate and blood pressure in patients who have hypertension, including even mild hypertension, because drug may increase blood pressure and cause arrhythmias, including tachycardia. Report abnormal findings, including exertional chest pain, unexplained syncope, or other symptoms suggestive of cardiac disease, to prescriber.
- Assess patient with history of Tourette's syndrome, motor or vocal tics, or psychological disorders for worsening of these conditions during methyphenidate therapy.
- Monitor blood pressure and pulse rate to detect hypertension and signs of excessive stimulation. Notify prescriber if you detect such signs. For patient with hypertension, expect to increase antihypertensive dosage or add another antihypertensive to existing regimen.
- **WARNING** Monitor patient for signs and symptoms of physi-

cal or psychological dependence. Methylphenidate's abuse potential is similar to that of amphetamines; use it cautiously if patient has a history of drug abuse.

• Monitor growth in children. Inform prescriber about failure to grow or gain weight; expect methylphenidate to be discontinued if growth suppression is present.

• Be aware that drug shouldn't be abruptly discontinued after long-term therapy; doing so may unmask dysphoria, paranoia, severe depression, or suicidal thoughts.

• Expect patient currently taking methylphenidate tablets b.i.d. or t.i.d., or E.R. tablets at doses of 20 to 60 mg daily, to be switched to E.R. once-daily tablets, as prescribed.

PATIENT TEACHING

• Stress importance of taking drug exactly as prescribed because misuse of this drug may cause serious adverse cardiovascular reactions, including sudden death.

• Instruct patient not to chew or crush E.R. tablets.

• Suggest that patient take tablets at least 6 hours before bedtime to avoid insomnia. Instruct her to take E.R. once-daily tablets in the morning.

• Advise patient taking E.R. once-daily tablets (Concerta) not to be alarmed if she notices intact tablet in stool. Inform her that drug is slowly released from nonabsorbable tablet shell.

• If patient will use transdermal patch, instruct him to apply it to clean, dry skin in his hip area 2 hours before an effect is needed and to remove it 9 hours after application. Stress importance of not applying patch to skin that is oily, damaged, or irritated and to avoid the waistline because movement with clothing may dislodge the patch. Tell patient to rotate application sites between both hips.

• Also tell patient to apply the transdermal patch immediately after opening the pouch and removing the protective liner. Instruct him to press the patch firmly in place with the palm of his hand for about 30 seconds. Reassure patient that, after application, exposing the site to water shouldn't cause patch to fall off. If a patch inadvertently comes off, tell patient to apply a new patch but to limit total exposure time for the day to 9 hours.

• Direct patient to notify prescriber about excessive nervousness, fever, insomnia, palpitations, rash, or vomiting.

• Warn patient with seizure disorder that drug may cause seizures.

• Inform parents of children on long-term therapy that drug has the potential to delay growth.

midazolam hydrochloride
Versed

Class, Category, and Schedule
Chemical class: Benzodiazepine
Therapeutic class: Sedative-hypnotic
Pregnancy category: D
Controlled substance schedule: IV

Indications and Dosages
▶ *To induce preoperative sedation or amnesia, to control preoperative anxiety*
ORAL SOLUTION
Children ages 6 months to 16 years. 0.25 to 0.5 mg/kg as a single dose 30 to 45 min before surgery. *Usual:* 0.5 mg/kg. *Maximum:* 20 mg.
I.V. INJECTION
Adults age 60 and over. 1.5 mg over 2 min immediately before procedure. After 2-min waiting period, dosage adjusted to desired level in 25% increments, as ordered. *Maximum:* 1 mg in 2 min.
Adults under age 60 and adolescents. Up to 2.5 mg over 2 min immediately before procedure. After 2-min waiting period, dosage adjusted to desired level in 25% increments, as ordered. *Maximum:* 5 mg.
Children ages 6 to 12. *Initial:* 0.025 to 0.05 mg/kg, up to 0.4 mg/kg, if needed. *Maximum:* 10 mg.
Children ages 6 months to 5 years. *Initial:* 0.05 to 0.1 mg/kg, up to 0.6 mg/kg, if needed. *Maximum:* 6 mg.
I.M. INJECTION
Adults age 60 and over. 0.02 to 0.05 mg/kg as a single dose 30 to 60 min before surgery.
Adults under age 60 and adolescents. 0.07 to 0.08 mg/kg as a single dose 30 to 60 min before surgery.
Children ages 6 months to 12 years. 0.1 to 0.15 mg/kg, up to 0.5 mg/kg for more anxious patients. *Maximum:* 10 mg.
▶ *To relieve agitation and anxiety in mechanically ventilated patients*
I.V. INFUSION
Adults. *Initial:* 0.01 to 0.05 mg/kg infused over several min, repeated at 10- to 15-min intervals until adequate sedation occurs. *Maintenance:* 0.02 to 0.1 mg/kg/hr initially, adjusted to desired

level in 25% to 50% increments, as ordered. After achieving desired level of sedation, infusion rate decreased by 10% to 25% every few hr, as ordered, until minimum effective infusion rate is determined.

Children. *Initial:* 50 to 200 mcg/kg over 2 to 3 min followed by 1 to 2 mcg/kg/min by continuous infusion. *Maintenance:* 0.4 to 6 mcg/kg/min.

Infants over age 32 weeks. 1 mcg/kg/min by continuous infusion.
Infants younger than age 32 weeks. 0.5 mcg/kg/min by continuous infusion.

Route	Onset	Steady State	Peak	Half-Life	Duration
I.V.*	1.5 to 5 min	Unknown	Rapid	1 to 12 hr	2 to 6 hr
I.M.*	5 to 15 min	Unknown	15 to 60 min	1 to 12 hr	2 to 6 hr
I.M.†	30 to 60 min	Unknown	Unknown	1 to 12 hr	Unknown

Mechanism of Action

May exert its sedating effect by increasing the activity of gamma-aminobutyric acid (GABA), a major inhibitory neurotransmitter in the brain. As a result, midazolam produces a calming effect, relaxes skeletal muscles, and—at high doses—induces sleep.

Contraindications

Acute angle-closure glaucoma; alcohol intoxication; coma; hypersensitivity to midazolam, other benzodiazepines, or their components; shock

Interactions

DRUGS

antihypertensives: Increased risk of hypotension
cimetidine, diltiazem, erythromycin, fluconazole, indinavir, itraconazole, ketoconazole, ranitidine, ritonavir, verapamil: Prolonged sedation caused by reduced midazolam metabolism
CNS depressants: Possibly increased CNS and respiratory depression and hypotension
rifampin: Decreased blood midazolam level

FOODS

grapefruit, grapefruit juice: Possibly increased blood midazolam level and risk of toxicity

---

* For sedation.
† For amnesia.

ACTIVITIES

alcohol use: Possibly increased CNS and respiratory depression and hypotension

Adverse Reactions

CNS: Agitation, delirium, or dreaming during emergence from anesthesia; anxiety; ataxia; chills; combativeness; confusion; dizziness; drowsiness; euphoria; excessive sedation; headache; insomnia; lethargy; nervousness; nightmares; paresthesia; prolonged emergence from anesthesia; restlessness; retrograde amnesia; sleep disturbance; slurred speech; weakness; yawning

CV: Cardiac arrest, hypotension, nodal rhythm, PVCs, tachycardia, vasovagal episodes

EENT: Blurred vision, diplopia, or other vision changes; increased salivation; laryngospasm; miosis; nystagmus; toothache

GI: Hiccups, nausea, retching, vomiting

RESP: Airway obstruction, bradypnea, bronchospasm, coughing, decreased tidal volume, dyspnea, hyperventilation, respiratory arrest, shallow breathing, tachypnea, wheezing

SKIN: Pruritus, rash, urticaria

Other: Injection site burning, edema, induration, pain, redness, and tenderness

Overdose

Monitor patient for signs and symptoms of overdose, including apnea, cardiac arrest, respiratory arrest, and respiratory depression.

Maintain open airway, monitor vital signs, and be prepared to assist with artificial respiration, as needed.

Anticipate the use of flumazenil to reverse the effects of midazolam. If patient has hypotension, administer I.V. fluids, place her in Trendelenburg's position, and administer a vasopressor, as prescribed. The effectiveness of forced diuresis and hemodialysis on midazolam overdose is unknown.

Nursing Considerations

- **WARNING** Be aware that I.V. midazolam is given only in hospital or ambulatory care settings that allow continuous monitoring of respiratory and cardiac function. Keep resuscitative drugs and equipment readily available.
- As needed, combine midazolam injection with D_5W, normal slaine solution, or lactated Ringer's solution. With D_5W and normal saline, solution is stable for 24 hours; with lactated Ringer's solution, 4 hours.
- As needed, mix injection in same syringe with atropine sulfate,

meperidine hydrochloride, morphine sulfate, or scopolamine hydrobromide. The resulting solution will be stable for 30 minutes.

• Expect child's dosage to be based on ideal body weight. This is especially important for an obese child.

• Expect neonates to have a higher risk of respiratory depression than other pediatric or adult patients.

• Assess patient's level of consciousness often because the range between sedation and unconsciousness or disorientation is narrower with midazolam than with other benzodiazepines.

• Be aware that recovery time is usually 2 hours but may take up to 6 hours.

PATIENT TEACHING

• Inform patient that she may not remember procedure because midazolam produces amnesia.

• Advise patient to avoid potentially hazardous activities until drug's adverse CNS effects, such as dizziness and drowsiness, have worn off.

• Instruct patient to avoid alcohol and other CNS depressants for 24 hours after receiving drug, unless directed otherwise by prescriber.

mirtazapine

Remeron, Remeron SolTab

Class and Category

Chemical class: Piperazinoazepine
Therapeutic class: Antidepressant
Pregnancy category: C

Indications and Dosages

▶ *To treat major depression*

DISINTEGRATING TABLETS, TABLETS

Adults. *Initial:* 15 mg daily, preferably at bedtime. Increased as needed and tolerated at 1- to 2-wk intervals. *Maximum:* 45 mg daily.

Route	Onset	Steady State	Peak	Half-Life	Duration
P.O.	1 to 2 wk	5 days	6 wk or longer	20 to 40 hr	Unknown

Contraindications

Hypersensitivity to mirtazapine or its components, use within 14 days of MAO inhibitor therapy

Mechanism of Action

May inhibit neuronal reuptake of norepinephrine and serotonin, increasing the action of these neurotransmitters in nerve cells. As a result, this tetracyclic antidepressant may elevate mood.

Interactions

DRUGS

antihypertensives: Increased hypotensive effects of these drugs or enhanced mirtazapine effects

anxiolytics, hypnotics, other CNS depressants (including sedatives): Increased CNS depression

MAO inhibitors: Possibly hyperpyrexia, hypertension, seizures

ACTIVITIES

alcohol use: Increased CNS depression

Adverse Reactions

CNS: Agitation, amnesia, anxiety, apathy, asthenia, ataxia, cerebral ischemia, chills, confusion, delirium, delusions, depersonalization, depression, dizziness, dream disturbances, drowsiness, dyskinesia, dystonia, emotional lability, euphoria, extrapyramidal reactions, fever, hallucinations, hostility, hyperkinesia, hyperreflexia, hypoesthesia, hypokinesia, lack of coordination, malaise, mania, migraine headache, neurosis, paranoia, paresthesia, seizures, somnolence, suicidal thinking, syncope, tremor, vertigo

CV: Angina, bradycardia, edema, hypercholesterolemia, hypertension, hypertriglyceridemia, hypotension, MI, orthostatic hypotension, peripheral edema, PVCs, vasodilation

EENT: Accommodation disturbances, conjunctivitis, dry mouth, earache, epistaxis, eye pain, glaucoma, gingival bleeding, glossitis, hearing loss, hyperacusis, keratoconjunctivitis, lacrimation, pharyngitis, sinusitis, stomatitis

ENDO: Breast pain

GI: Abdominal distention and pain, anorexia, cholecystitis, colitis, constipation, elevated ALT level, eructation, increased appetite, nausea, thirst, vomiting

GU: Amenorrhea, cystitis, dysmenorrhea, dysuria, hematuria, impotence, increased libido, leukorrhea, renal calculi, urinary frequency and incontinence, urine retention, UTI, vaginitis

HEME: Agranulocytosis, neutropenia

MS: Arthralgia, back pain, dysarthria, muscle twitching, myalgia, myasthenia, neck pain and rigidity

RESP: Asthma, bronchitis, cough, dyspnea, pneumonia
SKIN: Acne, alopecia, dry skin, exfoliative dermatitis, photosensitivity, pruritus, rash
Other: Dehydration, facial edema, flulike signs and symptoms, herpes simplex, weight gain or loss

Overdose

Monitor patient for signs and symptoms of overdose, including disorientation, drowsiness, memory loss, and tachycardia.

Maintain an open airway, monitor vital signs, and assess patient for tachycardia. When treating the patient for mirtazapine overdose, consider the possibility of multiple drug ingestion.

To decrease drug absorption, be prepared to induce vomiting or perform gastric lavage. Expect that oral activated charcoal may also be prescribed.

Institute suicide precautions according to facility policy, and anticipate psychiatric re-evaluation.

Nursing Considerations

- Administer mirtazapine before bedtime.
- Expect disintegrating tablet to dissolve on patient's tongue within 30 seconds.
- **WARNING** Don't give drug within 14 days of MAO inhibitor to avoid serious, possibly fatal, reaction.
- Supervise suicidal patient closely, especially when therapy starts or dosage changes; depression may temporarily worsen during these times.
- Monitor patient closely for signs of infection (such as fever, pharyngitis, and stomatitis), which may be linked to a low WBC count. If these signs occur, notify prescriber and expect to stop drug.
- Expect mirtazapine therapy to last 6 months or longer for acute depression.

PATIENT TEACHING

- Instruct patient not to swallow disintegrating tablet. Tell her to hold tablet on tongue and allow it to dissolve. Inform her that tablet will dissolve within 30 seconds.
- Instruct patient to avoid consuming alcohol and other CNS depressants during mirtazapine therapy and for up to 7 days afterward.
- Caution patient or caregiver about an increased risk of suicidal thinking, especially when mirtazapine therapy starts or dosage changes; tell them to report such thoughts immediately to prescriber.

- Advise patient to avoid potentially hazardous activities until she knows how the drug affects her.
- Direct patient to change position slowly to minimize effects of orthostatic hypotension.
- Suggest sugarless hard candy or gum to relieve dry mouth. Advise patient to notify prescriber if dry mouth persists longer than 2 weeks.
- Instruct patient to notify prescriber immediately about chills, fever, mouth irritation, sore throat, and other signs of infection.
- Encourage patient to visit prescriber regularly during therapy to monitor progress.

modafinil
Provigil

Class, Category, and Schedule
Chemical class: Benzhydryl sulfinylacetamide derivative
Therapeutic class: CNS stimulant
Pregnancy category: C
Controlled substance schedule: IV

Indications and Dosages
▶ *To improve daytime wakefulness in patients with narcolepsy, obstructive sleep apnea hypopnea syndrome, and shift-work sleep disorder*
TABLETS
Adults and adolescents age 16 and over. 200 mg daily in the morning or 1 hr before starting work. *Maximum:* 400 mg daily.
DOSAGE ADJUSTMENT Dosage reduced by 50% in patients with severe hepatic impairment.

Route	Onset	Steady State	Peak	Half-Life	Duration
P.O.	Unknown	2 to 4 days	Unknown	15 hr	Unknown

Mechanism of Action
May inhibit the release of gamma-aminobutyric acid (GABA), the most common inhibitory neurotransmitter, or CNS depressant, in the brain. Modafinil also increases the release of glutamate, an excitatory neurotransmitter, or CNS stimulant, in the thalamus and hippocampus. These two actions may improve wakefulness.

Contraindications
Hypersensitivity to modafinil or its components

Interactions
DRUGS
amitriptyline, citalopram, clomipramine, diazepam, imipramine, propranolol, tolbutamide, topiramate: Possibly prolonged elimination time and increased blood levels of these drugs
carbamazepine: Possibly decreased modafinil effectiveness and decreased blood carbamazepine level
cimetidine, clarithromycin, erythromycin, fluconazole, fluoxetine, fluvoxamine, itraconazole, ketoconazole, nefazodone, sertraline: Possibly inhibited metabolism, decreased clearance, and increased blood level of modafinil
contraceptive-containing implants or devices, oral contraceptives: Possibly contraceptive failure
cyclosporine: Possibly decreased blood cyclosporine level and increased risk of organ transplant rejection
dexamethasone, phenobarbital and other barbiturates, primidone, rifabutin, rifampin: Possibly decreased blood level and effectiveness of modafinil
dextroamphetamine: Possibly increased risk of adverse CNS stimulant effects
dextroamphetamine, methylphenidate: Possibly 1-hour delay in modafinil absorption
fosphenytoin, mephenytoin, phenytoin: Possibly decreased effectiveness of modafinil, increased blood phenytoin level, and increased risk of phenytoin toxicity
theophylline: Possibly decreased blood level and effectiveness of theophylline
triazolam: Possibly decreased triazolam effectiveness
warfarin: Possibly decreased warfarin metabolism and increased risk of bleeding
FOODS
all foods: 1-hour delay in modafinil absorption and possibly delayed onset of action
grapefruit juice: Possibly decreased modafinil metabolism

Adverse Reactions
CNS: Agitation, anxiety, confusion, depression, headache, insomnia, mania, nervousness, suicidal ideation
GI: Nausea
HEME: Agranulocytosis
SKIN: Drug rash with eosinophilia and systemic symptoms (DRESS), rash, Stevens-Johnson syndrome, toxic epidermal necrolysis

Other: Angioedema, infection, multi-organ hypersensitivity

Overdose

Monitor patient for signs and symptoms of overdose, including agitation, excitement, hypertension, insomnia, and tachycardia. Maintain open airway, and monitor cardiovascular function.

To decrease drug absorption, be prepared to induce vomiting or perform gastric lavage. The effectiveness of dialysis or drugs that change urine pH on modafinil overdose is unknown.

Institute suicide precautions according to facility policy, and anticipate psychiatric re-evaluation.

Nursing Considerations

- Be aware that modafinil shouldn't be given to patients with mitral valve prolapse syndrome or a history of left ventricular hypertrophy because drug may cause ischemic changes.
- Use cautiously in patients with a history of psychosis, depression, or mania because these conditions may worsen during modafinil therapy and may require therapy to be stopped.
- **WARNING** If patient has a history of alcoholism, stimulant abuse, or other substance abuse, monitor her for proper drug compliance during modafinil therapy. Observe for signs of misuse or abuse, including frequent prescription refill requests, increased frequency of dosing, or drug-seeking behavior. Monitor patient for signs and symptoms of excessive modafinil dosage, including aggressiveness, anxiety, confusion, decreased prothrombin time, diarrhea, irritability, nausea, nervousness, palpitations, sleep disturbances, and tremor.
- Be aware that modafinil, like other CNS stimulants, may produce alterations in mood, perception, thinking, judgment, feelings, and motor skills. It may also mask signs that the patient is physically in need of sleep.
- When administering modafinil to patient with a known history of psychosis, emotional instability, or psychological illness with psychotic features, be prepared to perform baseline behavioral assessments or frequent clinical observation.
- **WARNING** Monitor patient closely for evidence of multi-organ hypersensitivity, such as fever and rash, associated with organ dysfunction. Other signs and symptoms may include lymphadenopathy, hepatitis, liver function abnormalities, hematological abnormalities, pruritus, nephritis, oliguria, hepato-renal syndrome, arthralgia and asthenia. If suspected, notify prescriber and expect drug to be discontinued. Provide supportive care, as prescribed.

PATIENT TEACHING
• Inform patient that modafinil can help, but not cure, narcolepsy and that drug's full effects may not be immediately evident.
• Advise patient to avoid taking modafinil within 1 hour of eating because food may delay drug's absorption and onset of action. If she drinks grapefruit juice, encourage her to drink a consistent amount daily.
• Instruct patient to stop taking modafinil if a rash develops and to notify precriber.
•Urge patient to report chest pain, depression, anxiety, or evidence of psychosis or mania to prescriber.
• Inform patient that drug can affect her concentration and function and can hide signs of fatigue. Urge her not to drive or perform activities that require mental alertness until she knows how the drug affects her.
• Because alcohol may interfere with alertness, advise patient to avoid it while taking modafinil.
• Encourage patient to maintain a regular sleeping pattern.
• Caution patient to avoid excessive intake of foods, beverages, and OTC drugs that contain caffeine because caffeine may lead to increased CNS stimulation.
• Inform female patient that modafinil can decrease the effectiveness of certain contraceptives, including birth control pills and implantable hormonal contraceptives. If she uses such contraceptives, urge her to use an alternate birth control method during modafinil therapy and for up to 1 month after she stops taking the drug.
• Advise patient to keep follow-up appointments with prescriber so that her progress can be monitored.

molindone hydrochloride
Moban, Moban Concentrate

Class and Category
Chemical class: Dihydroindolone derivative
Therapeutic class: Antipsychotic drug
Pregnancy category: Not rated

Indications and Dosages
▶ *To manage symptoms of psychotic disorders*
ORAL SOLUTION, TABLETS
Adults and children older than age 12. *Initial:* 50 to 75 mg daily in divided doses t.i.d. or q.i.d. Dosage increased to 100 mg

daily in 3 to 4 days as needed. *Maintenance:* For mild psychosis, 5 to 15 mg t.i.d. or q.i.d.; for moderate psychosis, 10 to 25 mg t.i.d. or q.i.d.; for severe psychosis, 225 mg daily in divided doses. *Maximum:* 225 mg daily.

DOSAGE ADJUSTMENT Initial dosage reduced for elderly or debilitated patients.

Route	Onset	Steady State	Peak	Half-Life	Duration
P.O.	Unknown	Unknown	Unknown	2 hr	24 to 36 hr

Mechanism of Action

Occupies dopamine$_2$ (D$_2$) receptor sites in the reticular activating and limbic systems in the CNS. By blocking dopamine activity in these areas, molindone reduces the signs and symptoms of psychosis, helping the patient to think and behave more coherently.

Contraindications

Hypersensitivity to molindone, its components, or other antipsychotic drugs, including haloperidol, loxapine, phenothiazines, and thioxanthenes

Interactions

DRUGS

amphetamines: Decreased amphetamine effectiveness; decreased antipsychotic effectiveness of molindone

anesthetics, barbiturates, benzodiazepines, CNS depressants, opioid analgesics: Possibly prolonged and intensified CNS depressant effects

antacids, antidiarrheals: Decreased molindone absorption

anticholinergics, antidyskinetics, antihistamines: Possibly increased anticholinergic effects

beta blockers: Possibly increased effect of beta blocker

bromocriptine: Possibly decreased therapeutic effects of bromocriptine and increased serum prolactin level

extrapyramidal reaction-causing agents (amoxapine, haloperidol, loxapine, metoclopramide, olanzapine, phenothiazines, pimozide, rauwolfia alkaloids, risperidone, tacrine, thioxanthenes): Increased severity of extrapyramidal effects

levodopa: Inhibited antidyskinetic effects of levodopa; possibly decreased antipsychotic effects of molindone

lithium: Increased risk of neurotoxicity; increased extrapyramidal effects

MAO inhibitors, maprotiline, trazodone, tricyclic antidepressants: Possibly prolonged and intensified sedative or anticholinergic effects of all drugs

insulin, oral antidiabetic drugs: Possibly increased serum glucose level

phenytoin, tetracycline: Interference with absorption of phenytoin and tetracycline

ACTIVITIES

alcohol use: Prolonged and intensified CNS depression

Adverse Reactions

CNS: Drowsiness, euphoria, extrapyramidal reactions (such as dystonia, motor restlessness, pseudoparkinsonism, and tardive dyskinesia), headache, heatstroke, lack of coordination, mental depression, neuroleptic malignant syndrome, tiredness, twitching

CV: Orthostatic hypotension, tachycardia, unstable blood pressure

EENT: Blinking or eyelid spasm, blurred vision, dry mouth, inability to move eyes, nasal congestion

ENDO: Breast engorgement, lactation

GI: Constipation, nausea

GU: Decreased libido, menstrual irregularities, urine retention

MS: Muscle spasms of back, face, and neck; twisting movements of the body; weakness or stiffness of extremities

RESP: Dyspnea

SKIN: Diaphoresis, pale skin, rash

Overdose

Monitor patient for evidence of overdose, including coma, respiratory depression, sedation, and severe extrapyramidal reactions (dystonia, motor restlessness, pseudoparkinsonism, and tardive dyskinesia). Maintain an open airway, be prepared to assist with endotracheal intubation as needed, and institute continuous ECG monitoring.

To decrease absorption of drug in a conscious patient who isn't at risk for coma, be prepared to perform gastric lavage. For an unconscious patient, anticipate assisting with insertion of an endotracheal tube and gastric lavage. The inflated cuff of the endotracheal tube will help prevent aspiration of gastric contents into the lungs. Forced diuresis, hemodialysis, or peritoneal dialysis are ineffective for treating molindone overdose because only a small amount of the drug is excreted in urine. Expect to give an antidyskinetic (such as diphenhydramine or amantadine) or a synthetic anticholinergic antidyskinetic (such as benztropine, biperiden, or trihexyphenidyl) for extrapyramidal reactions.

Institute suicide precautions according to facility policy, and anticipate psychiatric re-evaluation.

Nursing Considerations

- **WARNING** Assess patient for signs and symptoms of neuroleptic malignant syndrome (such as diaphoresis, dyspnea, fatigue, fever, incontinence, pale skin, severe muscle stiffness, tachycardia, and unstable blood pressure), and notify prescriber immediately if they occur. Expect to discontinue drug and begin intensive medical treatment. If patient resumes antipsychotic therapy, monitor her carefully for recurrence.
- Molindone shouldn't be given to a patient who has severe CNS depression or is comatose because of CNS depressant effects.
- Monitor elderly patients for orthostatic hypotension and signs of tardive dyskinesia (including blinking or spasms of eyelids, involuntary movements of the extremities, and unusual facial expressions), because these patients may be sensitive to the drug's anticholinergic and extrapyramidal effects. Expect to reduce dosage or discontinue drug.
- Assess patient for evidence of heatstroke—such as confusion, hot and dry skin, inability to sweat, and weakness—because drug may suppress temperature regulation and increase anticholinergic effects. Notify prescriber immediately if they occur.
- Administer oral solution undiluted or mixed with carbonated beverage, fruit juice, milk, or water.

PATIENT TEACHING

- Instruct patient to follow treatment regimen and to notify her prescriber before discontinuing drug because gradual dosage reduction may be needed.
- Instruct patient not to take drug within 2 hours of taking an antacid. Advise her to take drug with food or a full glass of milk or water to reduce gastric irritation.
- Instruct patient to take oral solution undiluted or mixed with carbonated beverage, fruit juice, milk, or water.
- Advise the patient to avoid potentially hazardous activities until she knows how the drug affects her because of possible blurred vision, dizziness, and drowsiness.
- Urge patient to avoid alcohol because of possible additive effects and hypotension.
- Advise patient, especially if elderly, to rise slowly from a supine or seated position to avoid dizziness, light-headedness, and fainting.

• Explain that drug may reduce the body's response to heat; tell patient to avoid temperature extremes (such as a hot shower, hot tub, or sauna), and urge her to use caution during exercise.
• Warn patient not to take OTC drugs for cold or allergies; they can increase the risk of heatstroke and increase anticholinergic effects, such as blurred vision, constipation, dry mouth, and urine retention.
• If patient reports dry mouth, suggest sugarless chewing gum, hard candy, ice chips, and fluids.
• Inform patient and family members that it may take several weeks or months to see maximum improvement in signs and symptoms.

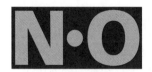

nalmefene hydrochloride
Revex

Class and Category
Chemical class: 6-Methylene analogue of naltrexone
Therapeutic class: Opioid antagonist
Pregnancy category: B

Indications and Dosages
▶ *To treat known or suspected opioid overdose*
I.V. , I.M., OR SUBCUTANEOUS INJECTION
Adults. 500 mcg/70 kg (154 lb); then second dose of 1,000 mcg/70 kg in 2 to 5 min, as indicated. *Maximum:* 1,500 mcg/70 kg.

Route	Onset	Steady State	Peak	Half-Life	Duration
I.V.	2 to 5 min	Unknown	Unknown	5½ to 16 hr	30 to 60 min*
I.M., SubQ	5 to 15 min	Unknown	Unknown	Unknown	Several hr

Mechanism of Action
Antagonizes mu, kappa, and sigma receptors in the CNS, thus reversing the analgesia, hypotension, respiratory depression, and sedation caused by most opioids. Mu receptors are responsible for analgesia, euphoria, miosis, and respiratory depression; kappa receptors, for analgesia and sedation. Sigma receptors control dysphoria and other delusional states.

Contraindications
Hypersensitivity to nalmefene or its components

Interactions
DRUGS
opioid analgesics (including alfentanil, fentanyl, and sufentanil): Reversal of these drugs' analgesic and adverse effects, possibly withdrawal signs and symptoms in opioid-dependent patients

---

* For partial reversal of opioid effects; up to several hr for full reversal.

Adverse Reactions

CNS: Agitation, chills, confusion, depression, dizziness, fever, hallucinations, headache, nervousness, somnolence, tremor

CV: Arrhythmias, hypertension, hypotension, tachycardia, vasodilation

EENT: Dry mouth, pharyngitis

GI: Diarrhea, nausea, vomiting

GU: Urine retention

SKIN: Pruritus

Other: Withdrawal signs and symptoms

Overdose

Patients given an overdose of nalmefene in the absence of opioid agonists have had no serious adverse reactions. Treatment of overdose should be symptomatic and supportive. Be aware that opioid-dependent patients may have withdrawal reactions (see WARNING under *Nursing Considerations*) and that using opioids to treat the withdrawal could result in respiratory and cardiovascular adverse reactions.

Nursing Considerations

- Use nalmefene cautiously in patients with hepatic or renal dysfunction because drug is metabolized by liver and excreted by kidneys.
- Also use drug cautiously in patients who have received a cardiotoxic drug and in those at increased risk for cardiovascular complications.
- **WARNING** Monitor patient for withdrawal effects, especially when patient is opioid-dependent. Signs and symptoms may include abdominal cramps, anorexia, anxiety, backache, bone or joint pain, confusion, depression, diaphoresis, dysphoria, erythema, fear, fever, irritability, labile blood pressure and pulse, lacrimation, muscle spasms, myalgia, mydriasis, nasal congestion, nausea, opioid craving, piloerection, restlessness, rhinorrhea, sensation of crawling skin, sleep disturbances, tremor, uneasiness, vomiting, and yawning.
- Be prepared to provide mechanical or assisted ventilation if reversal of opioid-induced respiratory depression is incomplete.

PATIENT TEACHING

- Urge opioid-dependent patient to seek drug rehabilitation.

Other Therapeutic Uses

Nalmefene hydrochloride is also indicated for the following:

- To treat postoperative opioid-induced respiratory depression

naloxone hydrochloride

Narcan

Class and Category

Chemical class: Thebaine derivative
Therapeutic class: Opioid antagonist
Pregnancy category: B

Indications and Dosages

▶ *To treat known or suspected opioid overdose*

I.V. INJECTION

Adults and children age 5 and over weighing more than 20 kg (44 lb). 0.4 to 2 mg repeated every 2 to 3 min, p.r.n. If no response after 10 mg, patient may not have opioid-induced toxicity.

Infants and children under age 5. 0.01 mg/kg as a single dose; if no improvement, another 0.1 mg/kg, as prescribed. Or, 0.1 mg/kg repeated every 2 to 3 min, as needed.

I.V., I.M., OR SUBCUTANEOUS INJECTION

Neonates. 0.01 mg/kg repeated I.V. every 2 to 3 min, as prescribed, until desired response occurs. Or, initial I.V. dose of 0.1 mg/kg.

Route	Onset	Steady State	Peak	Half-Life	Duration
I.V.	1 to 2 min	Unknown	5 to 15 min	About 1 hr*	45 min or longer
I.M., SubQ	2 to 5 min	Unknown	5 to 15 min	About 1 hr*	45 min or longer

Mechanism of Action

Briefly and competitively antagonizes mu, kappa, and sigma receptors in the CNS, thus reversing the analgesia, hypotension, respiratory depression, and sedation caused by most opioids. Mu receptors are responsible for analgesia, euphoria, miosis, and respiratory depression. Kappa receptors are responsible for analgesia and sedation. Sigma receptors control dysphoria and other delusional states.

Incompatibilities

Don't mix naloxone with any other solution unless you verify that drugs are compatible; drug is incompatible with alkaline, bisulfite, and metabisulfite solutions.

---

* For adults. Half-life is about 3 hr for neonates.

Contraindications
Hypersensitivity to naloxone or its components

Interactions
DRUGS

butorphanol, nalbuphine, pentazocine: Reversal of the analgesic and adverse effects of these drugs

opioid analgesics: Reversal of the analgesic and adverse effects of these drugs, possibly withdrawal signs and symptoms in opioid-dependent patients

Adverse Reactions
CNS: Seizures, tremor
CV: Hypertension (severe), tachycardia
GI: Nausea, vomiting
RESP: Hyperventilation
SKIN: Diaphoresis
Other: Withdrawal signs and symptoms

Overdose
When naloxone is given to a patient who hasn't taken opioids, the drug has no pharmacologic activity. However, it can cause withdrawal effects in opioid-dependent patients, including newborns of opioid-dependent mothers (see WARNING under *Nursing Considerations*).

Nursing Considerations
- Keep resuscitation equipment readily available during naloxone administration.
- Give drug by I.V. route whenever possible.
- Give repeat doses as prescribed, depending on patient's response.
- Anticipate that rapid reversal of opioid effects can cause diaphoresis, nausea, and vomiting.
- **WARNING** Monitor patient for withdrawal effects, especially when giving naloxone to opioid-dependent patient. Signs and symptoms may include abdominal cramps, anorexia, anxiety, backache, bone or joint pain, confusion, depression, diaphoresis, dysphoria, erythema, fear, fever, irritability, labile blood pressure and pulse, lacrimation, muscle spasms, myalgia, mydriasis, nasal congestion, nausea, opioid craving, piloerection, restlessness, rhinorrhea, sensation of crawling skin, sleep disturbances, tremor, uneasiness, vomiting, and yawning.
- Expect patient with hepatic or renal dysfunction to have increased circulating blood naloxone level.

PATIENT TEACHING
- Inform patient or family that naloxone will reverse opioid-induced adverse reactions.
- Urge opioid-dependent patient to seek drug rehabilitation.

Other Therapeutic Uses
Naloxone hydrochloride is also indicated for the following:
- To treat postoperative opioid-induced respiratory depression
- To reverse opioid-induced asphyxia
- As adjunct to treat hypotension caused by septic shock

naltrexone hydrochloride
ReVia, Vivitrol

Class and Category
Chemical class: Thebaine derivative
Therapeutic class: Opioid antagonist
Pregnancy category: C

Indications and Dosages
▶ *To treat opioid dependence*
TABLETS (REVIA)
Adults. *Initial:* 25 mg, repeated within 1 hr, if needed and if no withdrawal signs or symptoms occur. *Maintenance:* 50 mg daily or 350 mg/wk by intermittent dosing regimen.
▶ *As adjunct to treat alcoholism*
TABLETS (REVIA)
Adults. 50 mg daily for 12 wk.
I.M. INJECTION (VIVITROL)
Adults. 380 mg every mo

Route	Onset	Steady State	Peak	Half-Life	Duration
P.O.	15 to 30 min	Unknown	In 12 hr	4 hr*	24 hr†

Mechanism of Action
Displaces opioid agonists from—or blocks them from binding with—mu, kappa, and delta receptors. Opioid receptor blockade reverses the euphoric effect of opioids. Naltrexone also inhibits the effects of endogenous opioids, thus reducing alcohol craving.

---

* 13 hr for major metabolite, 6-beta-naltrexol.
† For 50 mg; 48 hr for 100 mg; 72 hr for 150 mg.

Contraindications

Acute hepatitis, acute opioid withdrawal, concurrent use of an opioid analgesic, hepatic failure, hypersensitivity to naltrexone or its components, opioid dependence

Interactions

DRUGS

opioid analgesics: Reversal of these drugs' analgesic and adverse effects, possibly withdrawal effects in opioid-dependent patients
thioridazine: Increased somnolence and lethargy

Adverse Reactions

CNS: Anxiety, chills, confusion, depression, dizziness, fatigue, fever, hallucinations, headache, insomnia, irritability, nervousness, restlessness
CV: Chest pain, edema, hypertension, tachycardia
EENT: Blurred vision, burning eyes, eyelid swelling, hoarseness, pharyngitis, rhinitis, sneezing, tinnitus
GI: Abdominal cramps, anorexia, constipation, diarrhea, GI ulceration, nausea, thirst, vomiting
GU: Difficult ejaculation, urinary frequency
MS: Arthralgia, myalgia
RESP: Cough, dyspnea
SKIN: Pruritus, rash
Other: Injection site reactions

Overdose

Limited information is available about naltrexone overdose. If an overdose occurs, expect to decrease drug absorption by inducing vomiting or performing gastric lavage. Patients undergoing naltrexone therapy should be closely monitored, and signs and symptoms should be treated, as needed.

Nursing Considerations

- To avoid withdrawal signs and symptoms, wait 7 to 10 days after last opioid dose, as prescribed, before starting patient on naltrexone.
- Give drug with food or antacids to decrease adverse GI reactions.
- Monitor baseline and periodic liver function test results, and observe patient for signs and symptoms of hepatotoxicity—including abdominal pain, dark urine, light-colored stools, and yellowing of eyes and skin—because drug may cause hepatocellular damage. Expect drug to be discontinued if abnormalities occur.
- Anticipate that some patients may need treatment for up to 1 year.

PATIENT TEACHING
- **WARNING** Caution patient against taking opioids again because he'll be more sensitive to them. In fact, taking previous doses could be fatal.
- Urge patient to undergo comprehensive rehabilitation along with naltrexone therapy.
- Instruct patient to tell his prescriber immediately if he develops evidence of hepatotoxicity, including abdominal pain, dark urine, light-colored stools, or yellowing of his eyes or skin.
- Inform patient about nonopioid treatments for cough, diarrhea, and pain.
- Instruct patient to carry medical identification that lists naltrexone therapy.

naratriptan hydrochloride

Amerge

Class and Category

Chemical class: Selective 5-hydroxytryptamine$_1$ (5-HT$_1$) receptor agonist
Therapeutic class: Antimigraine drug
Pregnancy category: C

Indications and Dosages

▶ *To relieve acute migraine*
TABLETS
Adults. 1 to 2.5 mg as a single dose, repeated in 4 hr p.r.n. if only partial relief obtained. *Maximum:* 5 mg daily.
DOSAGE ADJUSTMENT For patients with mild to moderate renal or hepatic impairment, maximum dosage reduced to 2.5 mg daily.

Route	Onset	Steady State	Peak	Half-Life	Duration
P.O.	Unknown	Unknown	Unknown	6 hr	Unknown

Mechanism of Action

Binds to receptors on intracranial blood vessels and sensory nerves in the trigeminal-vascular system to stimulate negative feedback, which halts the release of serotonin. In this way, naratriptan selectively constricts inflamed and dilated cranial vessels in the carotid circulation and inhibits the production of proinflammatory neuropeptides.

Contraindications

Basilar or hemiplegic migraine; cerebrovascular, peripheral vascular, or coronary artery disease (ischemic or vasospastic); hypersensitivity to naratriptan or its components; hypertension (uncontrolled); severe hepatic or renal dysfunction; use within 24 hours of another $5-HT_1$ agonist or an ergotamine-containing or ergottype drug, such as dihydroergotamine or methysergide

Interactions
DRUGS

ergotamine-containing drugs: Possibly prolonged or additive vasospastic reactions

fluoxetine, fluvoxamine, paroxetine, sertraline: Possibly weakness, hyperreflexia, and incoordination

oral contraceptives: Possibly reduced clearance and increased blood level of naratriptan

other selective $5-HT_1$ receptor agonists (including rizatriptan, sumatriptan, and zolmitriptan): Possibly additive effects

Adverse Reactions

CNS: Dizziness, drowsiness, fatigue, malaise, paresthesia
CV: Chest pain, pressure, or heaviness
EENT: Decreased salivation, otitis media, pharyngitis, photophobia, rhinitis, throat tightness
GI: Nausea, vomiting

Overdose

Monitor patient for evidence of overdose, including angina, hypertension, loss of coordination, neck tension, and tiredness. Maintain an open airway, monitor vital signs, and expect to continue ECG monitoring for at least 24 hours after overdose. Maintain fluid and electrolyte balance, and treat hypertension, as needed and prescribed. The effect of dialysis on naratriptan overdose is unknown.

Institute suicide precautions according to facility policy, and anticipate psychiatric re-evaluation.

Nursing Considerations

• **WARNING** Because naratriptan therapy can cause coronary artery vasospasm, monitor patient with coronary artery disease during therapy for signs and symptoms of angina. Because naratriptan may also cause peripheral vasospastic reactions, such as ischemic bowel disease, monitor patient for abdominal pain and bloody diarrhea.

- Monitor patient for hypertension during naratriptan therapy because drug may increase systolic blood pressure by up to 32 mm Hg.
- Be prepared to perform a complete neurovascular assessment in any patient who reports an unusual headache or who fails to respond to first dose of naratriptan.

PATIENT TEACHING
- Inform patient that naratriptan is used to treat acute migraine attacks but that it doesn't prevent or reduce the number of them.
- Advise patient not to take more than maximum prescribed dosage during any 24-hour period.
- If patient experiences no relief from initial dose of naratriptan, instruct him to notify prescriber rather than taking another dose in 4 hours because he may need a different drug.
- Advise patient to consult prescriber if he has more than four headaches during any 30-day period while taking naratriptan.

nefazodone hydrochloride

Class and Category
Chemical class: Phenylpiperazine derivative
Therapeutic class: Antidepressant
Pregnancy category: C

Indications and Dosages
▶ *To treat major depression*
TABLETS
Adults. *Initial:* 100 mg b.i.d., increased by 100 to 200 mg daily every wk, as prescribed. *Maintenance:* 150 to 300 mg b.i.d. *Maximum:* 600 mg daily.
DOSAGE ADJUSTMENT Initial dosage possibly reduced to 50 mg b.i.d. for elderly or debilitated patients; then dosage adjusted as ordered, based on patient response.

Route	Onset	Steady State	Peak	Half-Life	Duration
P.O.	Several wk	4 to 5 days	Unknown	2 to 4 hr	Unknown

Contraindications
Concurrent use of cisapride; hypersensitivity to nefazodone, other phenylpiperazine antidepressants, or their components; use within 14 days of MAO inhibitor therapy

Mechanism of Action

May inhibit serotonin reuptake at presynaptic neurons, increasing the neuronal level of serotonin, an inhibitory neurotransmitter that can regulate mood. Nefazodone also may act as a postsynaptic serotonin receptor antagonist, further increasing synaptic serotonin availability.

Interactions

DRUGS

alprazolam, buspirone, carbamazepine, cyclosporine, modafinil, triazolam: Increased blood levels of these drugs

antihypertensives: Increased risk of hypotension

cilostazol: Decreased cilostazol clearance, increased adverse effects of cilostazol, such as headache

cisapride: Increased blood levels of these drugs; prolonged QT interval; and, possibly, serious cardiovascular effects, including death from ventricular tachycardia

dextromethorphan, sibutramine, tramadol, trazodone: Increased risk of serotonin syndrome

digoxin: Increased blood digoxin level, increased risk of digitalis toxicity

haloperidol: Decreased haloperidol clearance

indinavir: Inhibited indinavir metabolism

levobupivacaine: Increased blood levobupivacaine level, possibly toxicity

lovastatin, simvastatin: Increased risk of rhabdomyolysis and myositis

MAO inhibitors: Possibly fatal reactions, including autonomic instability (with rapidly fluctuating vital signs), hyperthermia, mental status changes (such as severe agitation progressing to delirium and coma), muscle rigidity, and myoclonus

methadone: Increased blood level and adverse effects of methadone, additive CNS effects

nevirapine: Increased nefazodone metabolism, inhibited nevirapine metabolism

ritonavir: Inhibited nefazodone and ritonavir metabolism

sildenafil: Decreased sildenafil clearance

tacrolimus: Decreased tacrolimus clearance and increased adverse effects, including delirium and renal failure

ACTIVITIES

alcohol use: Increased risk of CNS depression

Adverse Reactions

CNS: Abnormal gait, apathy, asthenia, ataxia, chills, confusion, decreased concentration, delusions, depersonalization, dizziness, dream disturbances, euphoria, fever, hallucinations, headache, hostility, hypotonia, insomnia, light-headedness, malaise, memory loss, myoclonic jerks, neuralgia, paranoia, paresthesia, somnolence, suicidal ideation, syncope, tremor, vertigo

CV: Angina, hypertension, hypotension, peripheral edema, orthostatic hypotension, tachycardia, vasodilation, ventricular arrhythmias

EENT: Abnormal vision, blurred vision, conjunctivitis, diplopia, dry eyes and mouth, earache, epistaxis, eye pain, gingivitis, halitosis, hyperacusis, laryngitis, mydriasis, neck rigidity, periodontal abscess, pharyngitis, photophobia, stomatitis, taste perversion, tinnitus, visual field defects

ENDO: Breast pain, gynecomastia, lymphadenopathy

GI: Abdominal distention, colitis, constipation, diarrhea, dyspepsia, elevated liver function test results, eructation, esophagitis, gastritis, gastroenteritis, hernia, hiccups, increased appetite, nausea, peptic ulcer, rectal bleeding, thirst, vomiting

GU: Abnormal ejaculation; amenorrhea; cystitis; hematuria; hypermenorrhea; impotence; libido changes; nocturia; pelvic pain; polyuria; renal calculi; urinary frequency, incontinence, or urgency; urine retention; UTI; vaginal bleeding; vaginitis

HEME: Anemia, leukopenia

MS: Arthralgia, arthritis, bursitis, dysarthria, gout, muscle stiffness, tenosynovitis

RESP: Asthma, bronchitis, cough, dyspnea, pneumonia

SKIN: Acne, alopecia, dry skin, ecchymosis, eczema, maculopapular rash, photosensitivity, pruritus, rash, urticaria

Other: Allergic reaction, dehydration, infection, serotonin syndrome, weight loss

Overdose

Monitor patient for evidence of overdose, including bradycardia, hypotension, nausea, somnolence, vomiting, or an increase in frequency or severity of the adverse reactions listed above.

Maintain an open airway, monitor vital signs, and provide symptomatic and supportive treatment, as needed and prescribed. Be aware that the patient also may have ingested other drugs. To decrease drug absorption, be prepared to perform gastric lavage.

Institute suicide precautions according to facility policy, and anticipate psychiatric re-evaluation.

Nursing Considerations

• **WARNING** Be aware that nefazodone shouldn't be given with cisapride or MAO inhibitors; serious or fatal reactions may occur.

• Follow facility policy during initial nefazodone therapy if patient is at high risk for suicide.

• Assess patient for signs and symptoms of serotonin syndrome, such as abdominal cramps, aggressive behavior, agitation, chills, diarrhea, headache, insomnia, lack of coordination, nausea, palpitations, paresthesia, poor concentration, restlessness, and worsening of obsessive thoughts or compulsive behaviors.

• Monitor patient closely for suicidal tendencies, especially when therapy starts or dosage changes; depression may worsen temporarily during these times.

PATIENT TEACHING

• Instruct patient to take nefazodone exactly as prescribed and not to alter dosage without consulting prescriber.

• Inform patient that antidepressant effects may not occur for several weeks and that treatment may last 6 months or longer.

• Caution patient to avoid alcohol during nefazodone therapy.

• Advise patient to avoid potentially hazardous activities until he knows how the drug affects him.

• Suggest that patient try sugarless gum or hard candy for dry mouth. Urge him to notify prescriber if dry mouth persists for longer than 2 weeks.

• Urge caregivers to monitor patient closely for suicidal tendencies, especially when therapy starts or dosage changes because depression may worsen temporarily during these times.

nicotine for inhalation
Nicotrol Inhaler

nicotine nasal solution
Nicotrol NS

nicotine polacrilex
Nicorette, Nicorette Plus (CAN)

nicotine transdermal system
Habitrol, Nicoderm, NicoDerm CQ, Nicotrol, ProStep, Thrive

Class and Category
Chemical class: Pyridine alkaloid
Therapeutic class: Smoking cessation adjunct

Pregnancy category: C (nicotine polacrilex), D (other forms of nicotine)

Indications and Dosages

▶ *To relieve nicotine withdrawal symptoms, including craving*
CHEWING GUM
Adults. *Initial:* 2 or 4 mg p.r.n. or every 1 to 2 hr, adjusted to complete withdrawal by 4 to 6 mo. *Maximum:* 30 pieces of 2-mg gum daily or 20 pieces of 4-mg gum daily.
NASAL SOLUTION
Adults. 1 or 2 sprays (1 to 2 mg) in each nostril/hr. *Maximum:* 5 mg/hr or 40 mg daily for up to 3 mo.
ORAL INHALATION
Adults and adolescents. 6 to 16 cartridges (24 to 64 mg) daily for up to 12 wk; then dosage gradually reduced over 12 wk or less. *Maximum:* 16 cartridges (64 mg) daily for 6 mo.
TRANSDERMAL SYSTEM
Adults. *Initial:* 14 to 22 mg daily, adjusted to lower-dose systems over 2 to 5 mo.

DOSAGE ADJUSTMENT For adolescents and for adults who weigh less than 45 kg (100 lb) and who smoke less than 10 cigarettes daily or have heart disease, initial dosage reduced to 11 to 14 mg daily and adjusted to lower-dose systems over 2 to 5 mo.

Route	Onset	Steady State	Peak	Half-Life	Duration
Nasal spray	Unknown	Unknown	Unknown	1 to 3 hr	Unknown
Oral inhalation	Unknown	Unknown	Unknown	1 to 2 hr	Unknown
Transdermal system	Unknown	Unknown	Unknown	3 to 4 hr	Unknown

Mechanism of Action

Binds selectively to nicotinic-cholinergic receptors at autonomic ganglia, in the adrenal medulla, at neuromuscular junctions, and in the brain. By providing a lower dose of nicotine than cigarettes, this drug reduces nicotine craving and withdrawal signs and symptoms.

Contraindications

Hypersensitivity to nicotine, its components, or components of transdermal system; life-threatening arrhythmias; nonsmokers; recovery from an acute MI; severe angina pectoris; skin disorders (transdermal); temporomandibular joint disease (chewing gum)

Interactions
DRUGS

acetaminophen, beta blockers, imipramine, insulin, oxazepam, pentazo-cine, theophylline: Possibly increased therapeutic effects of these drugs (chewing gum, nasal spray, transdermal system)

alpha blockers, bronchodilators: Possibly increased therapeutic effects of these drugs (chewing gum, transdermal system)

bupropion: Potentiated therapeutic effects of nicotine, possibly increased risk of hypertension

sympathomimetics: Possibly decreased therapeutic effects of these drugs (chewing gum, transdermal system)

theophylline, tricyclic antidepressants: Possibly altered pharmacologic actions of these drugs (oral inhalation)

FOODS

acidic beverages (citrus juices, coffee, soft drinks, tea, wine): Decreased nicotine absorption from gum if beverages consumed within 15 minutes before or while chewing gum

caffeine: Increased effects of caffeine (chewing gum, nasal spray, transdermal system)

Adverse Reactions
CNS: Dizziness, dream disturbances, drowsiness, headache, irritability, light-headedness, nervousness (chewing gum, transdermal system); amnesia, confusion, difficulty speaking, headache, migraine headache, paresthesia (nasal spray); chills, fever, headache, paresthesia (oral inhalation)

CV: Arrhythmias (all forms); hypertension (chewing gum, transdermal system); peripheral edema (nasal spray)

EENT: Increased salivation, injury to teeth or dental work, mouth injury, pharyngitis, stomatitis (chewing gum); altered taste, dry mouth (chewing gum, transdermal system); altered smell and taste, burning eyes, dry mouth, earache, epistaxis, gum disorders, hoarseness, lacrimation, mouth and tongue swelling, nasal blisters, nasal irritation or ulceration, pharyngitis, rhinitis, sinus problems, sneezing, vision changes (nasal spray); altered taste, lacrimation, pharyngitis, rhinitis, sinusitis, stomatitis (oral inhalation)

GI: Eructation (chewing gum); abdominal pain, constipation, diarrhea, flatulence, increased appetite, indigestion, nausea, vomiting (chewing gum, transdermal system); abdominal pain, constipation, diarrhea, flatulence, hiccups, indigestion, nausea (nasal spray); diarrhea, flatulence, hiccups, indigestion, nausea, vomiting (oral inhalation)

GU: Dysmenorrhea (chewing gum, transdermal system); menstrual irregularities (nasal spray)
MS: Jaw and neck pain (chewing gum); arthralgia, myalgia (chewing gum, transdermal system); arthralgia, back pain, myalgia (nasal spray); back pain (oral inhalation)
RESP: Cough (chewing gum, transdermal system); bronchitis, bronchospasm, chest tightness, cough, dyspnea, increased sputum production (nasal spray); chest tightness, cough, dyspnea, wheezing (oral inhalation)
SKIN: Diaphoresis, erythema, pruritus, rash, urticaria (chewing gum, transdermal system); acne, flushing of face, pruritus, purpura, rash (nasal spray); pruritus, rash, urticaria (oral inhalation)
Other: Allergic reaction (chewing gum, transdermal system); physical dependence (nasal spray); flulike signs and symptoms, generalized pain, withdrawal signs and symptoms (oral inhalation)

Overdose

Monitor patient for evidence of overdose, including abdominal pain, altered hearing and vision, bradycardia, cardiac arrest, cold sweat, confusion, diarrhea, dizziness, fatigue, headache, hypotension, nausea, pale skin, respiratory failure, salivation, seizures, tremor, vomiting, and weakness.

Maintain an open airway, and be prepared to assist with artificial respiration, as needed. Expect to treat hypotension with I.V. fluids, a vasopressor, or atropine, as prescribed. Atropine may also be prescribed to treat bradycardia, diarrhea, excessive secretions, and hypotension. To treat seizures, expect to give lorazepam or a barbiturate; institute seizure precautions according to facility policy.

To decrease drug absorption if the patient ingested an inhaler cartridge, expect to administer activated charcoal orally in a conscious patient who isn't at risk for seizures. For an unconscious patient, anticipate assisting with insertion of an endotracheal tube. The tube's inflated cuff will help prevent aspiration of gastric contents into the lungs. Plan to give activated charcoal through a nasogastric tube. Know that multiple doses of activated charcoal may be needed as long as the cartridge remains in the GI system because it will continue to release nicotine. Expect to also give a saline cathartic or sorbitol to enhance elimination of the cartridge. The cartridge will be visible on X-ray.

If nasal solution comes in contact with patient's eyes, flush them with a gentle stream of water for 20 minutes to decrease drug absorption.

Overdose may occur if the patient chews multiple pieces of the gum at one time. Be aware that if the gum is swallowed without being chewed it won't release nicotine in significant amounts because of the acid pH of the stomach. To decrease absorption of the gum in a conscious patient who isn't at risk for seizures, induce vomiting with ipecac syrup. For an unconscious patient, anticipate assisting with insertion of an endotracheal tube. The tube's inflated cuff will help prevent aspiration of gastric contents into the lungs. Plan to perform gastric lavage and then give activated charcoal through a nasogastric tube. Give a saline cathartic, as prescribed, to enhance GI elimination of the gum.

Overdose may occur if the patient wears several transdermal systems at one time. Remove the patch and flush the skin with water. Avoid using soap because it will increase absorption of the nicotine. If the patient ingested the patch, administer activated charcoal, as prescribed, and plan to repeat these doses as long as the patch remains in the GI system. To speed passage of the patch, give a saline cathartic or sorbitol, as prescribed.

Institute suicide precautions according to facility policy, and anticipate psychiatric re-evaluation.

Nursing Considerations

- When administering nicotine by oral inhalation, expect optimal effect to result from continuous puffing for 20 minutes.
- Remove patch before patient has an MRI study to avoid possible burns.

PATIENT TEACHING

- Instruct patient to read and follow package instructions to obtain best results with nicotine product.
- Advise patient to notify prescriber about other drugs he takes.
- Stress that patient must stop smoking as soon as treatment starts to avoid toxicity.
- For chewing gum therapy, instruct patient to wait at least 15 minutes after drinking coffee, juice, soft drink, tea, or wine. Advise him to chew gum until he detects a tingling sensation or peppery taste and then to place the gum between his cheek and gum until tingling or peppery taste subsides. Then direct him to move the gum to a different site until tingling or taste subsides, repeating until he no longer feels the sensation—usually about 30 minutes. Caution against swallowing the gum.
- For nasal spray therapy, instruct patient to tilt his head back and spray into a nostril. Caution against sniffing, swallowing, or inhaling spray because nicotine is absorbed through nasal mucosa.

- Caution that prolonged use of nasal form may cause dependence.
- For oral inhalation therapy, instruct patient to use 6 to 16 cartridges per day to prevent or relieve withdrawal signs and symptoms and craving. Starting with 1 or 2 cartridges per day yields poor success. Direct patient to inhale through device just like a cigarette, puffing frequently for 20 minutes for best results.
- For transdermal patch therapy, instruct patient not to open package until immediately before use because nicotine will be lost in the air. Advise him to apply patch to clean, hairless, dry site on the upper outer arm or upper body. Instruct him to change patches and rotate sites every 24 hours and not to use the same site within 7 days. Advise patient to remove patch before undergoing an MRI procedure to avoid possible burns.
- **WARNING** Urge patient to keep all unused nicotine forms safely away from children and pets and to discard used forms carefully. (Enough nicotine may remain in used systems to poison children and pets.) Instruct him to contact a poison control center immediately if he suspects that a child has ingested nicotine.
- Explain to patient with asthma or COPD that nicotine may cause bronchospasm.
- Inform patient that it may take several attempts to successfully stop smoking. Urge him to join a smoking cessation program.

nortriptyline hydrochloride
Aventyl, Pamelor

Class and Category
Chemical class: Dibenzocycloheptene derivative
Therapeutic class: Antidepressant
Pregnancy category: C

Indications and Dosages
▶ *To treat depression*
CAPSULES, ORAL SOLUTION
Adults. *Initial:* 25 mg t.i.d. or q.i.d. *Maximum:* 150 mg daily.
Adolescents. 25 to 50 mg daily or 1 to 3 mg/kg daily in divided doses.
Children ages 6 to 12. 10 to 20 mg daily or 1 to 3 mg/kg daily in divided doses.
DOSAGE ADJUSTMENT Dosage possibly reduced to 30 to 50 mg daily (in divided doses or at bedtime) for elderly patients.

Route	Onset	Steady State	Peak	Half-Life	Duration
P.O.	2 to 3 wk	4 to 19 days	Unknown	18 to 44 hr	Unknown

Mechanism of Action
May interfere with reuptake of serotonin (and possibly other neurotransmitters) at presynaptic neurons, thus enhancing serotonin's effects at postsynaptic receptors. By restoring normal neurotransmitter levels at nerve synapses, this tricyclic antidepressant may elevate mood.

Contraindications
Acute recovery phase of a CVA or an MI; hypersensitivity to nortriptyline, other tricyclic antidepressants, or their components; use within 14 days of MAO inhibitor therapy

Interactions
DRUGS

amantadine, anticholinergics, antidyskinetics, antihistamines: Possibly increased anticholinergic effects, confusion, hallucinations, nightmares; increased CNS depression

anticonvulsants: Possibly increased CNS depression and risk of seizures, possibly decreased anticonvulsant effectiveness

antithyroid drugs: Possibly agranulocytosis

barbiturates, carbamazepine: Possibly decreased blood level and effectiveness of nortriptyline

bupropion, clozapine, cyclobenzaprine, haloperidol, loxapine, maprotiline, molindone, phenothiazines, thioxanthenes: Possibly increased sedative and anticholinergic effects of these drugs, possibly increased risk of seizures

cimetidine, fluoxetine: Possibly increased blood nortriptyline level and risk of toxicity

clonidine: Possibly decreased antihypertensive effect of clonidine, increased CNS depression

disulfiram: Possibly delirium

ethchlorvynol: Possibly delirium, increased CNS depression

guanadrel, guanethidine: Possibly decreased antihypertensive effect of these drugs

MAO inhibitors: Increased risk of hypertensive crisis, severe seizures, and death

oral anticoagulants: Possibly increased anticoagulant activity

pimozide, probucol: Possibly arrhythmias

sympathomimetics (including ophthalmic epinephrine and vasoconstrictive

local anesthetics): Increased risk of arrhythmias, hyperpyrexia, hypertension, and tachycardia
thyroid hormones: Possibly increased therapeutic and toxic effects of both drugs
ACTIVITIES
alcohol use: Increased CNS and respiratory depression, hypertension, and alcohol effects

Adverse Reactions

CNS: Ataxia, confusion, CVA, delirium, dizziness, drowsiness, excitation, hallucinations, headache, insomnia, nervousness, nightmares, parkinsonism, suicidal ideation, tremor
CV: Arrhythmias, orthostatic hypotension
EENT: Blurred vision, dry mouth, increased intraocular pressure, taste perversion
GI: Constipation, diarrhea, heartburn, ileus, increased appetite, nausea, vomiting
GU: Sexual dysfunction, urine retention
HEME: Bone marrow depression
RESP: Wheezing
SKIN: Diaphoresis, urticaria
Other: Weight gain

Overdose

Monitor patient for evidence of overdose, including agitation, arrhythmias, confusion, disturbed concentration, drowsiness, dyspnea, fever, hallucinations, irregular heartbeat, mydriasis, restlessness, seizures, unusual fatigue, vomiting, and weakness.

Maintain an open airway, institute continuous ECG monitoring (for at least 5 days), and closely observe patient's blood pressure, respiratory rate, and temperature. Be prepared to treat arrhythmias with lidocaine and sodium bicarbonate, as prescribed. Anticipate possible digitalization to prevent heart failure. Institute seizure precautions according to facility protocol, and administer anticonvulsant therapy, as prescribed.

Be prepared to perform gastric lavage to decrease drug absorption. Expect to administer activated charcoal followed by a bowel stimulant to enhance drug elimination. Tricyclic antidepressants are highly protein bound; therefore, dialysis, exchange transfusions, and forced diuresis are ineffective for treating overdose.

Be aware that use of I.V. physostigmine isn't routinely recommended, but it may be prescribed for comatose patients with respiratory depression, serious arrhythmias, severe hypertension, or uncontrollable seizures to reverse the anticholinergic effects of nortriptyline.

Institute suicide precautions according to facility policy, and anticipate psychiatric re-evaluation.

Nursing Considerations
- Expect to discontinue MAO inhibitor therapy 10 to 14 days before starting nortriptyline therapy.
- **WARNING** Monitor patients, especially adolescents and children, closely for suicidal thinking and behavior because nortriptyline increases the risk of suicidal ideation.
- Be aware that nortriptyline oral solution (10 mg/5 ml) contains 4% alcohol.
- Give drug with food to reduce adverse GI reactions.
- Monitor blood nortriptyline level; therapeutic range is 50 to 150 ng/ml.
- Monitor ECG tracing as appropriate to detect arrhythmias.

PATIENT TEACHING
- **WARNING** Urge caregiver and parents to watch the patient for evidence of abnormal thinking or behavior, including an increase in aggression or hostility. If unusual changes occur, stress importance of notifying prescriber.
- Inform patient that nortriptyline oral solution contains alcohol, in case he has a history of alcohol abuse.
- Discourage patient from drinking alcohol during nortriptyline therapy.
- Inform patient that improvement may not occur for several weeks.
- Advise patient to avoid potentially hazardous activities until he knows how the drug affects him.
- Instruct patient to change position slowly to minimize effects of orthostatic hypotension.
- Suggest that patient minimize constipation by drinking plenty of fluids (if allowed), eating high-fiber foods, and exercising regularly.

olanzapine
Zyprexa, Zyprexa Zydis

Class and Category
Chemical class: Thienobenzodiazepine derivative
Therapeutic class: Antipsychotic drug
Pregnancy category: C

Indications and Dosages

▶ *To treat psychosis*

DISINTEGRATING TABLETS, TABLETS

Adults. *Initial:* 5 to 10 mg daily *Usual:* 10 mg daily. *Maximum:* 20 mg daily.

▶ *To treat manic phase of acute bipolar disorder*

DISINTEGRATING TABLETS, TABLETS

Adults. *Initial:* 10 to 15 mg daily; may be increased or decreased by 5 mg every 24 hr as needed and prescribed. *Usual:* 5 to 20 mg daily for 3 to 4 wk. *Maximum:* 20 mg daily.

▶ *As adjunct in treating acute bipolar disorder*

ORALLY DISINTEGRATING TABLETS, TABLETS

Adults. *Initial:* 10 mg daily with lithium or valproate sodium; may be increased or decreased by 5 mg every 24 hr, as needed and prescribed. *Usual:* 5 to 20 mg daily for 6 wk. *Maximum:* 20 mg daily.

DOSAGE ADJUSTMENT Initial dosage possibly reduced to 5 mg for debilitated patients, those prone to hypotension, and nonsmoking women older than age 65.

▶ *To treat agitation in schizophrenia and bipolar I mania*

I.M. INJECTION

Adults. 5 to 10 mg p.r.n. Repeat as needed every 2 to 4 hr.

DOSAGE ADJUSTMENT Dosage decreased to 2.5 mg for debilitated patients, those prone to hypotension, and female nonsmokers over age 65. Dosage decreased to 5 mg for elderly patients.

Route	Onset	Steady State	Peak	Half-Life	Duration
P.O.	1 wk	1 wk	Unknown	21 to 54 hr	Unknown
I.M.	Unknown	1 wk	Unknown	21 to 54 hr	Unknown

Mechanism of Action

May achieve its antipsychotic effects by antagonizing dopamine and serotonin receptors. Anticholinergic effects may result from competitive binding to and antagonism of muscarinic receptors M_1 through M_5.

Contraindications

Blood dyscrasias, bone marrow depression, cerebral arteriosclerosis, coma, coronary artery disease, hepatic dysfunction, high-dose therapy with a CNS depressant, hypersensitivity to olanzapine or its components, hypertension, hypotension, myeloproliferative disorders, severe CNS depression, subcortical brain damage

Interactions

DRUGS

anticholinergics: Increased anticholinergic effects, altered thermo-regulation

antihypertensives: Increased effects of both drugs and risk of hypotension

benzodiazepines (parenteral): Increased risk of excessive sedation and cardiorespiratory depression

carbamazepine, omeprazole, rifampin: Increased olanzapine clearance

CNS depressants: Additive CNS depression, potentiated orthostatic hypotension

diazepam: Increased CNS depressant effects

fluvoxamine: Decreased olanzapine clearance

levodopa: Decreased levodopa efficacy

lorazepam (parenteral form): Possibly increased somnolence with I.M. injection of olazapine

ACTIVITIES

alcohol use: Additive CNS depression, potentiated orthostatic hypotension

smoking: Decreased blood olanzapine level

Adverse Reactions

CNS: Abnormal gait, agitation, akathisia, altered thermoregulation, amnesia, anxiety, asthenia, dizziness, euphoria, fever, headache, hypertonia, insomnia, nervousness, neuroleptic malignant syndrome, restlessness, somnolence, stuttering, suicidal ideation, tardive dyskinesia, tremor

CV: Bradycardia, chest pain, hypertension, hypotension, orthostatic hypotension, peripheral edema, tachycardia

EENT: Amblyopia, dry mouth, increased salivation, pharyngitis, rhinitis

ENDO: Hyperglycemia, ketoacidosis

GI: Abdominal pain, constipation, dysphagia, increased appetite, nausea, thirst, vomiting

GU: Urinary incontinence

HEME: Neutropenia

MS: Arthralgia; back, joint, or extremity pain; muscle spasms; twitching

RESP: Cough, hypoventilation (parenteral form)

SKIN: Ecchymosis, photosensitivity, pruritus, urticaria

Other: Anaphylaxis, angioedema, flulike signs and symptoms, weight gain

Overdose

Monitor patient for evidence of overdose, including drowsiness and slurred speech. Maintain open airway, monitor patient for arrhythmias, and maintain temperature. Institute seizure precautions, as needed, according to facility protocol.

To decrease drug absorption in a conscious patient who isn't at risk for coma or seizures, be prepared to perform gastric lavage. Expect that oral activated charcoal and a laxative may also be prescribed. Be aware that vomiting shouldn't be induced because of the potential for dystonic reactions of the head and neck or seizures. For an unconscious patient, anticipate assisting with the insertion of an endotracheal tube and then performing gastric lavage. The inflated cuff of the endotracheal tube will help prevent aspiration of gastric contents into the lungs.

Anticipate the use of a sympathomimetic to treat hypotension, as prescribed. Avoid dopamine, epinephrine, and other agents that have beta-agonist activity because these drugs may exacerbate hypotension.

Institute suicide precautions according to facility policy, and anticipate psychiatric re-evaluation.

Nursing Considerations

- Be aware that olanzapine may increase risk of death in elderly patients with dementia-related psychosis and worsen such conditions as angle-closure glaucoma, benign prostatic hyperplasia, and seizures.
- Use cautiously in patients with cardiovascular or cerebrovascular disease or any condition that would predispose patient to hypotension. Also use cautiously in patients receiving treatment with other drugs that may induce hypotension, bradycardia, or respiratory or CNS depression.
- Reconstitute parenteral olanzapine by dissolving contents of vial in 2.1 ml of sterile water to yield 5 mg/ml. Solution should be clear yellow. Use within 1 hour.
- Inject I.M. olanzapine slowly and deep into muscle mass.
- If drowsiness or dizziness occurs after I.M. injection of olanzapine, keep patient recumbent until postural hypotension, bradycardia, and hypoventilation have been relieved. Don't let patient sit or stand up until blood pressure and heart rate have returned to baseline.
- Monitor patient's blood pressure routinely during therapy because olanzapine may cause orthostatic hypotension.
- Assess daily weight to detect fluid retention.

- Notify prescriber if patient develops tardive dyskinesia or urinary incontinence.
- Be alert for evidence of neuroleptic malignant syndrome—such as altered mental status, autonomic instability, hyperpyrexia, and muscle rigidity—and immediately report them to prescriber.
- Monitor patient for suicidal tendencies. If you detect them, notify prescriber and implement suicide precautions according to facility policy.
- Monitor patient's blood glucose level routinely because the risk of hyperglycemia may increase with olanzapine use and may become severe. The risk may include ketoacidosis, coma, and death.

PATIENT TEACHING

- Instruct patient to peel back the foil on the disintegrating tablet blister pack rather than push the tablet through the foil. Tell him to remove the tablet with dry hands, place it on his tongue to dissolve it, and then swallow it with his saliva.
- Advise patient to avoid alcohol and smoking during olanzapine therapy.
- Urge patient to avoid potentially hazardous activities until he knows how the drug affects him.
- Instruct patient to change position slowly to minimize effects of orthostatic hypotension.
- Urge patient to avoid strenuous exercise and temperature extremes and to drink plenty of fluids.
- Instruct patient to avoid excessive sun exposure and to wear sunscreen and protective clothing while outdoors.
- Advise patient with diabetes to monitor blood glucose level closely and to report persistent hyperglycemia.
- Urge caregivers to monitor patient for suicidal tendencies, especially when therapy begins or dosages changes.

olanzapine and fluoxetine hydrochloride
Symbyax

Class and Category
Chemical class: Thienobenzodiazepine derivative (olanzapine) and selective serotonin reuptake inhibitor (fluoxetine)
Therapeutic class: Antipsychotic
Pregnancy category: C

Indications and Dosages
▶ *To treat depression in bipolar disorder*

CAPSULES

Adults. *Initial:* 6 mg olanzapine and 25 mg fluoxetine daily in the evening and then dosage increased as needed. *Maximum:* 12 mg olanzapine and 50 mg fluoxetine.

Route	Onset	Peak	Duration
P.O. (fluoxetine)	Unknown	6 to 8 hr	Unknown
P.O. (olanzapine)	Unknown	6 hr	Unknown

Mechanism of Action
May activate the monoaminergic neural system's serotonin, norepinephrine, and dopamine release in the prefrontal cortex to produce an enhanced antidepressant effect.

Contraindications
Hypersensitivity to olanzapine, fluoxetine, or other selective serotonin reuptake inhibitors or their components; pimozide therapy; tryptophan therapy; use within 14 days of an MAO inhibitor or within 5 weeks of thioridazine

Interactions
DRUGS

almotriptan: Increased risk of weakness, hyperreflexia, and incoordination

alprazolam, diazepam: Possibly prolonged half-life of these drugs

anticholinergics: Increased anticholinergic effects, altered thermoregulation

antihypertensives: Increased effects of both drugs

aspirin, NSAIDS, warfarin: Increased risk of bleeding

astemizole: Increased risk of serious arrhythmias

benzodiazepines (parenteral): Increased risk of excessive sedation and cardiorespiratory depression

buspirone: Decreased buspirone effects

carbamazepine, omeprazole, rifampin: Increased olanzapine clearance

clozapine, fluphenazine, haloperidol, maprotiline, trazodone: Increased risk of adverse effects

CNS depressants: Additive CNS depression, potentiated orthostatic hypotension

diazepam: Increased CNS depressant effects

fluvoxamine: Decreased olanzapine clearance

levodopa: Decreased levodopa efficacy

lithium: Increased or decreased blood lithium level
MAO inhibitors, serotonergic drugs, triptans: Increased risk of serotinin syndrome
phenytoin: Increased blood phenytoin level and risk of toxicity
pimozide: Increased risk of QT-interval prolongation
serotonergics (such as amphetamines and other psychostimulants, antidepressants, dopamine agonists, linezolid, lithium, St. John's wort, tramadol, triptans, and tryptophan): Serotonin syndrome
thioridazine: Increased risk of serious ventricular arrhythmias
tricyclic antidepressants: Increased risk of adverse effects, including seizures

ACTIVITIES
alcohol use: Additive CNS depression, potentiated orthostatic hypotension
smoking: Decreased blood olanzapine level

Adverse Reactions
CNS: Amnesia, asthenia, chills, fever, hyperkinesia, migraine, neuroleptic malignant syndrome, personality changes, seizures, serotonin syndrome, sleep disturbance, somnolence, speech alteration, suicidal ideation, tardive dyskinesia, tremor
CV: Bradycardia, chest pain, edema, hypertension, orthostatic hypotension, tachycardia, vasodilation
EENT: Abnormal vision, amblyopia, dry mouth, ear pain, increased salivation, otitis media, pharyngitis, taste perversion, tinnitus
ENDO: Breast pain, hyperglycemia, increased prolactin level, ketoacidosis, menorrhagia
GI: Diarrhea, elevated liver function test results, increased appetite, thirst
GU: Abnormal ejaculation, anorgasmia, decreased libido, impotence, urinary frequency or incontinence, UTI
MS: Arthralgia, muscle twitching, neck pain or rigidity,
RESP: Bronchitis, dyspnea
SKIN: Ecchymosis, erythema multiforme, photosensitivity, rash, urticaria
Other: Anaphylaxis, angioedema, hyponatremia, infection, weight gain or loss

Overdose
Olanzapine and fluoxetine overdose has no specific antidote. Monitor patient for evidence of overdose, including agitation, arrthymias, ataxia, coma, confusion, drowsiness, hypomania (talk-

ing or acting with uncontrolled excitement), impaired consciousness, lethargy, nausea, restlessness, seizures, slurred speech, somnolence, tachycardia, tremor, and vomiting.

Maintain an open airway, institute continuous ECG monitoring, and maintain patient's temperature. Expect to treat seizures with an anticonvulsant, such as diazepam, as prescribed, and institute seizure precautions according to facility protocol.

To decrease absorption of drug, be prepared to perform gastric lavage with appropriate airway protection. For an unconscious patient, anticipate assisting with insertion of an endotracheal tube and then performing gastric lavage. The inflated cuff of the endotracheal tube will help prevent aspiration of gastric contents into the lungs.

Do not induce vomiting because of possible dystonic reactions of the head and neck or possible seizures. Expect that activated charcoal with sorbitol also may be prescribed. Be aware that dialysis, forced diuresis, exchange transfusions, and hemoperfusion are ineffective for treating drug overdose because the drug is highly protein bound and has a large volume of distribution in the body.

Expect to give intravenous fluids and a sympathomimetic to treat hypotension, as prescribed. Avoid dopamine, epinephrine, and other drugs with beta-agonist activity because they may worsen hypotension.

If the patient also ingested a tricyclic antidepressant, watch for evidence of tricyclic antidepressant toxicity, including constipation, dry mouth, light-headedness, memory loss, slowed thinking and acting, and sedation. Fluoxetine inhibits metabolism of the tricyclic antidepressant, so these effects may last 3 weeks or more.

Institute suicide precautions according to facility policy, and anticipate psychiatric re-evaluation.

Nursing Considerations

• **WARNING** Monitor patient closely during olanzapine and fluoxetine therapy for potentially life-threatening serotonin syndrome. Signs and symptoms include agitation, coma, hallucinations, tachycardia, labile blood pressure, hyperthermia, hyperreflexia, incoordination, nausea, vomiting, and diarrhea. Be aware that concurrent therapy with serotonergic drugs or MAO inhibitors increases risk. If present, notify prescriber; expect to discontinue drug and provide supportive care.

• Use with caution in patients with cardiovascular or cerebrovascular disease or conditions that would predispose patients to hypotension because of olanzapine and fluoxetine's potential to cause orthostatic hypotension.

- Be aware that olanzapine should not be used in patients with dementia-related psychosis because of increased risk of cerebrovascular adverse effects and possibly death.
- Monitor patient's blood glucose level routinely because risk of hyperglycemia may increase with olanzapine use and may become severe. Risk includes ketoacidosis, coma, and death.
- Monitor patient closely for neuroleptic malignant syndrome (hyperthermia, muscle rigidity, altered level of consciousness, irregular pulse or blood pressure, tachycardia, diaphoresis, and arrhythmias), a rare but potentially fatal adverse effect.
- Monitor hepatic function, as ordered, in patients with hepatic disease because olanzapine and fluoxetine combination can elevate hepatic enzyme levels.
- Watch closely for abnormal behavior or thought patterns, especially in children, adolescents, and young adults, because risk of suicide is increased in patients receiving psychotropic drugs such as olanzapine and fluoxetine.

PATIENT TEACHING
- Advise patient to avoid exercise in hot weather to reduce the risk of dehydration and hypotension. Also instruct him to notify prescriber if he has prolonged diarrhea, nausea, or vomiting.
- Caution patient to avoid potentially hazardous activities until drug's CNS effects are known.
- Instruct patient to change position slowly to minimize effects of orthostatic hypotension.
- Caution patient to avoid using aspirin or NSAIDs while taking olanzapine and fluoxetine because concomitant use can increase the risk of bleeding.
- Advise patient to avoid alcohol and smoking during therapy because of increased risk of adverse effects.
- Tell patient to notify prescriber if he develops a rash or hives.
- Urge caregivers to monitor patient closely for abnormal behavior or thought patterns, especially if patient is a child, an adolescent, or a young adult.

orlistat
Xenical

Class and Category
Chemical class: Lipase inhibitor

Therapeutic class: Antiobesity drug
Pregnancy category: B

Indications and Dosages

▶ *To promote weight loss in patients with a body mass index above 30 kg (66 lb)/m², or, if patient has diabetes mellitus, hyperlipidemia, or hypertension, 27 kg (59 lb)/m²*

GELCAPS

Adults. 120 mg t.i.d. with fat-containing meals. *Maximum:* 360 mg daily.

Route	Onset	Steady State	Peak	Half-Life	Duration
P.O.	Unknown	Unknown	Unknown	1 to 2 hr	Unknown

Contraindications

Cholestasis, chronic malabsorption syndrome, hypersensitivity to orlistat or its components

Interactions

DRUGS

anticoagulants: Possibly decreased PT, increased INR, and unbalanced anticoagulant treatment
cyclosporine: Decreased plasma cyclosporine level
fat-soluble vitamins: Decreased vitamin absorption, especially vitamin E and beta-carotene
pravastatin: Potentiated lipid-lowering effect of pravastatin

Adverse Reactions

CNS: Anxiety, depression, dizziness, fatigue, headache, sleep disturbance
CV: Pedal edema
EENT: Gingival or tooth disorder
ENDO: Hypoglycemia
GI: Abdominal distention or pain, cholelithiasis, diarrhea (infectious), fatty or oily stool, fecal incontinence or urgency, flatulence with discharge, hepatitis, increased frequency of bowel movements, nausea, pancreatitis, rectal pain, vomiting
GU: Menstrual irregularities, UTI, vaginitis
MS: Arthralgia, arthritis, back pain, leg pain, myalgia, tendinitis
RESP: Bronchospasm, respiratory tract infection
SKIN: Dry skin, rash
Other: Flulike signs and symptoms

Overdose

Information regarding orlistat overdose isn't available. However,

Mechanism of Action

In the GI tract, orlistat binds with and inactivates gastric and pancreatic enzymes known as lipases, as shown. Normally, lipase enzymes convert ingested triglycerides into absorbable free fatty acids and monoglycerides. By inactivating lipase, orlistat allows undigested triglycerides to pass through the GI tract and exit the body in feces. Blocking the absorption of some of these fats lowers the number of calories the person receives from food, which promotes weight loss.

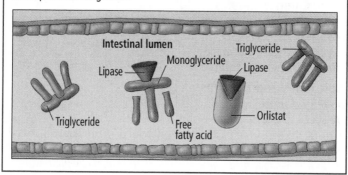

no significant adverse reactions were noted when normal-weight and obese subjects were given high doses of the drug in research studies. If an overdose occurs, monitor the patient for 24 hours and provide symptomatic and supportive treatment as needed. Expect that systemic effects of drug will be rapidly reversible.

Institute suicide precautions according to facility policy, and anticipate psychiatric re-evaluation.

Nursing Considerations
• Give orlistat with or up to 1 hour after meals that contain fat.
• Consult prescriber if you think patient has an eating disorder, such as anorexia nervosa or bulimia.

PATIENT TEACHING
• Instruct patient to take orlistat with or shortly after meals that contain fat.
• Advise patient to take a multivitamin that contains fat-soluble vitamins and beta-carotene at least 2 hours before or after taking drug, if indicated.
• Inform patient about drug's adverse GI effects, but explain that reducing dietary fat may decrease them. Instruct him to notify prescriber if they become too unpleasant.
• Help patient plan a reduced-fat diet (less than 30% of daily

calories) and an exercise program to promote weight loss.
• Advise patient to weigh himself daily, at the same time of day and wearing similar clothes, to check his progress in losing weight.

oxazepam

Apo-Oxazepam (CAN), Novoxapam (CAN), Serax

Class, Category, and Schedule

Chemical class: Benzodiazepine
Therapeutic class: Antianxiety drug, sedative-hypnotic
Pregnancy category: Not rated
Controlled substance schedule: IV

Indications and Dosages

▶ *To treat anxiety*

CAPSULES, TABLETS

Adults. 10 to 15 mg t.i.d. or q.i.d. for mild to moderate anxiety; up to 30 mg t.i.d. or q.i.d. for severe anxiety.

▶ *To help manage signs and symptoms of acute alcohol withdrawal*

CAPSULES, TABLETS

Adults. 15 to 30 mg t.i.d. or q.i.d.

DOSAGE ADJUSTMENT For elderly or debilitated patients, initial dose of 10 mg t.i.d. increased cautiously to 15 mg t.i.d. or q.i.d.

Route	Onset	Steady State	Peak	Half-Life	Duration
P.O.	Unknown	2 to 3 days	Unknown	5 to 20 hr	Unknown

Mechanism of Action

May potentiate the effects of gamma-aminobutyric acid (GABA) and other inhibitory neurotransmitters by binding to specific benzodiazepine receptors in the limbic and cortical areas of the CNS. GABA inhibits excitatory stimulation, which helps control emotional behavior. The limbic system contains highly dense areas of benzodiazepine receptors, which may explain oxazepam's antianxiety effects.

Contraindications

Acute angle-closure glaucoma; concurrent use of itraconazole or ketoconazole; hypersensitivity to oxazepam, benzodiazepines, or their components; psychoses

Interactions
DRUGS
cimetidine, oral contraceptives: Impaired metabolism and elimination of oxazepam
clozapine: Increased risk of respiratory depression and arrest
CNS depressants: Increased risk of apnea and CNS depression
levodopa: Decreased therapeutic effects of levodopa
probenecid: Increased therapeutic effects of oxazepam and risk of oversedation
ACTIVITIES
alcohol use: Increased risk of apnea and CNS depression

Adverse Reactions
CNS: Anxiety (in daytime), ataxia, confusion, depression, dizziness, drowsiness, fatigue, headache, insomnia, nightmares, sleep disturbance, slurred speech, syncope, talkativeness, tremor, vertigo
GI: Nausea
Other: Drug tolerance, physical and psychological dependence, withdrawal signs and symptoms

Overdose
Monitor patient for evidence of overdose, including bradycardia, coma, confusion, dyspnea, hyporeflexia, seizures, severe drowsiness, shakiness, slurred speech, staggering, and weakness.

Maintain an open airway, initiate continuous ECG monitoring, and administer I.V. fluids, as prescribed, to maintain blood pressure and promote diuresis. Institute seizure precautions according to facility protocol.

To decrease drug absorption in a conscious patient who isn't at risk for coma or seizures, be prepared to induce vomiting or perform gastric lavage. Expect that oral activated charcoal may also be prescribed. For an unconscious patient, anticipate assisting with the insertion of an endotracheal tube and then performing gastric lavage. The inflated cuff of the endotracheal tube will help prevent aspiration of gastric contents into the lungs.

Anticipate the use of a benzodiazepine receptor antagonist such as flumazenil to reverse oxazepam's sedative effects. Be aware that flumazenil may induce seizures, especially in a patient who has been on long-term benzodiazepine therapy or who has also ingested a cyclic antidepressant. If excitation occurs, a barbiturate shouldn't be used because it may increase excitement and prolong CNS depression. Dialysis is ineffective for treating benzodiazepine overdose.

Institute suicide precautions according to facility policy, and anticipate psychiatric re-evaluation.

Nursing Considerations

- **WARNING** Be aware that oxazepam may cause physical and psychological dependence.
- Be aware that drug shouldn't be stopped abruptly after prolonged use; doing so may cause seizures or withdrawal signs and symptoms, such as insomnia, irritability, and nervousness.
- Be aware that withdrawal signs and symptoms can occur when therapy is discontinued after only 1 to 2 weeks.
- **WARNING** If patient has a pulmonary disease (such as severe COPD), respiratory depression, or sleep apnea, monitor his respiratory status because drug may worsen ventilatory failure.
- Expect an increased risk of falls among elderly patients from impaired cognition and motor function. Take safety precautions according to facility policy.
- Be aware that drug may worsen acute intermittent porphyria, myasthenia gravis, and severe renal impairment, possibly resulting in nephrotoxicity.
- Expect patient with late-stage Parkinson's disease to experience decreased cognition or coordination and, possibly, increased psychosis when given oxazepam.

PATIENT TEACHING
- Instruct patient to take oxazepam exactly as prescribed and not to stop taking it without consulting prescriber.
- Caution patient about possible drowsiness and reduced coordination, and advise him to avoid potentially hazardous activities until he knows how the drug affects him.
- Urge patient to avoid alcohol, which increases sedative effects.
- Instruct patient to notify prescriber about excessive drowsiness or nausea.

oxcarbazepine

Trileptal

Class and Category

Chemical class: Tricyclic iminostilbene derivative
Therapeutic class: Anticonvulsant
Pregnancy category: C

Indications and Dosages

▶ *As adjunct to treat partial seizures*
ORAL SUSPENSION, TABLETS
Adults and adolescents over age 16. *Initial:* 300 mg b.i.d. Dosage increased by 600 mg daily every wk. *Usual:* 1,200 mg daily. *Maximum:* 2,400 mg daily.
Children ages 2 to 16. *Initial:* 4 to 5 mg/kg b.i.d. up to maximum initial dose of 600 mg daily. *Usual:* For children who weigh 20 to 29 kg (44 to 64 lb), 900 mg daily; 29.1 to 39 kg (64 to 86 lb), 1,200 mg daily; more than 39 kg (86 lb), 1,800 mg daily. *Maximum:* 1,800 mg daily.
Children ages 2 to 4 weighing less than 20 lb. *Initial:* 8 to 10 mg/kg b.i.d. up to maximum initial dose of 60 mg/kg daily.
DOSAGE ADJUSTMENT For patients with creatinine clearance of less than 30 ml/min/1.73 m², usual initial dosage reduced by 50%.
▶ *As monotherapy to treat partial seizures*
ORAL SUSPENSION, TABLETS
Adults and adolescents over age 16. *Initial:* 300 mg b.i.d. Dosage increased by 300 mg daily every 3 days as needed. *Usual:* 1,200 mg daily. *Maximum:* 2,400 mg daily.
Children ages 4 to 16. *Initial:* 4 to 5 mg/kg b.i.d., increased by 5 mg/kg daily every third day to maximum maintenance dosage, as needed. *Maximum:* For children weighing 20 to 24.9 kg (44 to 55 lb), 900 mg daily; for those weighing 25 to 34.9 kg (55 to 77 lb), 1,200 mg daily; for those weighing 35 to 49.9 kg (77 to 110 lb), 1,500 mg daily; for those weighing 50 to 59.9 kg (110 to 132 lb), 1,800 mg daily; for those weighing 60 to 70 kg (132 to 154 lb), 2,100 mg daily.
▶ *To convert to monotherapy in treating partial seizures*
ORAL SUSPENSION, TABLETS
Adults and adolescents over age 16. *Initial:* 300 mg b.i.d. Dosage increased by 600 mg daily every wk over 2 to 4 wk, as needed, while dosage of other anticonvulsant is reduced. *Usual:* 1,200 mg daily. *Maximum:* 2,400 mg daily.
Children ages 4 to 16. *Initial:* 4 to 5 mg/kg b.i.d., increased by 10 mg/kg daily weekly as needed to maximum maintenance dosage while dosage of other anticonvulsant is reduced over 3 to 6 wk. Maximum: For children who weigh 20 to 24.9 kg (44 to 55 lb), 900 mg daily; for 25 to 34.9 kg (55 to 77 lb), 1,200 mg daily; for 35 to 49.9 kg (77 to 110 lb), 1,500 mg daily; for 50 to

59.9 kg (110 to 132 lb), 1,800 mg daily; for 60 to 70 kg (132 to 154 lb), 2,100 mg daily.

Route	Onset	Steady State	Peak	Half-Life	Duration
P.O.	Unknown	Unknown	Unknown	2 hr*	Unknown

Mechanism of Action
May prevent or halt seizures by closing or blocking sodium channels in the neuronal cell membrane. By preventing sodium from entering the cell, oxcarbazepine may slow nerve impulse transmission, thus decreasing the rate at which neurons fire.

Contraindications
Hypersensitivity to carbamazepine, oxcarbazepine, or their components

Interactions
DRUGS
carbamazepine, phenobarbital, phenytoin, valproic acid: Decreased blood oxcarbazepine level, possibly increased blood levels of phenobarbital and phenytoin
felodipine, verapamil: Decreased blood levels of these drugs
oral contraceptives: Decreased effectiveness of oral contraceptives
ACTIVITIES
alcohol use: Possibly additive CNS depressant effects

Adverse Reactions
CNS: Abnormal gait, ataxia, difficulty concentrating, dizziness, fatigue, fever, headache, psychomotor slowing, speech impairment, somnolence, tremor
EENT: Abnormal vision, diplopia, nystagmus, rhinitis
GI: Abdominal pain, indigestion, nausea, vomiting
SKIN: Rash, Stevens-Johnson syndrome, toxic epidermal necrolysis
Other: Anaphylaxis, angioedema, hyponatremia

Overdose
Oxcarbazepine overdose has no specific antidote, and limited information is available about such overdose. Maintain open airway, and expect to provide symptomatic and supportive care, as

---

* 9 hr for the active metabolite 10-monohydroxy (MHD). Half-life is 19 hr for patients with severe renal impairment.

needed. To decrease drug absorption, expect to perform gastric lavage, followed by the administration of activated charcoal, as prescribed.

Institute suicide precautions according to facility policy, and anticipate psychiatric re-evaluation.

Nursing Considerations

- Before beginning oxcarbazepine therapy, ask patient if he has ever had an allergic reaction to carbamazepine; such a reaction would increase his risk of developing hypersensitivity to oxcarbazepine.
- Monitor serum sodium level for signs of hyponatremia, especially during first 3 months of therapy. Assess patient for signs and symptoms of hyponatremia, including confusion, headache, lethargy, and nausea.
- Be prepared to monitor therapeutic drug levels of oxcarbazepine during initiation and adjustment of drug therapy, and expect to adjust dosage accordingly.
- Implement seizure precautions, as appropriate, according to facility policy.
- Monitor patient closely for skin reactions. If such a reaction develops, notify prescriber immediately because serious skin reactions may be life threatening with oxcarbazepine.
- **WARNING** Monitor patient closely for evidence of multiorgan hypersensitivity, such as fever and rash, associated with organ dysfunction. Other signs and symptoms may include lymphadenopathy, hepatitis, liver function abnormalities, hematological abnormalities, pruritus, nephritis, oliguria, hepato-renal syndrome, arthralgia and asthenia. If suspected, notify prescriber and expect drug to be discontinued. Provide supportive care, as prescribed.

PATIENT TEACHING
- Instruct patient or caregiver about using the medicine dispensing system that's supplied by the manufacturer to prepare the oxcarbazepine dose. Tell him to shake the oral suspension bottle well and dilute the drug with a small amount of water or swallow it from the syringe and to rinse the syringe with warm water and allow it to dry after taking drug.
- Alert patient to possibility of hypersensitivity or serious skin reactions developing and to notify prescriber, if present.
- Warn patient to notify prescriber immediately if he develops a fever and rash with other symptoms because drug may need to be discontinued and emergency medical care may be required.

- Inform patient that he may experience dizziness, double vision, and unsteady gait while taking drug.
- Advise patient to avoid driving and other activities that require a high level of alertness until he knows how the drug affects him.
- Instruct patient not to drink alcohol while taking oxcarbazepine.
- Inform female patient who uses oral contraceptives that oxcarbazepine decreases their effectiveness; suggest that she use another form of contraception during therapy.
- Advise patient to keep scheduled appointments with prescriber so that his progress can be monitored.

paliperidone
Invega

Class and Category
Chemical class: Benzisoxazole derivative
Therapeutic class: Antipsychotic (atypical)
Pregnancy category: C

Indications and Dosages
▶ *To treat schizophrenia*
E.R. TABLETS
Adults. *Initial:* 6 mg once daily in the morning; then increased or decreased by 3 mg daily every 6 or more days, as needed. *Maximum:* 12 mg daily.
DOSAGE ADJUSTMENT For patients with mild renal impairment (creatinine clearance of 50 to 79 ml/min/1.73 m^2), maximum dosage is 6 mg daily. For patients with moderate to severe renal impairment (creatinine clearance less than 50 ml/min/1.73 m^2), maximum dosage is 3 mg daily.

Route	Onset	Peak	Duration
P.O.	Unknown	24 hr	Unknown

Mechanism of Action
Suppresses psychotic symptoms by selectively blocking serotonin and dopamine receptors in the mesocortical tract of the CNS. Paliperidone is the main active metabolite of risperidone.

Contraindications
AV block, cardiac arrhythmias, congenital heart disease, history of congenital long-QT syndrome; hypersensitivity to paliperidone, risperidone, or its components

Interactions
DRUGS
antiarrhythmics of class IA (such as quinidine, procainamide) and class

III (such as amiodarone, sotalol), antibiotics (such as gatifloxacin, moxi-floxacin), antipsychotics (such as chlorpromazine, thioridazine): Increased risk of QT-interval prolongation

antihypertensives: Increased antihypertensive effects

bromocriptine, levodopa, pergolide: Possibly antagonized effects of these drugs

CNS depressants: Additive CNS depression

Adverse Reactions

CNS: Agitation, akathisia, anxiety, asthenia, dizziness, dyskinesia, dystonia, extrapyramidal disorder, fatigue, fever, headache, hyperkinesia, hypertonia, parkinsonism, somnolence, syncope, tardive dyskinesia, tremor

CV: Bundle branch block, first-degree heart block, hypertension, orthostatic hypotension, palpitations, prolonged QT interval, tachycardia, venous thrombosis

EENT: Blurred vision, dry mouth, salivary hypersecretion, swollen tongue

ENDO: Hyperglycemia

GI: Dyspepsia, nausea, upper abdominal pain

HEME: Thrombocytopenia

MS: Back or limb pain

RESP: Cough, dyspnea

Other: Anaphylaxis, weight gain

Overdose

Watch for evidence of overdose, including drowsiness, ECG changes (such as prolonged QT interval), electrolyte imbalances, extrapyramidal reactions, hypotension, seizures, and tachycardia.

Maintain an open airway, give oxygen as needed, monitor vital signs, and implement continuous ECG monitoring and seizure precautions. Obtain blood to monitor electrolyte levels. For a conscious patient, be prepared to perform gastric lavage to decrease drug absorption. Expect that oral activated charcoal, followed by a laxative, may also be prescribed. For an unconscious patient, anticipate assisting with insertion of an endotracheal tube and then performing gastric lavage. The endotracheal tube's inflated cuff will help prevent aspiration of gastric contents. Vomiting shouldn't be induced because of the risk of sedation, seizures, and dystonic reactions of the head and neck.

Be prepared to treat arrhythmias, as needed and prescribed; however, be aware that drugs that prolong the QT interval—such as disopyramide, procainamide, and quinidine—shouldn't be used. If bretylium is prescribed, use it with caution because it may worsen the hypotensive effects of paliperidone. Expect to treat hypotension with I.V. fluids and a sympathomimetic; keep in mind that epinephrine and dopamine may worsen hypotension. To treat severe extrapyramidal reactions, expect to use an antidyskinetic, as prescribed.

Institute suicide precautions according to facility policy, and anticipate psychiatric re-evaluation.

Nursing Considerations

- Be aware that paliperidone shouldn't be given to any patient with a condition that severely narrows the GI tract because tablet doesn't change shape as it passes and could cause a blockage.
- **WARNING** Immediately notify prescriber and expect to stop drug if patient shows signs of neuroleptic malignant syndrome (such as altered mental status, autonomic instability, hyperpyrexia, muscle rigidity), which can be fatal.
- Monitor patient for involuntary, dyskinetic movements. Notify prescriber if present, and expect to stop therapy. In some cases, therapy may need to continue despite tardive dyskinesia.
- Monitor blood glucose level, as ordered, because drug increases the risk of hyperglycemia and possible ketoacidosis or hyperosmolar coma.

PATIENT TEACHING

- Instruct patient to take the tablet whole with liquid. Caution against chewing, splitting, or crushing the tablet because it's designed to release drug at a controlled rate.
- Explain that shell of tablet will pass in stool and that patient need not worry if he sees the tablet in his stool.
- Urge patient to rise from a sitting or lying position slowly to minimize effects of orthostatic hypotension.
- Caution patient to avoid hazardous activities until CNS effects of drug are known.
- Advise patient to avoid activities that may cause overheating, such as exercising strenuously, being exposed to extreme heat, or becoming dehydrated.

paraldehyde
Paral

Class, Category, and Schedule
Chemical class: Acetaldehyde polymer
Therapeutic class: Anticonvulsant

Pregnancy category: C
Controlled substance schedule: IV

Indications and Dosages

▶ *To manage seizures unresponsive to other drugs*

ORAL LIQUID, RECTAL LIQUID

Adults. Up to 12 ml oral liquid diluted to a 10% solution, every 4 hr, as needed. Or, 10 to 20 ml rectal liquid, diluted.

Children. 0.3 ml/kg P.O. or P.R. Or, 12 ml/m² of body surface.

Route	Onset	Steady State	Peak	Half-Life	Duration
P.O.	15 min	Unknown	Unknown	3 to 10 hr	8 to 12 hr

Mechanism of Action

Acts as a depressant at many levels of the CNS, including the ascending reticular activating system, producing an imbalance between facilitatory and inhibitory mechanisms.

Incompatibilities

Don't use plastic containers, syringes, tubing, or utensils when administering paraldehyde.

Contraindications

Bronchopulmonary disease, gastroenteritis (P.O.), hepatic dysfunction, hypersensitivity to paraldehyde or its components

Interactions

DRUGS

CNS depressants: Increased CNS depressant effects

disulfiram: Inhibition of acetaldehyde dehydrogenase and decreased metabolism of paraldehyde, which may increase blood levels of paraldehyde and acetaldehyde

ACTIVITIES

alcohol use: Increased CNS depressant effects

Adverse Reactions

CNS: Clumsiness, dizziness, drowsiness, hangover
EENT: Unpleasant breath odor
GI: Abdominal pain, hepatitis, nausea, vomiting
SKIN: Jaundice, rash

Overdose

Monitor patient for signs and symptoms of overdose, including abdominal cramps, bradycardia, cloudy urine, confusion, decreased urine output, dyspnea, hypotension, irritability, nausea, nervousness, respiratory depression, restlessness, tachypnea, tremor, vomiting, and weakness.

Maintain an open airway, and be prepared to treat hypotension. Assess patient for metabolic acidosis, and anticipate administering sodium bicarbonate or sodium lactate, as prescribed. Dialysis may be used to treat acidosis and support renal function.

To decrease absorption of oral liquid, perform gastric lavage, taking precautions to prevent aspiration. Expect to also administer mineral oil to relieve gastric irritation. To decrease drug absorption of rectal liquid, perform rectal lavage, as prescribed.

Institute suicide precautions according to facility policy, and anticipate psychiatric re-evaluation.

Nursing Considerations

- Dilute oral form of paraldehyde in milk or iced fruit juice to mask the odor and taste and to lessen gastric irritation.
- When administering drug P.R., dilute it with 1 or 2 parts olive oil, cottonseed oil, or normal saline solution to lessen irritation to mucous membranes.
- If patient is unable to take drug by mouth, administer it by nasogastric tube, as ordered.
- Be aware that paraldehyde is incompatible with many plastics.
- Don't give drug if it has a brownish color or smells like acetic acid (vinegarlike smell). Discard any unused portion, and don't give it if the container has been open for more than 24 hours.
- Expect to withdraw drug slowly because prolonged use may result in tolerance and psychological or physical dependence. Assess patient for signs and symptoms of withdrawal, such as delirium tremens and hallucinations.

PATIENT TEACHING

- Instruct patient to dilute P.O. form of paraldehyde in milk or iced fruit juice to mask the smell and taste and to lessen gastric irritation.
- Advise patient not to use plastic containers or utensils to administer drug.
- Instruct patient not to take drug if it has a brownish color or a strong vinegar-like odor.
- Advise patient not to change her dosage or stop taking paraldehyde without consulting her prescriber because withdrawal signs and symptoms may occur.
- Caution patient to avoid getting drug in her eyes or on her clothing or skin.

- Instruct patient to avoid alcohol and other sedatives because they may cause additive CNS depressant effects.
- Urge patient to avoid potentially hazardous activities until she knows how the drug affects her.
- Inform patient that her breath will have a strong, unpleasant odor and that this is a normal adverse effect of the drug.

paroxetine hydrochloride
Paxil, Paxil CR

paroxetine mesylate
Pexeva

Class and Category
Chemical class: Phenylpiperidine derivative
Therapeutic class: Antianxiety drug, antidepressant, antiobsessional drug, antipanic drug
Pregnancy category: D

Indications and Dosages
▶ *To treat major depression*
C.R. TABLETS
Adults. *Initial:* 25 mg daily, increased as prescribed and tolerated by 12.5 mg daily every wk. *Maximum:* 62.5 mg daily.
ORAL SUSPENSION, TABLETS
Adults. *Initial:* 20 mg daily, increased as prescribed and tolerated by 10 mg daily every wk. *Maximum:* 50 mg daily.
▶ *To treat obsessive-compulsive disorder*
ORAL SUSPENSION, TABLETS
Adults. *Initial:* 20 mg daily, increased as prescribed and tolerated by 10 mg daily every wk. *Usual:* 20 to 60 mg daily. *Maximum:* 60 mg daily.
▶ *To treat panic disorder*
C.R. TABLETS
Adults. *Initial:* 12.5 mg daily, increased as needed by 12.5 mg daily every wk. *Maximum:* 75 mg daily.
ORAL SUSPENSION, TABLETS
Adults. *Initial:* 10 mg daily, increased as prescribed and tolerated by 10 mg daily every wk. *Usual:* 10 to 60 mg daily *Maximum:* 60 mg daily.
▶ *To treat social anxiety disorder*
C.R. TABLETS
Adults. *Initial:* 12.5 mg daily, increased as needed by 12.5 mg daily every wk. *Maximum:* 37.5 mg daily.

▶ *To treat social anxiety disorder*
ORAL SUSPENSION, TABLETS (HYDROCHLORIDE)
Adults. *Initial:* 20 mg daily, increased as prescribed and tolerated by 10 mg daily every wk. *Usual:* 20 to 60 mg daily *Maximum:* 60 mg daily.
▶ *To treat generalized anxiety disorder*
ORAL SUSPENSION, TABLETS (HYDROCHLORIDE)
Adults. *Initial:* 20 mg daily, increased as prescribed and tolerated by 10 mg daily every wk. *Usual:* 20 to 50 mg daily *Maximum:* 60 mg daily.
▶ *To treat posttraumatic stress disorder*
ORAL SUSPENSION, TABLETS (HYDROCHLORIDE)
Adults. *Initial:* 20 mg daily, increased as prescribed and tolerated by 10 mg daily every wk. *Usual:* 20 to 50 mg daily. *Maximum:* 50 mg daily.
▶ *To treat premenstrual dysphoric disorder*
C.R. TABLETS
Adults. *Initial:* 12.5 mg daily in the morning, increased as needed after 1 wk to 25 mg daily. Or, 12.5 mg daily in the morning only during luteal phase of menstrual cycle (2-wk period before onset of monthly cycle), increased as needed after 1 wk to 25 mg daily in the morning during the luteal phase.
DOSAGE ADJUSTMENT For patients who are elderly, debilitated, or have creatinine clearance of less than 30 ml/min/ 1.73 m², initially 10 mg daily with maximum of 40 mg daily. Avoid C.R. form. For patients taking C.R. tablets who have creatinine clearance of less than 30 ml/min/1.73 m², initially 12.5 mg daily with maximum of 50 mg daily.

Route	Onset	Steady State	Peak	Half-Life	Duration
P.O.	1 to 4 wk	7 to 14 days	Unknown	3 to 65 hr	Unknown

Mechanism of Action
Potentiates serotonin activity in the CNS and inhibits serotonin reuptake at the presynaptic neuronal membrane. Reduced serotonin uptake causes increased levels and prolonged activity of serotonin at synaptic receptor sites and yields antianxiety, antidepressant, antiobsessional, and antipanic effects.

Contraindications
Hypersensitivity to paroxetine or its components, pimozide or thioridazine therapy, use within 14 days of an MAO inhibitor

Interactions
DRUGS

antacids: Hastened release of paroxetine C.R. form

aspirin, NSAIDs, warfarin: Increased anticoagulant activity and risk of bleeding

atomoxetine, risperidone, other drugs metabolized by CYP2D6: Increased plasma levels of these drugs

barbiturates, primidone: Decreased blood paroxetine level

cimetidine: Possibly increased blood paroxetine level

cisapride, isoniazid, MAO inhibitors, procarbazine: Possibly serotonin syndrome

codeine, haloperidol, metoprolol, perphenazine, propranolol, risperidone, thioridazine: Decreased metabolism and increased effects of these drugs

cyproheptadine: Decreased effects of paroxetine

dextromethorphan: Decreased dextromethorphan metabolism and increased risk of toxicity

digoxin: Possibly decreased digoxin effects

encainide, flecainide, propafenone, quinidine: Potentiated toxicity of these drugs

fosamprenavir, ritonavir: Decreased blood levels of paroxetine

linezolid, lithium, serotonin reuptake inhibitors, tramadol, triptans, tryptophan, St. John's wort: Increased risk of serotonin syndrome

lithium: Possibly increased blood paroxetine level

methadone: Decreased methadone metabolism, increased risk of adverse effects

phenytoin: Possibly phenytoin toxicity

pimozide: Increased blood pimozide level and risk of prolonged QT interval

procyclidine: Increased blood procyclidine level and anticholinergic effects

theophylline: Possibly increased blood theophylline level and risk of toxicity

thioridazine: Increased risk of prolonged QT interval

tramadol: Increased risk of seizures

tricyclic antidepressants: Increased metabolism and blood antidepressant levels; increased risk of toxicity, including seizures

Adverse Reactions
CNS: Agitation, akathesia, asthenia, confusion, dizziness, drowsiness, emotional lability, hallucinations, headache, impaired concentration, insomnia, mania, restlessness, serotonin syndrome, somnolence, suicidal ideation, tremor

CV: Palpitations, tachycardia
EENT: Blurred vision, dry mouth, rhinitis, taste perversion
GI: Abdominal cramps or pain, constipation, decreased appetite, diarrhea, flatulence, nausea, vomiting
GU: Decreased libido, difficult ejaculation, impotence, sexual dysfunction, urine retention
MS: Back pain, myalgia, myasthenia, myopathy
SKIN: Diaphoresis, rash
Other: Weight gain or loss

Overdose

Monitor patient for evidence of overdose, including dizziness, drowsiness, dry mouth, facial flushing, irritability, mydriasis, nausea, tachycardia, and tremor. Maintain an open airway, obtain baseline ECG, and institute continuous ECG monitoring.

To decrease drug absorption, be prepared to perform gastric lavage. Give activated charcoal, 20 to 30 g, every 4 to 6 hours for the first 2 days, as prescribed. If the patient also ingested a tricyclic antidepressant, paroxetine may inhibit its metabolism and cause toxic levels. Because paroxetine is widely distributed in the body, exchange transfusions, forced diuresis, hemodialysis, and hemoperfusion are ineffective for treating overdose.

Institute suicide precautions according to facility policy, and anticipate psychiatric re-evaluation.

Nursing Considerations

• Shake paroxetine oral suspension well before using. Measure with an oral syringe or calibrated measuring device.
• Make sure that patient swallows C.R. tablets whole. Don't let her cut, crush, or chew them.
• Monitor patient closely for GI bleeding, especially if she takes a drug known to cause it, such as aspirin, NSAIDs, or warfarin.
• To minimize adverse reactions, expect to taper dosage as ordered when drug is no longer needed.
• If patient experiences adverse GI reactions, give drug with food.
• Avoid giving enteric-coated tablets with antacids.
• **WARNING** Watch for evidence of worsening depression or suicidal ideation in patients taking paroxetine for depression, especially young adults and especially when therapy starts or dosage changes; depression may worsen during these times. Be aware that patients taking paroxetine for a condition other than depression may have an increased risk of suicidal thinking or behavior if they have a history of these problems.
• **WARNING** Monitor patient for evidence of life-threatening

serotonin syndrome, such as altered mental status (agitation, hallucinations, coma), autonomic instability (tachycardia, labile blood pressure, hyperthermia), neuromuscular aberrations (hyperreflexia, incoordination) and GI symptoms (nausea, vomiting, diarrhea). If present, notify prescriber immediately and expect to discontinue paroxetine and provide supportive care.

- Observe patient for sudden development of mania; all antidepressants can precipitate mania if patient is predisposed to it.
- Inquire about adverse reactions, particularly sexual dysfunction, and notify prescriber as needed.
- Be aware that paroxetine may precipitate serotonin syndrome, which may cause arrhythmias, coma, disseminated intravascular coagulation, renal and respiratory failure, seizures, and severe hypertension along with such milder signs and symptoms as abdominal cramps, aggressive behavior, agitation, chills, confusion, diarrhea, headache, insomnia, nausea, palpitations, paresthesia, poor coordination, restlessness, and worsening of obsessive thoughts or compulsive behaviors.

PATIENT TEACHING

- Advise patient to take paroxetine in the morning to minimize insomnia and with food if adverse GI reactions develop.
- Instruct patient to avoid taking C.R. paroxetine within 2 hours of an antacid.
- Instruct patient to swallow C.R. tablets whole. Don't let her cut, crush, or chew them.
- Suggest that patient avoid potentially hazardous activities until she knows how the drug affects her.
- Inform patient that drug may not achieve full effects for 4 weeks.
- Urge patient to avoid alcohol during paroxetine therapy because its effects on drug are unknown.
- Advise patient to notify prescriber immediately if she has trouble sleeping.
- Inform patient that episodes of acute depression may persist for months or longer and that they require continued follow-up.
- Instruct patient to avoid taking aspirin or NSAIDs while taking paroxetine because of an increased risk of bleeding if taken together. If patient takes warfarin, caution her to take bleeding precautions and to notifiy prescriber if bleeding occurs.
- If patient takes paroxetine for depression, urge caregivers or family to watch closely for increased depression or suicidal thinking, especially if the patient is a child or adolescent and especially when therapy starts or stops or when dosage changes.

- Instruct patient not to stop drug abruptly but to taper dosage as instructed to help prevent adverse reactions.
- Alert female patients of childbearing age that paroxetine may cause congenital malformations if taken during the first trimester of pregnancy. Stress the need to use effective contraceptive methods during paroxetine therapy and to notify prescriber immediately about possible, confirmed, or intended pregnancy.
- Tell patient to notify all health care professionals about paroxetine therapy because drug interactions could be serious.

pentobarbital sodium
Nembutal, Nova Rectal (CAN), Novopentobarb (CAN)

Class, Category, and Schedule
Chemical class: Barbiturate
Therapeutic class: Anticonvulsant, sedative-hypnotic
Pregnancy category: D
Controlled substance schedule: II (oral, parenteral), III (rectal)

Indications and Dosages
▶ *To provide daytime sedation*
ELIXIR
Adults. 20 mg t.i.d. or q.i.d.
Children. 2 to 6 mg/kg daily.
SUPPOSITORIES
Adults. 30 mg b.i.d. to q.i.d.
Children. 2 mg/kg t.i.d.
▶ *To provide short-term treatment of insomnia*
CAPSULES, ELIXIR
Adults. 100 mg at bedtime.
I.V. INJECTION
Adults. *Initial:* 100 mg, with additional small doses at 1-min intervals, as prescribed. *Maximum:* 500 mg.
I.M. INJECTION
Adults. 150 to 200 mg at bedtime.
SUPPOSITORIES
Adults and adolescents over age 14. 120 to 200 mg at bedtime.
Children ages 12 to 14. 60 to 120 mg at bedtime.
Children ages 5 to 12. 60 mg at bedtime.
Children ages 1 to 4. 30 to 60 mg at bedtime.
Infants ages 2 months to 1 year. 30 mg at bedtime.

▶ *To provide emergency treatment of seizures with eclampsia, meningitis, status epilepticus, tetanus, or toxic reaction to a local anesthetic or strychnine*

I.V. INJECTION

Adults. 100 mg, with additional small doses at 1-min intervals, as prescribed. *Maximum:* 500 mg.

Children. 50 mg, with additional small doses at 1-min intervals, as prescribed, until desired effect occurs.

I.M. INJECTION

Children. 50 mg, with additional small doses at 1-min intervals, as prescribed, until desired effect occurs.

DOSAGE ADJUSTMENT Dosage possibly reduced for elderly or debilitated patients and those with hepatic dysfunction.

Route	Onset	Steady State	Peak	Half-Life	Duration
P.O., P.R.	15 to 60 min	Unknown	1 to 4 hr	15 to 50 hr	3 to 4 hr
I.V.	1 min	Unknown	Unknown	15 to 50 hr	15 min
I.M.	10 to 25 min	Unknown	Unknown	15 to 50 hr	3 to 4 hr

Mechanism of Action

Inhibits ascending conduction in the reticular formation, which controls CNS arousal to produce drowsiness, hypnosis, and sedation. Pentobarbital also decreases the spread of seizure activity in the cortex, thalamus, and limbic system. It promotes an increased threshold for electrical stimulation in the motor cortex, which may contribute to its anticonvulsant properties.

Contraindications

Hepatic disease; history of addiction to hypnotics or sedatives; hypersensitivity to pentobarbital, barbiturates, or their components; nephritis; porphyria; severe respiratory disease with airway obstruction or dyspnea

Interactions

DRUGS

acetaminophen: Possibly decreased effects of acetaminophen (with long-term pentobarbital use)

carbamazepine, chloramphenicol, corticosteroids, cyclosporine, dacarbazine, disopyramide, doxycycline, griseofulvin, metronidazole, oral contraceptives, phenylbutazone, quinidine, theophyllines, vitamin D: Decreased effectiveness of these drugs

CNS depressants: Increased CNS depression and risk of habituation *divalproex sodium, valproic acid:* Increased risk of CNS toxicity and neurotoxicity

guanadrel, guanethidine: Possibly increased risk of orthostatic hypotension

halogenated hydrocarbon anesthetic: Increased risk of hepatotoxicity (with long-term pentobarbital use)

haloperidol: Possibly decreased blood haloperidol level, possibly altered seizure pattern or frequency

hydantoins: Possibly interference with hydantoin metabolism

leucovorin: Possibly decreased anticonvulsant effect of pentobarbital

maprotiline: Possibly enhanced CNS depression and decreased therapeutic effects of pentobarbital

mexiletine: Possibly decreased blood mexiletine level

oral anticoagulants: Possibly decreased therapeutic effects of these drugs, possibly increased risk of bleeding when pentobarbital is discontinued

tricyclic antidepressants: Possibly decreased therapeutic effects of these drugs

ACTIVITIES

alcohol use: Increased CNS depression

Adverse Reactions

CNS: Agitation, anxiety, ataxia, confusion, delusions, depression, dizziness, drowsiness, fever, hallucinations, headache, insomnia, irritability, nervousness, nightmares, paradoxical stimulation, seizures, syncope, tremor
CV: Orthostatic hypotension
EENT: Vision changes
GI: Anorexia, constipation, hepatic dysfunction, nausea, vomiting
HEME: Agranulocytosis
MS: Arthralgia, bone pain, muscle twitching or weakness
RESP: Respiratory depression
SKIN: Exfoliative dermatitis, rash, Stevens-Johnson syndrome
Other: Physical and psychological dependence, weight loss

Overdose

Monitor patient for evidence of overdose, including bradycardia, Cheyne-Stokes respiration, coma, confusion, decreased or absent reflexes, dyspnea, fever, hypothermia, miosis or mydriasis, oliguria, severe drowsiness, severe weakness, shock, slurred speech, staggering, tachycardia, and unusual eye movements. Consider chronic overdose if patient has continued irritability, insomnia, poor judgment, and severe confusion. Maintain an open airway, and carefully monitor blood pressure and temperature.

If the patient is conscious, be prepared to give ipecac syrup, as prescribed, to induce vomiting. Expect to give activated charcoal, 30 to 60 g, with water or sorbitol to prevent further absorption and to enhance drug elimination. For an unconscious patient, anticipate assisting with insertion of an endotracheal tube and then performing gastric lavage. The endotracheal tube's inflated cuff will help prevent aspiration of gastric contents into the lungs.

Be prepared to give a urine-alkalizing drug to increase elimination of pentobarbital. Administer I.V. fluids and a vasopressor, as prescribed. For severe cases, anticipate the need for hemodialysis or hemoperfusion. Be aware that, in cases of extreme barbiturate overdose, the patient may have a flat EEG because all electrical activity in the brain has ceased; however, this effect may be reversible.

Institute suicide precautions according to facility policy, and anticipate psychiatric re-evaluation.

Nursing Considerations

- Use pentobarbital with extreme caution in patients with depression, a history of drug abuse, or suicidal tendencies.
- Use drug cautiously in elderly or debilitated patients and those with acute or chronic pain because it may induce paradoxical stimulation.
- When using I.V. route, inject drug at 50 mg/minute or less to avoid adverse respiratory and circulatory reactions.
- If patient shows premonitory signs of hepatic coma, withhold drug and notify prescriber immediately.
- Monitor I.V. site closely, and take care to avoid extravasation. Drug is highly alkaline and may cause local tissue damage and necrosis.

PATIENT TEACHING

- Inform patient that pentobarbital is habit-forming, and stress the importance of taking it exactly as prescribed.
- Instruct patient who takes elixir form to use a calibrated measuring device and to close container tightly after use.
- Instruct patient who uses suppositories to refrigerate them.
- Advise patient to avoid potentially hazardous activities until she knows how the drug affects her.
- Urge patient to avoid alcohol and other CNS depressants because they may increase drug's adverse CNS effects.

Other Therapeutic Uses

Pentobarbital sodium is also indicated for the following:
- To provide preoperative sedation

perphenazine

Apo-Perphenazine (CAN), PMS Perphenazine (CAN), Trilafon, Trilafon Concentrate

Class and Category

Chemical class: Piperazine phenothiazine
Therapeutic class: Antipyschotic drug
Pregnancy category: Not rated

Indications and Dosages

▶ *To treat psychotic disorders*
ORAL SOLUTION
Hospitalized adults and adolescents. 8 to 16 mg b.i.d. to q.i.d., adjusted as prescribed and tolerated. *Maximum:* 64 mg daily.
TABLETS
Adults and adolescents. 4 to 16 mg b.i.d. to q.i.d., adjusted as prescribed and tolerated. *Maximum:* 24 mg daily for outpatients; 64 mg daily for hospitalized patients.
I.M. INJECTION
Adults and adolescents. 5 to 10 mg every 6 hr, adjusted as prescribed and tolerated. *Maximum:* 15 mg daily for outpatients; 30 mg daily for hospitalized patients.
DOSAGE ADJUSTMENT Initial dose possibly reduced and gradually increased for elderly, emaciated, or debilitated patients. Lower end of adult dosage range possibly needed for adolescents.

Route	Onset	Steady State	Peak	Half-Life	Duration
P.O.	Several wk	4 to 7 days	6 wk to 6 mo	Unknown	Unknown
I.M.	Unknown	Unknown	1 to 2 hr	Unknown	6 hr

Incompatibilities

Don't mix perphenazine oral solution with beverages that contain caffeine or tannins (such as coffee, colas, and teas) or pectinates (such as apple juice) because they're physically incompatible.

Contraindications

Blood dyscrasias; bone marrow depression; cerebral arteriosclerosis; coma; concurrent use of a CNS depressant (large doses); coronary artery disease; hepatic impairment; hypersensitivity to perphenazine, other phenothiazines, or their components; myeloproliferative disorders; prolonged QT interval; severe CNS depression; severe hypertension or hypotension; subcortical brain damage

Mechanism of Action

Blocks specific postsynaptic dopamine receptors to reduce signs and symptoms of psychosis, which may result from increased dopamine neurotransmission in brain areas—such as cerebral cortex, hypothalamus, and limbic system—that control motor activity, behavior, and emotion. Normally, when dopamine is released from presynaptic dopaminergic neurons in these areas, it engages with postsynaptic dopamine receptors, as shown top right. Several types of dopamine receptors have been identified; however, inhibition of the dopamine$_2$ (D$_2$) receptor is associated with a relief of psychotic signs and symptoms.

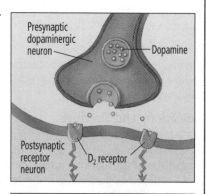

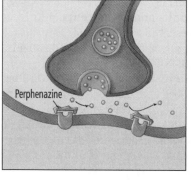

Like all phenothiazines, perphenazine primarily blocks postsynaptic D$_2$ receptors, an action that inhibits dopamine neurotransmission, as shown bottom right, and helps to control agitation, delusions, and hallucinations. The drug also has alpha-adrenergic blocking effects, which may be calming and sedating.

Interactions

DRUGS

antacids (aluminum- and magnesium-containing), antidiarrheals (adsorbent): Decreased absorption of oral perphenazine

amantadine, anticholinergics, antidyskinetics, antihistamines: Increased adverse anticholinergic effects

amphetamines: Decreased therapeutic effects of both drugs

anticonvulsants: Decreased seizure threshold, inhibited metabolism and toxicity of anticonvulsant

antithyroid drugs: Increased risk of agranulocytosis

apomorphine: Additive CNS depression, decreased emetic response to apomorphine if perphenazine is given first *appetite suppressants (except phenmetrazine):* Antagonized anorectic effect of appetite suppressants

beta blockers: Increased blood levels of both drugs and risk of arrhythmias, hypotension, irreversible retinopathy, and tardive dyskinesia

bromocriptine: Possibly interference with bromocriptine's effects

CNS depressants: Increased CNS and respiratory depression, increased hypotensive effects

dopamine: Antagonized peripheral vasoconstriction with high doses of dopamine

ephedrine: Decreased vasopressor response to ephedrine

epinephrine: Blocked alpha-adrenergic effects of epinephrine, possibly causing severe hypotension and tachycardia

hepatotoxic drugs: Increased risk of hepatotoxicity

hypotension-causing drugs: Increased risk of severe orthostatic hypotension

levodopa: Inhibited antidyskinetic effects of levodopa

lithium: Possibly neurotoxicity (disorientation, extrapyramidal signs and symptoms, unconsciousness)

maprotiline, tricyclic antidepressants: Prolonged and intensified sedative and anticholinergic effects of these drugs or perphenazine

metrizamide: Decreased seizure threshold

opioid analgesics: Increased CNS and respiratory depression, increased risk of orthostatic hypotension and severe constipation

ototoxic drugs, especially antibiotics: Possibly masking of some signs and symptoms of ototoxicity, such as dizziness, tinnitus, and vertigo

probucol, other drugs that prolong QT interval: Prolonged QT interval, which may increase risk of ventricular tachycardia

thiazide diuretics: Possibly hyponatremia and water intoxication

ACTIVITIES

alcohol use: Increased CNS and respiratory depression, hypotensive effects, and risk of heatstroke

Adverse Reactions

CNS: Behavioral changes, cerebral edema, dizziness, drowsiness, extrapyramidal reactions (such as akathisia, dystonia, pseudoparkinsonism), fever, headache, neuroleptic malignant syndrome, seizures, syncope, tardive dyskinesia (persistent)

CV: Bradycardia, cardiac arrest, hypertension, hypotension, orthostatic hypotension, prolonged QT interval, tachycardia, torsades de pointes

EENT: Blurred vision, dry mouth, glaucoma, laryngeal edema, miosis, mydriasis, nasal congestion, ocular changes (corneal opacification, retinopathy)

ENDO: Decreased libido, galactorrhea, gynecomastia, syndrome of inappropriate ADH secretion

GI: Anorexia, constipation, diarrhea, fecal impaction, nausea, vomiting

GU: Bladder paralysis, ejaculation failure, menstrual irregularities, polyuria, urinary frequency, urinary incontinence, urine retention

HEME: Agranulocytosis, eosinophilia, hemolytic anemia, leukopenia, pancytopenia, thrombocytopenic purpura

RESP: Asthma

SKIN: Diaphoresis, eczema, erythema, exfoliative dermatitis, hyperpigmentation, jaundice, pallor, photosensitivity, pruritus, urticaria

Other: Anaphylaxis, angioedema

Overdose

Watch for evidence of overdose, including agitation, areflexia or hyperreflexia, arrhythmias, blurred vision, cardiac arrest, coma, confusion, disorientation, drowsiness, dry mouth, dyspnea, heart failure, hyperpyrexia, hypotension, hypothermia, mydriasis, pulmonary edema, QRS complex changes, respiratory depression, seizures, shock, stupor, tachycardia, ventricular fibrillation, and vomiting.

Maintain an open airway, watch for arrhythmias, and maintain the patient's temperature. Institute seizure precautions according to facility protocol. Perform gastric lavage and give activated charcoal, as prescribed. Don't induce vomiting because of the potential for impaired consciousness or dystonic reactions of the head and neck.

To treat arrhythmias, don't give a drug that may prolong the QT interval—such as disopyramide, procainamide, or quinidine—because such drugs may have an additive effect with perphenazine. Expect to give phenytoin to control arrhythmias and norepinephrine or phenylephrine and I.V. fluids to treat hypotension, as prescribed. Epinephrine shouldn't be used because of risk of paradoxical hypotension. Anticipate digitalizing patient for heart failure, as prescribed. Expect to treat electrolyte imbalance and maintain acid-base balance, as prescribed. To manage seizures, expect to give diazepam followed by phenytoin. Avoid giving a barbiturate because it may potentiate CNS and respiratory depression.

Anticipate giving benztropine or diphenhydramine, as prescribed, to manage acute dyskinetic effects. Dialysis is ineffective. Expect to continue ECG monitoring for at least 5 days. Be aware that phenothiazine tablets are visible on X-ray.

Institute suicide precautions according to facility policy, and anticipate psychiatric re-evaluation.

Nursing Considerations
- Use perphenazine cautiously in patients with depression or hepatic, pulmonary, or renal dysfunction.
- Obtain blood samples for CBC and liver and renal function tests, as ordered, to detect adverse reactions.
- Monitor temperature frequently, and notify prescriber if it rises; a significant increase suggests drug intolerance.
- Monitor blood pressure of patient who takes large doses of perphenazine, especially if surgery is indicated, because of the increased risk of hypotension.

PATIENT TEACHING
- Instruct patient to take perphenazine exactly as prescribed to ensure optimal effectiveness and minimize possible adverse reactions.
- Remind patient who takes oral solution to use a calibrated measuring device.
- Instruct patient taking oral solution to dilute every 5 ml (teaspoon) of drug in 2 fluid oz of carbonated beverage, fruit juice (except apple), milk, soup, tomato juice, or water. Caution her not to mix drug in beverages that contain caffeine or tannins, such as coffee, cola, and tea.
- Caution patient not to spill oral solution on skin or clothing because it can cause contact dermatitis and damage clothing.
- Urge patient to avoid alcohol and other CNS depressants during perphenazine therapy and to avoid potentially hazardous activities until she knows how the drug affects her.
- Advise patient to avoid excessive sun exposure and to protect skin when outdoors.
- Stress the importance of notifying prescriber about persistent or severe adverse reactions.
- Urge patient to comply with long-term follow-up appointments to detect adverse reactions and determine if dosage should be adjusted.

Other Therapeutic Uses
Perphenazine is also indicated for the following:
- To treat severe nausea and vomiting

perphenazine and amitriptyline hydrochloride

Elavil Plus (CAN), Etrafon, Etrafon-A, Etrafon-D (CAN),
Etrafon-F (CAN), Etrafon-Forte, PMS Levazine (CAN), Triavil

Class and Category

Chemical class: Piperazine phenothiazine (perphenazine), dibenzo-
cycloheptadiene derivative (amitriptyline hydrochloride)
Therapeutic class: Antipsychotic-antidepressant
Pregnancy category: Not rated

Indications and Dosages

▶ *To treat anxiety associated with depression*
TABLETS
Adults and adolescents. 2 to 4 mg perphenazine and 10 to
50 mg amitriptyline t.i.d. or q.i.d., adjusted as needed and tolerated. *Maximum:* 32 mg perphenazine and 200 mg amitriptyline
daily.
DOSAGE ADJUSTMENT Expect to use a lower initial dose in
adolescents and debilitated and elderly patients.

Route	Onset	Steady State	Peak	Half-Life	Duration
P.O.	Several wk*;	4 to 7 days*;	6 wk to 6 mo*;	Unknown*;	Unknown*;
	14 to 21 days†	4 to 10 days†	Unknown†	1 to 46 hr†	Unknown†

Mechanism of Action

Both perphenazine and amitriptyline act on the CNS. Perphenazine, an antipsychotic drug, may block postsynaptic dopamine$_2$ (D$_2$) receptors in areas of
the brain that control activity and aggression—including the cerebral cortex,
hypothalamus, and limbic system—causing an improvement in psychotic conditions. Amitriptyline, a tricyclic antidepressant, blocks serotonin and norepinephrine reuptake by adrenergic nerves, which raises serotonin and norepinephrine levels at nerve synapses, elevating mood and reducing depression.

Contraindications

Acute recovery phase after an MI; bone marrow depression; concurrent use of a CNS depressant; hypersensitivity to amitriptyline,
phenothiazines, or their components; MAO inhibitor therapy
within 14 days

---

* For perphenazine.
† For amitriptyline.

Interactions

DRUGS

antacids (aluminum- and magnesium-containing), antidiarrheals (adsor-bent): Decreased absorption of perphenazine

analgesics, antihistamines, atropine, barbiturates, opioids: Increased CNS depressant effects

anticholinergics: Increased risk of hyperpyrexia

cimetidine, flecainide, fluoxetine, other antidepressants, paroxetine, pheno-thiazines, propafenone, quinidine, sertraline: Increased blood amitrip-tyline level

epinephrine: Blocked alpha-adrenergic effects of epinephrine, pos-sibly causing severe hypotension and tachycardia

ethchlorvynol: Possibly transient delirium

guanethidine, other antihypertensives: Decreased antihypertensive effects

ACTIVITIES

alcohol use: Enhanced CNS depression

Adverse Reactions

CNS: Anxiety, ataxia, behavioral changes, coma, delusions, dis-orientation, drowsiness, extrapyramidal reactions (such as aka-thisia, dystonia, pseudoparkinsonism), fatigue, fever, headache, hyperreflexia, insomnia, neuroleptic malignant syndrome, night-mares, peripheral neuropathy, psychoses, sedation, seizures, stroke, tardive dyskinesia, tremor

CV: Arrhythmias (bradycardia, heart block, prolonged AV conduc-tion, tachycardia), ECG changes, hypertension, hypotension, or-thostatic hypotension, MI, palpitations, peripheral edema

EENT: Abnormal taste, black tongue, blurred vision, dry mouth, increased salivation, laryngeal edema, nasal congestion, ocular changes (pigmentation of the cornea and lens), tinnitus

ENDO: Galactorrhea, gynecomastia, increased or decreased serum glucose level, syndrome of inappropriate ADH secretion

GI: Anorexia, biliary stasis, constipation, nausea, vomiting

GU: Libido changes, menstrual irregularities, testicular swelling, urinary frequency, urinary incontinence

HEME: Agranulocytosis, eosinophilia, leukopenia, pancytopenia, thrombocytopenic purpura

MS: Muscle weakness

RESP: Asthma

SKIN: Alopecia, eczema, erythema, exfoliative dermatitis, jaun-dice, photosensitivity, pruritus, urticaria

Other: Anaphylaxis, angioedema, weight gain or loss

Overdose

Monitor patient for evidence of overdose, including agitation, arrhythmias, drowsiness, heart failure, hyperpyrexia, hyperreflexia, hypertension, hypothermia, muscle rigidity, mydriasis, oculomotor disturbances, seizures, stupor, tachycardia, and vomiting.

Maintain an open airway, initiate continuous ECG monitoring, and closely observe the patient's blood pressure, respiratory rate, and temperature. Institute seizure precautions according to facility protocol. To decrease drug absorption, be prepared to induce vomiting or perform gastric lavage. Give activated charcoal, 20 to 30 g, every 4 to 6 hours for the first 24 to 48 hours, as ordered.

Expect to treat hypotension with norepinephrine but not epinephrine because the alpha-adrenergic effects of epinephrine may be blocked, resulting in hypotension and tachycardia. Be prepared to treat arrhythmias with neostigmine, propranolol, or pyridostigmine, as prescribed. Be aware that physostigmine, 1 to 3 mg, I.V., may also be prescribed to reverse signs and symptoms caused by amitriptyline, especially if arrhythmias, deep coma, or seizures occur. Expect that patient may need digitalization to treat heart failure. Plan to use continuous ECG monitoring for at least 5 days.

Expect to treat seizures with an inhalation anesthetic, diazepam, or paraldehyde but not a barbiturate because of the risk of increased CNS depression. Know that signs and symptoms of parkinsonism may be treated with benztropine or diphenhydramine, as prescribed. Amitriptyline is highly protein bound, so dialysis is ineffective for treating overdose.

Institute suicide precautions according to facility policy, and anticipate psychiatric re-evaluation.

Nursing Considerations

• Because of amitriptyline's atropine-like effects, use it cautiously in patients with a history of angle-closure glaucoma, seizures, or urine retention.

• If patient has a cardiovascular disorder, monitor her closely because amitriptyline may cause arrhythmias, such as prolonged conduction times and sinus tachycardia.

• Monitor patient's blood pressure, and assess her for hypertension or hypotension.

• Obtain blood samples for CBC and liver function tests, as ordered, to detect adverse effects.

• Monitor temperature frequently, and notify prescriber if it rises because a significant increase suggests drug intolerance. Expect that the drug may be discontinued if this occurs.

- Stay alert for behavior changes, such as decreased interest in personal appearance and obvious hallucinations. Be aware that schizophrenic patients may develop psychosis and paranoid patients may develop increased signs and symptoms.
- Avoid abrupt withdrawal of drug after prolonged therapy because headache, malaise, and nausea may occur.

PATIENT TEACHING

- Instruct patient to take perphenazine and amitriptyline exactly as prescribed to ensure optimal effectiveness and minimize adverse reactions.
- Advise patient to take drug after meals or with food to reduce GI discomfort.
- Explain to patient that it may take several weeks before she notices the full effect of the drug.
- Instruct patient to avoid using an antacid or antidiarrheal within 2 hours of taking the drug.
- Urge patient to avoid alcohol and other CNS depressants because they can enhance the CNS-depressant effects of perphenazine and amitriptyline.
- Caution the patient against driving or performing hazardous activities because perphenazine and amitriptyline can cause drowsiness and blurred vision.
- Advise the patient to avoid excessive heat because of the increased risk of heatstroke and to avoid excessive sun exposure because of possible photosensitivity.
- Caution patient to rise slowly from a lying or sitting position to minimize effects of orthostatic hypotension.
- Stress the importance of notifying prescriber about persistent or severe adverse reactions.
- Urge patient to comply with long-term follow-up to detect adverse reactions and determine possible need for dosage adjustments.

phendimetrazine tartrate

Adipost, Bontril PDM, Bontril Slow-Release, Melfiat, Obezine, Phendiet, Phendiet-105, Plegine, Prelu-2, PT 105

Class, Category, and Schedule

Chemical class: Phenylalkylamine
Therapeutic class: Appetite suppressant
Pregnancy category: Not rated
Controlled substance schedule: III

Indications and Dosages

▶ *As adjunct to treat exogenous obesity with behavior modification, caloric restriction, and exercise*

E.R. CAPSULES

Adults and adolescents age 16 and over. 105 mg daily 30 to 60 min before breakfast.

TABLETS

Adults and adolescents age 16 and over. 17.5 to 35 mg b.i.d. or t.i.d. 1 hr before meals. *Maximum:* 210 mg daily.

Route	Onset	Steady State	Peak	Half-Life	Duration
P.O.	Unknown	Unknown	Unknown	2 hr	Unknown
P.O. (E.R)	Unknown	Unknown	Unknown	10 hr	Unknown

Mechanism of Action

Stimulates the release of norepinephrine and dopamine from adrenergic nerve terminals in the lateral hypothalamic feeding center of the cerebral cortex and reticular activating system, which reduces appetite. By stimulating the CNS, phendimetrazine causes other effects, including reduced gastric acid production and increased metabolism, which may be effective in treating obesity.

Contraindications

Advanced arteriosclerosis; agitation; cerebral ischemia; glaucoma; history of alcohol or drug abuse; hypersensitivity to phendimetrazine, other sympathomimetic amines, or their components; hyperthyroidism; MAO inhibitor therapy within 14 days; moderate to severe hypertension; symptomatic cardiovascular disease

Interactions

DRUGS

antacids (calcium- and magnesium-containing), carbonic anhydrase inhibitors, citrates, sodium bicarbonate: Increased blood phendimetrazine level

amphetamines, other appetite suppressants, selective serotonin reuptake inhibitors: Possibly increased risk of cardiac valve dysfunction

anesthetics (inhaled): Increased risk of arrhythmias

antihypertensives (especially clonidine, guanadrel, guanethidine, methyldopa, rauwolfia alkaloids): Decreased hypotensive effect of these drugs

ascorbic acid: Increased excretion of phendimetrazine, causing decreased blood phendimetrazine level

CNS stimulants, thyroid hormones: Additive CNS stimulation
insulin, oral antidiabetic drugs: Altered blood glucose level
MAO inhibitors: Potentiated effects of phendimetrazine; possibly hypertensive crisis
phenothiazines: Reduced anorectic effect of phendimetrazine
tricyclic antidepressants: Possibly potentiated adverse cardiovascular effects
urinary acidifiers (including ammonium chloride and potassium or sodium phosphates): Decreased blood phendimetrazine level
vasopressors (especially catecholamines): Possibly potentiated vasopressor effect of these drugs
ACTIVITIES
alcohol use: Increased adverse CNS effects

Adverse Reactions

CNS: Cerebral ischemia, CNS stimulation, depression, dizziness, headache, insomnia, light-headedness, nervousness, mania, psychosis, syncope, tremor
CV: Chest pain, hypertension, palpitations, peripheral edema
EENT: Dry mouth
GI: Abdominal pain, constipation, nausea, vomiting
GU: Dysuria
RESP: Dyspnea
SKIN: Hives, rash
Other: Exercise intolerance

Overdose

Phendimetrazine overdose has no specific antidote. Monitor patient for signs and symptoms of overdose, including abdominal cramps, arrhythmias, coma, confusion, diarrhea, dyspnea, hallucinations, hostility, hyperreflexia, hyperthermia, labile blood pressure, nausea, panic reaction, restlessness, seizures, shock, tachypnea, tremor, and vomiting. Anticipate depression and fatigue to follow CNS excitement.

Maintain an open airway, monitor the patient's vital signs, and protect the patient from self-injury. Institute seizure precautions according to facility protocol. To decrease phendimetrazine absorption, perform gastric lavage or induce vomiting. Administer activated charcoal, as prescribed. Expect to administer a drug to promote urine acidification and I.V. fluids, as prescribed, to increase drug excretion.

Be prepared to administer a drug such as a barbiturate, diazepam, or phenytoin to control CNS stimulation and seizures. Anticipate administering drugs such as lidocaine to control arrhythmias, phentolamine or a nitrate to manage hypertension, and a beta blocker to control tachycardia. Be aware that the effectiveness of treating phendimetrazine overdose with hemodialysis or peritoneal dialysis is unknown.

Institute suicide precautions according to facility policy, and anticipate psychiatric re-evaluation.

Nursing Considerations

- **WARNING** Be aware that phendimetrazine should only be used for the short-term (few weeks) treatment of exogenous obesity and that the drug shouldn't be used in combination with other anorexigenics because cardiac valve dysfunction or pulmonary hypertension may occur.
- **WARNING** Monitor patient for chest pain, dyspnea, exercise intolerance, peripheral edema, and syncope, which may indicate cardiac valve dysfunction or pulmonary hypertension.
- Expect to monitor blood pressure in patients with mild hypertension because phendimetrazine may cause an increase blood pressure.
- **WARNING** Expect to taper drug gradually before discontinuing it to prevent withdrawal and increased rebound appetite. Monitor patient for withdrawal signs and symptoms, including abdominal cramps, depression, insomnia, nausea, nightmares, severe fever, and tremor. Notify prescriber immediately if signs or symptoms persist or worsen.
- Be aware that drug may cause physical and psychological dependence. Monitor patient for effects of chronic abuse, including hyperactivity, insomnia, personality changes, psychosis, severe dermatoses, and severe irritability.

PATIENT TEACHING

- Advise patient to notify prescriber immediately if she develops chest pain, dyspnea, exercise intolerance, peripheral edema, or syncope.
- Instruct patient to swallow the E.R. capsule whole.
- Instruct patient taking tablet form to take last dose at least 4 to 6 hours before bedtime to prevent insomnia.
- Instruct patient to take drug exactly as prescribed because of the risk of addiction. Caution her that tolerance to drug's therapeutic effects may develop in a few weeks and that long-term use may cause psychological or physical dependence. Inform her that the drug will be gradually reduced to avoid withdrawal signs and symptoms.
- Explain to patient that behavior changes are needed for long-

term weight loss. Stress the importance of maintaining a reduced caloric intake and routine exercise program.
- Instruct patient to avoid alcohol because of the risk of increased confusion, dizziness, light-headedness, and syncope.
- Advise patient to avoid driving and potentially hazardous activities until she knows how the drug affects her.
- Teach patient ways to relieve dry mouth, such as sucking on ice chips or using sugarless candy or gum.
- Caution patient that drug may cause a false-positive result in urine drug screen for amphetamines.
- Advise patient to notify prescriber immediately if she knows or suspects she's pregnant.

phenelzine sulfate
Nardil

Class and Category
Chemical class: Hydrazine derivative
Therapeutic class: Antidepressant
Pregnancy category: C

Indications and Dosages
▶ *To treat depression*
TABLETS
Adults. *Initial:* 1 mg/kg daily, increased gradually as prescribed and tolerated. *Maintenance:* 45 mg daily. *Maximum:* 90 mg daily.
DOSAGE ADJUSTMENT For elderly patients, initial dosage possibly reduced to 0.8 to 1 mg/kg daily in divided doses and increased as prescribed and tolerated to maximum of 60 mg daily.

Route	Onset	Steady State	Peak	Half-Life	Duration
P.O.	7 to 10 days	Unknown	4 to 8 wk	Unknown	10 days

Contraindications
Cardiovascular disease; cerebrovascular disease; heart failure; hepatic disease; history of headaches; hypersensitivity to phenelzine or its components; hypertension; pheochromocytoma; severe renal impairment; use of an anesthetic, an antihypertensive, bupropion, buspirone, carbamazepine, a CNS depressant, cyclobenzaprine, dextromethorphan, meperidine, a selective serotonin reuptake inhibitor, a sympathomimetic, or a tricyclic antidepressant; use within 14 days of another MAO inhibitor

Mechanism of Action

Relieves signs and symptoms of unipolar depressive disorders by inhibiting the enzyme MAO. Normally, MAO breaks down monoamine neurotransmitters, such as serotonin, as shown top right. By inhibiting this enzyme, phenelzine increases the concentration of serotonin in the vesicles of monoamine nerve endings, allowing more serotonin to be released and engage with receptors on postsynaptic cells, as shown bottom right. A serotonin deficiency may be responsible in part for endogenous depression.

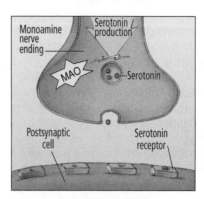

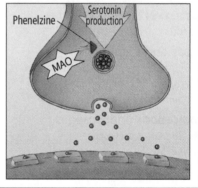

Interactions

DRUGS

anticholinergics, antidyskinetics, antihistamines: Increased anticholinergic effect, prolonged CNS depression (antihistamines)

anticonvulsants: Increased CNS depression, possibly altered pattern of seizures

beta blockers: Increased risk of bradycardia

bromocriptine: Possibly interference with bromocriptine's effects

bupropion: Increased risk of bupropion toxicity

buspirone: Increased risk of hypertension

caffeine-containing drugs: Increased risk of dangerous arrhythmias and severe hypertension

carbamazepine, cyclobenzaprine, maprotiline, other MAO inhibitors: Increased risk of hyperpyretic crisis, hypertensive crisis, severe seizures, and death; altered pattern of seizures (carbamazepine)

CNS depressants: Increased CNS depression

dextromethorphan: Increased risk of excitation, hypertension, and hyperpyrexia

diuretics: Increased hypotensive effect

doxapram: Increased vasopressor effects of either drug

fluoxetine: Increased risk of agitation, confusion, GI signs and symptoms, hyperpyretic episodes, hypertensive crisis, potentially fatal serotonin syndrome, restlessness, and severe seizures

guanadrel, guanethidine: Increased risk of hypertension

haloperidol, loxapine, molindone, phenothiazines, pimozide, thioxanthenes: Prolonged and intensified anticholinergic, hypotensive, and sedative effects of these drugs or phenelzine

insulin, oral antidiabetic drugs: Increased hypoglycemic effects

levodopa: Increased risk of sudden, moderate to severe hypertension

local anesthetics (with epinephrine or levonordefrin): Possibly severe hypertension

meperidine, other opioid analgesics: Increased risk of coma, hyperpyrexia, hypotension, immediate excitation, rigidity, seizures, severe hypertension, severe respiratory depression, sweating, vascular collapse, and death

methyldopa: Increased risk of hallucinations, headache, hyperexcitability, and severe hypertension

methylphenidate: Increased CNS stimulant effect of methylphenidate

metrizamide: Decreased seizure threshold, increased risk of seizures

oral anticoagulants: Increased anticoagulant activity

paroxetine, sertraline, trazodone, tricyclic antidepressants: Increased risk of potentially fatal serotonin syndrome

phenylephrine (nasal or ophthalmic): Potentiated vasopressor effect of phenylephrine

rauwolfia alkaloids: Increased risk of moderate to severe hypertension, CNS depression (when phenelzine is added to rauwolfia alkaloid therapy), CNS excitation and hypertension (when rauwolfia alkaloid is added to phenelzine therapy)

spinal anesthetics: Increased risk of hypotension

succinylcholine: Possibly increased neuromuscular blockade of succinylcholine

sympathomimetics: Prolonged and intensified cardiac stimulant and vasopressor effects

tryptophan: Increased risk of confusion, disorientation, hyperreflexia, hyperthermia, hyperventilation, mania or hypomania, and shivering

FOODS

foods and beverages high in tyramine or other pressor amines, such as aged cheese; beer; fava beans or other broad beans; cured meat or sausage; liqueurs; overripe fruit; red and white wine; reduced-alcohol and alcohol-free beer and wine; sauerkraut; sherry; smoked or pickled fish, meats, and poultry; yeast or protein extracts: Increased risk of sudden, severe hypertension

ACTIVITIES

alcohol use: Increased CNS depressant effects and hypertensive crisis

Adverse Reactions

CNS: Agitation, dizziness, drowsiness, headache, overstimulation, restlessness, sedation, sleep disturbance, suicidal ideation, weakness

CV: Bradycardia, edema, hypertensive crisis, orthostatic hypotension, palpitations, tachycardia

EENT: Blurred vision, dry mouth, photophobia

ENDO: Hypoglycemia (diabetic patients)

GI: Abdominal pain, constipation, diarrhea, elevated liver function test results, increased appetite, nausea

GU: Impotence, priapism, sexual dysfunction, urinary frequency, urine retention

MS: Muscle twitching

SKIN: Diaphoresis, rash

Other: Hypernatremia, weight gain

Overdose

Monitor patient for signs and symptoms of overdose, including anxiety, confusion, cool and clammy skin, diaphoresis, dizziness, drowsiness, dyspnea, fever, hallucinations, headache, hyperreflexia or hyporeflexia, hypertension or hypotension, insomnia, irritability, muscle stiffness, respiratory depression, seizures, and tachycardia. Signs and symptoms may be minimal for the first 12 hours and reach a maximum by 24 to 48 hours, so monitor patientopften during this time.

Maintain an open airway, administer oxygen as prescribed, and be prepared to assist with endotracheal intubation if the patient develops respiratory failure. Institute seizure precautions according to facility protocol. Monitor temperature, and expect to treat hyperpyrexia with an antipyretic and a cooling blanket, as prescribed. Be prepared to induce vomiting or perform gastric lavage, followed by administration of activated charcoal, as prescribed, to decrease absorption of phenelzine. Take precautions to protect patient's airway against aspiration. Hemodialysis, hemo-perfusion, and peritoneal dialysis may be effective for treating phenelzine overdose.

To treat hypotension, anticipate the use of I.V. fluids and a va-sopressor, such as norepinephrine. To treat hypertension, antici-pate the use of an alpha adrenergic blocker, such as phentol-amine or phenoxybenzamine. Expect to treat seizures with diazepam, and be aware that phenothiazines shouldn't be used because of possible hypotensive effects.

To treat signs and symptoms of a hypermetabolic state—such as coma, hyperpyrexia, hyperreflexia, muscle rigidity, respiratory failure, tachycardia, and tremor—expect to administer dantrolene, 2.5 mg/kg daily in divided doses, as prescribed. Monitor patient for hepatotoxicity and pleural and pericardial effusion.

Institute suicide precautions according to facility policy, and anticipate psychiatric re-evaluation.

Nursing Considerations

- Use phenelzine cautiously in patients with epilepsy because drug may alter seizure threshold.
- Use phenelzine cautiously in patients with diabetes mellitus be-cause insulin sensitivity may increase, increasing risk of hypo-glycemia.
- Expect to observe some therapeutic effect within 7 to 10 days, but keep in mind that full effect may not occur for 4 to 8 weeks.
- Monitor patient's cardiovascular status closely for changes in heart rate (especially if patient receives more than 30 mg daily) and signs and symptoms of life-threatening hypertensive crisis. Question patient frequently about headaches and palpitations. If either occurs, notify prescriber and expect to discontinue phenelzine.
- Expect to treat hypertensive crisis with phentolamine and use external cooling measures to manage fever, as prescribed.
- To avoid hypertensive crisis, expect to wait 10 to 14 days, as prescribed, when switching patient from one MAO inhibitor to another or when switching from a chemically related drug, such as amitriptyline or perphenazine.
- Watch patient (particularly a child, an adolescent, or a young adult) closely for suicidal tendencies, especially when therapy starts or dosage changes.

PATIENT TEACHING
- Inform patient and family members that therapeutic effects of

phenelzine may take several weeks to appear and that she should continue taking drug as prescribed.

- Caution patient to rise slowly from a lying or sitting position to minimize effects of orthostatic hypotension.
- **WARNING** Instruct patient to avoid these substances during phenelzine therapy and for 2 weeks afterward: alcohol-free and reduced-alcohol beer and wine; appetite suppressants; beer; broad beans; cheese (except cottage and cream cheese); chocolate and caffeine in large quantities; dry sausage (including Genoa salami, hard salami, pepperoni, and Lebanon bologna); hay fever drugs; inhaled asthma drugs; liver; meat extract; OTC cold and cough preparations (including those containing dextromethorphan); nasal decongestants (tablets, drops, or sprays); pickled herring; products that contain tryptophan; protein-rich foods that may have undergone protein changes by aging, pickling, fermenting, or smoking; sauerkraut; sinus drugs; weight-loss aids; yeast extracts (including brewer's yeast in large quantities); yogurt; and wine.
- Advise patient to inform all health care providers (including dentists) that she takes an MAO inhibitor, because certain drugs are contraindicated within 2 weeks of therapy.
- Urge patient to avoid potentially hazardous activities until she knows how the drug affects her.
- Stress the importance of reporting headaches and other unusual, persistent, or severe signs or symptoms.
- If patient has diabetes mellitus and is taking insulin or an oral antidiabetic drug, urge her to monitor blood glucose level often during therapy because phenelzine may affect glucose control.
- Tell family or caregiver to observe patient (particularly a child, an adolescent, or a young adult) closely for suicidal tendencies, especially when therapy starts or dosage changes.

phenobarbital
Ancalixir (CAN), Barbita, Solfoton
phenobarbital sodium
Luminal

Class, Category, and Schedule
Chemical class: Barbiturate
Therapeutic class: Anticonvulsant, sedative-hypnotic
Pregnancy category: D
Controlled substance schedule: IV

Indications and Dosages

▶ *To treat seizures*

CAPSULES, ELIXIR, TABLETS

Adults. 60 to 250 mg daily as a single dose or in divided doses.

Children. 1 to 6 mg/kg daily as a single dose or in divided doses.

I.V. INJECTION

Adults. 100 to 320 mg, repeated as needed and as prescribed. *Maximum:* 600 mg daily.

Children. *Initial:* 10 to 20 mg/kg as a single dose. *Maintenance:* 1 to 6 mg/kg daily.

▶ *To treat status epilepticus*

I.V. INFUSION OR INJECTION

Adults. 10 to 20 mg/kg given slowly and repeated as needed and as prescribed.

Children. 15 to 20 mg/kg over 10 to 15 min.

▶ *To provide short-term treatment of insomnia*

CAPSULES, ELIXIR, TABLETS

Adults. 100 to 320 mg at bedtime.

I.V., I.M., OR SUBCUTANEOUS INJECTION

Adults. 100 to 325 mg at bedtime.

▶ *To provide daytime sedation*

CAPSULES, ELIXIR, TABLETS

Adults. 30 to 120 mg daily in divided doses b.i.d. or t.i.d.

Children. 2 mg/kg t.i.d.

I.V., I.M., OR SUBCUTANEOUS INJECTION

Adults. 30 to 120 mg daily in divided doses b.i.d. or t.i.d.

DOSAGE ADJUSTMENT Dosage possibly reduced for elderly or debilitated patients to minimize confusion, depression, and excitement.

Route	Onset	Steady State	Peak	Half-Life	Duration
P.O.	20 to 60 min	Unknown	Unknown	53 to 118 hr*	Unknown
I.V.	5 min	Unknown	30 min	53 to 118 hr*	4 to 6 hr
I.M., SubQ	5 to 20 min	Unknown	Unknown	53 to 118 hr*	4 to 6 hr

Contraindications

Hepatic disease; history of addiction to hypnotics or sedatives; hypersensitivity to phenobarbital, other barbiturates, or their components; nephritis; porphyria; severe respiratory disease with airway obstruction or dyspnea

---

* For adults. Half-life is 60 to 180 hr for children; 48 hr for neonates.

Mechanism of Action

Inhibits ascending conduction of impulses in the reticular formation, which controls CNS arousal to produce drowsiness, hypnosis, and sedation. Phenobarbital also decreases the spread of seizure activity in the cortex, thalamus, and limbic system. It promotes an increased threshold for electrical stimulation in the motor cortex, which may contribute to its anticonvulsant properties.

Interactions

DRUGS

acetaminophen: Decreased acetaminophen effectiveness with long-term phenobarbital therapy

amphetamines: Delayed intestinal absorption of phenobarbital

anesthetics (halogenated hydrocarbon): Possibly hepatotoxicity

anticonvulsants (hydantoin): Unpredictable effects on metabolism of anticonvulsant

anticonvulsants (succinimide), including carbamazepine: Decreased blood levels and elimination half-lives of these drugs

calcium channel blockers: Possibly excessive hypotension

carbonic anhydrase inhibitors: Enhanced osteopenia induced by phenobarbital

chloramphenicol, corticosteroids, cyclosporine, dacarbazine, metronidazole, quinidine: Decreased effectiveness of these drugs from enhanced metabolism

CNS depressants: Additive CNS depression

cyclophosphamide: Possibly reduced half-life and increased leukopenic activity of cyclophosphamide

disopyramide: Possibly ineffectiveness of disopyramide

doxycycline, fenoprofen: Shortened half-life of these drugs

griseofulvin: Possibly decreased absorption and effectiveness of griseofulvin

guanadrel, guanethidine: Possibly increased orthostatic hypotension

haloperidol: Decreased seizure threshold, decreased blood haloperidol level

ketamine (high doses): Increased risk of hypotension and respiratory depression

leucovorin: Interference with phenobarbital's anticonvulsant effect

levothyroxine, oral contraceptives, phenylbutazone, tricyclic antidepressants: Decreased effectiveness of these drugs

loxapine, phenothiazines, thioxanthenes: Decreased seizure threshold

MAO inhibitors: Prolonged phenobarbital effects, possibly altered pattern of seizure activity

maprotiline: Increased CNS depression, decreased seizure threshold at high doses, decreased phenobarbital effectiveness

methoxyflurane: Possibly hepatotoxicity and nephrotoxicity

methylphenidate: Increased risk of phenobarbital toxicity

mexiletine: Decreased blood mexiletine level

oral anticoagulants: Decreased anticoagulant activity, increased risk of bleeding when phenobarbital is discontinued

pituitary hormones (posterior): Increased risk of arrhythmias and coronary insufficiency

primidone: Altered pattern of seizures, increased CNS effects of both drugs

valproate, valproic acid: Decreased phenobarbital metabolism, increased risk of barbiturate toxicity

vitamin D: Decreased phenobarbital effectiveness

xanthines: Increased xanthine metabolism, antagonized hypnotic effect of phenobarbital

ACTIVITIES

alcohol use: Additive CNS depression

Adverse Reactions

CNS: Anxiety, depression, dizziness, drowsiness, headache, irritability, lethargy, mood changes, paradoxical stimulation, sedation, vertigo

CV: Hypotension, sinus bradycardia

EENT: Miosis, ptosis

GI: Constipation, diarrhea, nausea, vomiting

GU: Decreased libido, impotence, sexual dysfunction

MS: Arthralgia, bone tenderness

RESP: Bronchospasm, respiratory depression

SKIN: Dermatitis, photosensitivity, rash, urticaria

Other: Injection site phlebitis (I.V.), physical and psychological dependence

Overdose

Monitor patient for signs and symptoms of overdose, including absent or decreased reflexes, bradycardia, Cheyne-Stokes respiration, coma, confusion, dyspnea, fever, hypothermia, miosis or mydriasis, oliguria, severe drowsiness, severe weakness, shock, slurred speech, staggering, tachycardia, and unusual eye movements. Consider chronic overdose if such signs and symptoms as continued insomnia, irritability, poor judgment, and severe confusion occur. Maintain an open airway, and carefully monitor blood pressure and temperature.

If the patient is conscious, be prepared to administer ipecac syrup, as prescribed, to induce vomiting. Expect to administer activated charcoal, 30 to 60 g, with water or sorbitol, to prevent further absorption and enhance drug elimination. For an unconscious patient, anticipate assisting with the insertion of an endotracheal tube and then performing gastric lavage. The inflated cuff of the endotracheal tube will help prevent aspiration of gastric contents into the lungs.

Be prepared to give a urine-alkalizing drug to increase phenobarbital elimination. Administer I.V. fluids and a vasopressor, as prescribed. For severe cases, anticipate the need for hemodialysis or hemoperfusion. Be aware that, in cases of extreme overdose, the patient may have a flat EEG because all electrical activity in the brain has ceased; however, this effect may be reversible.

Institute suicide precautions according to facility policy, and anticipate psychiatric re-evaluation.

Nursing Considerations

- Be aware that phenobarbital shouldn't be given during third trimester of pregnancy because repeated use can cause dependence in neonate. It also shouldn't be given to breast-feeding women because it may cause CNS depression in infants.
- Use I.V. route cautiously in patients with cardiovascular disease, hypotension, pulmonary disease, or shock because drug may cause adverse hemodynamic or respiratory effects.
- Because drug can cause respiratory depression, assess respiratory rate and depth before use, especially in patient with bronchopneumonia, pulmonary disease, respiratory tract infection, or status asthmaticus.
- Give elixir undiluted or mix with fruit juice, milk, or water. Use a calibrated device to measure doses.
- If necessary, crush tablets and mix with food or fluids.
- Reconstitute sterile powder with at least 10 ml of sterile water for injection. Don't use reconstituted solution if it fails to clear within 5 minutes. Further dilute prescribed dose with normal saline solution or D_5W, and infuse over 30 to 60 minutes.
- Don't give more rapidly than 60 mg/minute by I.V. injection.
- During I.V. use, monitor blood pressure, respiratory rate, and heart rate and rhythm. Anticipate increased risk of hypotension, even when giving drug at recommended rate. Keep resuscitation equipment readily available.

- During I.M. use, don't inject more than 5 ml into any one I.M. site to prevent sterile abscess formation.
- Be aware that drug may cause physical and psychological dependence.
- Anticipate that phenobarbital's CNS effects may exacerbate major depression, suicidal tendencies, or other mental disorders.
- Take safety precautions for elderly patients, as appropriate, because they're more likely to experience confusion, depression, and excitement as adverse CNS reactions.
- Watch for possible paradoxical stimulation in children.
- Be aware that drug may trigger signs and symptoms in patients with acute intermittent porphyria.

PATIENT TEACHING
- Instruct patient to take phenobarbital elixir undiluted or to mix it with fruit juice, milk, or water. Advise her to use a calibrated device to measure doses.
- If patient has trouble swallowing tablets, suggest that she crush them and mix with food or fluid.
- Caution patient about possible drowsiness and reduced alertness. Advise her to avoid potentially hazardous activities until she knows how the drug affects her.
- Urge patient to avoid alcohol during therapy.
- Inform parents that a child may react with paradoxical excitement. Tell them to notify prescriber if this occurs.
- Instruct women to notify prescriber about suspected, known, or intended pregnancy. Discourage breast-feeding during therapy.

Other Therapeutic Uses
Phenobarbital is also indicated for the following:
- To provide preoperative sedation

phentermine
Ionamin
phentermine hydrochloride
Adipex-P, Fastin, Obinex, Phentercot, Phentride, Pro-Fast, Teramine, Zantryl

Class, Category, and Schedule
Chemical class: Phenylalkylamine
Therapeutic class: Appetite suppressant
Pregnancy category: C
Controlled substance schedule: IV

Indications and Dosages

▶ *As adjunct to treat exogenous obesity with behavior modification, caloric restriction, and exercise*

CAPSULES

Adults and adolescents age 16 and over. 15 to 37.5 mg daily before breakfast or 1 to 2 hr after breakfast.

RESIN CAPSULES

Adults and adolescents age 16 and over. 15 to 30 mg daily before breakfast.

TABLETS

Adults and adolescents age 16 and over. 15 to 37.5 mg daily before breakfast or 1 to 2 hr after breakfast. Or, 8 mg t.i.d. 30 min before meals.

Route	Onset	Steady State	Peak	Half-Life	Duration
P.O.	Unknown	Unknown	Unknown	19 to 20 hr	12 to 14 hr

Mechanism of Action

Stimulates the release of dopamine and norepinephrine from adrenergic nerve terminals in the lateral hypothalamic feeding center of the cerebral cortex and reticular activating system, which reduces appetite. By stimulating the CNS, phentermine causes other effects, including reduced gastric acid production and increased metabolism, which may be effective in treating obesity.

Contraindications

Advanced arteriosclerosis; agitation; cerebral ischemia; glaucoma; history of alcohol or drug abuse; hypersensitivity to phentermine, other sympathomimetic amines, or their components; hyperthyroidism; MAO inhibitor therapy within 14 days; moderate to severe hypertension; symptomatic cardiovascular disease

Interactions

DRUGS

antacids (calcium- and magnesium-containing), carbonic anhydrase inhibitors, citrates, sodium bicarbonate: Increased blood phentermine level

amphetamines, other appetite suppressants, selective serotonin reuptake inhibitors: Possibly increased risk of cardiac valve dysfunction

anesthetics (inhaled): Increased risk of arrhythmias

antihypertensives (especially clonidine, guanadrel, guanethidine, methyldopa, rauwolfia alkaloids): Decreased hypotensive effect

ascorbic acid: Increased excretion of phentermine, causing decreased blood phentermine level
CNS stimulants, thyroid hormones: Additive CNS stimulation
insulin, oral antidiabetic drugs: Altered blood glucose level
MAO inhibitors: Potentiated effects of phentermine; possibly hypertensive crisis
phenothiazines: Reduced anorectic effect of phentermine
tricyclic antidepressants: Possibly potentiated adverse cardiovascular effects
urinary acidifiers (including ammonium chloride and potassium or sodium phosphates): Decreased blood phentermine level
vasopressors (especially catecholamines): Possibly potentiated vasopressor effect of these drugs
ACTIVITIES
alcohol use: Increased adverse CNS effects

Adverse Reactions

CNS: Cerebral ischemia, CNS stimulation, depression, dizziness, headache, insomnia, light-headedness, mania, nervousness, psychosis, syncope, tremor
CV: Chest pain, hypertension, palpitations, peripheral edema
EENT: Dry mouth
GI: Abdominal pain, constipation, nausea, vomiting
GU: Dysuria
RESP: Dyspnea
SKIN: Hives, rash
Other: Exercise intolerance

Overdose

Phentermine overdose has no specific antidote. Monitor patient for signs and symptoms of overdose, including abdominal cramps, arrhythmias, coma, confusion, diarrhea, dyspnea, hallucinations, hostility, hyperreflexia, hyperthermia, labile blood pressure, nausea, panic reaction, restlessness, seizures, shock, tachypnea, tremor, and vomiting. Anticipate depression and fatigue to follow CNS excitement.

Maintain an open airway, monitor vital signs, and protect patient from self-injury. Institute seizure precautions according to facility protocol. To decrease drug absorption, perform gastric lavage or induce vomiting, and administer activated charcoal, as prescribed. Expect to administer a drug to promote urine acidification and I.V. fluids, as prescribed, to increase drug excretion.

Be prepared to administer a drug such as a barbiturate, diazepam, or phenytoin to control CNS stimulation and seizures. Anticipate administering drugs such as lidocaine to control arrhythmias, phentolamine or a nitrate to manage hypertension, and a beta blocker to control tachycardia. Be aware that the effectiveness of hemodialysis or peritoneal dialysis is unknown.

Institute suicide precautions according to facility policy, and anticipate psychiatric re-evaluation.

Nursing Considerations

* **WARNING** Be aware that phentermine should be used only for short-term (few weeks) treatment of exogenous obesity and that it shouldn't be used with selective serotonin reuptake inhibitors or MAO inhibitors because cardiac valve dysfunction may occur.
* **WARNING** Monitor patient for chest pain, dyspnea, exercise intolerance, peripheral edema, and syncope, which may indicate cardiac valve dysfunction or pulmonary hypertension. Notify prescriber immediately if these signs or symptoms occur, and expect to discontinue the drug.
* Expect to monitor blood pressure in patients with mild hypertension because phentermine may increase blood pressure.
* **WARNING** Expect to taper drug gradually before discontinuing to prevent withdrawal and increased rebound appetite. Monitor patient for withdrawal effects, including abdominal cramps, depression, insomnia, nausea, nightmares, severe fever, and tremor. Notify prescriber immediately if these signs or symptoms persist or worsen.
* Be aware that drug may cause physical and psychological dependence. Monitor patient for effects of chronic abuse, including hyperactivity, insomnia, personality changes, psychosis, severe dermatoses, and severe irritability.

PATIENT TEACHING

* Advise patient to notify prescriber immediately about chest pain, dyspnea, exercise intolerance, peripheral edema, or syncope.
* Instruct patient to swallow the resin capsule whole and to take it in the morning or 10 to 14 hours before bedtime.
* Instruct patient taking tablet form to take last dose at least 4 to 6 hours before bedtime to prevent insomnia.
* Instruct patient to take drug exactly as prescribed because of the risk of addiction. Caution that tolerance to drug's therapeutic effects may develop in a few weeks and that long-term use may cause psychological or physical dependence. Explain that the dose will be gradually reduced to avoid withdrawal effects.

- Explain to patient that behavior changes are needed for long-term weight loss. Stress the importance of maintaining a reduced caloric intake and routine exercise program.
- Instruct patient to avoid alcohol because of the risk of increased confusion, dizziness, light-headedness, and syncope.
- Advise patient to avoid potentially hazardous activities until she knows how the drug affects her.
- Teach patient ways to relieve dry mouth, such as sucking on ice chips or using sugarless candy or gum.
- Caution patient that drug may cause a false-positive result in urine drug screen for amphetamines.
- Advise patient to notify prescriber immediately if she knows or suspects that she's pregnant.

phenytoin
Dilantin-30 (CAN), Dilantin-125, Dilantin Infatabs
phenytoin sodium
Dilantin, Dilantin Kapseals, Phenytex
Class and Category
Chemical class: Hydantoin derivative
Therapeutic class: Anticonvulsant
Pregnancy category: C
Indications and Dosages
▶ *To treat tonic-clonic, simple, or complex partial seizures in patients who have had no prior treatment*
CHEWABLE TABLETS, ORAL SUSPENSION (PHENYTOIN)
Adults and adolescents. *Initial:* 125 mg suspension or 100 to 125 mg tablet t.i.d., adjusted every 7 to 10 days as needed and tolerated.
Children. *Initial:* 5 mg/kg daily in divided doses b.i.d. or t.i.d., adjusted as needed and tolerated. *Maintenance:* 4 to 8 mg/kg daily in divided doses b.i.d. or t.i.d. *Maximum:* 300 mg daily.
EXTENDED CAPSULES (PHENYTOIN SODIUM)
Adults and adolescents. *Initial:* 100 mg t.i.d., adjusted every 7 to 10 days as needed and tolerated. *Maintenance:* Once seizures are controlled, adjusted dosage given daily if needed and tolerated.
DOSAGE ADJUSTMENT For hospitalized patients without hepatic or renal disease, oral loading dose of 400 mg followed in 2 hr by 300 mg and then in 2 more hr by another 300 mg for a total of 1 g.

Children. *Initial:* 5 mg/kg daily in divided doses b.i.d. or t.i.d., adjusted as needed and tolerated. *Maintenance:* 4 to 8 mg/kg daily in divided doses b.i.d. or t.i.d. *Maximum:* 300 mg daily.

PROMPT CAPSULES (PHENYTOIN SODIUM)

Adults and adolescents. 100 mg t.i.d., adjusted every 7 to 10 days as needed and tolerated.

Children. *Initial:* 5 mg/kg daily in divided doses b.i.d. or t.i.d., adjusted as needed and tolerated. *Maintenance:* 4 to 8 mg/kg daily in divided doses b.i.d. or t.i.d. *Maximum:* 300 mg daily.

▶ *To treat status epilepticus*

I.V. INJECTION (PHENYTOIN SODIUM)

Adults and adolescents. *Initial:* 15 to 20 mg/kg by slow push in 50 ml of sodium chloride for injection at a rate not to exceed 50 mg/min. *Maintenance:* Beginning within 12 to 24 hr of initial dose, 5 mg/kg daily P.O. in divided doses b.i.d. to q.i.d., or 100 mg I.V. every 6 to 8 hr.

Children. 15 to 20 mg/kg at no more than 1 mg/kg/min. *Maximum:* 50 mg/min.

DOSAGE ADJUSTMENT For elderly or very ill patients and those with cardiovascular or hepatic disease, dosage reduced and rate slowed to 25 mg/min, as prescribed, or possibly as low as 5 to 10 mg/min to reduce the risk of adverse reactions.

▶ *To prevent or treat seizures during neurosurgery*

I.V. INJECTION (PHENYTOIN SODIUM)

Adults. 100 to 200 mg every 4 hr at a rate not to exceed 50 mg/min during or immediately after neurosurgery.

Mechanism of Action

Limits the spread of seizure activity and the start of new seizures by regulating voltage-dependent sodium and calcium channels in neurons, inhibiting calcium movement across neuronal membranes, and enhancing sodium-potassium ATP activity in neurons and glial cells. These actions all help stabilize the neurons.

Incompatibilities

Don't mix phenytoin in same syringe with any other drugs or with any I.V. solutions other than sodium chloride for injection because precipitate will form.

Contraindications

Adams-Stokes syndrome, hypersensitivity to phenytoin or its

components, SA block, second- or third-degree heart block, sinus bradycardia

Interactions

DRUGS

acetaminophen: Possibly hepatoxicity, decreased acetaminophen effects

activated charcoal, antacids, calcium salts, enteral feedings, sucralfate: Decreased absorption of oral phenytoin

allopurinol, benzodiazepines, chloramphenicol, cimetidine, disulfiram, fluconazole, isoniazid, itraconazole, methylphenidate, metronidazole, miconazole, omeprazole, phenacemide, ranitidine, sulfonamides, trazodone, trimethoprim: Decreased metabolism and increased effects of phenytoin

amiodarone, ticlopidine: Possibly increased blood phenytoin level

antifungals (azoles): Increased blood phenytoin level, decreased blood antifungal level

antineoplastics, nitrofurantoin, pyridoxine: Decreased phenytoin effects

barbiturates: Variable effects on blood phenytoin level

bupropion, clozapine, loxapine, MAO inhibitors, maprotiline, molindone, phenothiazines, pimozide, thioxanthenes, tricyclic antidepressants: Decreased seizure threshold, decreased anticonvulsant effect of phenytoin

calcium channel blockers: Increased metabolism and decreased effects of these drugs, possibly increased blood phenytoin level

carbamazepine: Decreased blood level and effects of carbamazepine, possibly phenytoin toxicity

carbonic anhydrase inhibitors: Increased risk of osteopenia from phenytoin

chlordiazepoxide, diazepam: Possibly increased blood phenytoin level, decreased effects of these drugs

clonazepam: Possibly decreased blood level and effects of clonazepam, possibly phenytoin toxicity

corticosteroids, cyclosporine, dicumarol, digoxin, disopyramide, doxycycline, estrogens, furosemide, lamotrigine, levodopa, methadone, metyrapone, mexiletine, oral contraceptives, quinidine, sirolimus, tacrolimus, theophylline: Increased metabolism and decreased effects of these drugs

dopamine: Increased risk of severe hypotension and bradycardia (with I.V. phenytoin)

fluoxetine: Increased blood phenytoin level and risk of phenytoin toxicity *folic acid, leucovorin:* Decreased blood phenytoin level, increased risk of seizures

haloperidol: Decreased effects of haloperidol, decreased anticonvulsant effect of phenytoin

halothane anesthetics: Increased risk of hepatotoxicity and phenytoin toxicity

ifosfamide: Decreased phenytoin effects, possibly increased toxicity

influenza virus vaccine: Possibly decreased phenytoin effects

insulin, oral antidiabetic drugs: Possibly hyperglycemia, increased blood phenytoin level (with tolbutamide)

levonorgestrel, mebendazole, streptozocin, sulfonylureas: Decreased effects of these drugs

lidocaine, propranolol (possibly other beta blockers): Increased cardiac depressant effects (with I.V. phenytoin), possibly decreased blood level and increased adverse effects of phenytoin

lithium: Increased risk of lithium toxicity, increased risk of neurologic signs and symptoms with normal blood lithium level

meperidine: Increased metabolism and decreased effects of meperidine, possibly meperidine toxicity

methadone: Possibly increased metabolism of methadone and withdrawal signs and symptoms

neuromuscular blockers: Shorter duration of action and decreased effects of neuromuscular blockers

oral anticoagulants: Decreased metabolism and increased effects of phenytoin; early increase in anticoagulant effect followed by decrease

paroxetine: Decreased bioavailability of both drugs

phenylbutazone, salicylates: Increased phenytoin effects, possibly phenytoin toxicity

primidone: Increased primidone effects, possibly primidone toxicity

rifampin: Increased hepatic metabolism of phenytoin

valproic acid: Possibly decreased phenytoin metabolism, resulting in increased phenytoin effects; possibly decreased blood valproic acid level

vitamin D: Possibly decreased vitamin D effects, resulting in rickets or osteomalacia (with long-term use of phenytoin)

ACTIVITIES

alcohol use: Additive CNS depression, increased phenytoin clearance

Adverse Reactions

CNS: Ataxia, confusion, depression, dizziness, drowsiness, excitement, fever, headache, involuntary motor activity, lethargy, nervousness, peripheral neuropathy, restlessness, slurred speech, tremor, weakness

CV: Cardiac arrest, hypotension, vasculitis

EENT: Amblyopia, conjunctivitis, diplopia, earache, epistaxis, eye pain, gingival hyperplasia, hearing loss, loss of taste, nystagmus, pharyngitis, photophobia, rhinitis, sinusitis, taste perversion, tinnitus

ENDO: Gynecomastia, hyperglycemia

GI: Abdominal pain, anorexia, constipation, diarrhea, epigastric pain, hepatic dysfunction, hepatic necrosis, hepatitis, nausea, vomiting

GU: Glycosuria, priapism, renal failure

HEME: Acute intermittent porphyria (exacerbation), agranulocytosis, anemia, eosinophilia, leukopenia, pancytopenia, thrombocytopenia

MS: Arthralgia, arthropathy, bone fractures, muscle twitching, osteomalacia, polymyositis

RESP: Apnea, asthma, bronchitis, cough, dyspnea, hypoxia, increased sputum production, pneumonia, pneumothorax, pulmonary fibrosis

SKIN: Exfoliative dermatitis, jaundice, maculopapular or morbilliform rash, purpuric dermatitis, Stevens-Johnson syndrome, toxic epidermal necrolysis, unusual hair growth, urticaria

Other: Facial feature enlargement, injection site pain, lupuslike signs and symptoms, lymphadenopathy, polyarteritis, weight gain or loss

Overdose

Phenytoin overdose has no specific antidote. Monitor patient for signs and symptoms of overdose, including ataxia, blurred vision, confusion, dizziness, drowsiness, dysarthria, hyperreflexia, nausea, nystagmus, seizures, slurred speech, staggering, tiredness, tremor, and vomiting.

Maintain an open airway, and expect to administer oxygen and a vasopressor, as prescribed, to treat cardiovascular, CNS, and respiratory depression. Institute seizure precautions according to facility protocol.

Be prepared to induce vomiting or perform gastric lavage and to give activated charcoal and a cathartic, as prescribed, to decrease drug absorption. Be aware that dialysis, diuresis, exchange transfusions, and plasmapheresis are ineffective for phenytoin overdose because the drug isn't eliminated by the kidneys.

Monitor patient's hematologic status following recovery because phenytoin may cause agranulocytosis, leukopenia, and thrombocytopenia.

Institute suicide precautions according to facility policy, and anticipate psychiatric re-evaluation.

Nursing Considerations

- Be aware that preferred administration routes for phenytoin are oral and I.V. injection. With I.M. administration, phenytoin has a variable absorption rate.
- If patient has difficulty swallowing, open prompt (rapid-release) capsules and mix contents with food or fluid.
- Shake oral suspension before measuring dose, and use a calibrated measuring device.
- To minimize GI distress, give phenytoin with or just after meals.
- Inspect I.V. form for particles and discoloration before administering.
- **WARNING** Avoid rapid I.V. injection of phenytoin; it may cause cardiac arrest, CNS depression, or severe hypotension.
- To decrease vein irritation, follow I.V. injection with flush of sodium chloride for injection through same I.V. catheter.
- Continuously monitor ECG tracings and blood pressure when administering I.V. phenytoin.
- Frequently assess I.V. site for signs of extravasation because drug can cause tissue necrosis.
- If patient has an NG tube in place, dilute suspension threefold with sodium chloride for injection, D_5W, or sterile water, to minimize drug absorption by polyvinyl chloride tubing. After administration, flush tube with at least 20 ml of diluent.
- Separate oral phenytoin administration by at least 2 hours from antacids and calcium salts.
- Expect continuous enteral feedings to disrupt phenytoin absorption and, possibly, reduce blood phenytoin level. Discontinue tube feedings 1 to 2 hours before and after phenytoin administration, as prescribed. Anticipate giving increased phenytoin doses to compensate for reduced bioavailability during continuous tube feedings.
- Monitor blood phenytoin level. Therapeutic level ranges from 10 to 20 mcg/ml.
- **WARNING** Monitor hematologic status during therapy because phenytoin can cause blood dyscrasias. A patient with a history of agranulocytosis, leukopenia, or pancytopenia may have an increased risk of infection because phenytoin can cause myelosuppression.

- Keep in mind that phenytoin may worsen intermittent porphyria.
- If patient has diabetes mellitus, frequently monitor his blood glucose level because phenytoin can stimulate glucagon and impair insulin secretion, either of which can raise blood glucose level.
- If patient is receiving thyroid replacement therapy, monitor blood thyroid hormone levels as appropriate, because phenytoin may decrease circulating thyroid hormone levels and increase thyroid-stimulating hormone level.
- Be aware that long-term phenytoin therapy may increase patient's requirements for folic acid or vitamin D supplements. However, keep in mind that a diet high in folic acid may decrease seizure control.

PATIENT TEACHING

- Instruct patient to crush or thoroughly chew phenytoin chewable tablets before swallowing or to shake oral solution well before using.
- Advise patient to take drug exactly as prescribed and not to change brands or dosage or stop taking drug unless prescriber instructs her to do so.
- Instruct patient to avoid taking an antacid or calcium product within 2 hours of phenytoin.
- Urge patient to avoid alcohol during therapy.
- Caution patient to avoid potentially hazardous activities until she knows how the drug affects her.
- If patient has diabetes mellitus, inform her about the increased risk of hyperglycemia and the possible need for increased antidiabetic drug dosage during therapy. Advise her to monitor her blood glucose level frequently.
- Stress the importance of good oral hygiene, and encourage patient to inform her dentist that she's taking phenytoin.
- Encourage patient to wear or carry medical identification indicating her diagnosis and drug therapy.

physostigmine salicylate

Antilirium

Class and Category

Chemical class: Salicylic acid derivative
Therapeutic class: Anticholinergic antidote, cholinesterase inhibitor
Pregnancy category: C

Indications and Dosages

▶ *To counteract toxic anticholinergic effects (anticholinergic syndrome)*
I.V. OR I.M. INJECTION
Adults and adolescents. 0.5 to 2 mg at no more than 1 mg/min; then 1 to 4 mg, repeated every 20 to 30 min as needed and as prescribed.
Children. 0.02 mg/kg I.V. at a rate not to exceed 0.5 mg/min, repeated every 5 to 10 min as needed and as prescribed. *Maximum:* 2 mg/dose.

Route	Onset	Steady State	Peak	Half-Life	Duration
I.V.	3 to 8 min	Unknown	5 min	15 to 40 min	30 to 60 min
I.M.	3 to 8 min	Unknown	20 to 30 min	15 to 40 min	30 to 60 min

Mechanism of Action

Inhibits the destruction of acetylcholine by acetylcholinesterase. This action increases the concentration of acetylcholine at cholinergic transmission sites and prolongs and exaggerates the effects of acetylcholine that are blocked by toxic doses of anticholinergics.

Contraindications

Asthma; cardiovascular disease; diabetes mellitus; gangrene; GI or GU obstruction; hypersensitivity to physostigmine, sulfites, or their components

Interactions

DRUGS

choline esters: Enhanced effects of carbachol and bethanechol with concurrent use of physostigmine, and enhanced effects of acetylcholine and methacholine with previous use of physostigmine
succinylcholine: Prolonged neuromuscular paralysis

Adverse Reactions

CNS: CNS stimulation, fatigue, hallucinations, restlessness, seizures (with too-rapid I.V. administration), weakness
CV: Bradycardia (with too-rapid I.V. administration), irregular heartbeat, palpitations
EENT: Increased salivation, lacrimation, miosis
GI: Abdominal pain, diarrhea, nausea, vomiting
GU: Urinary urgency
MS: Muscle twitching

RESP: Bronchospasm, chest tightness, dyspnea (with too-rapid I.V. administration), increased bronchial secretions, wheezing
SKIN: Diaphoresis

Overdose

Physostigmine overdose may cause cholinergic crisis. Monitor patient for such signs and symptoms as bradycardia, coma, confusion, diaphoresis, diarrhea, hypertension or hypotension, increased salivation, miosis, muscle weakness, nausea, paralysis (including respiratory paralysis), seizures, and tachycardia.

Maintain an open airway, prepare for mechanical ventilation, and begin continuous ECG monitoring. Institute seizure precautions according to facility protocol. Expect to give the antidote—atropine—2 to 4 mg I.V. every 3 to 10 minutes in adults or 1 mg I.V. in children, as prescribed. Keep in mind that atropine counteracts only muscarinic cholinergic effects; paralytic effects may continue. Expect to give pralidoxime to counteract these effects.

Nursing Considerations

- Use physostigmine cautiously in patients with bradycardia, epilepsy, or Parkinson's disease.
- Avoid rapid I.V. administration because it may lead to bradycardia, respiratory distress, or seizures.
- Frequently monitor pulse and respiratory rates, blood pressure, and neurologic status during therapy.
- Monitor ECG tracing during I.V. administration.
- If patient has asthma, closely monitor her for asthma attack because drug may precipitate attack by causing bronchoconstriction.
- If patient has a history of seizures, monitor her for them because drug can induce seizures by causing CNS stimulation.

PATIENT TEACHING

- Reassure patient that her vital signs will be monitored frequently to help prevent or detect adverse reactions.
- Instruct patient to notify prescriber immediately about signs and symptoms of cholinergic crisis.

pimozide

Orap

Class and Category

Chemical class: Diphenylbutylpiperidine derivative
Therapeutic class: Antidyskinetic
Pregnancy category: C

Indications and Dosages

▶ *To manage signs and symptoms of Tourette's syndrome unresponsive to standard therapy*

TABLETS

Adults. *Initial:* 1 to 2 mg daily in divided doses, increased gradually every other day, as needed and tolerated. *Maximum:* The lesser of 0.2 mg/kg daily or 10 mg daily.

Children over age 12. *Initial:* 0.05 mg/kg daily at bedtime, increased gradually every 3 days, as needed and tolerated. *Maximum:* The lesser of 0.2 mg/kg or 10 mg daily.

Route	Onset	Steady State	Peak	Half-Life	Duration
P.O.	Unknown	Unknown	Unknown	54 to 168 hr*	Unknown

Mechanism of Action

Acts as a selective dopamine$_2$ (D$_2$) receptor antagonist in the CNS. Pimozide predominantly blocks postsynaptic D$_2$ receptors and may possibly block presynaptic D$_2$ receptors. This blockade alters central dopamine metabolism and function, which suppresses motor and vocal tics in patients with Tourette's syndrome.

Contraindications

Arrhythmias (including long QT syndrome); CNS depression; coma; concurrent therapy with another drug that prolongs QT interval, such as azithromycin, clarithromycin, dirithromycin, disopyramide, erythromycin, indinavir, itraconazole, ketoconazole, maprotiline, nefazodone, nelfinavir, a phenothiazine, probucol, procainamide, quinidine, ritonavir, saquinavir, a tricyclic antidepressant, troleandomycin, and zileuton; hypersensitivity to pimozide, its components, or other antipsychotic drugs; motor or vocal tics not caused by Tourette's syndrome

Interactions

DRUGS

amphetamines, methylphenidate, pemoline: Increased incidence of tics; possibly decreased stimulant effect of amphetamines
anticholinergics: Increased anticholinergic effects of pimozide
anticonvulsants: Possibly lowered seizure threshold
antidepressants: Possibly increased QT-interval prolongation

---

* For adults. Half-life is 17 to 115 hr for children.

CNS depressants: Increased CNS depressant effects
extrapyramidal reaction-causing drugs (such as amoxapine, haloperidol, loxapine, metoclopramide, molindone, olanzapine, phenothiazines, rauwolfia alkaloids, risperidone, tacrine, and thioxanthenes): Increased anticholinergic, CNS depressant, and extrapyramidal effects
MAO inhibitors: Increased anticholinergic, hypotensive, and sedative effects of both drugs

FOODS
grapefruit juice: Possibly inhibition of pimozide metabolism

ACTIVITIES
alcohol use: Increased CNS depressant effects

Adverse Reactions

CNS: Anxiety, behavior changes, depression, drowsiness, extrapyramidal reactions that may be irreversible (akathisia, dystonia, pseudoparkinsonism, tardive dyskinesia), headache, neuroleptic malignant syndrome, tiredness
CV: Arrhythmias, orthostatic hypotension, prolonged QT interval
EENT: Blurred vision, dry mouth
ENDO: Breast engorgement, galactorrhea
HEME: Leukopenia, thrombocytopenia
GI: Anorexia, constipation, diarrhea, nausea, vomiting
GU: Decreased libido, menstrual irregularities
SKIN: Rash, skin discoloration
Other: Weight loss

Overdose

Monitor patient for evidence of overdose, including coma, ECG changes, extrapyramidal reactions (such as muscle trembling, jerking, or stiffness), hypotension, respiratory depression, and seizures.

Maintain an open airway, institute continuous ECG monitoring and seizure precautions, and assess patient for prolonged QT interval and torsades de pointes. Be prepared to treat torsades de pointes with magnesium sulfate and correction of electrolyte imbalances, and anticipate possible cardiac pacing.

To decrease drug absorption, be prepared to perform gastric lavage. Be aware that vomiting shouldn't be induced because of the potential for dystonia and seizures. Expect to monitor patient for at least 4 days because pimozide has a long half-life.

To treat hypotension, administer albumin, I.V. fluids, plasma, or a vasopressor such as metaraminol, norepinephrine, or phenylephrine. Be aware that epinephrine shouldn't be used because it may cause paradoxical hypotension. Expect to treat seizures with diazepam, as prescribed. To manage dystonia, expect to administer benztropine or diphenhydramine.

Institute suicide precautions according to facility policy, and anticipate psychiatric re-evaluation.

Nursing Considerations

- **WARNING** Review patient's current and recent drug use to identify drugs that may interact with pimozide and cause life-threatening arrhythmias. As appropriate, discuss your findings with the prescriber.
- Pimozide shouldn't be used to treat simple tics because of the risk of severe cardiovascular or extrapyramidal effects.
- Don't administer pimozide with grapefruit juice because of risk of inhibiting metabolism of the drug.
- Obtain baseline ECG and periodic ECG tracings during therapy, especially during times of dosage adjustment, to assess patient for prolonged QT interval.
- Observe patient for evidence of tardive dyskinesia, such as wormlike tongue movements. Notify prescriber if these occur.
- Avoid stopping pimozide abruptly unless severe adverse reactions occur.
- Monitor patient for neuroleptic malignant syndrome, a rare but possibly fatal disorder that may occur with pimozide therapy. Signs and symptoms include altered mental status, arrhythmias, fever, and muscle rigidity.

PATIENT TEACHING
- Advise patient to take pimozide exactly as prescribed because of the cardiotoxic effects. Tell her not to abruptly stop taking the drug because withdrawal signs and symptoms may occur.
- Instruct patient not to take drug with grapefruit juice.
- Advise parent of a child taking pimozide that the drug should be taken at bedtime to minimize drowsiness and tiredness.
- Caution patient to rise slowly from a lying or sitting position to minimize effects of orthostatic hypotension.
- Urge patient not to drink alcohol during therapy.
- If sedation occurs, caution patient to avoid driving and other potentially hazardous activities.
- Suggest that patient use ice chips or sugarless gum or candy to relieve dry mouth.
- Instruct patient to report repetitive movements, tremor, and vision changes to her prescriber.

pralidoxime chloride
(2-PAM chloride, 2-pyridine aldoxime methochloride)

Protopam Chloride

Class and Category

Chemical class: Quaternary ammonium oxime
Therapeutic class: Anticholinesterase antidote
Pregnancy category: C

Indications and Dosages

▶ *As adjunct to reverse organophosphate pesticide toxicity*
I.V. INFUSION, I.M. OR SUBCUTANEOUS INJECTION

Adults. *Initial:* 1 to 2 g in 100 ml of normal saline solution infused over 15 to 30 min, given with atropine, 2 to 6 mg, every 5 to 60 min until muscarinic effects disappear; may be repeated in 1 hr and then every 3 to 8 hr if muscle weakness persists. If I.V. route isn't feasible, use I.M. or subcutaneous route.

Children. *Initial:* 20 mg/kg in 100 ml of normal saline solution infused over 15 to 30 min, given with atropine (dosage individualized). If muscle weakness persists, may be repeated in 1 hr and then every 3 to 8 hr. If I.V. route isn't feasible, use I.M. or subcutaneous route.

▶ *To treat anticholinesterase overdose secondary to myasthenic drugs (including ambenonium, neostigmine, and pyridostigmine)*
I.V. INJECTION

Adults. *Initial:* 1 to 2 g, followed by 250 mg every 5 min.

▶ *To treat exposure to nerve agents*
I.V. INJECTION

Adults. *Initial:* 1 atropine-containing autoinjector followed by 1 pralidoxime-containing autoinjector as soon as the effects of atropine are evident; both injections may be repeated every 15 min for 2 additional doses if nerve agent signs and symptoms persist.

DOSAGE ADJUSTMENT Dosage reduced for patients with renal insufficiency.

Route	Onset	Steady State	Peak	Half-Life	Duration
I.V., I.M.	Unknown	Unknown	Unknown	1 to 3 hr	Unknown

Contraindications

Hypersensitivity to pralidoxime chloride or its components

Mechanism of Action

Reverses muscle paralysis by removing the phosphoryl group from inhibited cholinesterase molecules at the neuromuscular junction of skeletal and respiratory muscles. Reactivation of cholinesterase restores the body's ability to metabolize acetylcholine, which is inhibited by the effects of organophosphate pesticides, anticholinesterase overdose, or nerve agent poisoning.

Interactions

DRUGS

aminophylline, morphine, phenothiazines, reserpine, succinylcholine, theophylline: Increased evidence of organophosphate poisoning
barbiturates: Potentiated barbiturate effects

Adverse Reactions

CNS: Dizziness, drowsiness, headache
CV: Increased systolic and diastolic blood pressure, tachycardia
EENT: Accommodation disturbances, blurred vision, diplopia
GI: Nausea, vomiting
MS: Muscle weakness
RESP: Hyperventilation
Other: Injection site pain

Overdose

Monitor patient for signs and symptoms of overdose, including accommodation disturbances, blurred vision, diplopia, dizziness, headache, nausea, and tachycardia. Keep in mind that it may be difficult to distinguish signs and symptoms of pralidoxime overdose from the adverse effects of the poison.

Maintain an open airway, be prepared to administer artificial respiration, and provide supportive and symptomatic care as needed.

Nursing Considerations

- Be aware that pralidoxime must be given within 36 hours of toxicity to be effective.
- Use drug with extreme caution in patients with myasthenia gravis who are being treated for organophosphate poisoning because pralidoxime may precipitate myasthenic crisis.
- Reconstitute drug according to manufacturer's guidelines and administration route.
- For intermittent infusion, further dilute with normal saline solution to a volume of 100 ml and infuse over 15 to 30 minutes.

- Avoid rapid administration, which may cause hypertension, laryngospasm, muscle spasms, neuromuscular blockade, and tachycardia. Also avoid intradermal injection.
- Closely monitor neuromuscular status during therapy.
- If patient has renal insufficiency, monitor BUN and serum creatinine levels, as appropriate, because pralidoxime is excreted in urine.
- When pralidoxime is administered with atropine, expect signs and symptoms of atropination—such as dry mouth and nose, flushing, mydriasis, and tachycardia—to occur earlier than might be expected when atropine is given alone.

PATIENT TEACHING
- Inform patient receiving I.M. pralidoxime that she'll experience pain at the injection site for 40 to 60 minutes afterward.
- Reassure patient that she'll be closely monitored throughout therapy.

pramipexole dihydrochloride
Mirapex

Class and Category
Chemical class: Benzothiazolamine derivative
Therapeutic class: Antidyskinetic
Pregnancy category: C

Indications and Dosages
▶ *To treat Parkinson's disease, with or without concurrent levodopa therapy*
TABLETS
Adults. *Initial:* 0.125 mg t.i.d. for 1 wk, increased weekly thereafter as follows: for week 2, 0.25 mg t.i.d.; for week 3, 0.5 mg t.i.d.; for week 4, 0.75 mg t.i.d.; for week 5, 1 mg t.i.d.; for week 6, 1.25 mg t.i.d.; and for week 7, 1.5 mg t.i.d. *Maintenance:* 1.5 to 4.5 mg daily in divided doses t.i.d. *Maximum:* 4.5 mg daily.
DOSAGE ADJUSTMENT For patients with renal impairment, dosage reduced as follows: for creatinine clearance of 35 to 59 ml/min/1.73 m^2, initial dose of 0.125 mg b.i.d. and maximum of 3 mg daily; for creatinine clearance of 15 to 34 ml/min/1.73 m^2, initial dose of 0.125 mg daily and maximum of 1.5 mg daily. Drug shouldn't be given to patients with creatinine clearance less than 15 ml/min/1.73 m^2.
▶ *To treat restless legs syndrome*

TABLETS

Adults. *Initial:* 0.125 mg once daily, 2 to 3 hours before bedtime. In 4 to 7 days, increased to 0.25 mg once daily, 2 to 3 hours before bedtime as needed. In 4 to 7 more days, further increased to 0.5 mg once daily, 2 to 3 hours before bedtime, as needed.

DOSAGE ADJUSTMENT For patients with moderate to severe renal impairment (creatinine clearance of 20 to 60 ml/min/ 1.73 m^2), dosage interval for titration increased to 14 days if needed.

Route	Onset	Steady State	Peak	Half-Life	Duration
P.O.	Unknown	2 days	Unknown	8 to 12 hr	Unknown

Mechanism of Action
May stimulate dopamine receptors in the brain, thereby easing signs and symptoms of Parkinson's disease, which may be caused by a dopamine deficiency.

Contraindications
Hypersensitivity to pramipexole or its components

Interactions
DRUGS

carbidopa, levodopa: Possibly increased peak blood levodopa level and potentiation of levodopa's dopaminergic adverse effects
cimetidine, diltiazem, quinidine, quinine, ranitidine, triamterene, verapamil: Decreased pramipexole clearance
CNS depressants: Additive sedative effects
haloperidol, metoclopramide, phenothiazines, thioxanthenes: Decreased pramipexole effectiveness

ACTIVITIES

alcohol use: Possibly additive sedative effects

Adverse Reactions
CNS: Amnesia, anxiety, asthenia, confusion, dream disturbances, drowsiness, dyskinesia, dystonia, fever, hallucinations, insomnia, malaise, paranoia, restlessness
CV: Edema, orthostatic hypotension
EENT: Diplopia, dry mouth, rhinitis, vision changes
GI: Anorexia, constipation, dysphagia, nausea
GU: Decreased libido, impotence, urinary frequency, urinary incontinence
MS: Arthralgia, myalgia, myasthenia

RESP: Pneumonia
SKIN: Diaphoresis, rash
Other: Weight loss

Overdose

Limited information is available about pramipexole overdose. Expect to provide supportive and symptomatic care, as needed. Maintain open airway, and institute continuous ECG monitoring. Be prepared to perform gastric lavage to decrease drug absorption. Expect to treat CNS stimulation with a phenothiazine or a butyrophenone antipsychotic drug, as prescribed.

Institute suicide precautions according to facility policy, and anticipate psychiatric re-evaluation.

Nursing Considerations

• Use pramipexole cautiously in patients with hallucinations, hypotension, or retinal problems (such as macular degeneration) because drug may exacerbate these conditions.
• Also use cautiously in patients with renal impairment because pramipexole elimination may be decreased.
• Take safety precautions according to facility policy until it's known how drug affects patient.
• Don't stop pramipexole therapy abruptly. Sudden withdrawal may cause a sign and symptom complex resembling neuroleptic malignant syndrome, consisting of hyperpyrexia, muscle rigidity, altered level of consciousness, and autonomic instability.

PATIENT TEACHING

• **WARNING Caution patient that she may suddenly fall asleep without warning while performing daily activities, such as driving, eating, or talking. Advise her to inform her prescriber if this occurs, and caution her against driving or performing hazardous activities.**
• Advise patient to take pramipexole with meals if nausea develops.
• Caution patient about possible dizziness or light-headedness, which may result from orthostatic hypotension. Advise her not to rise quickly from a lying or sitting position, to minimize these effects.
• Urge patient to avoid alcohol and other CNS depressants because they may increase sedation.
• Instruct patient to notify prescriber immediately about vision problems or urinary frequency or incontinence.
• Inform patient that improvement in motor performance and activities of daily living may take 2 to 3 weeks.

pregabalin
Lyrica

Class and Category
Chemical class: Structural derivative of gamma-aminobutyric acid
Therapeutic class: Analgesic, anticonvulsant
Pregnancy category: C

Indications and Dosages
▶ *To relieve neuropathic pain associated with diabetic peripheral neuropathy*
CAPSULES
Adults. *Initial:* 50 mg t.i.d., increased to 100 mg t.i.d. within 1 wk as needed.
▶ *To relieve postherpetic neuralgia; as adjunct therapy to manage partial onset seizures*
CAPSULES
Adults. *Initial:* 75 mg b.i.d. or 50 mg t.i.d., increased to 150 mg b.i.d. or 100 mg t.i.d. within 1 week as needed. Then increased to 300 mg b.i.d. or 200 mg t.i.d. in 2 to 4 weeks as needed.
▶ *To manage fibromyalgia*
CAPSULES
Adults. *Initial:* 75 mg b.i.d., increased to 150 mg b.i.d. in 1 wk, as needed, and then to 225 mg b.i.d. in 1 wk as needed. *Maximum:* 450 mg daily.
DOSAGE ADJUSTMENT If patient's creatinine clearance is 30 to 60 ml/min/1.73 m^2, daily dosage reduced by 50%. If creatinine clearance is 15 to 30 ml/min/1.73 m^2, daily dosage reduced by 75% and frequency reduced to daily or b.i.d. If creatinine clearance is less than 15 ml/min/1.73 m^2, daily dosage decreased to as low as 25 mg daily. If patient has hemodialysis, daily dosage is reduced and supplemental dose given immediately after every 4-hour hemodialysis session as follows: If reduced daily dosage is 25 mg daily, give supplemental dose of 25 to 50 mg. If reduced daily dosage is 25 to 50 mg daily, give supplemental dose of 50 to 75 mg. If reduced daily dosage is 75 mg, give supplemental dose of 100 to 150 mg.

Route	Onset	Peak	Duration
P.O.	Unknown	1.5 hr	Unknown

Contraindications
Hypersenstivity to pregabalin or its components

Mechanism of Action
Binds to the alpha$_2$-delta site, an auxiliary subunit of voltage calcium channels, in CNS tissue where it may reduce calcium-dependent release of several neurotransmitters, possibly by modulating calcium channel function. With fewer neurotransmitters present, pain sensation and seizure activity are reduced.

Interactions
DRUGS
angiotensin-converting enzyme inhibitors: Increased risk of pregabalin-induced angioedema
CNS depressants: Additive CNS effects such as somnolence
lorazepam, oxycodone: Additive effects on cognitive and gross motor function
thiazolidinedione antidiabetics: Possibly increased risk of peripheral edema and weight gain
ACTIVITIES
alcohol use: Additive effects on cognitive and gross motor function

Adverse Reactions
CNS: Abnormal gait, amnesia, anxiety, asthenia, ataxia, confusion, difficulty concentrating, dizziness, euphoria, extrapyramidal syndrome, fever, headache, hypertonia, hypesthesia, incoordination, intracranial hypertension, myoclonus, nervousness, neuropathy, paresthesia, psychotic depression, schizophrenic reaction, somnolence, stupor, tremor, twitching, vertigo
CV: Chest pain, heart failure, peripheral edema, ventricular fibrillation
EENT: Amblyopia, blurred vision, conjunctivitis, decreased visual acuity, diplopia, dry mouth, nystagmus, otitis media, tinnitus, visual field defect
ENDO: Hypoglycemia
GI: Abdominal pain, constipation, diarrhea, flatulence, gastroenteritis, gastrointestinal hemorrhage, increased appetite, nausea, vomiting
GU: Acute renal failure, anorgasmia; decreased libido; glomerulitis, impotence; nephritis; urinary frequency, incontinence, or retention
HEME: Decreased platelet count, leukopenia, thrombocytopenia

MS: Arthralgia, back pain, elevated creatine kinase levels, leg cramps, myalgia, myasthenia
RESP: Apnea, dyspnea
SKIN: Ecchymosis, exfoliative dermatitis, pruritus, Stevens-Johnson syndrome
Other: Anaphylaxis, angioedema, facial edema, hypersensitivity reaction, weight gain

Overdose

Pregabalin overdose has no specific antidote. Monitor patient for signs and symptoms of pregabalin overdose, which are similar to those experienced by patients receiving recommended doses of pregabalin.

Maintain an open airway, and monitor patient's vital signs closely and ECG continuously. Expect to induce vomiting or perform gastric lavage, as prescribed, to reduce amount of drug absorbed.

Be aware that hemodialysis may be helpful because it can clear about 50% of the drug from the body in 4 hours. Expect to give symptomatic and supportive care, as needed.

Institute suicide precautions according to facility policy, and anticipate psychiatric re-evaluation.

Nursing Considerations

• Be aware that pregabalin therapy should not be stopped abruptly but gradually over a minimum of 1 week to decrease the risk of seizure activity and avoid unpleasant symptoms such as diarrhea, headache, insomnia, and nausea.
• Monitor patient closely for adverse reactions, especially signs of hypersensitivity, such as skin redness, blisters, hives, rash, dyspnea, facial swelling, and wheezing. If present, discontinue drug immediately and notify prescriber. Be prepared to provide supportive care.

PATIENT TEACHING
• Warn patient not to stop taking pregabalin abruptly.
• Urge patient to avoid potentially hazardous activities until she knows how drug affects her.
• Instruct patient to notify prescriber if she has changes in vision or unexplained muscle pain, tenderness, or weakness, especially if these muscle symptoms are accompanied by malaise or fever.
• Alert patient that drug may cause edema and weight gain.
• If patient also takes a thiazolidinedione antidiabetic drug, tell her these effects may be intensified. If significant, tell patient to notify prescriber.

- Inform male patient who plans to father a child that pregabalin could impair his fertility.
- Instruct diabetic patients to inspect their skin while taking pregabalin.

primidone

Apo-Primidone (CAN), Myidone, Mysoline, PMS Primidone (CAN), Sertan (CAN)

Class and Category

Chemical class: Prodrug of phenobarbital
Therapeutic class: Anticonvulsant
Pregnancy category: Not rated

Indications and Dosages

▶ *To manage generalized tonic-clonic seizures, nocturnal myoclonic seizures, complex partial seizures, and simple partial seizures caused by epilepsy*

CHEWABLE TABLETS, ORAL SUSPENSION, TABLETS

Adults and children age 8 and over. *Initial:* 100 or 125 mg at bedtime for first 3 days; then increased to 100 or 125 mg b.i.d. for next 3 days, followed by 100 or 125 mg t.i.d. for next 3 days. On 10th day, expect to begin maintenance dosage as prescribed. *Maintenance:* 250 mg t.i.d. or q.i.d., adjusted as needed. *Maximum:* 2 g daily.

Children under age 8. *Initial:* 50 mg at bedtime for first 3 days; then increased to 50 mg b.i.d. for next 3 days, followed by 100 mg b.i.d. for next 3 days. On 10th day, begin maintenance dosage. *Maintenance:* 125 to 250 mg t.i.d., adjusted as needed.

Route	Onset	Steady State	Peak	Half-Life	Duration
P.O.	Unknown	Unknown	Unknown	3 to 23 hr*	Unknown

Mechanism of Action

Prevents seizures by decreasing the excitability of neurons and increasing the motor cortex's threshold of electrical stimulation. Primidone's active metabolites, phenobarbital and phenylethylmalonamide (PEMA), are synergistic and may add to the anticonvulsant action of the drug.

---

* 75 to 126 hr for phenobarbital metabolite and 10 to 25 hr for phenylethylmalonamide metabolite.

Contraindications

Hypersensitivity to primidone, phenobarbital, or their components; porphyria

Interactions

DRUGS

acetaminophen: Decreased acetaminophen effectiveness, increased risk of hepatotoxicity

adrenocorticoids, chloramphenicol, cyclosporine, dacarbazine, disopyramide, doxycycline, levothyroxine, metronidazole, mexiletine, oral anticoagulants, oral contraceptives (estrogen-containing), quinidine, tricyclic antidepressants: Decreased effectiveness of these drugs

amphetamines: Possibly delayed absorption of primidone

anticonvulsants: Possibly altered pattern of seizures

carbamazepine: Decreased effectiveness of primidone

carbonic anhydrase inhibitors: Increased risk of osteopenia

CNS depressants: Possibly enhanced CNS and respiratory depressant effects of both drugs

cyclophosphamide: Reduced half-life and increased leukopenic activity of cyclophosphamide

enflurane, halothane, methoxyflurane: Increased risk of hepatotoxicity; increased risk of nephrotoxicity (with methoxyflurane)

fenoprofen: Decreased elimination half-life of fenoprofen

folic acid: Increased folic acid requirements

griseofulvin: Decreased antifungal effects of griseofulvin

guanadrel, guanethidine: Possibly aggravated orthostatic hypotension

haloperidol, loxapine, maprotiline, molindone, phenothiazines, thioxanthenes: Possibly lowered seizure threshold and increased CNS depression

leucovorin: Possibly decreased anticonvulsant effects of primidone (with large doses)

MAO inhibitors: Possibly prolonged effects of primidone and altered pattern of seizures

methylphenidate: Possibly increased blood primidone level, resulting in toxicity

phenobarbital: Increased sedative effects of either drug, possibly altered pattern of seizures

phenylbutazone: Decreased primidone effectiveness, increased metabolism and decreased half-life of phenylbutazone

rifampin: Decreased blood primidone level

valproic acid: Increased blood primidone level, leading to increased CNS depression and neurotoxicity; decreased half-life of valproic

acid and enhanced risk of hepatotoxicity
vitamin D: Decreased effects of vitamin D
xanthines: Increased metabolism and clearance of xanthines (except dyphylline)
ACTIVITIES
alcohol use: Possibly increased CNS and respiratory depressant effects of primidone

Adverse Reactions

CNS: Ataxia, confusion, dizziness, drowsiness, excitement, mental changes, mood changes, restlessness
EENT: Diplopia, nystagmus
GI: Anorexia, nausea, vomiting
GU: Impotence
RESP: Dyspnea
Other: Folic acid deficiency

Overdose

Monitor patient for signs and symptoms of overdose, including absent or decreased reflexes, bradycardia, Cheyne-Stokes respirations, coma, confusion, dyspnea, fever, hypothermia, miosis or mydriasis, oliguria, primidone crystalluria, severe drowsiness, severe weakness, shock, slurred speech, staggering, tachycardia, and unusual eye movements. Consider chronic overdose if such signs and symptoms as continued irritability, insomnia, poor judgment, and severe confusion occur. Maintain open airway, and carefully monitor blood pressure and temperature.

If patient is conscious, be prepared to administer ipecac syrup, as prescribed, to induce vomiting. Expect to administer activated charcoal, 30 to 60 g, with water or sorbitol to prevent further absorption and to enhance drug elimination. For an unconscious patient, anticipate assisting with the insertion of an endotracheal tube and then performing gastric lavage. The inflated cuff of the endotracheal tube will help prevent aspiration of gastric contents into the lungs.

Be prepared to give a urine-alkalizing drug to increase drug elimination. Give I.V. fluids and a vasopressor, as prescribed. For severe cases, anticipate the need for hemodialysis or hemoperfusion. Be aware that, in cases of extreme primidone overdose, the patient may have a flat EEG because all electrical activity in the brain has ceased; however, this effect may be reversible.

Institute suicide precautions according to facility policy, and anticipate psychiatric re-evaluation.

Nursing Considerations

• Monitor blood levels of primidone and phenobarbital (its active metabolite), as ordered, to determine therapeutic level or detect toxic levels.

• Anticipate that drug may cause confusion, excitement, or mood changes in elderly patients and children.

• Assess patient for evidence of folic acid deficiency, including mental dysfunction, neuropathy, tiredness, and weakness.

PATIENT TEACHING

• Instruct patient to crush primidone tablets and mix them with foods or fluids, as needed.

• Advise patient taking oral suspension to shake the bottle well and measure doses with a calibrated device.

• Suggest that patient take drug with meals to minimize adverse GI reactions.

• Urge patient not to stop taking primidone abruptly because doing so can precipitate seizures.

• Caution patient about possible decreased alertness.

• Tell her to avoid hazardous activities until drug effects are clear.

• Urge patient to avoid alcohol and other CNS depressants during primidone therapy.

prochlorperazine
Compazine, Stemetil (CAN)

prochlorperazine edisylate
Compazine

prochlorperazine maleate
Compazine, Compazine Spansule, Nu-Prochlor (CAN), Stemetil (CAN)

Class and Category
Chemical class: Piperazine phenothiazine
Therapeutic class: Antianxiety drug, antipsychotic drug
Pregnancy category: Not rated

Indications and Dosages
▶ *To manage psychotic disorders, such as schizophrenia*
ORAL SOLUTION (PROCHLORPERAZINE EDISYLATE)
Adults and adolescents. 5 to 10 mg t.i.d. or q.i.d., increased gradually every 2 to 3 days, as needed and tolerated. *Maximum:* 150 mg daily.
Children ages 2 to 12. 2.5 mg b.i.d. or t.i.d. *Maximum:* On day

1, 10 mg for all children; thereafter, 25 mg daily for children ages 6 to 12, 20 mg daily for children ages 2 to 6.

TABLETS (PROCHLORPERAZINE MALEATE)

Adults and adolescents. 5 to 10 mg t.i.d. or q.i.d., increased gradually every 2 to 3 days, as needed and tolerated. *Maximum:* 150 mg daily.

I.M. INJECTION (PROCHLORPERAZINE EDISYLATE)

Adults and adolescents. *Initial:* 10 to 20 mg, repeated every 2 to 4 hr, as prescribed, to bring symptoms under control (usually 3 to 4 doses). *Maintenance:* 10 to 20 mg every 4 to 6 hr. *Maximum:* 200 mg daily.

Children ages 2 to 12. 132 mcg/kg/dose on day 1, then increased as needed. *Maximum:* On day 1, give 10 mg for all children; thereafter, 25 mg daily for children ages 6 to 12 and 20 mg daily for children ages 2 to 6.

SUPPOSITORIES (PROCHLORPERAZINE)

Adults and adolescents. 10 mg t.i.d. or q.i.d., increased by 5 to 10 mg every 2 to 3 days, as needed and tolerated.

Children ages 2 to 12. 2.5 mg b.i.d or t.i.d. *Maximum:* On day 1, give 10 mg for all children; thereafter, 25 mg daily for children ages 6 to 12 and 20 mg daily for children ages 2 to 6.

▶ *To provide short-term treatment of anxiety*

E.R. CAPSULES (PROCHLORPERAZINE MALEATE)

Adults and adolescents. 15 mg daily in the morning, or 10 mg every 12 hr. *Maximum:* 20 mg daily for no longer than 12 wk.

ORAL SOLUTION, TABLETS (PROCHLORPERAZINE EDISYLATE)

Adults and adolescents. 5 mg t.i.d. or q.i.d. *Maximum:* 20 mg daily for no longer than 12 wk.

DOSAGE ADJUSTMENT Initial dose usually reduced and subsequent dosage increased more gradually for elderly, emaciated, and debilitated patients.

Route	Onset	Steady State	Peak	Half-Life	Duration
P.O., I.M., P.R.	Up to several wk	4 to 7 days	Up to 6 mo	Unknown	Unknown

Incompatibilities

Don't mix prochlorperazine in same syringe with other drugs. A precipitate may form when prochlorperazine edisylate is mixed in same syringe with morphine sulfate.

Contraindications

Age less than 2 years, blood dyscrasias, bone marrow depression, cerebral arteriosclerosis, coma, coronary artery disease, hepatic dysfunction, hypersensitivity to phenothiazines, myeloproliferative disorders, pediatric surgery, severe CNS depression, severe hypertension or hypotension, subcortical brain damage, use of large quantities of CNS depressants, weight less than 9 kg (20 lb)

Mechanism of Action

Alleviates signs and symptoms of psychosis by possibly blocking postsynaptic dopamine$_2$ (D$_2$) receptors, depressing the release of selected hormones, and producing an alpha-adrenergic blocking effect in the brain.

Anticholinergic effects and alpha-adrenergic blockade reduce anxiety by decreasing arousal and filtering internal stimuli to the brain stem reticular activating system.

Interactions
DRUGS

antacids (aluminum- or magnesium-containing), antidiarrheals (adsorbent): Possibly inhibited absorption of oral prochlorperazine
amantadine, anticholinergics, antidyskinetics, antihistamines: Possibly intensified anticholinergic adverse effects, increased risk of prochlorperazine-induced hyperpyretic effect
amphetamines: Decreased stimulant effect of amphetamines, decreased antipsychotic effect of prochlorperazine
anticonvulsants: Lowered seizure threshold
antithyroid drugs: Increased risk of agranulocytosis
apomorphine: Possibly decreased emetic response to apomorphine, additive CNS depression
appetite suppressants: Possibly antagonized anorectic effect of appetite suppressants (except for phenmetrazine)
beta blockers: Increased risk of additive hypotensive effects, irreversible retinopathy, arrhythmias, and tardive dyskinesia
bromocriptine: Decreased effectiveness of bromocriptine
cisapride, disopyramide, erythromycin, pimozide, probucol, procainamide: Additive QT-interval prolongation, increased risk of ventricular tachycardia
CNS depressants: Additive CNS depression
dopamine: Possibly antagonized peripheral vasoconstriction (with high doses of dopamine)
ephedrine, epinephrine: Decreased vasopressor effects of these drugs
hepatotoxic drugs: Increased incidence of hepatotoxicity

hypotension-producing drugs: Possibly severe hypotension with syncope
levodopa: Inhibited antidyskinetic effect of levodopa
lithium: Reduced absorption of oral prochlorperazine, increased excretion of lithium, increased extrapyramidal effects, possibly masking of early signs and symptoms of lithium toxicity
MAO inhibitors, maprotiline, tricyclic antidepressants: Possibly prolonged and intensified anticholinergic and sedative effects, increased blood antidepressant levels, inhibited prochlorperazine metabolism, and increased risk of neuroleptic malignant syndrome
mephentermine: Possibly antagonized antipsychotic effect of prochlorperazine and vasopressor effect of mephentermine
metrizamide: Increased risk of seizures
opioid analgesics: Increased risk of CNS and respiratory depression, orthostatic hypotension, severe constipation, and urine retention
ototoxic drugs: Possibly masking of some symptoms of ototoxicity, such as dizziness, tinnitus, and vertigo
phenytoin: Possibly inhibited phenytoin metabolism and increased risk of phenytoin toxicity
thiazide diuretics: Possibly potentiated hyponatremia and water intoxication
ACTIVITIES
alcohol use: Additive CNS depression

Adverse Reactions
CNS: Akathisia, altered temperature regulation, dizziness, drowsiness, extrapyramidal reactions (such as dystonia, pseudoparkinsonism, tardive dyskinesia)
CV: Hypotension, orthostatic hypotension, tachycardia
EENT: Blurred vision, dry mouth, nasal congestion, ocular changes, pigmentary retinopathy
ENDO: Galactorrhea, gynecomastia
GI: Constipation, epigastric pain, nausea, vomiting
GU: Dysuria, ejaculation disorders, menstrual irregularities, urine retention
SKIN: Decreased sweating, photosensitivity, pruritus, rash
Other: Weight gain

Overdose
Monitor patient for signs and symptoms of overdose, including agitation, areflexia or hyperreflexia, arrhythmias, blurred vision, cardiac arrest, coma, confusion, disorientation, drowsiness, dry mouth, dyspnea, heart failure, hyperpyrexia, hypotension, hy-

pothermia, mydriasis, pulmonary edema, QRS complex changes, respiratory depression, seizures, shock, stupor, tachycardia, ventricular fibrillation, and vomiting.

Maintain an open airway, monitor patient for arrhythmias, and maintain temperature. Institute seizure precautions according to facility protocol. Perform gastric lavage, and administer activated charcoal, as prescribed. Expect to administer saline cathartic if patient ingested E.R. form. Be aware that vomiting shouldn't be induced because of the potential for impaired consciousness or dystonic reactions of the head and neck.

To treat arrhythmias, don't administer any drug that may prolong the QT interval—such as disopyramide, procainamide, and quinidine—because these drugs may have an additive effect with prochlorperazine. Expect to administer phenytoin to control arrhythmias and norepinephrine or phenylephrine and I.V. fluids to treat hypotension, as prescribed. Epinephrine shouldn't be used because of risk of paradoxical hypotension. Anticipate digitalizing patient for heart failure, as prescribed. Expect to treat electrolyte imbalance and maintain acid-base balance, as prescribed. To manage seizures, expect to administer diazepam, followed by phenytoin. Avoid giving a barbiturate because it may potentiate CNS and respiratory depression.

Anticipate administering benztropine or diphenhydramine, as prescribed, to manage acute dyskinetic effects. Dialysis is ineffective for treating phenothiazine overdose. Expect to continue ECG monitoring for at least 5 days and to treat patient who has overdosed on E.R. form for as long as signs and symptoms persist. Be aware that phenothiazine tablets are visible on X-ray.

Institute suicide precautions according to facility policy, and anticipate psychiatric re-evaluation.

Nursing Considerations

- Avoid contact between skin and solution forms of prochlorperazine because contact dermatitis could result.
- Inject I.M. form slowly and deeply into upper outer quadrant of buttocks. Keep patient lying down for 30 minutes after injection to minimize hypotensive effects.
- Rotate I.M. injection sites to prevent irritation and sterile abscesses.
- Protect prochlorperazine from light.
- Be aware that parenteral solution may develop a slight yellowing but that such discoloring doesn't affect potency. Don't use if discoloration is pronounced or precipitate is present.

- Expect antipsychotic effects to occur in 2 to 3 weeks, although the range is days to months.
- **WARNING** Because drug has numerous serious adverse effects, monitor patient closely.
- Be aware that adverse reactions may occur for up to 12 weeks after E.R. capsules have been discontinued.

PATIENT TEACHING

- Instruct patient to take prochlorperazine with food or a full glass of milk or water to minimize GI distress.
- Advise patient to swallow E.R. capsules whole, not to crush or chew them.
- Instruct patient using a suppository to refrigerate it for 30 minutes or hold it under running cold water before removing the wrapper if it softens during storage.
- Teach patient how to correctly administer the suppository form.
- Caution patient receiving long-term therapy not to stop taking prochlorperazine abruptly because doing so may lead to such adverse reactions as nausea, trembling, and vomiting.
- Urge patient to avoid alcohol and OTC drugs that may contain CNS depressants.
- Advise patient to rise slowly from lying and sitting positions, to minimize effects of orthostatic hypotension.
- Urge patient to avoid potentially hazardous activities because of the risk of drowsiness and impaired judgment and coordination.
- Instruct patient to avoid excessive sun exposure and to wear sunscreen when outdoors.
- Urge patient to notify prescriber about involuntary movements and restlessness.
- Inform patient that adverse reactions may occur for up to 12 weeks after discontinuing E.R. capsules.

Other Therapeutic Uses

Prochlorperazine is also indicated for the following:
- To control nausea and vomiting related to surgery
- To control severe nausea and vomiting

procyclidine hydrochloride

Kemadrin, PMS-Procyclidine (CAN), Procyclid (CAN)

Class and Category

Chemical class: Synthetic tertiary amine
Therapeutic class: Antidyskinetic
Pregnancy category: C

Indications and Dosages

▶ *To treat parkinsonism*
ELIXIR, TABLETS
Adults and adolescents. *Initial:* 2.5 mg t.i.d. after meals; may be increased gradually to 5 mg t.i.d., as needed. If needed, a fourth dose of 5 mg may be given at bedtime.

▶ *To treat drug-induced extrapyramidal signs and symptoms*
ELIXIR, TABLETS
Adults and adolescents. *Initial:* 2.5 mg t.i.d.; dosage increased in daily increments of 2.5 mg, as needed and tolerated.

Route	Onset	Steady State	Peak	Half-Life	Duration
P.O.	Unknown	Unknown	Unknown	Unknown	4 hr

Mechanism of Action

Competes with acetylcholine to block muscarinic cholinergic receptors in the CNS, which may decrease salivation and relax smooth muscle. Procyclidine also may block dopamine reuptake and storage in CNS cells, thus prolonging dopamine's effects.

Contraindications

Achalasia, angle-closure glaucoma, bladder neck obstructions, hypersensitivity to procyclidine or its components, megacolon, myasthenia gravis, prostatic hyperplasia, pyloric or duodenal obstruction, stenosing peptic ulcers

Interactions

DRUGS
amantadine, other anticholinergics, MAO inhibitors: Additive anticholinergic effects
antidiarrheals (adsorbent): Decreased therapeutic effect of procyclidine
carbidopa-levodopa, levodopa: Potentiated dopaminergic effects of levodopa
chlorpromazine: Decreased blood chlorpromazine level
CNS depressants: Increased sedative effects
digoxin: Increased risk of digitalis toxicity
haloperidol: Possibly worsening of schizophrenic signs and symptoms, decreased blood haloperidol level, tardive dyskinesia
ACTIVITIES
alcohol use: Increased sedative effects

Adverse Reactions

CNS: Drowsiness, euphoria, headache, memory loss, nervousness, paresthesia, unusual excitement
CV: Orthostatic hypotension, tachycardia
EENT: Blurred vision; dry mouth, nose, or throat
GI: Constipation, indigestion, nausea, vomiting
GU: Dysuria
MS: Muscle cramps
SKIN: Decreased sweating, photosensitivity

Overdose

Monitor patient for evidence of overdose, including clumsiness; dyspnea; hallucinations; insomnia; seizures; severe drowsiness; severe dryness of mouth, nose, or throat; tachycardia; toxic psychoses; unsteadiness; and unusually dry, flushed, warm skin.

Maintain open airway, monitor vital signs, and institute seizure precautions according to facility protocol. Expect to induce vomiting or perform gastric lavage to decrease absorption of drug, as prescribed, except in patients who may be convulsive, precomatose, or psychotic. If the patient is an adult, expect to administer physostigmine salicylate, 1 to 2 mg, I.M. or I.V., repeated in 2 hours, as needed, to reverse cardiovascular and CNS toxic effects. Be prepared to administer a short-acting barbiturate or diazepam, as prescribed, to control excitement. Pilocarpine 0.5% may be prescribed to treat mydriasis.

Institute suicide precautionary measures according to facility policy, and anticipate psychiatric re-evaluation.

Nursing Considerations

- Use procyclidine cautiously in patients with cardiac disorders because of drug's anticholinergic effects. Frequently monitor blood pressure and heart rate and rhythm.
- Monitor patient for drug abuse because procyclidine provides a false sense of well-being that may tempt patient to abuse it.

PATIENT TEACHING

- Instruct patient to take procyclidine after meals to minimize GI distress.
- Advise patient to avoid alcohol and OTC drugs that may contain CNS depressants because of potential for drug interactions.
- Urge patient to avoid potentially hazardous activities because of risk of drowsiness and reduced alertness.
- Caution patient not to stop taking procyclidine abruptly because doing so may cause sudden adverse reactions.

- If patient reports dry mouth, suggest sugarless hard candy or gum and increased fluid intake.
- Inform patient that exercise and increased fluid intake can help prevent constipation.
- Urge patient to avoid extreme temperatures because procyclidine may decrease sweating, thereby increasing the risk of heatstroke. Also, advise her to wear sunscreen when outdoors.
- If patient wears contact lenses, explain that drug may increase lens awareness or blur vision. Suggest using artificial tears.
- Instruct patient to notify prescriber about adverse reactions.

promethazine hydrochloride

Anergan 25, Anergan 50, Antinaus 50, Histantil (CAN), Pentazine, Phenazine 25, Phenazine 50, Phencen-50, Phenergan, Phenergan Fortis, Phenergan Plain, Phenerzine, Phenoject-50, Pro-50, Promacot, Pro-Med 50, Promet, Prorex-25, Prorex-50, Prothazine, Shogan, V-Gan-25, V-Gan-50

Class and Category

Chemical class: Phenothiazine derivative
Therapeutic class: Sedative-hypnotic
Pregnancy category: C

Indications and Dosages

▶ *To provide nighttime sedation*
SYRUP, TABLETS
Adults and adolescents. 25 to 50 mg at bedtime. *Maximum:* 150 mg daily.
Children age 2 and over. 0.5 to 1 mg/kg or 10 to 25 mg at bedtime.
I.V. INJECTION
Adults and adolescents. 25 to 50 mg at bedtime.
I.M. INJECTION, SUPPOSITORIES
Adults and adolescents. 25 to 50 mg at bedtime.
Children age 2 and over. 0.5 to 1 mg/kg or 12.5 to 25 mg at bedtime.
DOSAGE ADJUSTMENT Dosage usually decreased for elderly patients.

Contraindications

Angle-closure glaucoma; benign prostatic hyperplasia; bladder neck obstruction; bone marrow depression; breast-feeding; children under age 2; coma; hypersensitivity or history of an idiosyn-

cratic reaction to promethazine, its components, or other phenothiazines; hypertensive crisis; lower respiratory tract disorders, including asthma, when used as an antihistamine; pyloroduodenal
obstruction; stenosing peptic ulcer; use of large quantities of a
CNS depressant

Route	Onset	Steady State	Peak	Half-Life	Duration
P.O.	15 to 60 min	Unknown	Unknown	Unknown	4 to 6 hr
I.V.	3 to 5 min	Unknown	Unknown	9 to 16 hr	4 to 6 hr
I.M., P.R.	20 min	Unknown	Unknown	6 to 13 hr*	4 to 6 hr

Mechanism of Action
Crosses the blood-brain barrier and causes sedation and relief of anxiety by
blocking histaminergic receptors in the CNS and acting as an antagonist at
other receptor sites. The sedative effects of promethazine are also related to
its ability to indirectly reduce stimuli to the reticular activating system.

Interactions
DRUGS
amphetamines: Decreased stimulant effect of amphetamines
anticholinergics: Possibly intensified anticholinergic adverse effects
anticonvulsants: Lowered seizure threshold
appetite suppressants: Possibly antagonized anorectic effect of appetite suppressants
beta blockers: Increased risk of additive hypotensive effects, irreversible retinopathy, arrhythmias, and tardive dyskinesia
bromocriptine: Decreased effectiveness of bromocriptine
CNS depressants: Additive CNS depression
dopamine: Possibly antagonized peripheral vasoconstriction (with
high doses of dopamine)
ephedrine, metaraminol, methoxamine: Decreased vasopressor response to these drugs
epinephrine: Blocked alpha-adrenergic effects of epinephrine, increased risk of hypotension
guanadrel, guanethidine: Decreased antihypertensive effects of these
drugs
hepatotoxic drugs: Increased risk of hepatotoxicity
hypotension-producing drugs: Possibly severe hypotension with
syncope

* For I.M. dosage form.

levodopa: Inhibited antidyskinetic effects of levodopa
MAO inhibitors: Possibly prolonged and intensified anticholinergic and CNS depressant effects of promethazine
metrizamide: Increased risk of seizures
ototoxic drugs: Possibly masking of some signs and symptoms of ototoxicity, such as dizziness, tinnitus, and vertigo
quinidine: Additive cardiac effects
riboflavin: Increased riboflavin requirements
ACTIVITIES
alcohol use: Additive CNS depression

Adverse Reactions

CNS: Akathisia, CNS stimulation, confusion, dizziness, drowsiness, dystonia, euphoria, excitation, faintness, fatigue, hallucinations, hysteria, incoordination, insomnia, irritability, nervousness, neuroleptic malignant syndrome, paradoxical stimulation, pseudoparkinsonism, restlessness, sedation, seizures, somnolence, tardive dyskinesia, tremors
CV: Bradycardia, hypotension, hypertension, tachycardia
EENT: Blurred vision; diplopia; dry mouth, nose, and throat; nasal stuffiness; tinnitus; vision changes
ENDO: Hyperglycemia
GI: Anorexia, cholestatic jaundice, ileus, nausea, rectal burning or stinging (suppository form), vomiting
GU: Dysuria
HEME: Agranulocytosis, leukopenia, thrombocytopenia, thrombocytopenic purpura
RESP: Apnea, respiratory depression, tenacious bronchial secretions
SKIN: Dermatitis, diaphoresis, photosensitivity, rash, urticaria
Other: Angioneurotic edema, paradoxical reactions

Overdose

Monitor patient for signs and symptoms of overdose, including clumsiness; drowsiness; dry mouth, nose, or throat; dyspnea; facial flushing; hallucinations; hypotension; insomnia; muscle spasms of the back and neck; restlessness; seizures; tremor; and unconsciousness.

Maintain an open airway, administer oxygen as needed, and monitor vital signs. Institute seizure precautions according to facility protocol. To decrease drug absorption, expect to perform gastric lavage with 0.45NS and then give a saline cathartic, such as milk of magnesia, to enhance elimination. Be aware that vomiting shouldn't be induced because of the potential for impaired consciousness, seizures, and dystonic reactions of the head and neck.

Expect to treat hypotension with I.V. fluids, Trendelenburg positioning, or a vasopressor such as levarterenol or phenylephrine. Epinephrine shouldn't be used because of risk of paradoxical hypotension. Anticipate administering diphenhydramine or a barbiturate to treat extrapyramidal reactions. Stimulants shouldn't be used because of the risk of seizures. Dialysis is ineffective for treating promethazine overdose.

Institute suicide precautions according to facility policy, and anticipate psychiatric re-evaluation.

Nursing Considerations

- Use promethazine cautiously in children because they may be more sensitive to drug's effects, especially respiratory effects that may result in life-threatening respiratory depression and apnea regardless of weight-calculated dosage. In addition, use cautiously in elderly patients and patients with cardiovascular disease or hepatic dysfunction because of potential adverse effects.
- Also use drug cautiously in patients with asthma because of its anticholinergic effects and in patients with seizure disorders or who take medication that may affect seizure threshold because drug may lower patient's seizure threshold.
- Inject I.M. form deep into large muscle mass, and rotate injection sites.
- **WARNING** Avoid inadvertent intra-arterial injection of promethazine because it can cause arteriospasm; gangrene may develop from impaired circulation.
- Administer I.V. injection at a rate not to exceed 25 mg/minute; rapid I.V. administration may produce a transient fall in blood pressure.
- **WARNING** Monitor respiratory function because drug may suppress cough reflex and cause thickening of bronchial secretions, aggravating such conditions as asthma, chronic bronchitis, and emphysema. Although uncommon, it may depress respirations to the point of apnea.
- Monitor patient's hematologic status as ordered because promethazine may cause bone marrow depression, especially when used with other known marrow-toxic agents. Assess patient for signs and symptoms of infection or bleeding.
- **WARNING** Monitor patient for signs and symptoms of neuroleptic malignant syndrome, such as fever, hypertension or

hypotension, involuntary motor activity, mental changes, muscle rigidity, tachycardia, and tachypena. Be prepared to provide supportive treatment and additional drug therapy, as prescribed.
• Be aware that patient shouldn't undergo intradermal allergen tests within 72 hours of receiving promethazine because drug may significantly alter flare response.

PATIENT TEACHING
• Instruct patient to use a calibrated measuring device when using promethazine syrup, to ensure accurate dose.
• Teach patient how to correctly administer the suppository form, if necessary.
• Advise patient to avoid OTC drugs unless approved by prescriber.
• Instruct patient to notify prescriber immediately if she experiences involuntary movements and restlessness.
• Urge patient to avoid alcohol and other CNS depressants while taking promethazine.
• Instruct patient to avoid potentially hazardous activities until she knows how the drug affects her.
• Suggest that patient relieve dry mouth with frequent rinsing and use of sugarless gum or hard candy.
• Advise patient to avoid excessive sun exposure and to use sunscreen when outdoors.

Other Therapeutic Uses
Promethazine hydrochloride is also indicated for the following:
• To prevent or treat motion sickness
• To treat vertigo
• To prevent or treat nausea and vomiting associated with certain types of anesthesia and surgery
• To treat signs and symptoms of allergic response
• To provide preoperative or postoperative sedation
• To relieve apprehension and promote sleep the night before surgery
• To provide obstetrical sedation

propofol
(disoprofol)
Diprivan

Class and Category
Chemical class: 2,6-diisopropylphenol derivative

Therapeutic class: Sedative-hypnotic
Pregnancy category: B

▶ *To provide sedation for critically ill patients in intensive care*
I.V. INFUSION
Adults. 2.8 to 130 mcg/kg/min. *Usual:* 27 mcg/kg/min.
DOSAGE ADJUSTMENT For elderly, debilitated, or ASA-PS III or IV patients, induction dose is decreased and maintenance rate of administration is slower.

Route	Onset	Steady State	Peak	Half-Life	Duration
I.V.	Within 40 sec	Unknown	Unknown	3 to 12 hr*	3 to 5 min

Mechanism of Action

Decreases cerebral blood flow, cerebral metabolic oxygen consumption, and intracranial pressure and increases cerebrovascular resistance, which may play a role in propofol's hypnotic effects.

Incompatibilities

Don't mix propofol with other drugs before administering it. Don't administer propofol through same I.V. line as blood or plasma products because globular component of emulsion will aggregate.

Contraindications

Hypersensitivity to propofol or its components, to eggs or egg products, or to soybeans or soy products

Interactions

DRUGS
CNS depressants: Additive CNS depressant, respiratory depressant, and hypotensive effects; possibly decreased emetic effects of opioids
droperidol: Possibly decreased control of nausea and vomiting
ACTIVITIES
alcohol use: Additive CNS depressant, respiratory depressant, and hypotensive effects

Adverse Reactions

CV: Bradycardia, hypotension
GI: Nausea, vomiting
MS: Involuntary muscle movements (transient)

---

* For terminal phase; however, 70% of the drug is eliminated in 30 to 60 min.

RESP: Apnea

Other: Anaphylaxis; injection site burning, pain, or stinging

Overdose

Propofol overdose may cause cardiovascular and respiratory depression, characterized by apnea, bradycardia, and hypotension. If overdose occurs, discontinue propofol infusion immediately. Be prepared to treat respiratory depression with artificial ventilation and oxygen. Expect to treat cardiovascular depression by administering I.V. fluids, placing the patient in Trendelenburg's position, and administering a vasopressor or anticholinergic.

Nursing Considerations

* Use propofol cautiously in patients with cardiac disease, peripheral vascular disease, impaired cerebral circulation, or increased intracranial pressure because the drug may aggravate these disorders.
* To dilute drug, use only D_5W to yield 2 mg/ml or more.
* Consult prescriber about pretreating injection site with 1 ml of 1% lidocaine to minimize pain, burning, or stinging from propofol. (However, be aware that lidocaine shouldn't be added to propofol solution at more than 20 mg/200 mg propofol because emulsion may become unstable.) Giving drug through a larger vein in the forearm or antecubital fossa may also minimize injection site discomfort.
* Shake vial well before using, and give drug promptly after opening. Use vial for only one patient. Use prefilled syringes within 6 hours of opening.
* Use a drop counter, syringe pump, or volumetric pump to safely control infusion rate. Don't infuse drug through filter with a pore size of less than 5 microns because doing so could cause emulsion to break down.
* Discard all unused portions of propofol solution as well as reservoirs, I.V. tubing, and solutions immediately after or within 12 hours of administration (6 hours if propofol was transferred from original container) to prevent bacterial growth in stagnant solution. Also, protect solution from light.
* Expect patient to recover from sedation within 8 minutes.
* **WARNING** Esepcially in patients receiving prolonged high-dose infusions, watch for propofol infusion syndrome, which may cause severe metabolic acidosis, hyperkalemia, lipemia, rhabdomyolysis, hepatomegaly, and cardiac and renal failure. Alert prescriber immediately, and be prepared to provide emergency supportive care as ordered.

PATIENT TEACHING
• Encourage patient and family to voice concerns and ask questions before propofol administration.
• Reassure patient that she'll be closely monitored throughout drug administration and that her vital functions, including breathing, will be supported as needed.

Other Therapeutic Uses
Propofol is also indicated for the following:
• To induce or maintain anesthesia

propranolol hydrochloride
Apo-Propranolol (CAN), Detensol (CAN), Inderal, Inderal LA, Novopranol (CAN), pms Propranolol (CAN)

Class and Category
Chemical class: Beta blocker
Therapeutic class: Antimigraine drug, antitremor drug
Pregnancy category: C

Indications and Dosages
▶ *To control tremor*
ORAL SOLUTION, TABLETS
Adults. *Initial:* 40 mg b.i.d., adjusted as needed and prescribed. *Maximum:* 320 mg daily.
▶ *To prevent vascular migraine headaches*
E.R. TABLETS
Adults. *Initial:* 80 mg daily, increased gradually, as needed. *Maximum:* 240 mg daily.
ORAL SOLUTION, TABLETS
Adults. *Initial:* 20 mg q.i.d., increased gradually, as needed. *Maximum:* 240 mg daily.
DOSAGE ADJUSTMENT Dosage increased or decreased for elderly patients, depending on sensitivity to propranolol.

Route	Onset	Steady State	Peak	Half-Life	Duration
P.O.	Unknown	Unknown	1 to 1.5 hr	3 to 5 hr	Unknown
E.R.	Unknown	Unknown	Unknown	8 to 11 hr	Unknown

Contraindications
Asthma, cardiogenic shock, greater than first-degree AV block, heart failure (unless secondary to tachyarrhythmia that's responsive to propranolol), hypersensitivity to propranolol or its components, sinus bradycardia

---

Mechanism of Action

May prevent migraine headaches by inhibiting vasodilation of the blood vessels in the brain and arteriolar spasms in the cortex. Propranolol's antitremor effect may be related to the drug's ability to block peripheral beta$_2$ receptors, causing a reduction in the amplitude of the tremor.

Interactions

DRUGS

allergen immunotherapy, allergenic extracts for skin testing: Increased risk of serious systemic adverse reactions or anaphylaxis

amiodarone: Additive depressant effects on conduction, negative inotropic effects

anesthetics (hydrocarbon inhalation): Increased risk of myocardial depression and hypotension

beta blockers: Additive beta blockade effects

calcium channel blockers, clonidine, diazoxide, guanabenz, reserpine, other hypotension-producing drugs: Additive hypotensive effect and, possibly, other beta blockade effects

cimetidine: Possibly interference with propranolol clearance

estrogens: Decreased antihypertensive effect of propranolol

fentanyl, fentanyl derivatives: Possibly increased risk of initial bradycardia after induction doses of fentanyl or a derivative (with long-term propranolol use)

glucagon: Possibly blunted hyperglycemic response

insulin, oral antidiabetic drugs: Possibly impaired glucose control, masking of tachycardia in response to hypoglycemia

lidocaine: Decreased lidocaine clearance, increased risk of lidocaine toxicity

MAO inhibitors: Increased risk of significant hypertension

neuromuscular blockers: Possibly potentiated and prolonged action of these drugs

NSAIDs: Possibly decreased hypotensive effects

phenothiazines: Increased blood levels of both drugs

propafenone: Increased blood level and half-life of propranolol

sympathomimetics, xanthines: Possibly mutual inhibition of therapeutic effects

ACTIVITIES

nicotine chewing gum, smoking cessation, smoking deterrents: Increased therapeutic effects of propranolol

Adverse Reactions

CNS: Anxiety, depression, dizziness, drowsiness, fatigue, fever, insomnia, lethargy, nervousness, weakness
CV: AV conduction disorders, cold extremities, heart failure, hypotension, sinus bradycardia
EENT: Laryngospasm, nasal congestion, pharyngitis, sore throat
GI: Abdominal pain, constipation, diarrhea, nausea, vomiting
GU: Sexual dysfunction
HEME: Agranulocytosis
MS: Muscle weakness
RESP: Bronchospasm, dyspnea, respiratory distress, wheezing
SKIN: Erythema multiforme, erythematous rash, exfoliative dermatitis, Stevens-Johnson syndrome, toxic epidermal necrolysis, urticaria
Other: Anaphylaxis, flulike syndrome

Overdose

Monitor patient for signs and symptoms of overdose, including bluish discoloration of the nail beds and palms of the hands, bradycardia, dizziness, dyspnea, hypotension, irregular heartbeat, seizures, and syncope. Maintain an open airway, and institute continuous ECG monitoring and seizure precautions according to facility protocol. Be prepared to perform gastric lavage, followed by the administration of activated charcoal.

To treat bradycardia that occurs with hypotension, administer atropine or glucagon, as prescribed. Expect to administer a catecholamine—such as dobutamine, dopamine, epinephrine, isoproterenol, or norepinephrine—to give chronotropic and inotropic support and also to treat hypotension. Calcium chloride may be effective in improving myocardial contractility because overdose with propranolol may cause hypocalcemia. Keep in mind that transvenous pacing may be needed for heart block.

If the patient develops pulmonary edema or cardiac failure, anticipate the use of digoxin, furosemide, or a $beta_2$ agonist, such as isoproterenol. To treat bronchospasm, anticipate the need for a theophylline derivative. Be prepared to treat seizures with diazepam or lorazepam, as prescribed.

Nursing Considerations

• Monitor blood pressure, apical and radial pulses, fluid intake and output, daily weight, respiration, and circulation in extremities before and during propranolol therapy.

- If patient has heart failure, particularly if she has severely compromised left ventricular dysfunction, monitor her cardiac output because propranolol's negative inotropic effect can depress it.
- Be aware that propranolol can mask tachycardia that occurs with hyperthyroidism and that abrupt withdrawal of drug in patients with hyperthyroidism or thyrotoxicosis can precipitate thyroid storm.
- If patient has diabetes and is taking an antidiabetic drug, monitor her because propranolol can prolong hypoglycemia or promote hyperglycemia. It also can mask some signs and symptpoms of hypoglycemia—especially tachycardia, palpitations, and tremor—but it doesn't suppress diaphoresis or hypertensive response to hypoglycemia.
- **WARNING** Be aware that stopping drug abruptly can cause MI, myocardial ischemia, severe hypertension, or ventricular arrhythmias, particularly if patient has cardiac disease.

PATIENT TEACHING
- Instruct patient to take propranolol at the same time every day.
- Caution patient not to change dosage without consulting prescriber and not to stop taking drug abruptly.
- Advise patient to notify prescriber immediately if she experiences shortness of breath.
- If patient is diabetic, instruct her to regularly monitor blood glucose level and test urine for ketones.
- Advise patient to consult prescriber before taking any OTC drug, especially cold remedies.
- Urge patient to avoid potentially hazardous activities until she knows how the drug affects her.
- Advise smoker to notify prescriber immediately if she stops smoking because smoking cessation may decrease drug metabolism, calling for dosage adjustments.

Other Therapeutic Uses
Propranolol hydrochloride is also indicated for the following:
- To manage hypertension
- To treat chronic angina
- To treat supraventricular arrhythmias and ventricular tachycardia
- As adjunct to treat hypertrophic cardiomyopathy
- As adjunct to manage pheochromocytoma
- To prevent an MI

protriptyline hydrochloride
Triptil (CAN), Vivactil

Class and Category
Chemical class: Dibenzocycloheptene derivative
Therapeutic class: Antidepressant
Pregnancy category: Not rated

Indications and Dosages
▶ *To treat depression*
TABLETS
Adults. *Initial:* 5 to 10 mg t.i.d. or q.i.d., increased every wk by 10 mg daily, as needed. *Maximum:* 60 mg daily.
Children age 12 and over. *Initial:* 5 mg t.i.d., increased as needed.
DOSAGE ADJUSTMENT For elderly patients, initial dosage limited to 5 mg t.i.d., then adjusted as needed.

Route	Onset	Steady State	Peak	Half-Life	Duration
P.O.	2 to 3 wk	14 to 19 days	Unknown	67 to 89 hr	Unknown

Mechanism of Action
May block the reuptake of norepinephrine and serotonin (and possibly other neurotransmitters) at neuronal membranes, thus enhancing their effects at postsynaptic receptors. These neurotransmitters may play a role in relieving signs and symptoms of depression.

Contraindications
Acute recovery phase after an MI, hypersensitivity to protriptyline or its components, use within 14 days of MAO inhibitor therapy

Interactions
DRUGS
amantadine, anticholinergics, antidyskinetics, antihistamines: Additive anticholinergic effects, potentiated effects of antihistamines or protriptyline, possibly impaired detoxification of atropine and related drugs
anticonvulsants: Possibly lowered seizure threshold and decreased anticonvulsant effectiveness; enhanced CNS depression
antithyroid drugs: Possibly agranulocytosis
barbiturates, carbamazepine: Decreased therapeutic effects of protriptyline

bupropion, clozapine, cyclobenzaprine, haloperidol, loxapine, maprotiline, molindone, phenothiazines, thioxanthenes: Prolonged and intensified anticholinergic and sedative effects, lowered seizure threshold, increased risk of neuroleptic malignant syndrome; increased blood protriptyline level and inhibited phenothiazine metabolism (with phenothiazine use)

cimetidine: Increased risk of protriptyline toxicity

clonidine, guanadrel, guanethidine: Decreased hypotensive effects of these drugs; increased CNS depression (with clonidine use)

CNS depressants: Possibly serious potentiation of CNS and respiratory depression and hypotensive effect

disulfiram, ethchlorvynol: Possibly transient delirium; increased CNS depression (with ethchlorvynol use)

fluoxetine: Increased blood protriptyline level

MAO inhibitors: Increased risk of hyperpyretic crisis, severe seizures, and death

methylphenidate: Possibly antagonized effects of methylphenidate and increased blood protriptyline level

metrizamide: Increased risk of seizures

naphazoline, oxymetazoline, phenylephrine, xylometazoline: Possibly increased vasopressor effects of these drugs

oral anticoagulants: Possibly increased anticoagulant activity

pimozide, probucol: Possibly prolonged QT interval and ventricular tachycardia

sympathomimetics: Possibly potentiated cardiovascular effects, decreased vasopressor effects of ephedrine and mephentermine

thyroid hormones: Increased therapeutic and toxic effects of both drugs

ACTIVITIES

alcohol use: Possibly increased response to alcohol

Adverse Reactions

CNS: Agitation, ataxia, confusion, dizziness, drowsiness, exacerbation of psychosis, extrapyramidal reactions, fatigue, lack of coordination, paresthesia, peripheral neuropathy, tremor, weakness
CV: Arrhythmias, including heart block and tachycardia; CVA; hypertension; hypotension; MI; orthostatic hypotension; palpitations
EENT: Black tongue, blurred vision, dry mouth, increased intraocular pressure, lacrimation, stomatitis, tongue swelling
ENDO: Hyperglycemia, hypoglycemia
GI: Abdominal cramps, anorexia, constipation, diarrhea, epigastric discomfort, hepatic dysfunction, nausea, vomiting

GU: Impotence, libido changes, nocturia, urinary frequency and hesitancy, urine retention

SKIN: Diaphoresis, petechiae, photosensitivity, rash, urticaria

Other: Facial edema, weight gain or loss

Overdose

Monitor patient for signs and symptoms of overdose, including agitation, arrhythmias, confusion, disturbed concentration, drowsiness, dyspnea, fever, hallucinations, irregular heartbeat, mydriasis, restlessness, seizures, unusual fatigue, vomiting, and weakness.

Maintain open airway, institute continuous ECG monitoring (for at least 5 days), and closely observe patient's blood pressure, respiratory rate, and temperature. Be prepared to treat arrhythmias with lidocaine and sodium bicarbonate, as prescribed. Anticipate that patient may need digitalization to prevent heart failure. Institute seizure precautions according to facility protocol, and administer anticonvulsant drug therapy, as prescribed.

Be prepared to perform gastric lavage to decrease drug absorption. Expect to administer activated charcoal, followed by a bowel stimulant, to enhance drug elimination. Protriptyline is highly protein bound; therefore, dialysis, exchange transfusions, and forced diuresis are ineffective for treating overdose.

Be aware that use of I.V. physostigmine isn't routinely recommended, but it may be prescribed to reverse the anticholinergic effects of protriptyline if patient is comatose and has respiratory depression, serious arrhythmias, severe hypertension, or uncontrollable seizures.

Institute suicide precautions according to facility policy, and anticipate psychiatric re-evaluation.

Nursing Considerations

- Use protriptyline cautiously in patients with a history of seizures because drug can lower seizure threshold.
- Use drug cautiously in patients with a history of urine retention or increased intraocular pressure because of drug's autonomic activity.
- **WARNING** Avoid administering protriptyline with an MAO inhibitor. If patient is being switched from an MAO inhibitor to protriptyline, make sure that MAO inhibitor has been discontinued for 14 days before starting protriptyline.

PATIENT TEACHING

- Inform patient that protriptyline therapy may take several weeks to reach full effect.

- Instruct patient to avoid potentially hazardous activities until she knows how the drug affects her.
- Advise patient to change position slowly to minimize effects of orthostatic hypotension.
- Urge patient to avoid alcohol while taking drug.
- Suggest that patient drink water and use sugarless gum or hard candy to relieve dry mouth.
- Advise patient to avoid sunlight and tanning booths and to wear protective clothing, a hat, and sunscreen when outdoors.
- If patient is diabetic, instruct her to check blood glucose level frequently during first few weeks of protriptyline therapy.

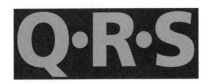

quazepam
Doral

Class, Category, and Schedule
Chemical class: Benzodiazepine
Therapeutic class: Sedative-hypnotic
Pregnancy category: X
Controlled substance schedule: IV

Indications and Dosages
▶ *To treat insomnia*
TABLETS
Adults. 15 mg at bedtime.
DOSAGE ADJUSTMENT In elderly and debilitated patients, dosage possibly reduced to 7.5 mg at bedtime after 1 or 2 nights of therapy.

Route	Onset	Steady State	Peak	Half-Life	Duration
P.O.	Unknown	7 to 13 days	Unknown	25 to 41 hr	Unknown

Mechanism of Action
May antagonize mu receptors at limbic, thalamic, and hypothalamic regions of the brain, blocking release of such inhibitory neurotransmitters as gamma-aminobutyric acid (GABA) and acetylcholine. Central receptors interact with GABA receptors, allowing for greater influx of chloride into the neuron, thereby suppressing neuronal excitability. GABA effects may inhibit spinal afferent pathways and block the cortical and limbic arousal that normally occurs when reticular pathways are stimulated. These effects result in various levels of CNS depression, including sleep.

Contraindications
Hypersensitivity to quazepam or its components, pregnancy, sleep apnea (known or suspected)

Interactions

DRUGS

addictive drugs: Possibly habituation

carbamazepine: Decreased blood quazepam level, possibly increased blood carbamazepine level

cimetidine, diltiazem, disulfiram, erythromycin, fluoxetine, fluvoxamine, isoniazid, itraconazole, ketoconazole, nefazodone, oral contraceptives, propoxyphene, ranitidine, verapamil: Possibly potentiated effects of quazepam

clozapine: Possibly syncope, with respiratory depression or arrest

CNS depressants, tricyclic antidepressants: Increased CNS depression

digoxin: Possibly increased blood digoxin level and risk of digitalis toxicity

levodopa: Possibly decreased therapeutic effects of levodopa

phenytoin: Increased risk of phenytoin toxicity

theophyllines: Possibly antagonized effects of quazepam

zidovudine: Increased risk of zidovudine toxicity

FOODS

grapefruit juice: Increased blood quazepam level

ACTIVITIES

alcohol use: Additive CNS depression

smoking: Possibly decreased effectiveness of quazepam

Adverse Reactions

CNS: Amnesia (anterograde), anxiety, ataxia, confusion, depression, dizziness, drowsiness, euphoria, fatigue, headache, lightheadedness, paresthesia, sleep-driving, slurred speech, tremor, weakness

CV: Chest pain, palpitations, tachycardia

EENT: Blurred vision, dry mouth, hyperacusis, photophobia, worsening of glaucoma

GI: Abdominal cramps, constipation, diarrhea, heartburn, nausea, thirst, vomiting

GU: Renal dysfunction, urinary incontinence, urine retention

MS: Muscle spasms

RESP: Increased tracheobronchial secretions

Other: Anaphylaxis, angioedema

Overdose

Monitor patient for signs and symptoms of overdose, including bradycardia, coma, confusion, dyspnea, hyporeflexia, seizures, severe drowsiness, shakiness, slurred speech, staggering, and weakness.

Maintain an open airway, institute continuous ECG monitoring, and administer I.V. fluids, as prescribed, to maintain blood pressure and promote diuresis. Institute seizure precautions according to facility protocol.

To decrease drug absorption in a conscious patient who isn't at risk for coma or seizures, be prepared to induce vomiting or perform gastric lavage. Expect that oral activated charcoal may also be prescribed. For an unconscious patient, anticipate assisting with the insertion of an endotracheal tube and then performing gastric lavage. The inflated cuff of the endotracheal tube will help prevent aspiration of gastric contents into the lungs.

Anticipate the use of a benzodiazepine receptor antagonist such as flumazenil to reverse the sedative effects. Be aware that flumazenil may induce seizures, especially if patient has undergone long-term quazepam therapy or has also ingested a cyclic antidepressant. If excitation occurs, a barbiturate shouldn't be used because it may increase excitement and prolong CNS depression. Dialysis is ineffective for treating quazepam overdose.

Institute suicide precautions according to facility policy, and anticipate psychiatric re-evaluation.

Nursing Considerations

- Use quazepam cautiously in patients with angle-closure glaucoma because of drug's anticholinergic effects; in patients with hepatic dysfunction because this condition may prolong quazepam's half-life; in patients with myasthenia gravis because drug may worsen condition; in patients with severe COPD because adverse effects of quazepam may compromise respiratory function; in patients with renal dysfunction because accumulation of metabolites may result in toxicity; and in elderly patients because of age-related decreases in hepatic, renal, and cardiac function.
- **WARNING** Monitor patient closely after giving quazepam because anaphylaxis or angioedema, although rare, may occur with the first dose or later doses. Notify prescriber immediately, and be prepared to provide supportive emergency care.
- **WARNING** If eye pain develops in patient with angle-closure glaucoma, notify prescriber immediately.
- **WARNING** Be aware that quazepam may intensify signs and symptoms of depression. Monitor patient closely for suicidal ideation. Institute suicide precautions, as appropriate, according to facility policy.

PATIENT TEACHING
• Urge patient to avoid alcohol during quazepam therapy because it may increase drug's sedative effects.
• Inform patient that quazepam may cause daytime drowsiness. Advise him not to drive or perform other activities that require alertness until he knows how the drug affects him.
• Instruct patient not to discontinue drug abruptly after prolonged use (6 weeks or longer).
• Instruct female patient of childbearing age to use effective contraception during therapy and to notify prescriber immediately if she knows or suspects she's pregnant.
• Tell family to report sleep-driving episodes, in which the patient drives while not fully awake and usually has no recall of the event.
• Instruct patient to seek immediate medical attention for hypersensitivity reactions including facial swelling, throat tightness, or difficulty breathing.

quetiapine fumarate

Seroquel, Seroquel XR

Class and Category

Chemical class: Dibenzothiazepine derivative
Therapeutic class: Antipsychotic drug
Pregnancy category: C

Indications and Dosages

▶ *To treat schizophrenia*
TABLETS
Adults. *Initial:* 25 mg b.i.d. on day 1. Dosage increased by 25 to 50 mg b.i.d. or t.i.d. on days 2 and 3. *Usual:* 300 to 400 mg daily by day 4, in divided doses b.i.d. or t.i.d. Dosage increased every 2 days in increments of 25 to 50 mg b.i.d., as needed. *Maximum:* 800 mg daily.
E.R. TABLETS
Adults. *Initial:* 300 mg once daily in evening. Dosage increased daily in increments up to 300 mg, as needed. *Maximum:* 800 mg daily.

▶ *To manage psychotic disorders other than schizophrenia*
TABLETS
Adults. *Initial:* 25 mg b.i.d. on day 1. Increased by 25 to 50 mg b.i.d. or t.i.d. on days 2 and 3. *Usual:* 300 to 400 mg daily by day 4, in divided doses b.i.d. or t.i.d. Increased every 2 days in incre-

ments of 25 to 50 mg b.i.d., as needed. *Maximum:* 800 mg daily.
▶ *To treat depressive episodes in bipolar disorder*
TABLETS
Adults. *Initial:* 50 mg daily at bedtime on day 1, followed by
100 mg daily at bedtime on day 2, 200 mg daily at bedtime on
day 3, and 300 mg daily at bedtime thereafter. *Maintenance:*
300 mg at bedtime.
▶ *To treat acute manic episodes in bipolar I disorder*
TABLETS
Adults. 50 mg b.i.d., increased to 200 mg b.i.d. on day 4 (in
increments no greater than 100 mg daily) and then further in-
creased to 400 mg b.i.d. on day 6 (in increments no greater than
200 mg daily), as needed.
▶ *As adjunct to lithium or divalproex in maintaining stabilization in
bipolar I disorder*
E.R. TABLETS
Adults. 200 to 400 mg b.i.d.

Route	Onset	Steady State	Peak	Half-Life	Duration
P.O.	Unknown	2 days	Unknown	6 hr	Unknown

Mechanism of Action
May produce antipsychotic effects by interfering with dopamine binding
to dopamine$_2$ (D$_2$) receptor sites in the brain and by antagonizing serotonin
5-HT$_2$, dopamine$_1$ (D$_1$), histamine H$_1$, and alpha$_1$- and alpha$_2$-adrenergic
receptors.

Contraindications
Hypersensitivity to quetiapine or its components

Interactions
DRUGS
antihypertensives: Possibly enhanced antihypertensive effects of
these drugs
cimetidine, erythromycin, fluconazole, itraconazole, ketoconazole: Decreased clearance and possibly increased effects of quetiapine
CNS depressants: Possibly increased CNS depression
lorazepam: Possibly increased effects of lorazepam
phenytoin, thioridazine: Increased clearance and possibly decreased
effectiveness of quetiapine
ACTIVITIES
alcohol use: Possibly enhanced CNS depression

Adverse Reactions

CNS: Dizziness, drowsiness, extrapyramidal reactions, hypertonia, seizures, suicidal ideation, tardive dyskinesia
CV: Hypercholesterolemia, orthostatic hypotension, palpitations
EENT: Dry mouth, pharyngitis, rhinitis
ENDO: Hyperglycemia
GI: Anorexia, constipation, indigestion
HEME: Agranulocytosis, leukopenia, neutropenia
MS: Dysarthria, muscle weakness
RESP: Cough, dyspnea
SKIN: Diaphoresis
Other: Flulike signs and symptoms, weight gain

Overdose

Monitor patient for signs and symptoms of overdose, including bradycardia, drowsiness, hypokalemia (assess patient for weakness), hypotension, irregular heartbeat, prolonged QT interval, and tachycardia.

Maintain an open airway, administer oxygen as needed, monitor vital signs, and institute continuous ECG monitoring. To decrease drug absorption in a conscious patient, be prepared to perform gastric lavage. Expect that oral activated charcoal, followed by a laxative, may also be prescribed. For an unconscious patient, anticipate assisting with insertion of an endotracheal tube and then performing gastric lavage. The inflated cuff of the endotracheal tube will help prevent aspiration of gastric contents into the lungs. Be aware that vomiting shouldn't be induced because of the risk of dystonic reactions of the head and neck.

Be prepared to treat arrhythmias, as needed and prescribed; however, be aware that drugs that prolong the QT interval—such as disopyramide, procainamide, and quinidine—shouldn't be used. If bretylium is prescribed, use it with caution because it may increase the hypotensive effects of quetiapine. Expect to treat hypotension with I.V. fluids and a sympathomimetic; keep in mind that dopamine and epinephrine may increase hypotension. To treat severe extrapyramidal reactions, expect to use an antidyskinetic, as prescribed.

Institute suicide precautions according to facility policy, and anticipate psychiatric re-evaluation.

Nursing Considerations

• Be aware that quetiapine may increase the risk of death in elderly patients with dementia-related psychosis.
• **WARNING** During treatment, monitor patient for predispos-

ing factors for neuroleptic malignant syndrome; these include heat stress, physical exhaustion, dehydration, and organic brain disease. The syndrome is characterized by altered mental status, autonomic instability (which may include arrhythmias, diaphoresis, irregular blood pressure or pulse, and tachycardia), hyperpyrexia, and muscle rigidity.

- Assess patient for tardive dyskinesia—a potentially irreversible complication characterized by involuntary, dyskinetic movements of the tongue, mouth, jaw, eyelids, or face. Notify prescriber if such signs develop because quetiapine therapy may need to be discontinued.
- If patient has a low white blood cell count or a history of drug-induced leukopenia or neutropenia, check his complete blood count often during first few months of therapy, as ordered. If white blood cell count declines during quetiapine therapy, notify prescriber and expect drug to be discontinued.
- Monitor patient for orthostatic hypotension, especially during initial dosage adjustment period. Be prepared to correct underlying conditions, such as dehydration and hypovolemia, before starting therapy, as prescribed.
- Watch patient closely for suicidal tendencies, especially when therapy starts or dosage changes and especially if patient is a child, an adolescent, or a young adult.
- Watch for signs and symptoms of hypothyroidism during treatment because drug can cause dose-dependent decreases in total and free thyroxine (T_4) levels.
- Monitor laboratory results during first 3 weeks of therapy for transient elevations in hepatic enzyme levels. Notify prescriber if elevations persist or become progressively worse.
- Monitor patient's blood glucose and lipid levels routinely, as ordered, because the risk of hyperglycemia and hypercholesterolemia is increased during quetiapine therapy.

PATIENT TEACHING

- Instruct patient to take quetiapine with food to reduce stomach upset.
- Advise patient not to stop taking quetiapine suddenly because doing so may worsen his signs and symptoms.
- Tell family or caregiver to watch patient closely for suicidal tendencies, especially when therapy starts or dosage changes and especially if patient is a child, a teenager, or a young adult.
- Inform patient that drug may cause dizziness or drowsiness. Advise him not to drive or perform other activities that require alertness until he knows how the drug affects him.

- Instruct patient to rise slowly from a seated or lying position to reduce the risk of dizziness or fainting.
- Urge patient to avoid consuming alcoholic beverages because they can increase dizziness and drowsiness.
- Encourage patient on long-term therapy to have regular eye examinations so that cataracts can be detected.

ramelteon
Rozerem

Class and Category
Chemical class: Melatonin receptor agonist
Therapeutic class: Hypnotic
Pregnancy category: C

Indications and Dosages
▶ *To treat insomnia in patients having trouble falling asleep*
TABLETS
Adults. 8 mg 30 min before bedtime.

Route	Onset	Peak	Duration
P.O.	Unknown	0.5 to 1.5 hr	Unknown

Mechanism of Action
Binds to melatonin receptors MT1 and MT2 in the suprachiasmatic nucleus (SCN) of the hypothalamus. The SCN regulates the sleep-wake cycle, and endogenous melatonin probably is involved in maintaining the circadian rhythm underlying that cycle.

Contraindications
Hypersensitivity to ramelteon or its components, severe hepatic dysfunction

Interactions
DRUGS
benzodiazepines, melatonin, other sedative-hypnotics: Possible additive sedative effects
fluconazole, fluvoxamine, ketoconazole: Increased plasma ramelteon levels
rifampin: Decreased ramelteon effectiveness
ACTIVITIES
alcohol use: Possibly additive CNS effect

Adverse Reactions

CNS: Depression, dizziness, fatigue, headache, insomnia exacerbation, somnolence
ENDO: Decreased testosterone levels, increased prolactin levels
GI: Diarrhea, dysgeusia, nausea
MS: Arthralgia, myalgia
RESP: Upper respiratory tract infection

Overdose

No case of ramelteon has been documented. Ramelteon overdose has no specific antidote. Monitor the patient for signs and symptoms that could be caused by ramelteon overdose.

Maintain an open airway, and monitor vital signs. Perform gastric lavage, as ordered, to decrease the amount of drug absorbed. Give I.V. fluids, as needed and ordered. Expect to provide symptomatic and supportive therapy, as indicated. Be aware that hemodialysis is not effective in treating ramelteon overdose.

Institute suicide precautions according to facility policy, and anticipate psychiatric re-evaluation.

Nursing Considerations

- Be aware that ramelteon therapy is not recommended for patients with severe sleep apnea or COPD because its effects have not been studied in these patient populations.
- Use cautiously in patients with mild to moderate hepatic dysfunction. Drug is contraindicated in severe hepatic dysfunction.
- Ramelteon is the first approved hypnotic not classified as a controlled substance.
- Monitor depressed patient closely for evidence of worsening of depression. Athough depression has not been identified as an adverse reaction of ramelteon, the drug is a hypnotic and hypnotics worsen depression, including causing suicidal ideation.

PATIENT TEACHING

- Instruct patient not to take ramelteon with or immediately after a high-fat meal.
- Caution patient to avoid hazardous activities after taking ramelteon; drug's intended effect is to decrease alertness.
- Advise limiting alcohol intake during therapy.
- Tell patient to notify prescriber if insomnia worsens or new signs or symptoms occur.
- Inform patient that drug may affect reproductive hormones; urge patient to report cessation of menses or galactorrhea (women) or decreased libido or problems with infertility.

rasagiline
Azilect

Class and Category
Chemical class: Propargylamine
Therapeutic class: Irreversible MAO inhibitor
Pregnancy category: C

Indications and Dosages
▶ *To treat idiopathic Parkinson's disease as initial monotherapy in early-stage disease*
TABLETS
Adults. 1 mg once daily.
▶ *As adjunct to levodopa or levodopa and carbidopa in treatment of later-stage idiopathic Parkinson's disease*
TABLETS
Adults. 0.5 mg once daily increased to 1 mg once daily, as needed.
DOSAGE ADJUSTMENT For patients with mild hepatic failure, dosage shouldn't exceed 0.5 mg daily.

Route	Onset	Peak	Duration
P.O.	Unknown	1 hr	Unknown

Mechanism of Action
Inhibits metabolic degradation of catecholamines and serotonin in the CNS and peripheral tissues, increasing extracellular dopamine level in the striatum. The increased dopamine level helps control alterations in voluntary muscle movement (such as tremors and rigidity) in Parkinson's disease because dopamine, a neurotransmitter, is essential for normal motor function. By stimulating peripheral and central dopaminergic 2 (D2) receptors on postsynaptic cells, dopamine inhibits firing of striatal neurons (such as cholineric neurons), improving motor function.

Contraindications
Acute MI; angina; cardiac arrhythmias; coronary artery disease; cerebrovascular disease; CVA; elective surgery that requires general anesthesia; hypersensitivity to rasagiline or its components; moderate to severe hepatic impairment; pheochromocytoma; use within 14 days of cyclobenzaprine, dextromethorphan, MAO inhibitors, meperidine, methadone, mirtazapine, propoxyphene, St. John's wort, sympathomimetic amines, or tramadol

Interactions
DRUGS
ciprofloxacin and other CYP1A2 inhibitors: Increased rasagiline plasma level
dextromethorphan: Increased risk of psychosis or bizarre behavior
levodopa, levodopa and carbidopa: Increased risk of dyskinesias
MAO inhibitors, sympathomimetics: Increased risk of hypertensive crisis
meperidine, methadone, propoxyphene, tramadol: Increased risk of life-threatening adverse reactions characterized by coma, severe hypertension or hypotension, severe respiratory depression, seizures, malignant hyperpyrexia, excitation, and peripheral vascular collapse
selective serotonin reuptake inhibitors, tetracyclic antidepressants, tricyclic antidepressants: Increased risk of severe CNS toxicity characterized by hyperpyrexia, behavioral and mental changes, diaphoresis, muscular rigidity, hypertension, syncope, and death

Adverse Reactions
CNS: Abnormal dreams, amnesia, anxiety, asthenia, ataxia, cerebral ischemia, coma, confusion, CVA, depression, difficulty thinking, dizziness, dyskinesia, dystonia, fever, hallucinations, headache, malaise, manic-depressive reaction, nightmares, paresthesia, seizures, somnolence, stupor, syncope, vertigo
CV: Angina, bundle branch heart block, chest pain, heart failure, hypertensive crisis, MI, orthostatic hypotension, thrombophlebitis, ventricular tachycardia or fibrillation
EENT: Blurred vision, conjunctivitis, dry mouth, gingivitis, hemorrhage, laryngeal edema, retinal detachment or hemorrhage, rhinitis
GI: Abdominal pain, anorexia, constipation, diarrhea, dyspepsia, dysphagia, epistaxis, gastroenteritis, GI hemorrhage, intestinal obstruction or perforation, liver function test abnormalities, nausea, vomiting
GU: Acute renal failure, albuminuria, decreased libido, hematuria, impotence, incontinence, priapism
HEME: Anemia, leukopenia, thrombocytopenia
MS: Arthralgia, arthritis, bone necrosis, bursitis, leg cramps, myasthenia, neck pain or stiffness, tenosynovitis
RESP: Apnea, asthma, cough, dyspnea, pleural effusion, pneumothorax, interstitial pneumonia
SKIN: Alopecia, carcinoma, diaphoresis, ecchymosis, exfoliative dermatitis, pruritus, ulcer, vesiculobullous rash

Other: Angioedema, flu syndrome, hypersensitivity reaction, hypocalcemia, weight loss

Overdose

Rasagiline overdose hasn't been reported. If it occurs, monitor patient for signs and symptoms, which may not appear until up to 12 hours later and will involve mainly the CNS and cardiovascular systems. Monitor patient for drowsiness, dizziness, faintness, irritability, hyperactivity, agitation, severe headache, hallucinations, trismus, opisthotonos, convulsions, coma, rapid and irregular pulse, hypertension, hypotension and vascular collapse, precordial pain, respiratory depression or failure, hyperpyrexia, diaphoresis, and cool, clammy skin.

Rasagiline overdose has no specific antidote. Provide symptomatic, supportive care. Support respiration through airway mangement, use of supplemental oxygen, and mechanical ventilation, as needed. Monitor body temperature closely. Intensive management of hyperpyrexia may be needed. Also maintain fluid and electrolyte balance, as needed.

Implement suicide precautions according to facility policy, and anticipate psychiatric re-evaluation.

Nursing Considerations

- **WARNING** Notify prescriber immediately if patient has evidence of hypertensive crisis, such as blurred vision, chest pain, difficulty thinking, stupor or coma, seizures, severe headache, neck stiffness, nausea, vomiting, palpitations or signs and symptoms suggesting a CVA. Expect to stop drug immediately if these occur.
- Keep phentolamine readily available to treat hypertensive crisis. Give 5 mg by slow I.V. infusion, as prescribed, to reduce blood pressure without causing excessive hypotension. Use external cooling measures, as prescribed, to manage fever.
- Maintain tyramine restriction and avoid amine-containing medications for at least 2 weeks after stopping rasagiline because of the irreversible inhibition of MAO and the need for new MAO enzyme synthesis.
- If patient has a dyskinesia and receives rasagiline as an adjunct to levodopa, watch for worsening of the dyskinesia. If it occurs, notify prescriber and expect levodopa dosage to be decreased.

PATIENT TEACHING
- **WARNING** Instruct patient to avoid the following food, beverages, and drugs during rasagiline therapy and for 2 weeks afterward: alcohol-free and reduced-alcohol beer and wine;

appetite suppressants; beer; broad beans; cheese (except cottage and cream cheese); chocolate and caffeine in large quantities; dry sausage (including Genoa salami, hard salami, Lebanon bologna, and pepperoni); hay fever drugs; inhaled asthma drugs; liver; meat extract; OTC cold and cough preparations (including those containing dextromethorphan); nasal decongestants (tablets, drops, or sprays); pickled herring products that contain tryptophan; protein-rich foods that may have undergone protein changes by aging, fermenting, pickling, or smoking; sauerkraut; sinus drugs; weight-loss preparations; yeast extracts (including brewer's yeast in large quantities); yogurt; and wine.

- Advise patient to stop taking rasagiline and to notify prescriber immediately if he develops blurred vision, chest pain, trouble thinking, stupor or coma, seizures, severe headache, stiff neck, nausea, vomiting, palpitations, or evidence of CVA.
- Suggest that patient change position slowly to minimize effects of orthostatic hypotension.
- Alert patient that drug may cause hallucinations. If they occur, tell patient to notify prescriber promptly.

risperidone
Risperdal Consta, Risperdal

Class and Category
Chemical class: Benzisoxazole derivative
Therapeutic class: Antipsychotic drug
Pregnancy category: C

Indications and Dosages
▶ *To manage psychotic disorders*
ORAL SOLUTION, TABLETS
Adults. 1 mg b.i.d. on day 1; 2 mg b.i.d. on day 2; 3 mg b.i.d. on day 3. Or, 2 mg once on first day, 4 mg once on second day; and 6 mg once on third day. Daily dosage then increased by 1 to 2 mg at 1- to 2-wk intervals, as needed. *Maximum:* 16 mg daily.
I.M. INJECTION
Adults. *Initial:* 25 mg every 2 wk, increased as needed every 4 wk to 37.5 mg or 50 mg. *Maximum:* 50 mg every 2 wk.
▶ *To treat bipolar mania*
ORAL SOLUTION, ORALLY DISINTEGRATING TABLETS, TABLETS
Adults. *Initial:* 2 or 3 mg daily, increased as needed by 1 mg daily up to 6 mg. *Maximum:* 6 mg daily, not to exceed 3 wk.

DOSAGE ADJUSTMENT Initial dose limited to 0.5 mg b.i.d. for elderly or debilitated patients, those with renal or hepatic impairment, and those at increased risk for hypotension, then increased by 0.5 mg b.i.d. every wk, as needed. Dosage given once daily after target dosage has been maintained for 2 or 3 days. Maximum for patients with severe hepatic dysfunction, 4 mg daily; for elderly patients, 3 mg daily.

▶ *To manage irritability in autistic disorder*

ORALLY DISINTEGRATING TABLETS

Children age 5 and over weighing less than 20 kg. *Initial:* 0.25 mg once daily or 0.125 mg b.i.d., increased after 4 days to 0.5 mg once daily or 0.25 mg b.i.d. After 14 days, dosage may be increased in increments of 0.25 mg daily every 2 wk, as needed.

Adolescents and children age 5 and over weighing 20 kg or more. *Initial:* 0.5 mg once daily or 0.25 mg b.i.d., increased after 4 days to 1 mg once daily or 0.5 mg b.i.d. After 14 days, dosage may be increased in increments of 0.5 mg daily every 2 wk, as needed.

Route	Onset	Steady State	Peak	Half-Life	Duration
P.O.	Unknown	5 to 6 days	Unknown	20 to 24 hr	Unknown

Mechanism of Action

Selectively blocks serotonin and dopamine receptors in the mesocortical tract of the CNS to suppress signs and symptoms of psychosis.

Incompatibilities

Don't mix risperidone oral solution with cola or tea.

Contraindications

Hypersensitivity to risperidone or its components

Interactions

DRUGS

antihypertensives: Increased antihypertensive effects

bromocriptine, levodopa, pergolide: Possibly antagonized effects of these drugs

carbamazepine: Increased risperidone clearance with long-term concurrent use

clozapine: Decreased risperidone clearance with long-term concurrent use

CNS depressants: Additive CNS depression

fluoxetine, paroxetine: Increased plasma risperidone level

ACTIVITIES
alcohol use: Additive CNS depression

Adverse Reactions

CNS: Aggressiveness, agitation, anxiety, asthenia, decreased concentration, dizziness, dream disturbances, drowsiness, dystonia, fatigue, headache, lassitude, memory loss, nervousness, neuroleptic malignant syndrome, parkinsonism, restlessness, somnolence
CV: Chest pain, hypercholesterolemia, orthostatic hypotension, palpitations, prolonged QT interval, tachycardia
EENT: Decreased or increased salivation, dry mouth, pharyngitis, rhinitis, sinusitis, vision changes
ENDO: Benign pituitary adenomas, galactorrhea, hyperglycemia
GI: Abdominal pain, constipation, diarrhea, indigestion, nausea, vomiting
GU: Amenorrhea, decreased libido, dysmenorrhea, dysuria, hypermenorrhea, polyuria, sexual dysfunction
MS: Arthralgia, back pain
RESP: Cough, dyspnea
SKIN: Diaphoresis, dry skin, hyperpigmentation, photosensitivity, pruritus, rash, seborrhea
Other: Local injection site reactions (induration, pain, redness, or swelling), weight gain or loss

Overdose

Watch for signs and symptoms of overdose, including drowsiness, ECG changes (such as prolonged QT interval), electrolyte imbalances, extrapyramidal reactions, hypotension, seizures, and tachycardia.

Maintain an open airway, administer oxygen as needed, monitor vital signs, and institute continuous ECG monitoring and seizure precautions. Obtain blood to monitor electrolyte levels. To decrease drug absorption in a conscious patient, be prepared to perform gastric lavage. Expect that oral activated charcoal, followed by a laxative, may also be prescribed. For an unconscious patient, anticipate assisting with insertion of an endotracheal tube and then performing gastric lavage. The endotracheal tube's inflated cuff will help prevent aspiration of gastric contents into the lungs. Vomiting shouldn't be induced because of the risk of sedation, seizures, and dystonic reactions of the head and neck.

Be prepared to treat arrhythmias, as needed and prescribed; however, be aware that drugs that prolong the QT interval—such as disopyramide, procainamide, and quinidine—shouldn't be used. If bretylium is prescribed, use it with caution because it

PATIENT TEACHING
• Instruct patient to dilute risperidone oral solution with coffee, low-fat milk, orange juice, or water but not with cola or tea.
• If patient will be taking orally disintegrating tablets, tell him to open the blister pack using dry hands to peel back the foil and expose the tablet. Caution him not to push the tablet through the foil because doing so could damage the tablet. Tell him to immediately place the tablet on his tongue, where it will dissolve within seconds. Caution against chewing the tablet or trying to spit it out after placing it in his mouth.
• Advise patient to avoid hazardous activities until he knows how the drug affects him and to rise slowly from a lying or sitting position to minimize effects of orthostatic hypotension.
• Urge patient to avoid alcohol because of its additive CNS effects.
• If patient has diabetes, caution him to monitor his glucose level closely while taking risperidone because it may increase his blood glucose level.

rivastigmine tartrate
Exelon

Class and Category
Chemical class: Carbamate derivative
Therapeutic class: Antidementia drug
Pregnancy category: B

Indications and Dosages
▶ *To treat mild to moderate Alzheimer's-type dementia*
CAPSULES
Adults. *Initial:* 1.5 mg b.i.d. with meals, morning and evening. Dosage increased by 1.5 mg daily every 2 wk, as needed. *Maximum:* 6 mg b.i.d.
▶ *To treat mild to moderate dementia in Parkinson's disease*
CAPSULES
Adults. *Initial:* 1.5 mg b.i.d. with meals, morning and evening. Dosage increased by 1.5 mg daily every 4 wk, as needed. *Maximum:* 6 mg b.i.d.
DOSAGE ADJUSTMENT If patient develops nausea or vomiting, treatment should be discontinued for several doses, as prescribed, and restarted at same or next-lowest dose.

Route	Onset	Steady State	Peak	Half-Life	Duration
P.O.	Unknown	Unknown	6 hr	1 hr	12 hr

Mechanism of Action

May slow the decline of cognitive function in Alzheimer's disease by increasing acetylcholine levels at cholinergic transmission sites. This action prolongs and exaggerates acetylcholine effects that are otherwise blocked by toxic levels of anticholinergics. Cognitive decline is partly related to cholinergic deficits along neuronal pathways, projecting from the basal forebrain to the cerebral cortex and hippocampus, that are involved in memory, attention, learning, and cognition. Rivastigmine, a cholinesterase inhibitor, may inhibit destruction of acetylcholine by cholinesterase, thereby slowing the disease.

Contraindications

Hypersensitivity to carbamate derivatives, rivastigmine, or their components

Interactions

DRUGS

anticholinergics: Possibly decreased effectiveness of anticholinergics
bethanechol, succinylcholine: Possibly synergistic effects

Adverse Reactions

CNS: Aggression, agitation, anxiety, asthenia, bradykinesia, confusion, depression, dizziness, dyskinesia, extrapyramidal symptoms, fatigue, fever, hallucinations, headache, insomnia, malaise, restlessness, seizures, somnolence, transient ischemic attack, tremor, worsening of Parkinson's diease, parkinsonism, vertigo
CV: Chest pain, hypertension
EENT: Rhinitis
GI: Abdominal pain, anorexia, constipation, diarrhea, dyspepsia, flatulence, indigestion, nausea, vomiting
GU: UTI
MS: Back pain
RESP: Dyspnea
SKIN: Diaphoresis, Stevens-Johnson syndrome
Other: Dehydration, flulike signs and symptoms, weight loss

Overdose

Monitor patient for signs and symptoms of overdose, including bradycardia, diaphoresis, hypotension, increased salivation, muscle weakness, nausea, seizures, shock, and vomiting.

Limited information is available about rivastigmine overdose. Expect to maintain an open airway and institute seizure precautions according to facility protocol. Provide symptomatic and supportive care, as needed. If patient develops severe nausea and vomiting, administer an antiemetic, as prescribed.

Institute suicide precautions according to facility policy, and anticipate psychiatric re-evaluation.

Nursing Considerations
• Administer rivastigmine with food to reduce adverse GI effects.
• Avoid stopping drug abruptly because doing so may increase behavioral disturbances and decline in cognitive function.
• Monitor patient for extrapyramidal symptoms because drug may cause or worsen them.
• Monitor weight daily because rivastigmine may cause anorexia and weight loss.
• Monitor respiratory status of patients with pulmonary disease—including asthma, chronic bronchitis, and emphysema—because rivastigmine has a weak affinity for peripheral cholinesterase, which may increase bronchoconstriction and bronchial secretions.
• Ensure adequate urine output; cholinomimetics such as rivastigmine may cause or worsen urinary tract or bladder obstruction.
• If patient has Parkinson's disease, monitor him for exaggerated parkinsonian signs and symptoms, which may result from drug's increased cholinergic effects on CNS.
• If patient has just had surgery and is taking rivastigmine, watch for possibly exaggerated muscle relaxation and extended respiratory depression due to prolonged neuromuscular blockade.

PATIENT TEACHING
• Explain that rivastigmine can't cure Alzheimer's disease but may slow the progressive deterioration of memory and improve patient's ability to perform activities of daily living.
• Advise patient and family that drug should be taken with food to reduce adverse GI effects.
• Instruct family to supervise patient's self-administration of drug.
• Instruct patient and family to monitor dietary intake because gastritis may lead to decreased appetite.

rizatriptan benzoate
Maxalt, Maxalt-MLT

Class and Category
Chemical class: Selective 5-hydroxytryptamine$_1$ (5-HT$_1$) receptor agonist
Therapeutic class: Antimigraine drug
Pregnancy category: C

Indications and Dosages

▶ *To relieve acute migraine headache*
DISINTEGRATING TABLETS, TABLETS
Adults. 5 to 10 mg when migraine starts; repeated every 2 hr,
p.r.n. *Maximum:* 30 mg daily.
DOSAGE ADJUSTMENT For patients taking propranolol, initial dosage reduced to 5 mg, then repeated every 2 hr, p.r.n., up
to maximum of 15 mg daily.

Route	Onset	Steady State	Peak	Half-Life	Duration
P.O.	Unknown	Unknown	Unknown	2 to 3 hr	Unknown

Mechanism of Action

Binds to selective 5-HT$_1$ receptor sites on cerebral blood vessels, causing vessels to constrict. This may decrease the characteristic pulsing sensation and thus relieve the pain of migraines. Rizatriptan may also relieve pain by inhibiting the release of proinflammatory neuropeptides and reducing transmission of trigeminal nerve impulses from sensory nerve endings during a migraine attack.

Contraindications

Basilar or hemiplegic migraine, hypersensitivity to rizatriptan or
its components, ischemic coronary artery disease, uncontrolled
hypertension, use within 14 days of MAO inhibitor therapy, use
within 24 hours of other 5-HT$_1$ receptor agonists or ergotamine-
containing or ergot-type drugs

Interactions

DRUGS
ergotamine-containing drugs: Prolonged vasospastic reactions
MAO inhibitors, propranolol: Increased blood rizatriptan level
other selective 5-HT$_1$ receptor agonists (including naratriptan, sumatriptan, and zolmitriptan): Additive vasospastic effects
selective serotonin reuptake inhibitors: Increased risk of weakness, hyperreflexia, and lack of coordination

Adverse Reactions

CNS: Altered temperature sensation, anxiety, asthenia, ataxia,
chills, confusion, depression, disorientation, dizziness, dream disturbances, drowsiness, euphoria, fatigue, hangover, headache, hypoesthesia, insomnia, mental impairment, nervousness, paresthesia, somnolence, tremor, vertigo

CV: Arrhythmias, such as bradycardia and tachycardia; chest pain; hot flashes; hypertension; palpitations
EENT: Blurred vision; burning eyes; dry eyes, mouth, and throat; earache; eye pain or irritation; lacrimation; nasal congestion and irritation; pharyngitis; tinnitus; tongue swelling
GI: Abdominal distention, constipation, diarrhea, dysphagia, flatulence, heartburn, indigestion, nausea, thirst, vomiting
GU: Menstrual irregularities, polyuria, urinary frequency
MS: Arthralgia; dysarthria; muscle spasms, stiffness, or weakness; myalgia
RESP: Dyspnea, upper respiratory tract infection
SKIN: Diaphoresis, flushing, pruritus, rash, urticaria
Other: Dehydration, facial edema

Overdose

Monitor patient for evidence of overdose, including angina, bradycardia, dizziness, headache, hypertension, somnolence, and vomiting. Maintain an open airway, monitor vital signs, and expect to continue ECG monitoring for at least 12 hours after overdose.

To decrease drug absorption, be prepared to perform gastric lavage and give activated charcoal, as prescribed. Maintain fluid and electrolyte balance, and treat hypertension, as prescribed. The effect of dialysis on rizatriptan overdose is unknown.

Institute suicide precautions according to facility policy, and anticipate psychiatric re-evaluation.

Nursing Considerations

• Use rizatriptan cautiously in patients with renal or hepatic dysfunction because of impaired drug metabolism or excretion. Monitor BUN and serum creatinine levels and liver function test results, as appropriate.
• Use cautiously in patients with peripheral vascular disease because drug may cause vasospastic reactions leading to vascular and colonic ischemia with abdominal pain and bloody diarrhea. Assess peripheral circulation and bowel sounds often.
• If patient has cardiovascular risk factors, assess his cardiovascular status and institute continuous ECG monitoring, as ordered, immediately after giving rizatriptan because of possible asymptomatic cardiac ischemia.
• If patient has hypertension, check blood pressure regularly because rizatriptan may cause transient increase in blood pressure.

PATIENT TEACHING

• Instruct patient taking disintegrating tablets to remove tablet from blister pack with dry hands, place it immediately on

tongue, let it dissolve, and swallow it with saliva.
- If patient is phenylketonuric, advise him not to use disintegrating tablet form because it contains phenylalanine.
- Instruct patient to seek emergency care immediately if cardiac symptoms, such as chest pain, occur after administration.
- Caution patient about possible adverse CNS reactions, and advise him to avoid potentially hazardous activities until he knows how the drug affects him.

ropinirole hydrochloride
Requip

Class and Category
Chemical class: Dipropylaminoethyl indolone derivative
Therapeutic class: Antidyskinetic
Pregnancy category: C

Indications and Dosages
▶ *To treat signs and symptoms of Parkinson's disease*
TABLETS
Adults. *Initial:* 0.25 mg t.i.d. Dosage increased every wk according to the following schedule: 0.25 mg t.i.d. in wk 1; 0.5 mg t.i.d. in wk 2; 0.75 mg t.i.d. in wk 3; 1 mg t.i.d. in wk 4. After wk 4, dosage increased by 1.5 mg daily every wk up to 9 mg daily, then by 3 mg daily every wk up to 24 mg daily. *Maximum:* 24 mg daily.
▶ *To treat moderate to severe primary restless legs syndrome*
TABLETS
Adults. *Initial:* 0.25 mg 1 to 3 hr before bedtime. Increased to 0.5 mg after 2 days and then to 1 mg at end of first week. If needed, increased further in 0.5-mg increments every wk. *Maximum:* 4 mg daily.

Route	Onset	Steady State	Peak	Half-Life	Duration
P.O.	Unknown	2 days	Unknown	6 hr	Unknown

Mechanism of Action
Directly stimulates postsynaptic dopamine$_2$ (D$_2$) receptors in the brain and acts as an agonist at peripheral D$_2$ receptors. These actions inhibit firing of striatal cholinergic neurons, thus helping control alterations in voluntary muscle movement (such as tremors and rigidity) in Parkinson's disease.

Contraindications
Hypersensitivity to ropinirole or its components

Interactions
DRUGS

carbamazepine, cimetidine, ciprofloxacin, clarithromycin, diltiazem, enoxacin, erythromycin, fluvoxamine, mexiletine, norfloxacin, omeprazole, phenobarbital, phenytoin, rifampin, ritonavir, troleandomycin: Altered drug clearance and increased blood level of ropinirole

chlorprothixene, domperidone, droperidol, haloperidol, metoclopramide, phenothiazines, thiothixene: Possibly decreased effectiveness of ropinirole

CNS depressants: Additive effects

ethinyl estradiol: Possibly reduced clearance of ropinirole

levodopa: Increased risk of hallucinations

ACTIVITIES

alcohol use: Additive effects

Adverse Reactions
CNS: Asthenia, confusion, dizziness, falling asleep during activities of daily living, fatigue, hallucinations, headache, hypoesthesia, paresthesia, malaise, neuralgia, rigors, somnolence, syncope, transient ischemic attack, vertigo

CV: Acute coronary syndrome, angina, bradycardia, cardiac failure, chest pain, hypertension, MI, orthostatic hypotension, palpitations, peripheral edema, sick sinus syndrome, tachycardia

EENT: Abnormal vision, dry mouth, nasal congestion, nasopharyngitis, pharyngitis, rhinitis, toothache

ENDO: Hot flashes

GI: Abdominal pain, constipation, diarrhea, dyspepsia, gastric hemorrhage, gastroenteritis, indigestion, intestinal obstruction, ischemic hepatitis, nausea, pancreatitis, vomiting

GU: Elevated BUN level, erectile dysfunction, UTI

HEME: Anemia

MS: Arthralgia; arthritis; muscle cramps, spasms, or stiffness; myalgia; neck pain; osteoarthritis; pain in extremity; tendinitis; worsening of restless leg syndrome in early morning hours

RESP: Asthma, bronchitis, cough, upper respiratory tract infection

SKIN: Diaphoresis, flushing, night sweats, rash

Other: Influenza, viral infection, weight loss

Overdose
Monitor patient for evidence of overdose, including agitation, angina, confusion, dyskinesia, nausea, orthostatic hypotension,

sedation, and vomiting. Maintain an open airway, monitor vital signs, and administer symptomatic and supportive care, as needed. To decrease drug absorption, be prepared to perform gastric lavage.

Institute suicide precautions according to facility policy, and anticipate psychiatric re-evaluation.

Nursing Considerations

- **WARNING** Expect to reassess patient periodically during ropinirole treatment for excessive sedation. Patient may develop excessive and acute drowsiness as late as 1 year after beginning therapy.
- When ropinirole is given as adjunct to levodopa, expect levodopa dosage to be gradually decreased as tolerated.
- Expect to discontinue ropinirole gradually over a 7-day period, as follows: Over first 4 days, frequency should be reduced from t.i.d. to b.i.d.; during last 3 days, frequency should be reduced to daily, followed by complete withdrawal of drug.
- **WARNING** Monitor patient for altered mental status during drug withdrawal. Rapid dosage reduction may lead to a sign and symptom complex resembling neuroleptic malignant syndrome (altered level of consciousness, autonomic instability, fever, and muscle rigidity).
- Watch for hallucinations, especially if patient has Parkinson's disease, is elderly, or takes levodopa because this adverse effect is more likely in these patients.
- Monitor patient for orthostatic hypotension, especially if he has early Parkinson's disease. Orthostatic hypotension can occur more than 4 weeks after start of therapy or after a dosage reduction because ropinirole may impair systemic regulation of blood pressure.
- Monitor patient for worsening of existing dyskinesia because ropinirole may potentiate dopaminergic adverse effects of levodopa.
- Avoid using CNS depressants, sleep aids, and other drugs that affect the CNS during ropinirole therapy because they increase the risk of somnolence.

PATIENT TEACHING
- Inform patient with Parkinson's disease that ropinirole helps to improve muscle control and movement but doesn't cure Parkinson's disease.
- Encourage patient to take ropinirole with food to decrease risk of adverse GI effects.

- Caution patient to avoid performing hazardous activities until CNS effects of drug are known, including whether sedating effects occur at any time during therapy.
- Alert patient with restless leg syndrome that symptoms might appear in early morning hours with ropinirole use and could be worse or spread to other limbs. Tell patient to notify prescriber if this occurs.
- Instruct patient to change positions slowly to minimize drug effect on blood pressure.
- If patient falls asleep during normal activities, advise him to notify prescriber.
- Instruct patient to stand or rise slowly from a seated position to reduce the risk of dizziness or fainting.
- Encourage patient to avoid consuming alcohol or sedating medication (such as sleep aides) during ropinirole therapy because doing so may enhance drug's CNS depressant effects.
- Inform patient that chewing sugarless gum, sucking hard candy, and drinking plenty of water may help relieve drug-related dry mouth.

secobarbital sodium

Novo-Secobarb (CAN), Seconal

Class, Category, and Schedule

Chemical class: Barbiturate
Therapeutic class: Sedative-hypnotic
Pregnancy category: D
Controlled substance schedule: II

Indications and Dosages

▶ *To provide short-term treatment of insomnia*
CAPSULES
Adults. 100 mg at bedtime.
▶ *To relieve apprehension, daytime anxiety, and tension*
CAPSULES
Adults. 30 to 50 mg t.i.d. or q.i.d.
Children. 2 mg/kg t.i.d.
DOSAGE ADJUSTMENT Reduced dosage required for elderly or debilitated patients and those with renal or hepatic dysfunction.

Route	Onset	Steady State	Peak	Half-Life	Duration
P.O.	10 to 15 min	Unknown	15 to 30 min	15 to 40 hr	1 to 4 hr

Mechanism of Action

Inhibits upward conduction of nerve impulses to the reticular formation of the brain, thereby disrupting impulse transmission to the cortex. This action depresses the CNS, producing drowsiness, hypnosis, and sedation.

Contraindications

History of barbiturate addiction; hypersensitivity to secobarbital, other barbiturates, or their components; nephritis; porphyria; severe hepatic or respiratory impairment

Interactions

DRUGS

acetaminophen, adrenocorticoids, beta blockers, chloramphenicol, cyclosporine, dacarbazine, disopyramide, estrogens, metronidazole, oral anticoagulants, oral contraceptives, quinidine, thyroid hormones, tricyclic antidepressants: Decreased effectiveness of these drugs

addictive drugs: Increased risk of addiction

calcium channel blockers: Possibly excessive hypotension

carbamazepine, succinimide anticonvulsants: Decreased blood levels and increased elimination of these drugs

carbonic anhydrase inhibitors: Increased risk of osteopenia

CNS depressants: Increased CNS depressant effects

cyclophosphamide: Increased risk of leukopenic activity and reduced half-life of cyclophosphamide

divalproex sodium, valproic acid: Increased CNS depression and neurologic toxicity

doxycycline, fenoprofen: Increased elimination of these drugs

general anesthetics (enflurane, halothane, methoxyflurane): Increased risk of hepatotoxicity; increased risk of nephrotoxicity (with methoxyflurane)

griseofulvin: Decreased griseofulvin absorption

guanadrel, guanethidine: Possibly increased orthostatic hypotension

haloperidol: Decreased blood haloperidol level

MAO inhibitors: Possibly prolonged CNS depressant effects of secobarbital

maprotiline: Increased CNS depressant effect

methylphenidate: Increased risk of barbiturate toxicity

mexiletine: Decreased blood mexiletine level

phenylbutazone: Decreased effectiveness of secobarbital

posterior pituitary hormones: Increased risk of arrhythmias and coronary insufficiency

primidone: Increased sedative effect of either drug
vitamin D: Decreased vitamin D effects
xanthines (aminophylline, oxtriphylline, theophylline): Increased metabolism of xanthines (except dyphylline), decreased hypnotic effect of secobarbital
FOODS
caffeine: Increased caffeine metabolism, decreased hypnotic effect of secobarbital
ACTIVITIES
alcohol use: Increased CNS depression

Adverse Reactions

CNS: Anxiety, clumsiness, confusion, depression, dizziness, drowsiness, hangover, headache, insomnia, irritability, lethargy, nervousness, nightmares, paradoxical stimulation, syncope
CV: Hypotension
GI: Anorexia, constipation, nausea, vomiting
MS: Arthralgia, muscle weakness
RESP: Hypoventilation
SKIN: Exfoliative dermatitis, hives, jaundice, rash, Stevens-Johnson syndrome
Other: Angioedema, drug dependence, weight loss

Overdose

Monitor patient for evidence of overdose, including absent or decreased reflexes, bradycardia, Cheyne-Stokes respiration, coma, confusion, dyspnea, fever, hypothermia, miosis or mydriasis, oliguria, severe drowsiness, severe weakness, shock, slurred speech, staggering, tachycardia, and unusual eye movements. Consider chronic overdose if patient has continued irritability, insomnia, poor judgment, and severe confusion. Maintain an open airway, and carefully monitor blood pressure and temperature.

If patient is conscious, be prepared to give ipecac syrup, as prescribed, to induce vomiting. Expect to give activated charcoal, 30 to 60 g, with water or sorbitol to prevent further absorption and to enhance drug elimination. For an unconscious patient, anticipate assisting with insertion of an endotracheal tube and then performing gastric lavage. The endotracheal tube's inflated cuff will help prevent aspiration of gastric contents into the lungs.

Be prepared to administer a urine-alkalizing drug to increase drug elimination. Administer I.V. fluids and a vasopressor, as prescribed. For severe cases, anticipate the need for hemodialysis or hemoperfusion.

Be aware that, in extreme secobarbital overdose, the patient may have a flat EEG because all electrical activity in the brain has ceased; however, this effect may be reversible.

Institute suicide precautions according to facility policy, and anticipate psychiatric re-evaluation.

Nursing Considerations

- When secobarbital is used to treat insomnia, be aware that it should only be used for a short time because the drug loses its effectiveness after 2 weeks.
- Assess patient for evidence of exfoliative dermatitis, such as fever and red, scaly, or thickened skin. If this occurs, notify prescriber and expect to discontinue drug immediately because this may indicate a potentially fatal hypersensitivity reaction.
- **WARNING** To avoid withdrawal signs and symptoms, expect to taper drug after long-term therapy. Such signs and symptoms usually appear 8 to 12 hours after stopping drug and may include anxiety, insomnia, muscle twitching, nausea, orthostatic hypotension, vomiting, weakness, and weight loss. Severe signs and symptoms may include delirium, hallucinations, and seizures. Generalized tonic-clonic seizures may occur within 16 hours or up to 5 days after last dose.

PATIENT TEACHING

- Caution patient not to take secobarbital more often than prescribed because of the risk of addiction.
- Inform patient that taking drug with food may reduce adverse GI effects.
- Advise patient to avoid alcohol and caffeine and potentially hazardous activities during therapy.
- Inform patient about possible hangover effect.
- If patient takes an oral contraceptive, recommend using an additional form of birth control during therapy.
- Caution patient not to abruptly stop taking drug.
- Instruct patient to notify prescriber of bone pain, muscle weakness, rash, skin lesions, or unexplained weight loss during therapy.
- Encourage patient to use other nondrug therapies to treat insomnia. Offer suggestions for improved sleep, such as getting moderate exercise during the day, setting regular sleep habits, and using relaxation techniques.

Other Therapeutic Uses

Secobarbital sodium is also indicated for the following:
- To induce sedation before surgery

secobarbital sodium and amobarbital sodium
Tuinal

Class, Category, and Schedule
Chemical class: Barbiturate
Therapeutic class: Sedative-hypnotic
Pregnancy category: D
Controlled substance schedule: II

Indications and Dosages
▶ *To provide short-term treatment of insomnia*
CAPSULES
Adults. 100 mg (50 mg each of secobarbital sodium and amobarbital sodium) to 200 mg (100 mg each of secobarbital sodium and amobarbital sodium) at bedtime.
DOSAGE ADJUSTMENT Possibly reduced for elderly or debilitated patients and those with renal or hepatic dysfunction.

Route	Onset	Steady State	Peak	Half-Life	Duration
P.O.	10 to 15 min*	Unknown*	15 to 30 min*	15 to 40 hr*	1 to 4 hr*
	45 to 60 min†	Unknown†	Unknown†	16 to 40 hr†	6 to 8 hr†

Mechanism of Action
Acts nonselectively on the CNS to alter cerebral function, decrease motor activity, depress the sensory cortex, and produce drowsiness, hypnosis, and sedation. Secobarbital and amobarbital combine to reduce wakefulness and alertness by acting in the thalamus to depress reticular activating system and interfere with impulse transmission from periphery to cortex. They produce CNS-depressant effects ranging from mild sedation and anxiety reduction to anesthesia and coma, depending on dosage, route, and individual patient response. Secobarbital and amobarbital have different rates of action and dissipation. The combination provides a balanced sedative-hypnotic effect.

Contraindications
History of barbiturate addiction; hypersensitivity to secobarbital, amobarbital, or their components; nephritis; porphyria; severe hepatic or respiratory dysfunction

---

* For secobarbital.
† For amobarbital.

Interactions
DRUGS
antihistamines, CNS depressants: Additive CNS depressant effects
corticosteroids, oral anticoagulants: Increased metabolism of these drugs, causing decreased anticoagulant response
doxycycline: Shortened half-life and increased elimination of doxycycline
estradiol, estrone, progesterone, other steroidal hormones: Increased metabolism of these hormones, leading to decreased effectiveness
griseofulvin: Decreased absorption of griseofulvin
MAO inhibitors: Inhibited metabolism of secobarbital and amobarbital, causing prolonged CNS depressant effects
phenytoin: Possibly accelerated metabolism of phenytoin
sodium valproate, valproic acid: Decreased metabolism of secobarbital and amobarbital
vitamin D: Decreased effects of vitamin D
FOODS
caffeine: Increased metabolism of caffeine; decreased hypnotic effect of secobarbital and amobarbital
ACTIVITIES
alcohol use: Increased CNS depressant effects

Adverse Reactions
CNS: Anxiety, clumsiness, CNS depression, confusion, dizziness, drowsiness, hallucinations, hangover, headache, insomnia, irritability, light-headedness, nervousness, nightmares, paradoxical stimulation, syncope, unsteadiness
CV: Bradycardia, hypotension
GI: Constipation, hepatic dysfunction, nausea, vomiting
HEME: Agranulocytosis, megaloblastic anemia, thrombocytopenia
MS: Osteopenia, rickets
RESP: Apnea, hypoventilation
SKIN: Exfoliative dermatitis, rash, Stevens-Johnson syndrome
Other: Angioedema, physical and psychological dependence, potentially fatal withdrawal syndrome, tolerance

Overdose
Monitor patient for signs and symptoms of overdose, including absent or decreased reflexes, bradycardia, Cheyne-Stokes respiration, coma, confusion, dyspnea, fever, hypothermia, miosis or mydriasis, oliguria, severe drowsiness, severe weakness, shock, slurred speech, staggering, tachycardia, and unusual eye movements. Consider chronic overdose if patient has continued irri-

tability, insomnia, poor judgment, and severe confusion. Maintain an open airway, and carefully monitor patient's blood pressure and temperature.

If the patient is conscious, be prepared to administer ipecac syrup, as prescribed, to induce vomiting. Expect to administer activated charcoal, 30 to 60 g, with water or sorbitol to prevent further absorption and to enhance drug elimination. For an unconscious patient, anticipate assisting with the insertion of an endotracheal tube and then performing gastric lavage. The inflated cuff of the endotracheal tube will help prevent aspiration of gastric contents into the lungs.

Be prepared to administer a urine-alkalizing drug to increase elimination of secobarbital and amobarbital. Administer I.V. fluids and a vasopressor, as prescribed. For severe cases, anticipate the need for hemodialysis or hemoperfusion.

Be aware that, in cases of extreme overdose, the patient may have a flat EEG because all electrical activity in the brain has ceased; however, this effect may be reversible.

Institute suicide precautions according to facility policy, and anticipate psychiatric re-evaluation.

Nursing Considerations

- Be aware that secobarbital and amobarbital is used for short-term treatment of insomnia because the drug loses its effectiveness after 2 weeks.
- Monitor patient for paradoxical reactions to the drug—such as confusion, excitement, or mental depression—especially if he's elderly.
- Be aware that drug has the potential to exaggerate depression, suicidal tendencies, and other mental disorders.
- Be aware that drug shouldn't be discontinued abruptly because withdrawal signs and symptoms can occur.
- Assess patient for signs and symptoms of exfoliative dermatitis, such as fever and red, scaly, or thickened skin. If this occurs, notify prescriber and expect to discontinue drug immediately because this may indicate a potentially fatal hypersensitivity reaction.
- Be aware that drug may cause physical and psychological dependence.

PATIENT TEACHING

- Instruct patient to take secobarbital and amobarbital exactly as prescribed because of the risk of addiction.
- Instruct patient to report severe dizziness, persistent drowsiness, rash, or skin lesions.

- Advise patient to use caution when driving or performing tasks that require alertness.
- Instruct patient not to use alcohol or other CNS depressants (unless prescribed) because they increase drug's effects.
- If patient is female and takes an oral contraceptive, suggest an additional form of birth control during therapy. Advise her to notify prescriber immediately if she knows or suspects she's pregnant. Caution against breast-feeding while taking drug.
- Encourage patient to use other nondrug therapies to treat insomnia. Offer suggestions for improved sleep, such as getting moderate exercise during the day, setting regular sleep habits, and using relaxation techniques.

Other Therapeutic Uses
Secobarbital sodium and amobarbital sodium is also indicated for the following:
- To induce sedation before surgery

selegiline hydrochloride
Apo-Selegiline (CAN), Carbex, Eldepryl, Gen-Selegiline (CAN), Novo-Selegiline (CAN), Nu-Selegiline (CAN), SD Deprenyl (CAN), Selegiline-5 (CAN), Zelapar

selegiline transdermal system
EMSAM

Class and Category
Chemical class: Phenethylamine derivative
Therapeutic class: Antidepressant (EMSAM), antidyskinetic
Pregnancy category: C

Indications and Dosages
▶ *As adjunct to carbidopa and levodopa to treat Parkinson's disease*
CAPSULES, TABLETS
Adults. 10 mg once daily or 5 mg b.i.d. with breakfast and lunch.
DOSAGE ADJUSTMENT For patient with levodopa-induced adverse reactions, 2.5 mg q.i.d.
▶ *As adjunct to carbidopa-levodopa therapy to treat Parkinson's disease in patients whose response to therapy has deteriorated*
ORALLY DISINTEGRATING TABLETS (ZELAPAR)
Adults. *Initial:* 1.25 mg daily before breakfast and without liquids for at least 6 weeks; then increased to 2.25 mg daily, if needed and tolerated.

▶ *To treat depression*
TRANSDERMAL SYSTEM (EMSAM)
Adults. *Initial:* 6 mg/24 hr with patch applied to upper torso, upper thigh, or outer surface of upper arm daily Dosage increased
every 2 wk in increments of 3 mg/24 hr, as needed. *Maximum:*
12 mg/24 hr.

Route	Onset	Steady State	Peak	Half-Life	Duration
P.O.	Unknown	Unknown	Unknown	16 to 69 hr	Unknown

Mechanism of Action

Reduces dopamine metabolism by noncompetitively inhibiting the brain enzyme monoamine oxidase type B. This increases the amount of dopamine
available to relieve signs and symptoms of parkinsonism. Selegiline's
metabolites may also enhance dopamine transmission by inhibiting its reuptake at synapses.

Selegiline also inhibits intracellular monamine oxidase in the outer membrane of mitochrondira of nerve cells in the CNS. This prevents catabolism of
neurotransmitter amines such as norephinephrine, dopamine, and serotonin,
as well as neuromodulators such as phenylethylamine, and increases
monoamine neurotransmitter activity. Mood elevation may result from increased monoamine neurotransmitter activity in the brain.

Contraindications

Hypersensitivity to selegiline or its components; pheochromocytoma; use within 14 days of meperidine; use within 10 days of
general anesthesia; use with carbamazepine, oxcarbazepine, selective serotonin reuptake inhibitors (fluoxetine, paraxetine, sertraline), dual serotonin and norephinephrine reuptake inhibitors
(duloxetine, venlafaxine), tricyclic antidepressants (amitriptyline,
bupropion, imipramine), analgesics (tramadol, propoxyphene),
dextromethorphan; use with St. John's wort, mirtazapine, cyclobenzaprine, oral selegline, other MAO inhibitors, sympathomi-
imetic amines (EMSAM only)

Interactions
DRUGS
carbamazepine, oxcarbazepine: Increased blood selegiline level
fluoxetine, fluvoxamine, nefazodone, paroxetine, sertraline, venlafaxine:
Increased risk of adverse reactions similar to those of serotonin
syndrome (confusion, hypomania, restlessness, myoclonus), auto-

nomic instability, delirium, muscle rigidity, and severe agitation
levodopa: Increased risk of confusion, dyskinesia, hallucinations, nausea, and orthostatic hypotension
meperidine, possibly other opioid agonists: Increased risk of diaphoresis, excitation, muscle rigidity, and severe hypertension
sympathomimetics: Increased risk of severe hypertension
tricyclic antidepressants: Possibly serious CNS reactions, including decreased level of consciousness, hyperpyrexia, hypertension, muscle rigidity, seizures, and syncope

FOODS
caffeine: Increased risk of hypertension
foods that contain tyramine or other high-pressor amines: Increased risk of sudden and severe hypertension

ACTIVITIES
alcohol use: Increased risk of hypertension

Adverse Reactions

CNS: Anxiety, chills, confusion, dizziness, drowsiness, dyskinesia, euphoria, extrapyramidal reactions, fatigue, hallucinations, headache, insomnia, irritability, lethargy, memory loss, mood changes, nervousness, paresthesia, restlessness, suicidal ideation, syncope, tremor, weakness
CV: Arrhythmias, chest pain, hypertension, orthostatic hypotension, palpitations, peripheral edema
EENT: Altered taste, blepharospasm, blurred vision, burning lips or mouth, diplopia, dry mouth, pharyngitis, sinusitis, tinnitus
GI: Abdominal pain, anorexia, constipation, diarrhea, GI bleeding, heartburn, nausea, vomiting
GU: Dysuria, urinary hesitancy, urinary urgency, urine retention
MS: Arthralgia, back and leg pain, muscle fatigue and spasms, neck stiffness
RESP: Asthma
SKIN: Diaphoresis, photosensitivity, rash
Other: Application site reactions (EMSAM)

Overdose

Monitor patient for evidence of overdose, including agitation, angina, cool and clammy skin, diaphoresis, dizziness, fainting, hypertension or hypotension, hyperpyrexia, irregular heartbeat, irritability, opisthotonos, respiratory depression, seizures, tachycardia, and trismus (lockjaw). These effects may not be present or may be minimal in the first 24 hours after ingestion and will peak in 48 hours. Be prepared to monitor patient throughout this period.

Maintain an open airway, administer oxygen as prescribed,

and be prepared to assist with intubation and mechanical ventilation, as needed. Monitor vital signs, and institute continuous ECG monitoring and seizure precautions according to facility protocol.

To decrease drug absorption in a conscious patient who isn't at risk for coma or seizures, be prepared to induce vomiting or perform gastric lavage. Expect that oral activated charcoal may also be prescribed. For an unconscious patient, anticipate assisting with the insertion of an endotracheal tube and then performing gastric lavage. The inflated cuff of the endotracheal tube will help prevent aspiration of gastric contents into the lungs.

Be prepared to treat hypotension and shock with I.V. fluids and a vasopressor. An adrenergic shouldn't be used because it may increase the pressor response. Anticipate the use of diazepam to treat CNS stimulation, and know that phenothiazines should be avoided. To treat hyperpyrexia, administer an antipyretic and use a cooling blanket, as needed and prescribed.

Institute suicide precautions according to facility policy, and anticipate psychiatric re-evaluation.

Nursing Considerations

- Assess patient for mental status and mood changes because selegiline can exacerbate such conditions as dementia, severe psychosis, tardive dyskinesia, and tremor.
- Watch patient closely for suicidal tendencies, especially when therapy starts or dosage changes and especially if patient is a child, an adolescent, or a young adult.
- Monitor patient for decreased symptoms of Parkinson's disease or depression to evaluate drug's effectiveness.
- Monitor patient who is also taking levodopa for levodopa-induced adverse reactions, including confusion, dyskinesia, hallucinations, nausea, and orthostatic hypotension.
- Be aware that drug can reactivate gastric ulcers because it prevents breakdown of gastric histamine. Assess patient for related symptoms, such as abdominal pain.

PATIENT TEACHING

- Advise patient to avoid taking selegiline in the late afternoon or evening because it may interfere with sleep.
- Caution patient to take only prescribed amount because increased dosage may cause severe adverse reactions.
- If patient will use the transdermal form, explain how and where to apply the patch, stressing the need to rotate sites. Tell patient to wash his hands well after application and to dispose of removed patch immediately.

- Stress that only one patch can be worn at a time. If a patch falls off, tell patient to apply a new patch to a new site and to resume his previous schedule.
- Urge patient to avoid tyramine-rich foods and beverages during and for 2 weeks after stopping selegiline therapy unless patient is prescribed the lowest dosage of transdermal system (6 mg per 24 hours), which doesn't require diet modification. Review which foods are considered tyramine-rich.
- Instruct patient to immediately report a severe headache, neck stiffness, a racing heart, palpitations, or other sudden or unusual symptoms.
- Caution patient to avoid exposing transdermal patch to direct heat, such as in heating pads, electric blankets, heat lamps, saunas, hot tubs, and prolonged sunlight exposure.
- Tell patient not to cut the transdermal patch into smaller pieces.
- If patient will use orally disintegrating tablets, instruct him to take them before breakfast and without liquids.
- Tell patient to remove the tablet from the blister pack by peeling away the foil backing with dry hands and not by pushing the tablet through the foil, which can damage the tablet. He should then immediately place the tablet on top of his tongue, where it will disintegrate in seconds. Remind him not to eat or drink anything for 5 minutes before and after taking the tablet.
- Urge patient to avoid potentially hazardous activities until he knows how the drug affects him.
- Advise patient to change position slowly to minimize effects of orthostatic hypotension.
- Suggest that patient elevate his legs when sitting to reduce ankle swelling.
- Instruct patient to report possible evidence of overdose, including muscle twitching and eye spasms.
- Tell family or caregiver to observe patient closely for suicidal tendencies, especially when therapy starts or dosage changes and especially if patient is a child, a teenager, or a young adult.
- Urge patient to notify prescriber if dry mouth lasts longer than 2 weeks. Advise him to have routine dental checkups.

sertraline hydrochloride
Zoloft

Class and Category
Chemical class: Naphthylamine derivative

Therapeutic class: Antidepressant, antiobsessional, antipanic drug
Pregnancy category: C

Indications and Dosages

▶ *To treat major depression*
ORAL CONCENTRATE, TABLETS
Adults. *Initial:* 50 mg daily, increased after several wk in increments of 50 mg daily every wk, as needed. *Maximum:* 200 mg daily.

▶ *To treat obsessive-compulsive disorder*
ORAL CONCENTRATE, TABLETS
Adults and adolescents. *Initial:* 50 mg daily, increased after several wk in increments of 50 mg daily every wk, as needed. *Maximum:* 200 mg daily.
Children ages 6 to 13. *Initial:* 25 mg daily, increased every wk, as needed. *Maximum:* 200 mg daily.

▶ *To treat panic disorder, social anxiety disorder, and post-traumatic stress disorder*
ORAL CONCENTRATE, TABLETS
Adults. *Initial:* 25 mg daily, increased to 50 mg daily after 1 wk; then increased by 50 mg daily every wk, as needed. *Maximum:* 200 mg daily.
DOSAGE ADJUSTMENT Initial dosage reduction recommended for elderly patients and those with hepatic impairment.

Route	Onset	Steady State	Peak	Half-Life	Duration
P.O.	2 to 4 wk*	7 days	Unknown	26 hr	Unknown

Mechanism of Action

Inhibits reuptake of the neurotransmitter serotonin by CNS neurons, thereby increasing the amount of serotonin available in nerve synapses. An elevated serotonin level may result in elevated mood and reduced depression. This action may also relieve signs and symptoms of other psychiatric conditions attributed to serotonin deficiency.

Contraindications

Disulfiram therapy (oral concentrate only), hypersensitivity to sertraline or its components, use within 14 days of MAO inhibitor therapy

* For antidepressant and antipanic effects; for antiobsessional effect, onset is longer than 4 wk.

Interactions
DRUGS

aspirin, NSAIDs, warfarin: Increased anticoagulant activity and risk of bleeding
cimetidine: Increased sertraline half-life
MAO inhibitors: Possibly hyperpyretic episodes, hypertensive crisis, serotonin syndrome, and severe seizures
moclobemide, serotonergics: Increased risk of potentially fatal serotonin syndrome
tolbutamide: Possibly hypoglycemia
tricyclic antidepressants: Possibly impaired metabolism of tricyclic antidepressants, resulting in increased risk of toxicity

Adverse Reactions
CNS: Agitation, aggression, anxiety, dizziness, drowsiness, fatigue, fever, headache, hyperkinesias, insomnia, nervousness, paresthesia, serotonin syndrome, suicidal ideation, tremor, weakness, yawning
CV: Palpitations
EENT: Dry mouth, epistaxis, sinusitis, vision changes
ENDO: Syndrome of inappropriate ADH secretion
GI: Abdominal cramps, anorexia, constipation, diarrhea, flatulence, increased appetite, indigestion, nausea, vomiting
GU: Anorgasmy, decreased libido, ejaculation disorders, impotence, urinary incontinence
SKIN: Diaphoresis, flushing, purpura, rash
Other: Weight loss

Overdose
Monitor patient for signs and symptoms of overdose, including anxiety, ECG changes, mydriasis, nausea, somnolence, tachycardia, and vomiting.

Maintain open airway, monitor vital signs, and institute continuous ECG monitoring. Anticipate the possibility that the patient may also have ingested other drugs or alcohol.

To decrease drug absorption in a conscious patient who isn't at risk for coma or seizures, be prepared to perform gastric lavage. Expect that oral activated charcoal may also be prescribed. Be aware that inducing vomiting isn't recommended. For an unconscious patient, anticipate assisting with the insertion of an endotracheal tube and then performing gastric lavage. The inflated cuff of the endotracheal tube will help prevent aspiration of gastric contents into the lungs. Dialysis, exchange transfusions, forced diuresis, and hemoperfusion are ineffective for treating sertraline overdose because the drug has a large volume of distribution in the body.

Institute suicide precautions according to facility policy, and anticipate psychiatric re-evaluation.

Nursing Considerations

- Use sertraline cautiously in patients with hepatic or renal dysfunction. Monitor liver function test results and serum BUN and creatinine levels, as appropriate.
- **WARNING** Be aware that oral concentrate form of sertraline contains alcohol and shouldn't be given to a patient who takes disulfiram.
- To prepare the oral concentrate dose, use the dropper that's provided to measure the drug, and dilute it just before administration with 4 oz (120 ml) of ginger ale, lemonade, lemon lime soda, orange juice, or water. A slight haze may appear after mixing; this is normal.
- Because drug can cause weight loss, use cautiously in patients with anorexia nervosa or other condition that makes weight loss undesirable. Monitor weight during therapy, and notify prescriber of rapid weight loss.
- Monitor for hypo-osmolarity of serum and urine and for hyponatremia, which may indicate sertraline-induced syndrome of inappropriate ADH secretion.
- Check blood glucose level often in a diabetic patient who also takes tolbutamide. Tolbutamide dosage may need adjustment.
- Be aware that effective antidepressant therapy can promote mania in predisposed people. If evidence of mania develops, notify prescriber immediately and expect to withhold sertraline.
- Watch closely for suicidal tendencies, especially when therapy starts and dosage changes, and especially in children and adolescents.
- Monitor patient closely for evidence of GI bleeding, especially if patient also takes a drug known to cause GI bleeding, such as aspirin, an NSAID, or warfarin.
- Expect to taper dosage when drug is no longer needed, as ordered, to minimize adverse reactions.

PATIENT TEACHING
- Instruct patient to take sertraline with food if adverse GI reactions develop.
- Instruct patient taking oral concentrate to use the dropper that's provided to measure the drug and to dilute it properly.

- Warn family or caregiver to observe patient closely for suicidal tendencies, especially when therapy starts and dosage changes, and particularly if patient is a child or teenager.
- Advise patient to avoid potentially hazardous activities until he knows how the drug affects him.
- Inform patient that it may take 2 to 4 weeks or longer for drug effects to be apparent.
- Advise patient against using OTC products or herbal supplements during sertraline therapy unless approved by prescriber.
- Caution patient not to stop taking drug abruptly. Explain that gradual tapering helps to avoid withdrawal effects.
- If patient is diabetic and takes tolbutamide, advise him to monitor his blood glucose level often while taking sertraline.
- Instruct female patient to notify prescriber if she is or could be pregnant to discuss the benefits and risks of continuing sertraline therapy while pregnant.
- **WARNING** Inform patient that taking sertraline with certain other drugs increases the risk of serotonin syndrome, a rare but serious complication. Teach patient to recognize its signs and symptoms, and advise her to notify prescriber immediately if they occur.

sibutramine hydrochloride monohydrate
Meridia

Class, Category, and Schedule
Chemical class: Cyclobutanemethanamine
Therapeutic class: Appetite suppressant
Pregnancy category: C
Controlled substance schedule: IV

Indications and Dosages
▶ *As adjunct to dieting to manage obesity*
CAPSULES
Adults. *Initial:* 10 mg daily, increased to 15 mg daily after 4 wk if weight loss is inadequate. *Maximum:* 15 mg daily.
DOSAGE ADJUSTMENT Reduction to 5 mg daily may be needed if patient can't tolerate 10-mg dose.

Route	Onset	Steady State	Peak	Half-Life	Duration
P.O.	Unknown	4 days	Unknown	1.1 hr*	Unknown

* 14 to 16 hr for active metabolites.

Mechanism of Action

Inhibits central reuptake of dopamine, norepinephrine, and serotonin primarily by the action of its active metabolites, thereby suppressing appetite and lowering food intake, leading to weight loss.

Contraindications

Anorexia nervosa, concomitant use of other centrally acting appetite suppressants, hypersensitivity to sibutramine or its components, use within 14 days of MAO inhibitor therapy

Interactions

DRUGS

certain allergy, cold and cough drugs, and decongestants; ephedrine; phenylpropanolamine; pseudoephedrine: Increased risk of elevated blood pressure or heart rate

certain opioid analgesics (dextromethorphan, fentanyl, meperidine, pentazocine), dihydroergotamine, lithium, MAO inhibitors, serotonergics, sumatriptan, tryptophan, zolmitriptan: Increased risk of potentially fatal serotonin syndrome

erythromycin, ketoconazole: Possibly decreased sibutramine clearance

Adverse Reactions

CNS: Anxiety, depression, dizziness, drowsiness, headache, insomnia, nervousness, paresthesia, somnolence

CV: Chest pain, edema, hypertension, palpitations, tachycardia

EENT: Dry mouth, earache, rhinitis, sinusitis, taste perversion

GI: Abdominal pain, anorexia, constipation, diarrhea, gastritis, increased appetite, indigestion, nausea, thirst, vomiting

GU: Dysmenorrhea, urine retention, UTI, vaginal candidiasis

HEME: Bleeding

MS: Arthralgia, back or neck pain, myalgia, tenosynovitis

SKIN: Acne, diaphoresis, ecchymosis, flushing, urticaria

Other: Anaphylaxis, angioedema, flulike signs and symptoms

Overdose

Information about sibutramine overdose is limited. Few serious adverse reactions have been known to occur, although one case of tachycardia has been reported.

Maintain open airway, monitor vital signs, and institute continuous ECG monitoring. Give supportive and symptomatic care, as needed. To treat hypertension and tachycardia, expect to administer a beta blocker, as prescribed. The benefits of treating the overdose with forced diuresis or dialysis are unknown.

Institute suicide precautionary measures according to facility policy, and anticipate psychiatric re-evaluation.

Nursing Considerations

* Use sibutramine cautiously in patients with a history of substance abuse. Observe patient for signs of misuse, including drug-seeking behavior, drug tolerance, and increasing dosage.
* Use cautiously in patients with mild to moderate renal impairment; drug shouldn't be used in patients with severe renal impairment, including those with end-stage renal disease undergoing dialysis.
* Measure blood pressure and pulse rate before and during sibutramine therapy.
* Because serotonin release from nerve terminals has been linked to cardiac valve dysfunction, assess patient for a third heart sound.
* **WARNING** If patient takes a drug for migraine headache, watch for evidence of serotonin syndrome, which may include agitation, anxiety, ataxia, chills, confusion, diaphoresis, disorientation, dysarthria, excitement, hemiballismus, hyperreflexia, hyperthermia, hypomania, lack of coordination, loss of consciousness, mydriasis, myoclonus, restlessness, tachycardia, tremor, vomiting, and weakness. Notify prescriber immediately if these occur.
* Because drug decreases salivary flow and causes dry mouth, monitor patient for signs and symptoms of dental caries, oral candidiasis, and periodontal disease.

PATIENT TEACHING

* Caution patient not to take sibutramine more often than prescribed.
* Teach patient how to measure his blood pressure and pulse rate during therapy.
* Emphasize that sibutramine is intended as an adjunct to a calorie-reducing diet, not a replacement for it.
* Advise patient against taking OTC products that may contain ephedrine because of the increased risk of hypertension.
* Urge patient to avoid potentially hazardous activities until he knows how the drug affects him.
* Advise patient to report unusual bleeding or unexplained appearance of ecchymosis.
* If patient reports dry mouth, suggest sugar-free hard candy or gum or a saliva substitute.

sildenafil citrate

Revatio, Viagra

Class and Category

Chemical class: Pyrazolopyrimidinone derivative
Therapeutic class: Anti-impotence drug
Pregnancy category: B

Indications and Dosages

▶ *To treat erectile dysfunction*

TABLETS

Adults. 50 mg daily, taken 1 hr before sexual activity; increased as prescribed, based on patient's response. *Maximum:* 100 mg daily.

DOSAGE ADJUSTMENT Initial dose reduced to 25 mg for elderly patients, those with hepatic cirrhosis or severe renal impairment (creatinine clearance less than 30 ml/min/1.73 m2), and those taking potent cytochrome P450 3A4 inhibitors or ritonavir. Maximum: 25 mg/48 hr. Dosage reduced to 25 mg if taken within 4 hr of an alpha blocker. Maximum: 25 mg/48 hr.

▶ *To treat pulmonary arterial hypertension and improve exercise ability in patients classified by World Health Organization as group 1*

TABLETS

Adults. 20 mg t.i.d.

Route	Onset	Steady State	Peak	Half-Life	Duration
P.O.	30 min	Unknown	Unknown	4 hr	4 hr

Mechanism of Action

Enhances effect of nitric oxide (released in the penis by sexual stimulation), which increases the cGMP level, relaxes smooth muscle, and increases blood flow into the corpus cavernosum, thus producing a penile erection.

Contraindications

Concomitant continuous or intermittent nitrate therapy, hypersensitivity to sildenafil or its components

Interactions

DRUGS

antihypertensives, alpha blockers: Increased risk of symptomatic hypotension

barbiturates, bosentan, carbamazepine, efavirenz, nevirapine, phenytoin, rifabutin, rifampin: Altered plasma levels of either drug

cimetidine, erythromycin, itraconazole, ketoconazole, mibefradil: Prolonged sildenafil effect
nitrates: Profound hypotension
protease inhibitors: Increased sildenafil effect
rifampin: Decreased sildenafil effect
FOODS
high-fat meals: Drug absorption delayed by up to 60 minutes

Adverse Reactions

CNS: Cerebrovascular, intracerebral, or subarachnoid hemorrhage; dizziness; headache; migraine; syncope; transient ischemic attack
CV: Heart failure, hypertension, hypotension, myocardial ischemia, orthostatic hypotension, palpitations, sudden cardiac death, tachycardia, ventricular arrhythmias
EENT: Abrupt reduction or loss of hearing; blurred vision; change in color perception; diplopia; epistaxis; increased intraocular pressure; nasal congestion; nonarteritic anterior ischemic optic neuropathy; ocular burning, pressure, redness, or swelling; paramacular edema; photophobia; retinal vascular bleeding or disease; tinnitus; visual decrease or temporary vision loss; vitreous detachment
ENDO: Uncontrolled diabetes mellitus
GI: Diarrhea, indigestion
GU: Cystitis, dysuria, painful erection, priapism, UTI
MS: Arthralgia, back pain
RESP: Pulmonary hemorrhage, upper respiratory tract infection
SKIN: Flushing, photosensitivity

Overdose

Monitor patient for signs and symptoms of overdose similar to the adverse reactions listed above; however, expect them to be more prevalent.

Be prepared to give supportive and symptomatic care, as needed and prescribed. Dialysis is ineffective for treating overdose because sildenafil is highly protein-bound and isn't eliminated by the kidneys.

Institute suicide precautions according to facility policy, and anticipate psychiatric re-evaluation.

Nursing Considerations

• Use sildenafil cautiously in patients with renal or hepatic dysfunction, in elderly patients, and in men with penile abnormalities that may predispose them to priapism.

- Also use cautiously in patients with left ventricular outflow obstruction, such as aortic stenosis and idiopathic hypertrophic subaortic stenosis, and those with severely impaired autonomic control of blood pressure because these conditions increase sensitivity to vasodilators such as sildenafil.
- Monitor vision, especially in patients over age 50; who have diabetes, hypertension, coronary artery disease, or hyperlipidemia; or who smoke because, although rare, sildenafil use has been linked to nonarteritic anterior ischemic optic neuropathy that may result in permanently decreased vision.
- Monitor blood pressure and heart rate and rhythm before and often during therapy.
- Monitor blood glucose level often in diabetic patient because sildenafil may alter glucose control.

PATIENT TEACHING
- Explain that sildenafil used to treat erectile dysfunction may be taken up to 4 hours before sexual activity but that taking it 1 hour beforehand provides the best results.
- Caution patient that he shouldn't take sildenafil more often than prescribed.
- **WARNING** Instruct patient not to take sildenafil if he takes any form of organic nitrate, either continuously or intermittently, because profound hypotension and death could result. Also caution patient taking sildenafil for erectile dysfunction not to take more than 25 mg within 4 hours of taking an alpha blocker, such as doxazosin, or other blood pressure–lowering drugs because symptomatic orthostatic hypotension may occur.
- Tell patient to stop taking sildenafil and notify prescriber if he develops a sudden loss of vision in one or both eyes.
- Advise patient taking drug for erectile dysfunction to seek sexual counseling to enhance drug's effects.
- Inform patient that drug won't protect him from sexually transmitted diseases, including HIV infection. Counsel him about protective measures, as needed.
- To avoid possible penile damage and permanent loss of erectile function, urge patient to notify prescriber immediately if erection is painful or lasts longer than 4 hours.
- If patient is diabetic, instruct him to frequently monitor his blood glucose level because drug may affect glucose control.
- Instruct patient to stop taking sildenafil immediately and to notify prescriber if he has a sudden reduction or loss of hearing.

sodium oxybate

Xyrem

Class and Category

Chemical class: Gamma hydroxybutyrate (GHB)
Therapeutic class: Antinarcoleptic
Pregnancy category: B
Controlled substance schedule: III

Indications and Dosages

▶ *To treat excessive daytime sleepiness and cataplexy in patients with narcolepsy*

ORAL SOLUTION

Adults. *Initial:* 2.25 g at bedtime, when patient is in bed, followed by 2.25 g 2.5 to 4 hr later (4.5 g every night). Dosage increased by 1.5 g/night (0.75 g/dose) every 2 wk. *Maximum:* 4.5 g at bedtime, when patient is in bed, followed by 4.5 g 2.5 to 4 hr later (9 g every night).

DOSAGE ADJUSTMENT For patients with hepatic insufficiency, initial dosage 1.125 g at bedtime, when patient is in bed, followed by 1.125 g 2.5 to 4 hr later (2.25 g every night).

Route	Onset	Peak	Duration
P.O.	15 to 45 min	0.75 to 1.5 hr	2 to 3 hr

Mechanism of Action

Probably acts as a neurotransmitter in the regulation of sleep cycles, blood flow, emotion, and memory, most likely through brain receptors specific for GHB and through binding to GABA-B receptors. At low doses, sodium oxybate inhibits presynaptic dopamine release; at high doses, it stimulates dopamine release. It may decrease symptoms of narcolepsy by inducing REM sleep and increasing delta sleep. The precise mechanism of anti-cataplectic activity in patients with narcolepsy isn't known.

Contraindications

Use with sedative-hypnotic drugs, hypersensitivity to sodium oxybate or its components, succinic semialdehyde dehydrogenase deficiency

Interactions

DRUGS

bupropion, tramadol: Increased risk of seizure

CNS depressants: Possible increased risk of additive CNS depression
ACTIVITIES
alcohol use: Possible increased risk of additive CNS depression

Adverse Reactions

CNS: Attention difficulty, confusion, depression, disorientation, dizziness, fatigue, hallucinations, headache, hypoesthesia, lethargy, nightmares, psychosis, sensation of drunkenness, seizures, sleep paralysis, sleep walking, somnolence, suicidal ideation, tremor, vertigo, weakness
CV: Bradycardia, hypertension, sinus tachycardia
EENT: Blurred vision, nasopharyngitis, pharyngolaryngeal pain, rhinitis, sinusitis, tinnitus
GI: Abdominal pain, diarrhea, dyspepsia, fecal incontinence, gastroenteritis, nausea, vomiting
GU: Enuresis, urinary incontinence
MS: Back pain, cataplexy, muscle weakness
RESP: Increased obstructive sleep apnea, respiratory depression, upper respiratory tract infection
SKIN: Excessive perspiration

Overdose

Sodium oxybate overdose has no specific antidote. Monitor the patient for evidence of overdose, including confusion, agitation, combative state, ataxia, coma, urinary incontinence, fecal incontinence, vomiting, diaphoresis, headache, impaired psychomotor skills, blurred vision, seizures, depressed respirations, Cheyne-Stokes respirations, apnea, bradycardia, hypothermia, and muscular hypotonia.

Maintain an open airway, and be prepared to perform endotracheal intubation if patient develops respiratory depression. Monitor vital signs, institute continuous ECG monitoring, and assess capillary refill, peripheral pulses, skin sensation, and warmth. Administer oxygen therapy and possibly mechanical ventilation, as needed. Institiue seizure precautions according to facility protocol, and expect to treat seiaures with an anticonvulsant, as prescribed.

Expect to administer oral activated charcoal, as prescribed. Hemodialysis isn't warranted because of the drug's rapid metabolism. Provide symptomatic and supportive therapy, as indicated and prescribed.

Institute suicide precautions according to facility policy, and anticipate psychiatric re-evaluation.

Nursing Considerations
- Use cautiously in patients with sleep apnea because sodium oxybate may worsen symptoms.
- Monitor patient's respiratory status closely because sodium oxybate can cause respiratory depression, especially in patients with impaired respiratory function.
- Use such safety measures as keeping the bed in low position and the siderails up after drug has been administered because of its potential adverse CNS effects, such as confusion and the sensation of being drunk.
- Monitor patient closely for depression because drug may worsen it.
- Monitor elderly patients closely for impaired motor or cognitive function; risk is increased in these patients.

PATIENT TEACHING
- Tell patient that he must be in bed before taking first nightly dose of sodium oxybate to prevent injuries because of the drug's rapid onset of action.
- Instruct patient to take first nightly dose at least 2 hours after eating and to maintain a similar relationship between eating and taking drug.
- Tell patient he should sleep between each of the two nightly doses; urge him to set an alarm so he can take the second dose at the prescribed time.
- Advise patient to avoid performing hazardous activities during the day until drug effects that extend into the day are known.
- Instruct patient to avoid consuming alcohol while taking drug.
- Inform patient that drug contains sodium, which should be considered if he needs to limit sodium intake.
- Warn patient that drug has been abused, especially by young adults, and that he should store it in a safe and secure spot.
- Instruct patient to take drug exactly as prescribed and not to increase dosage or frequency without consulting prescriber because drug has addictive properties.
- Tell patient that close follow-up with prescriber is essential.

sumatriptan succinate
Imitrex

Class and Category
Chemical class: Selective 5-hydroxytryptamine$_1$ (5-HT$_1$) receptor agonist

Therapeutic class: Antimigraine drug
Pregnancy category: C

Indications and Dosages

▶ *To relieve acute migraine headaches*

TABLETS

Adults. 25 to 100 mg as a single dose as soon as possible after onset of signs or symptoms, repeated every 2 hr, as needed and prescribed. *Maximum:* 300 mg daily.

DOSAGE ADJUSTMENT For patients with hepatic dysfunction, 50 mg maximum as single dose.

SUBCUTANEOUS INJECTION

Adults. *Initial:* 6 mg, repeated after 1 to 2 hr, if needed. *Maximum:* Two 6-mg injections/24 hr. If migraine signs and symptoms return after initial subcutaneous injection, 50 mg P.O. every 2 hr up to 200 mg daily.

NASAL SPRAY

Adults. 1 or 2 sprays (5 or 10 mg) into one nostril as a single dose or 1 spray (20 mg) into one nostril as a single dose. One additional dose may be taken if another attack occurs after at least 2 hr. *Maximum:* 40 mg daily.

Route	Onset	Steady State	Peak	Half-Life	Duration
P.O.	30 min	Unknown	2 to 4 hr	2.5 hr	Up to 24 hr
SubQ	10 min	Unknown	1 to 2 hr	2.5 hr	Up to 24 hr
Nasal	15 min	Unknown	Unknown	2 hr	Up to 24 hr

Mechanism of Action

May stimulate 5-HT$_1$ receptors, causing selective vasoconstriction of inflamed and dilated cranial blood vessels in carotid circulation, thus decreasing carotid arterial blood flow and relieving acute migraines.

Contraindications

Basilar or hemiplegic migraine, cardiovascular disease, concurrent use of ergotamine-containing drugs, hypersensitivity to sumatriptan or its components, ischemic heart disease, Prinzmetal's angina, use within 14 days of MAO inhibitor therapy, use within 24 hours of another selective 5-HT$_1$ receptor agonist

Interactions

DRUGS

antidepressants, lithium: Increased risk of serious adverse effects *ergotamine-containing drugs:* Possibly additive or prolonged vaso-constrictive effects

fluoxetine, fluvoxamine, paroxetine, sertraline: Possibly incoordination, hyperreflexia, and weakness

MAO inhibitors: Risk of decreased sumatriptan clearance, increased risk of serious adverse effects

Adverse Reactions

CNS: Anxiety, dizziness, drowsiness, fatigue, fever, headache, malaise, numbness, sedation, seizures, sensation of heaviness or pressure, sensation of warmth or heat, weakness, tight feeling in head, tingling, vertigo

CV: Arrhythmias; chest heaviness, pain, pressure, or tightness; coronary artery vasospasm; ECG changes; hypertension; hypotension; palpitations

EENT: Abnormal vision; nasal burning (P.O., subcutaneous); jaw or mouth discomfort; nasal irritation (nasal); nose or throat discomfort; photophobia (P.O., subcutaneous); taste perversion (nasal); tongue numbness or soreness

GI: Abdominal discomfort, dysphagia

MS: Jaw discomfort, muscle cramps, myalgia, neck pain or stiffness

SKIN: Dermatitis, diaphoresis, erythema, flushing, pallor, photosensitivity (P.O., subcutaneous), pruritus, rash, urticaria

Other: Injection site burning, pain, and redness

Overdose

Because overdose with sumatriptan hasn't been reported, expect to monitor patient for such signs and symptoms as angina; ataxia; cyanosis; desquamation, hair loss, and scab formation at injection site; erythema of extremities; mydriasis; paralysis; respiratory depression; seizures; sluggishness; and tremor.

Maintain an open airway, monitor patient's vital signs, and initiate continuous ECG monitoring to assess patient for ischemia. Expect to treat ischemia with a vasodilator, as needed and prescribed. Also, institute seizure precautions according to facility protocol.

To decrease drug absorption of the oral form of sumatriptan, be prepared to induce vomiting or perform gastric lavage. Monitor patient who has overdosed on the nasal spray for as long as signs and symptoms occur, which may be 10 hours.

Institute suicide precautionary measures according to facility policy, and anticipate psychiatric re-evaluation.

Nursing Considerations

• Assess patient for chest pain, and monitor blood pressure in those with coronary artery disease (CAD) before and for at least 1 hour after administering sumatriptan.

• Don't administer sumatriptan within 24 hours of another 5-HT$_1$ receptor agonist, such as naratriptan, rizatriptan, or zolmitriptan.

• Give tablets intact and with fluids to disguise unpleasant taste.

• After nasal administration, rinse tip of bottle with hot water (don't suction water into bottle) and dry with a clean tissue. Replace cap after cleaning.

• Inspect injection solution for particles and discoloration before administering. Discard solution if you detect these changes.

• Be aware that drug shouldn't be administered I.V. because this may precipitate coronary artery vasospasm.

• If patient has risk factors for CAD, assess him for arrhythmias, chest pain, and other signs and symptoms of heart disease.

• If patient has seizure disorder, institute seizure precautions according to facility protocol because sumatriptan may lower seizure threshold.

PATIENT TEACHING

• Instruct patient to read and follow manufacturer's instructions on how to use sumatriptan to ensure maximum therapeutic results.

• Advise patient to take drug as soon as possible after the onset of migraine signs or symptoms.

• Urge patient to contact prescriber and avoid taking sumatriptan if headache signs and symptoms aren't typical.

• Remind patient not to exceed prescribed daily dose.

• Advise patient to swallow tablets whole and drink fluids to disguise unpleasant taste.

• Show patient suitable sites for subcutaneous injection, and teach him how to load, administer, and discard autoinjector. Remind him to use the autoinjector only for 4- and 6-mg doses.

• Instruct patient to take no more than two subcutaneous doses in 24 hours and not to take a second dose if first dose doesn't provide significant relief.

• Inform patient that he may experience burning, pain, and redness for 10 to 30 minutes after subcutaneous injection. Suggest that he apply ice to relieve pain and redness.

• Teach patient how to use nasal form correctly.

• To avoid cross-contamination, advise patient not to use the

same nasal container for more than one person.
- Encourage patient to lie down in a dark, quiet room after taking drug to help relieve migraine.
- Instruct patient to seek emergency care for chest, jaw, or neck tightness after taking sumatriptan because drug may cause coronary artery vasospasm; subsequent doses may require ECG monitoring.
- Urge patient to report palpitations or rash to prescriber.
- Advise patient to avoid potentially hazardous activities until he knows how the drug affects him.
- If patient has seizure disorder, inform him that drug may lower seizure threshold.
- Encourage yearly ophthalmic examinations for any patient who requires prolonged drug therapy.

Other Therapeutic Uses
Sumatriptan succinate is also indicated for the following:
- To relieve cluster headaches (injection form only)

sumatriptan and naproxen sodium
Treximet

Class and Category
Chemical class: Serotonin 5-HT$_1$ receptor agonist (sumatriptan), propionic acid derivative (naproxen)
Therapeutic class: Antimigraine
Pregnancy category: C

Indications and Dosages
▶ *To treat acute migraine headache attacks*
TABLETS
Adults. 85 mg sumatriptan and 500 mg naproxen (1 tablet), repeated as needed after 2 hr. *Maximum:* 170 mg sumatriptan and 1,000 mg naproxen (2 tablets) in 24 hr.

Route	Onset	Peak	Duration
P.O. (sumatriptan)	20 min	2 to 4 hr	Up to 24 hr
P.O. (naproxen sodium)	30 min	1 hr	7 to 12 hr

Contraindications
Angioedema, asthma, bronchospasm, nasal polyps, rhinitis, or urticaria induced by aspirin, iodides, or other NSAIDs; basilar or hemilegic migraine; cardiac, cerebrovascular, or peripheral vascu-

lar disease including any type of ischemia; concurrent use of ergotamine-containing drugs; hepatic impairment; history of coronary artery bypass graft surgery; hypersensitivity to sumatriptan, naproxen or their components; uncontrolled hypertension; use within 14 days of MAO inhibitor therapy; use within 24 hours of another serotonin 5-HT$_1$ receptor agonist or any ergotamine-containing or ergot-type drugs such as dihydroergotamine or methysergide

Mechanism of Action
Sumatriptan may stimulate 5-HT$_1$ receptors, causing selective vasoconstriction of inflamed and dilated cranial blood vessels in carotid circulation, thus decreasing carotid arterial blood flow and relieving acute migraines.

Naproxen blocks cyclooxygenase, the enzyme needed to synthesize prostaglandins, which mediate the inflammatory response and cause local vasodilation, swelling, and pain. Thus, naproxen reduces symptoms of inflammation and provides added relief of migraine pain.

Interactions
DRUGS
sumatriptan component
antidepressants, lithium: Increased risk of serious adverse effects
ergotamine-containing drugs: Possibly additive or prolonged vasoconstrictive effects
fluoxetine, fluvoxamine, paroxetine, sertraline: Possibly incoordination, hyperreflexia, and weakness
MAO inhibitors: Risk of decreased sumatriptan clearance, increased risk of serious adverse effects
naproxen component
ACE inhibitors: Decreased antihypertensive effects; increased risk of renal dysfunction
acetaminophen: Increased risk of adverse renal effects with combined long-term use
anticoagulants, thrombolytics: Prolonged PT; increased risk of bleeding
antihypertensives: Decreased antihypertensive effectiveness
aspirin: Decreased aspirin effectiveness from lowered plasma and peak aspirin levels
beta blockers: Decreased antihypertensive effects of these drugs
bone marrow depressants, such as aldesleukin and cisplatin: Increased risk of leukopenia and thrombocytopenia

cefamandole, cefoperazone, cefotetan, plicamycin, valproic acid: Increased risk of hypoprothrombinemia and bleeding
cimetidine: Altered blood naproxen level
colchicine, glucocorticoids, NSAIDs, potassium supplements, salicylates: Increased GI irritability and bleeding
cyclosporine, gold compounds, nephrotoxic drugs: Increased risk of nephrotoxicity
digoxin: Increased blood digoxin level and risk of digitalis toxicity
diuretics: Decreased diuretic effectiveness
furosemide: Decreased natriuretic effect
insulin, oral antidiabetic drugs: Increased effectiveness of these drugs; risk of hypoglycemia
lithium: Increased risk of lithium toxicity
methotrexate: Increased risk of methotrexate toxicity
naproxen-containing products: Increased risk of toxicity
phenytoin: Increased blood phenytoin level
probenecid: Increased risk of naproxen toxicity

Adverse Reactions

CNS: Anxiety, asthenia, aseptic meningitis, atypical sensations, chills, cognitive impairment, CVA, decreased concentration, depression, dizziness, dream disturbances, drowsiness, fatigue, fever, headache, insomnia, light-headedness, malaise, paresthesia, seizures, somnolence, vertigo, weakness
CV: Arrhythmias; chest heaviness, pain, pressure, or tightness; coronary artery vasospasm; edema; ECG changes; heart failure; hypertension; hypotension; MI; palpitations; tachycardia; vasculitis
EENT: Dry mouth, jaw or mouth discomfort, nasal burning, nose or throat discomfort, photophobia, stomatitis, tinnitus, tongue numbness or soreness, vision or hearing changes
ENDO: Hyperglycemia, hypoglycemia
GI: Abdominal pain, anorexia, colitis, constipation, diarrhea, diverticulitis, dyspepsia, dysphagia, elevated liver function test results, esophagitis, flatulence, gastritis, gastroenteritis, gastroesophageal reflux disease, GI bleeding and ulceration, heartburn, hematemesis, indigestion, melena, nausea, pancreatitis, perforation of stomach or intestines, stomatitis, vomiting
GU: Glomerulonephritis, hematuria, interstitial nephritis, menstrual irregularities, nephrotic syndrome, renal failure, renal papillary necrosis
HEME: Agranulocytosis, anemia, aplastic anemia, eosinophilia, granulocytopenia, hemolytic anemia, leukopenia, neutropenia,

pancytopenia, thrombocytopenia

MS: Muscle cramps or weakness, myalgia, neck pain or stiffness

RESP: Asthma, dyspnea, eosinophilic pneumonitis, respiratory depression

SKIN: Alopecia, dermatitis, diaphoresis, ecchymosis, erythema multiforme, flushing, pallor, photosensitivity, pruritus, pseudoporphyria, purpura, rash, Stevens-Johnson syndrome, toxic epidermal necrolysis, urticaria

Other: Anaphylaxis, angioedema, hyperkalemia

Overdose

Monitor patient for evidence of overdose, such as lethargy, dizziness, drowsiness, epigastric pain, abdominal discomfort, heartburn, indigestion, nausea, transient alterations in liver function, hypoprothrombinemia, renal dysfunction, metabolic acidosis, apnea, disorientation, vomiting, or GI bleeding. Hypertension, acute renal failure, respiratory depression, and coma may occur, but are rare. Seizures and anaphylactoid reactions also may occur. Because naproxen sodium can be absorbed rapidly, expect early, high blood levels of this component. It isn't known what dose of this drug could be life-threatening.

Provide symptomatic, supportive care. No antidote is available for an overdose of sumatriptan and naproxen. Within 4 hours of ingestion or after a large overdose, expect to provide some combination of induced emesis, activated charcoal (60 to 100 g in adults, 1 to 2 g/kg in children), and an osmotic cathartic.

Expect that hemodialysis, forced diuresis, alkalinization of urine, and hemoperfusion won't be effective because of the degree to which one or both drugs are protein bound.

Nursing Considerations

- Be aware that sumatriptan and naproxen shouldn't be given to elderly patients because they're more likely to have decreased hepatic and renal function, coronary artery disease (CAD), and more pronounced blood pressure increases.
- Know that drug isn't recommended for patients with advanced renal disease.
- Use sumatriptan and naproxen with extreme caution in patients with a history of ulcer disease or GI bleeding because NSAIDs such as naproxen increase risk of GI bleeding and ulceration.
- Use drug cautiously in patients with a history of epilepsy or a lowered seizure threshold because sumatriptan may raise the risk of seizures. Institute seizure precautions in these patients.

- Use drug cautiously in patients with hypertension and monitor blood pressure closely throughout therapy because drug can start or worsen hypertension. Because of naproxen's sodium content, watch for fluid retention.
- Expect to give first dose of sumatriptan and naproxen in a medical setting. If patient has risk factors for CAD, assess him for chest pain and monitor blood pressure and ECG before administration and for at least 1 hour afterward.
- Don't give sumatriptan and naproxen within 24 hours of another 5-HT$_1$ receptor agonist, such as naratriptan, rizatriptan, or zolmitriptan.
- Be aware that serious GI tract ulceration, bleeding, and perforation can occur without warning or symptoms. Elderly patients are at greater risk. To minimize risk, give sumatriptan and naproxen with food. If GI distress occurs, withhold drug and notify prescriber immediately.
- Rehydrate a dehydrated patient before giving drug. If patient has renal disease, monitor renal function closely during therapy.
- **WARNING** Monitor patient closely for thrombotic events, including MI and CVA, because NSAIDs such as naproxen increase the risk.
- Monitor liver function test results because, in rare cases, elevations may progress to severe hepatic reactions, including fatal hepatitis, liver necrosis, and hepatic failure.
- Monitor BUN and serum creatinine levels in patients with heart failure, impaired renal function, or hepatic dysfunction; those who take diuretics or ACE inhibitors; and the elderly because drug may cause renal failure.
- Monitor CBC for decreased hemoglobin level and hematocrit because drug may worsen anemia.
- **WARNING** If patient has bone marrow suppression or is receiving chemotherapy, monitor laboratory results (including WBC count) and watch for evidence of infection because naproxen has anti-inflammatory and antipyretic actions that may mask signs and symptoms, such as fever and pain.
- Assess patient's skin routinely for rash or other hypersensitivity reactions because NSAIDs such as naproxen may cause serious skin reactions without warning, even in patients with no history of NSAID hypersensitivity. Discontinue drug at first sign of reaction and notify prescriber.
- If patient complains of vision changes, notify prescriber; patient may need an ophthalmic examination.

PATIENT TEACHING

• Advise patient to take sumatriptan and naproxen as soon as possible after migraine symptoms start.

• Urge patient to contact prescriber and to avoid taking sumatriptan and naproxen if headache symptoms aren't typical.

• Caution patient not to exceed recommended dose; serious adverse reactions may occur.

• Encourage patient to lie down in a dark, quiet room after taking drug to help relieve migraine.

• Advise patient to take drug with food to reduce GI distress.

• Tell patient to take drug with a full glass of water and to remain upright for 15 to 30 minutes afterward to prevent drug from lodging in esophagus and causing irritation.

• Caution patient to avoid hazardous activities until drug's CNS effects are known.

• Tell pregnant patient to avoid naproxen-containing products late in pregnancy.

• Explain that naproxen may increase the risk of serious adverse cardiovascular reactions; urge patient to seek immediate medical attention for such signs or symptoms as chest pain, shortness of breath, weakness, and slurred speech and to have yearly cardiovascular examinations if they have risk factors for heart disease.

• Tell patient that drug may also increase the risk of serious adverse GI reactions. Stress the need to seek immediate medical attention for epigastric or abdominal pain, indigestion, black or tarry stools, and vomiting blood or material that looks like coffee grounds.

• Alert patient to the possibility of rare but serious skin reactions, and urge him to seek immediate medical attention for rash, blisters, fever, or other evidence of hypersensitivity, such as itching.

• Caution patient with a seizure disorder that drug may lower the seizure threshold.

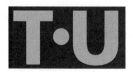

tacrine hydrochloride
(tetrahydroaminoacridine, THA)
Cognex

Class and Category
Chemical class: Monoamine acridine
Therapeutic class: Antidementia drug
Pregnancy category: C

Indications and Dosages
▶ *To treat mild to moderate dementia of Alzheimer's type*
CAPSULES
Adults. *Initial:* 10 mg q.i.d. for 4 wk, increased to 20 mg q.i.d. and adjusted every 4 wk as prescribed. *Maximum:* 160 mg daily in 4 divided doses.

Route	Onset	Steady State	Peak	Half-Life	Duration
P.O.	Unknown	Unknown	Unknown	1.5 to 4 hr	Unknown

Contraindications
Hypersensitivity to tacrine, other acridine derivatives, or their components; jaundice from previous tacrine use; serum bilirubin level that exceeds 3 mg/dl

Interactions
DRUGS
anticholinergics: Decreased effects of both drugs
cholinergics, other cholinesterase inhibitors: Increased effects of these drugs and tacrine, possibly leading to toxicity
cimetidine: Increased blood tacrine level, possibly leading to toxicity
neuromuscular blockers: Prolonged or exaggerated muscle relaxation
NSAIDs: Increased gastric acid secretion, possibly GI irritation and bleeding
theophylline: Increased blood theophylline level and possible toxicity
FOODS
all foods: Reduced tacrine bioavailability

ACTIVITIES
smoking: Possibly decreased tacrine effectiveness

Mechanism of Action

May relieve dementia in Alzheimer's disease by increasing the acetylcholine level in the CNS. In Alzheimer's disease, some cholinergic neurons lose their ability to function, which decreases the acetylcholine level. The remaining functioning cholinergic neurons release acetylcholine, but it's enzymatically broken down by cholinesterases into acetic acid and choline, as shown top right. Without acetylcholine to activate muscarinic (M) and nicotinic (N) receptors on postsynaptic cell membranes, nerve transmission and excitability decrease.

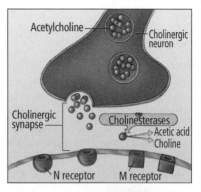

Tacrine binds with and inhibits cholinesterases, making more intact acetylcholine available in cholinergic synapses, as shown bottom right. This prolongs and enhances acetylcholine's effects, which increases nerve transmission and reduces signs and symptoms of dementia.

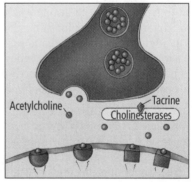

Adverse Reactions

CNS: Agitation, anxiety, asthenia, ataxia, confusion, depression, dizziness, fatigue, hallucinations, headache, hostility, insomnia, seizures, somnolence, syncope, tremor

CV: Arrhythmias, chest pain, conduction disturbances, hypertension, hypotension, palpitations, peripheral edema, sick sinus syndrome

EENT: Rhinitis
GI: Abdominal pain, anorexia, constipation, diarrhea, elevated liver function test results, flatulence, indigestion, nausea, vomiting
GU: Bladder obstruction, urinary frequency and incontinence, UTI
MS: Back pain, muscle stiffness, myalgia
RESP: Asthma, cough, upper respiratory tract infection, wheezing
SKIN: Flushing, jaundice, purpura, rash
Other: Weight loss

Overdose

Monitor patient for signs and symptoms of overdose, including bradycardia, diaphoresis, excessive salivation, hypotension, muscle weakness (which may include the respiratory muscles), nausea, seizures, shock, and vomiting.

Maintain an open airway, and institute continuous ECG monitoring and seizure precautions according to facility protocol.

Anticipate the use of an anticholinergic, such as atropine sulfate, to reverse the signs and symptoms of tacrine overdose. Expect to treat adults with atropine sulfate, 1 to 2 mg I.V., and to treat children with atropine sulfate, 0.05 mg/kg I.V. or I.M., every 10 to 30 minutes, as needed and prescribed. The effects of dialysis or hemoperfusion on tacrine overdose aren't known.

Institute suicide precautions according to facility policy, and anticipate psychiatric re-evaluation.

Nursing Considerations

- If patient has asthma, monitor her for wheezing and increased mucus production because drug may increase bronchoconstriction and bronchial secretions.
- Expect to monitor hepatic enzyme levels (specifically ALT), as ordered, every other week from at least week 4 to week 16 of tacrine therapy.
- If patient has elevated serum ALT level, monitor her for signs and symptoms of hepatitis, such as jaundice and right-upper-quadrant pain. ALT level should return to normal 4 to 6 weeks after therapy stops.
- Once ALT level returns to normal, expect to begin tacrine again (starting at 10 mg q.i.d.) as prescribed, and check hepatic enzyme levels weekly for 16 weeks, monthly for 2 months, and every 3 months thereafter, as ordered.
- Monitor patient for bradyarrhythmias, conduction disturbances, and sick sinus syndrome because tacrine may have a vagotonic effect on the heart rate.
- **WARNING** Be aware that tacrine's cholinergic effects may

worsen seizures or parkinsonian signs and symptoms.
- Monitor patient's urine output, and assess her for abdominal distention and abnormal bowel sounds because drug's cholinergic effects may exacerbate conditions involving urinary tract or GI obstruction or ileus.
- Be aware that patients with peptic ulcer disease and those receiving an NSAID are at increased risk for developing diarrhea, nausea, and vomiting because tacrine increases gastric acid secretion.
- Assess patient for increased Alzheimer's signs and symptoms because drug becomes less effective as the disease progresses and the number of intact cholinergic neurons declines.

PATIENT TEACHING
- Instruct patient to take tacrine on an empty stomach, and advise caregiver to make sure that drug is swallowed.
- If patient experiences GI distress, suggest taking drug with meals. Mention that drug's effects may be delayed.
- Urge patient to seek assistance when walking and changing position until she knows how the drug affects her. Instruct her to avoid potentially hazardous activities during this period.
- Advise patient not to smoke because it decreases drug's effectiveness.
- Caution patient not to abruptly stop taking drug. Doing so may impair cognitive ability.
- Inform caregiver that drug becomes less effective as Alzheimer's disease progresses.
- Urge caregiver to make sure patient returns regularly for follow-up visits and laboratory tests to monitor drug effectiveness.

tadalafil
Cialis

Class and Category
Chemical class: Phosphodiesterase inhibitor
Therapeutic class: Anti-impotence drug
Pregnancy category: B

Indications and Dosages
▶ *To treat erectile dysfunction*
TABLETS
Adults. *Initial:* 10 mg daily taken 1 hr before sexual activity; dosage decreased to 5 mg or increased to 20 mg, as prescribed, based on response. *Maximum:* 20 mg daily. Alternatively, 2.5 mg daily at

the same time of day regardless of anticipated sexual activity; dosage increased to 5 mg daily based on response.

DOSAGE ADJUSTMENT For patients taking potent CYP3A4 inhibitors such as ketoconazole, itraconazole, and ritonavir, dosage shouldn't exceed 10 mg every 72 hr if taken 1 hr before sexual activity or 2.5 mg if taken daily. For patients with moderate to severe renal insufficiency, dosage shouldn't exceed 5 mg daily if taken 1 hr before sexual activity. Patients with severe renal insufficiency shouldn't take tadalafil on a daily basis. For patients with mild to moderate hepatic impairment, dosage shouldn't exceed 10 mg daily.

Route	Onset	Peak	Duration
P.O.	Unknown	30 min to 6 hr	Unknown

Mechanism of Action
Enhances the effect of nitric oxide released in the penis during sexual stimulation. Nitric oxide activates the enzyme guanylate cyclase, which causes increased levels of cGMP in the corpus cavernosum. This leads to increased blood flow to the penis, thus producing an erection.

Contraindications
Continuous or intermittent nitrate therapy, hypersensitivity to tadalafil or its components, retinitis pigmentosa

Interactions
DRUGS
carbamazepine, phenytoin, phenobarbitol: Possibly decreased tadalafil effects
doxazosin, tamsulosin and other alpha blockers: Increased risk of symptomatic hypotension
erythromycin, itraconazole, ketoconazole, ritonavir: Prolonged tadalafil effects
nitrates: Profound hypotension
protease inhibitors (other than ritonavir): Possibly prolonged tadalafil effects
rifampin: Decreased tadalafil effects
FOODS
grapefruit juice: Possibly prolonged tadalafil effects
ACTIVITIES
alcohol use: Potentiated blood pressure lowering effects

Adverse Reactions

CNS: Asthenia, dizziness, fatigue, headache, hypesthesia, insomnia, migraine, paresthesia, seizures, somnolence, stroke, syncope, vertigo

CV: Angina pectoris, chest pain, hypotension, hypertension, MI, postural hypotension, palpitations, sudden cardiac death, tachycardia

EENT: Abrupt hearing reduction or loss, blurred vision, changes in color vision, conjunctivitis, dry mouth, epistaxis, eyelid swelling, eye pain, increased lacrimation, nasal congestion, nonarteritic anterior ishcemic optic neuropathy, pharyngitis, retinal artery or vein occlusion, visual field defects

GI: Abnormal liver function studies, diarrhea, dysphagia, dyspepsia, esophagitis, gastroesophageal reflux, gastritis, increased gamma-glutamyl transpeptidase levels, nausea, upper abdominal pain, vomiting

GU: Priapism, spontaneous penile erection

MS: Arthralgia, back or neck pain, extremity pain, myalgia

RESP: Dyspnea

SKIN: Diaphoresis, exfoliative dermatitis, flushing, pruritus, rash, Stevens-Johnson syndrome

Other: Facial edema, hypersensitivity reactions

Overdose

Tadalafil overdose has no specific antidote. Monitor the patient for adverse reactions to tadalafil therapy because overdose produces similar effects.

Maintain an open airway, and monitor patient's vital signs. Expect to provide symptomatic and supportive therapy as indicated. Be aware that hemodialysis is not effective in eliminating tadalafil from the body.

Institute suicide precautions according to facility policy, and anticipate psychiatric re-evaluation.

Nursing Considerations

• Know that patients with hereditary degenerative retinal disorders, including retinitis pigmentosa, should not receive tadalafil because of the risk of serious ophthalmic adverse reactions.

• Patients with severe hepatic impairment shouldn't take tadalafil because its effects in these patients are unknown. Patients with severe renal impairment shouldn't take tadafil on a daily basis because of their decreased ability to clear drug from the body.

• Use tadalafil cautiously in patients with left ventricular outflow obstruction, such as aortic stenosis and idiopathic hypertrophic subaortic stenosis, and those with severely impaired autonomic control of blood pressure because these conditions increase sensitivity to vasodilators such as tadalafil.

• Use tadalafil cautiously in patients with conditions that may predispose them to priapism, such as sickle cell anemia, multiple myeloma, leukemia, or penile deformities (such as angulation, cavernosal fibrosis, or Peyronie's disease).

• Monitor blood pressure and heart rate and rhythm before and during therapy.

PATIENT TEACHING

• Explain that tadalafil should be taken 1 hour before sexual activity to provide the most effective results.

• **WARNING** Tell patient not to take tadalafil if he takes any form of organic nitrate, either continuously or intermittently, because profound hypotension and death could result.

• **WARNING** Tell patient to seek immediate medical attention if he has a sudden loss of vision.

• Urge patient to seek sexual counseling to enhance drug effects.

• To avoid possible penile damage and permanent loss of erectile function, urge patient to notify prescriber immediately if erection is painful or lasts longer than 4 hours.

• Advise patient to limit alcohol consumption while taking tadalafil.

• Instruct patient to stop taking tadalafil immediately and notify prescriber if he has a sudden hearing reduction or loss.

temazepam

Apo-Temazepam (CAN), Novo-Temazepam (CAN), Restoril

Class, Category, and Schedule

Chemical class: Benzodiazepine
Therapeutic class: Sedative-hypnotic
Pregnancy category: X
Controlled substance schedule: IV

Indications and Dosages

▶ *To provide short-term management of insomnia*
CAPSULES
Adults. 7.5 to 30 mg 30 min before bedtime. *Maximum:* 30 mg daily.
DOSAGE ADJUSTMENT For elderly or debilitated patients, 7.5 mg 30 min before bedtime. Maximum is 15 mg daily.

Route	Onset	Steady State	Peak	Half-Life	Duration
P.O.	Unknown	3 days	Unknown	8 to 15 hr	Unknown

Mechanism of Action

May potentiate the effects of gamma-aminobutyric acid (GABA) and other inhibitory neurotransmitters by binding to specific benzodiazepine receptor sites in the limbic and cortical areas of the CNS. By binding to these receptor sites, temazepam increases GABA's inhibitory effects and blocks cortical and limbic arousal.

Contraindications

Hypersensitivity to temazepam, other benzodiazepines, or their components; pregnancy

Interactions

DRUGS

antihistamines (such as brompheniramine, carbinoxamine, chlorpheniramine, clemastine, cyproheptadine, diphenhydramine, trimeprazine), anxiolytics, barbiturates, general anesthetics, opioid analgesics, phenothiazines, promethazine, sedative-hypnotics, tramadol, tricyclic antidepressants: Increased sedation or respiratory depression

clozapine: Risk of respiratory depression or arrest

digoxin: Increased risk of elevated blood digoxin level and digitalis toxicity

flumazenil: Increased risk of withdrawal signs and symptoms

levodopa: Possibly decreased levodopa effects

oral contraceptives: Decreased response to temazepam

phenytoin: Possibly phenytoin toxicity

probenecid: Increased response to temazepam

zidovudine: Possibly zidovudine toxicity

Activities

alcohol use: Increased CNS depression and risk of apnea

smoking: Increased temazepam clearance

Adverse Reactions

CNS: Aggressiveness, anxiety (in daytime), ataxia, confusion, decreased concentration, depression, dizziness, drowsiness, euphoria, fatigue, headache, insomnia, nightmares, slurred speech, syncope, talkativeness, tremor, vertigo, wakefulness during last third of night

CV: Palpitations, tachycardia

EENT: Abnormal or blurred vision, increased salivation
GI: Abdominal pain, constipation, diarrhea, hepatic dysfunction, nausea, thirst, vomiting
GU: Decreased libido
HEME: Agranulocytosis, anemia, leukopenia, neutropenia, thrombocytopenia
MS: Muscle spasm or weakness
RESP: Increased bronchial secretions
SKIN: Diaphoresis, flushing, jaundice, pruritus, rash
Other: Physical and psychological dependence

Overdose

Monitor patient for evidence of overdose, including bradycardia, coma, confusion, dyspnea, hyporeflexia, seizures, severe drowsiness, shakiness, slurred speech, staggering, and weakness.

Maintain an open airway, institute continuous ECG monitoring, and administer I.V. fluids, as prescribed, to maintain blood pressure and promote diuresis. Institute seizure precautions according to facility protocol.

To decrease drug absorption in a conscious patient who isn't at risk for coma or seizures, be prepared to induce vomiting or perform gastric lavage. Expect that oral activated charcoal may also be prescribed. For an unconscious patient, anticipate assisting with the insertion of an endotracheal tube and then performing gastric lavage. The inflated cuff of the endotracheal tube will help prevent aspiration of gastric contents into the lungs.

Anticipate giving a benzodiazepine receptor antagonist such as flumazenil to reverse the sedative effects. Be aware that flumazenil may induce seizures, especially if patient has had long-term benzodiazepine therapy or has also ingested a cyclic antidepressant. If excitation occurs, a barbiturate shouldn't be used because it may increase excitement and prolong CNS depression. Dialysis is ineffective for treating benzodiazepine overdose.

Institute suicide precautions according to facility policy, and anticipate psychiatric re-evaluation.

Nursing Considerations

- Use temazepam cautiously in patients with a history of depression or suicidal thoughts.
- **WARNING Monitor patient for signs of physical and psychological dependence during therapy.**
- Implement safety precautions, according to facility policy, especially in elderly patients, because they're more sensitive to drug's CNS effects.

- If patient has respiratory depression, severe COPD, or sleep apnea, assess her for signs and symptoms of ventilatory failure.
- Be aware that temazepam can aggravate acute intermittent porphyria, myasthenia gravis, and severe renal impairment.
- Be aware that temazepam may cause worsening psychosis or deterioration of cognition or coordination in patients with late-stage Parkinson's disease.
- Be aware that drug shouldn't be stopped abruptly, even after only 1 to 2 weeks of therapy, because doing so may cause seizures or withdrawal symptoms, such as insomnia, irritability, and nervousness.

PATIENT TEACHING

- Instruct patient to take temazepam exactly as prescribed and not to stop taking it or change dosage without consulting prescriber.
- Explain the risks associated with abrupt cessation, including abdominal cramps, acute sense of hearing, confusion, depression, diaphoresis, nausea, numbness, perceptual disturbances, photophobia, tachycardia, tingling, trembling, and vomiting.
- Advise patient to avoid alcohol because it increases drug's sedative effects.
- Caution patient about possible drowsiness. Advise her to avoid hazardous activities until she knows how the drug affects her.
- Urge patient to notify prescriber immediately about excessive drowsiness, nausea, and known or suspected pregnancy.

thiamine hydrochloride
(vitamin B₁)

Betaxin (CAN), Bewon (CAN), Biamine

Class and Category

Chemical class: Water-soluble B-complex vitamin
Therapeutic class: Nutritional supplement
Pregnancy category: A (parenteral), Not rated (oral)

Indications and Dosages

▶ *To provide nutritional supplementation based on U.S. and Canadian recommended daily intake*

ELIXIR, TABLETS

Adult and adolescent males over age 10. 1.2 to 1.5 mg daily (0.8 to 1.3 mg daily Canadian).

Adult and adolescent females over age 10. 1 to 1.1 mg daily (0.8 to 0.9 mg daily Canadian).

Pregnant women. 1.5 mg daily (0.9 to 1 mg daily Canadian).
Breast-feeding women. 1.6 mg daily (1 to 1.2 mg daily Canadian).
Children ages 7 to 10. 1 mg daily (0.8 to 1 mg daily Canadian).
Children ages 4 to 6. 0.9 mg daily (0.7 mg daily Canadian).
Children ages 1 to 3. 0.3 to 0.7 mg daily (0.3 to 0.6 mg daily Canadian).

▶ *To treat beriberi*
ELIXIR, TABLETS
Adults. 5 to 10 mg t.i.d.
Children and infants. 10 mg daily.
I.V. OR I.M. INJECTION
Adults. *Initial:* 5 to 100 mg every 8 hr, switched to P.O. therapy as soon as possible and continued for total of 1 mo.
Children and infants. 10 to 25 mg daily.

▶ *To treat Wernicke's encephalopathy*
I.V. OR I.M. INJECTION
Adults. *Initial:* 100 mg I.V. *Maintenance:* 50 to 100 mg I.V. or I.M. daily until normal recommended daily intake is achieved.

Mechanism of Action
Replaces vitamin in thiamine deficiency, which can lead to beriberi or Wernicke's encephalopathy. Thiamine combines with ATP to produce thiamine pyrophosphate, which acts as a coenzyme in carbohydrate metabolism. Thiamine is needed for conversion of pyruvic acid to acetyl-CoA so it can enter the Krebs cycle; otherwise pyruvic acid accumulates in the blood, where it's converted to lactic acid.

Incompatibilities
Don't add parenteral thiamine to alkaline or neutral solutions or mix it with oxidizing and reducing agents, including barbiturates, carbonates, citrates, and copper ions.

Contraindications
Hypersensitivity to thiamine preparations or their components

Adverse Reactions
CNS: Restlessness, weakness
CV: Cyanosis, hypotension, shock, vasodilation
EENT: Sneezing, throat tightness
GI: GI bleeding, nausea, vomiting
RESP: Pulmonary edema, respiratory distress

SKIN: Diaphoresis, pruritus, sensation of warmth, urticaria
Other: Angioedema, injection site induration and tenderness

Overdose

Thiamine is considered to be nontoxic; however, be prepared to monitor patient for the adverse reactions listed above, which may occur after repeated doses of the parenteral form of thiamine. The most serious adverse reaction is hypersensitivity, which may progress to death. Expect to provide supportive and symptomatic care, as needed and prescribed.

Nursing Considerations

- Be aware that symptoms of thiamine deficiency may appear as a syndrome of nonspecific symptoms that include headache, malaise, myalgia, and nausea.
- **WARNING** Severe thiamine deficiency causes beriberi, which can affect the CNS and cardiovascular system. Monitor patient for neurologic effects, such as ataxia, confabulation, impaired ability to learn, neuropathy, and retrograde amnesia, as well as cardiovascular effects, such as biventricular failure, edema, and peripheral vasodilation.
- Expect an intradermal test dose to be prescribed before I.V. administration of thiamine.
- Use drug immediately if mixed in solutions that contain sodium bisulfite as an antioxidant or preservative because of poor stability.
- Be aware that a high-carbohydrate diet and dextrose-containing I.V. solutions may increase thiamine requirements and worsen signs and symptoms of thiamine deficiency.
- Assess patient for tenderness and induration at I.M. injection site. Reduce discomfort by applying cool compresses.
- Be aware that thiamine absorption is decreased in patients with alcoholism, cirrhosis, or GI disease.
- Assess laboratory test results and patient for signs of lactic acidosis. Without adequate thiamine, unconverted pyruvic acid can accumulate in blood and convert to lactic acid.
- Keep in mind that thiamine is a water-soluble vitamin that won't accumulate in the body.

PATIENT TEACHING
- Inform breast-feeding patient that she and infant must be treated with thiamine if infant has beriberi.
- Encourage patient to improve diet to prevent recurrence of thiamine deficiency.

thiopental sodium
Pentothal

Class, Category, and Schedule
Chemical class: Barbiturate
Therapeutic class: Anticonvulsant, sedative-hypnotic
Pregnancy category: C
Controlled substance schedule: III

Indications and Dosages
▶ *To control seizures following anesthesia or from other causes*
I.V. INJECTION
Adults. *Initial:* 75 to 125 mg (3 to 5 ml of 2.5% solution) as soon as possible after onset of seizure. *Maximum:* 250 mg given over 10 min.
▶ *To facilitate narcoanalysis*
I.V. INFUSION OR INJECTION
Adults. Dosage individualized based on patient's age, condition, sex, and weight; injected at 100 mg/min (4 ml/min of 2.5% solution) with patient counting backward from 100. Expect to discontinue injection once patient becomes confused with her counting but is still awake. Alternatively, use 0.2% concentration in D_5W for injection and infuse at 50 ml/min.

Route	Onset	Steady State	Peak	Half-Life	Duration
I.V.	10 to 40 sec	Unknown	Unknown	3 to 8 hr*	10 to 30 min

Mechanism of Action
Depresses the CNS and may inhibit the ascending transmission of impulses in the reticular formation. Thiopental may enhance or mimic the inhibitory action of gamma-aminobutyric acid (GABA), thereby having an anticonvulsant effect and producing sedation and hypnosis.

Incompatibilities
Don't mix thiopental with acidic I.V. medications or solutions, succinylcholine, or tubocurarine.

Contraindications
History of porphyria; hypersensitivity to thiopental, its components, or other barbiturates

---

* 10 to 12 hr with prolonged administration.

Interactions
DRUG

clonidine, CNS depressants, guanabenz, magnesium sulfate, methyldopa, metyrosine, pargyline, rauwolfia alkaloids: Additive CNS depressant effects

diazoxide, diuretics, guanadrel, guanethidine, mecamylamine, trimethaphan: Possibly additive hypotensive effect

ketamine: Increased risk of hypotension or respiratory depression; possibly countered hypnotic effect of thiopental

phenothiazines: Possibly increased CNS depression or excitation, increased hypotensive effect

ACTIVITIES

alcohol use: Additive CNS depressant effects

Adverse Reactions
CNS: Agitation, anxiety, seizures

CV: Bradycardia, hypotension, shock, tachycardia, thrombophlebitis

GI: Hiccups

RESP: Apnea, bronchospasm, cough, laryngospasm, respiratory depression, wheezing

SKIN: Hives, itching, rash, redness

Other: Angioedema

Overdose
Monitor patient for evidence of overdose, including apnea, CNS depression, hypotension, respiratory depression, and shock.

Maintain an open airway, administer oxygen as needed, and be prepared to assist with endotracheal intubation, as needed. Discontinue thiopental immediately, and monitor blood and tissue oxygenation, serum electrolyte levels, and vital signs. Be prepared to treat hypotension by administering I.V. fluids and placing the patient in Trendelenburg's position. Anticipate the need for a vasopressor or inotropic drug.

Nursing Considerations
- Before giving thiopental, expect to give an anticholinergic, such as atropine or glycopyrrolate, to minimize secretions.
- Be prepared to give a test dose of 25 to 75 mg (1 to 3 ml of 2.5% solution) to determine tolerance or sensitivity. Expect to observe patient for at least 1 minute after giving test dose.
- Dilute drug with a compatible I.V. solution before administering, such as D_5W for injection, normal saline solution for injection, or sterile water for injection. Be aware that sterile water

for injection shouldn't be used to prepare the 0.2% or 0.4% solution because it would result in a hypotonic solution and cause hemolysis.

- To prepare the 0.2% solution, dilute 1 g of thiopental with 500 ml of compatible diluent to produce a final concentration of 2 mg/ml.
- To prepare 0.4% solution, dilute 1 g of thiopental with 250 ml of compatible diluent or 2 g of thiopental with 500 ml of compatible diluent to produce a final concentration of 4 mg/ml.
- To prepare 2.5% solution, dilute 1 g of thiopental with 40 ml of compatible diluent or 5 g of thiopental with 200 ml of compatible diluent to produce a final concentration of 25 mg/ml.
- Inspect the solution for particles before giving it. Use solution within 24 hours of reconstitution, and discard unused portion after 24 hours.
- Monitor blood and tissue oxygenation and vital signs during I.V. administration. Keep emergency equipment and drugs nearby in case respiratory depression occurs.
- If patient has a history of cardiovascular disease or hypotension, monitor her for cardiovascular depressant effects, such as bradycardia, hypotension, or shock.
- If patient has a history of seizures, institute seizure precautions according to facility protocol.
- If patient is debilitated or has a history of respiratory disease, monitor respiratory rate, rhythm, and quality for signs of respiratory depression.

PATIENT TEACHING
- Explain the need for frequent hemodynamic monitoring.
- Advise patient to use caution for at least 24 hours after receiving thiopental when driving or performing tasks that require alertness.
- Instruct patient not to consume alcohol or other CNS depressant substances for at least 24 hours after thiopental administration (unless prescribed) because they increase the effects of thiopental.
- Instruct patient to report persistent drowsiness, rash, severe dizziness, or skin lesions to her prescriber.

Other Therapeutic Uses
Thiopental sodium is also indicated for the following:
- To induce general anesthesia
- As adjunct to general or local anesthesia
- To treat cerebral hypertension

thioridazine

Mellaril (CAN), Mellaril-S, Novo-Ridazine (CAN)

thioridazine hydrochloride

Apo-Thioridazine (CAN), Mellaril, Mellaril Concentrate, Novo-Ridazine (CAN), PMS Thioridazine

Class and Category

Chemical class: Piperidine phenothiazine
Therapeutic class: Antipsychotic drug
Pregnancy category: Not rated

Indications and Dosages

▶ *To treat schizophrenia in patients unresponsive to other antipsychotic drugs*

ORAL SOLUTION, ORAL SUSPENSION, TABLETS

Adults. *Initial:* 50 to 100 mg t.i.d., gradually increased, as needed and tolerated. *Maintenance:* 200 to 800 mg daily in 2 to 4 divided doses. *Maximum:* 800 mg daily.
Children ages 2 to 12. *Initial:* 0.5 mg/kg daily in divided doses, gradually increased, as prescribed. *Maximum:* 3 mg/kg daily.

Route	Onset	Steady State	Peak	Half-Life	Duration
P.O.	Up to several wk	4 to 7 days	6 wk to 6 mo	Unknown	Unknown

Mechanism of Action

Depresses the areas of the brain that control activity and aggression, including the cerebral cortex, hypothalamus, and limbic system by blocking postsynaptic dopamine$_2$ (D$_2$) receptors. The drug may relieve anxiety by indirectly reducing arousal and increasing filtration of internal stimuli to the brain stem reticular activating system.

Incompatibilities

Don't administer thioridazine oral suspension with carbamazepine oral suspension; a rubbery orange precipitate may form in stool.

Contraindications

Coma; concurrent use of drugs that prolong the QT interval or history of arrhythmias or prolonged QT interval; concurrent use of drugs that inhibit the metabolism of thioridazine, such as fluoxetine, fluvoxamine, paroxetine, pindolol, and propranolol; concurrent use of high doses of a CNS depressant; hypersensitivity to thioridazine, other phenothiazines, or their components; reduced cytochrome P450 2D6 activity; severe CNS depression; severe hypertensive or hypotensive cardiac disease

Interactions

DRUGS

amantadine, antihistamines, antimuscarinics, clozapine, cyclobenzaprine, diphenoxylate, disopyramide, maprotilene: Additive anticholinergic effects

amiodarone, bepridil, cisapride, disopyramide, erythromycin, flecainide, grepafloxacin, ibutilide, pimozide, probucol procainamide, quinidine, sotalol, sparfloxacin, tocainide: Possibly prolonged QT interval

amphetamine, dextroamphetamine, chlorpromazine: Possibly decreased effects of these drugs and thioridazine

antacids, antidiarrheals (adsorbent), kaolin, rifabutin, rifampin, rifapentine: Reduced bioavailability of thioridazine

anxiolytics, benzodiazepines, clonidine, dronabinol, guanabenz, guanfacine, opioid analgesics, phenothiazines, sedative-hypnotics: Possibly increased CNS effects or hypotension

barbiturates: Increased CNS depression and lowered seizure threshold

bromocriptine: Possibly decreased effectiveness of bromocriptine

carbamazepine: Possibly decreased blood thioridazine level

charcoal: Reduced thioridazine absorption

dopamine, droperidol, haloperidol, metoclopramide, metyrosine: Possibly increased adverse CNS effects

ephedrine, epinephrine, norepinephrine, phenylephrine: Possibly severe hypotension, MI, or tachycardia

fluoxetine, fluvoxamine, other cytochrome P450 2D6 inhibitors, paroxetine, pindolol: Inhibited metabolism of thioridazine, leading to elevated blood thioridazine level

fosphenytoin, phenytoin, valproic acid: Increased CNS effects, lowered seizure threshold

general anesthetics: Possibly potentiated CNS depression

guanadrel, guanethidine, methyldopa: Inhibited hypotensive effect of these drugs

levodopa, pergolide, pramipexole, ropinirole: Possibly inhibited antiparkinsonian response

lithium (high doses): Risk of encephalopathic syndrome (characterized by confusion, elevated liver function test results and fasting serum glucose level, extrapyramidal signs and symptoms, fever, lethargy, leukocytosis, and weakness)

MAO inhibitors: Possibly exaggerated extrapyramidal reactions

methoxsalen, oral contraceptives, porfimer, sulfonamides, sulfonylureas, tetracyclines, thiazide diuretics, vitamin A analogues: Possibly increased photosensitivity

propranolol: Increased blood propranolol and thioridazine levels, increased CNS effects, hypotension

tramadol: Increased blood tramadol level, possibly increased risk of seizures

trazodone: Possibly additive hypotension

ACTIVITIES

alcohol use: Additive CNS effects

Adverse Reactions

CNS: Akathisia, altered temperature regulation, depression, dizziness, drowsiness, extrapyramidal reactions (dystonia, laryngospasm, motor restlessness, pseudoparkinsonism), headache, insomnia

CV: ECG changes, hypertension, hypotension, prolonged QT interval, torsades de pointes, ventricular tachycardia

EENT: Blurred vision, change in color perception, dry mouth, impaired night vision, mydriasis, photophobia

ENDO: Breast engorgement, galactorrhea

GI: Constipation, ileus, nausea

GU: Amenorrhea, decreased libido, ejaculation disorders, impotence, menstrual irregularities, priapism, urine retention

HEME: Agranulocytosis, anemia, aplastic anemia, eosinophilia, leukocytosis, leukopenia, pancytopenia, thrombocytopenia

SKIN: Hyperpigmentation, jaundice, photosensitivity

Other: Weight gain

Overdose

Monitor patient for signs and symptoms of overdose, including agitation, areflexia and hyperreflexia, arrhythmias, blurred vision, cardiac arrest, coma, confusion, disorientation, drowsiness, dry mouth, dyspnea, heart failure, hyperpyrexia, hypotension, hypothermia, mydriasis, pulmonary edema, QRS complex changes, respiratory depression, seizures, shock, stupor, tachycardia, ventricular fibrillation, and vomiting.

Maintain an open airway, monitor patient for arrhythmias, and maintain temperature. Institute seizure precautions according to facility protocol. Perform gastric lavage, and administer activated charcoal, as prescribed. Be aware that vomiting shouldn't be induced because of the potential for impaired consciousness or dystonic reactions of the head and neck.

When treating arrhythmias, don't administer any drug that may prolong the QT interval—such as disopyramide, procainamide, or quinidine—because these drugs may have an additive effect with thioridazine. Expect to administer phenytoin to control arrhythmias and norepinephrine or phenylephrine and I.V. fluids to treat hypotension, as prescribed. Epinephrine shouldn't be used because of risk of paradoxical hypotension. Anticipate digitalizing patient for heart failure, as prescribed. Expect to treat electrolyte imbalance and maintain acid-base balance, as prescribed, and to administer diazepam, followed by phenytoin, to manage seizures. Avoid giving a barbiturate because it may potentiate CNS and respiratory depression.

Anticipate administering benztropine or diphenhydramine, as prescribed, to manage acute dyskinetic effects. Dialysis is ineffective for treating phenothiazine overdose. Expect to continue ECG monitoring for at least 5 days. Be aware that phenothiazine tablets are visible on X-ray.

Institute suicide precautions according to facility policy, and anticipate psychiatric re-evaluation.

Nursing Considerations
- **WARNING** Expect to give thioridazine only if patient hasn't responded to therapy with at least two other antipsychotic drugs because it may prolong the QT interval and has been linked to torsades de pointes and sudden death.
- Obtain baseline and serial ECG and serum potassium levels, as prescribed. Notify prescriber if QTc interval is greater than 450 milliseconds or if potassium level is abnormal, and expect to discontinue drug immediately.
- If patient has heart disease, frequently monitor blood pressure and assess her for chest pain, because thioridazine can cause hypotension and precipitate angina. If male patient has benign prostatic hyperplasia, monitor his urine output because drug can worsen urine retention.
- Be aware that if patient has a seizure disorder, high doses and large dosage changes may lower seizure threshold. Use seizure precautions, as appropriate, according to facility protocol.
- Administer drug with food, milk, or a full glass of water to minimize GI distress.
- Measure oral suspension using calibrated measuring device. Dilute with 2 to 4 oz (60 to 120 ml) of acidified tap water, distilled water, or fruit juice immediately before administration.
- Don't let oral solution come in contact with skin to prevent contact dermatitis.
- Administer antacid or adsorbent antidiarrheal at least 1 hour

before or 2 hours after thioridazine.

- **WARNING** Be aware that thioridazine can cause neuroleptic malignant syndrome—especially in male patients. Signs and symptoms include altered level of consciousness, altered mental status, autonomic instability (diaphoresis, hypertension or hypotension, sinus tachycardia), hyperthermia, and severe extrapyramidal dysfunction. Acute renal failure, increased serum creatine phosphokinase level, and leukocytosis also have occurred. Notify prescriber immediately if such signs and symptoms develop, and be prepared to discontinue therapy.
- Be aware that drug shouldn't be discontinued abruptly. Sudden withdrawal of thioridazine may produce transient dizziness, nausea, tremor, and vomiting.
- Assess patient for eye pain because drug's anticholinergic effects can worsen angle-closure glaucoma.
- Promptly investigate and report blurred vision, defective color perception, or impaired night vision because of the risk of pigmentary retinopathy.
- Expect prescriber to discontinue thioridazine and order CBC if patient experiences signs of infection. Also expect drug therapy to be stopped 48 hours before myelography and resumed 24 to 48 hours afterward.
- Monitor patient for signs and symptoms of tardive dyskinesia—such as uncontrollable movements of the arms, face, or legs—even after treatment stops. Notify prescriber if they develop.

PATIENT TEACHING

- Instruct patient to take thioridazine exactly as prescribed and not to stop taking drug without consulting prescriber because of the risk of withdrawal signs and symptoms.
- Instruct patient to notify prescriber immediately if she develops unusual signs and symptoms—such as dizziness, palpitations, and syncope—because they may reflect torsades de pointes.
- Advise patient not to take drug within 2 hours of an antacid.
- Caution patient to avoid alcohol use, which increases drug's sedative effects, and to avoid potentially hazardous activities if drowsiness occurs.
- Urge patient to notify prescriber immediately if she experiences blurred vision, defective color perception, difficulty with nighttime vision, excessive drowsiness, nausea, sore throat, or other symptoms of infection. Treatment may be discontinued.
- Advise female patient to use effective contraception while tak-

ing drug because of the high risk of fetal harm. Instruct her to inform prescriber immediately of known or suspected pregnancy.
• Because drug may alter temperature regulation, urge patient to avoid exposure to extreme temperatures during therapy.
• Advise patient to wear protective dark glasses to reduce risk of adverse vision reactions, and to have regular eye examinations.
• If patient requires long-term therapy, explain the risk of tardive dyskinesia, and urge her to notify prescriber immediately if she develops uncontrollable movements of her arms, face, or legs.
• Instruct patient to tell other prescribers that she's taking thioridazine before she takes any new drug.

thiothixene
Navane
thiothixene hydrochloride
Navane, Thiothixene HCl Intensol

Class and Category
Chemical class: Thioxanthene derivative
Therapeutic class: Antipsychotic drug
Pregnancy category: Not rated

Indications and Dosages
▶ *To manage the signs and symptoms of psychotic disorders*
CAPSULES (THIOTHIXENE), ORAL SOLUTION (THIOTHIXENE HYDROCHLORIDE)
Adults and children age 12 and over. *Initial:* 2 mg t.i.d. (for mild conditions) or 5 mg b.i.d. (for more severe conditions), increased every wk, as needed. *Usual:* 10 to 40 mg daily in divided doses. *Maximum:* 60 mg daily (for severe conditions).
DOSAGE ADJUSTMENT For elderly patients, lowest effective dosage used for maintenance therapy; maximum dosage limited to 30 mg daily. For some patients, one daily dose possibly used for maintenance therapy.
I.M. INJECTION (THIOTHIXENE HYDROCHLORIDE)
Adults. *Initial:* 4 mg b.i.d. to q.i.d. *Optimal:* 4 mg every 6 to 12 hr. *Usual:* 16 to 20 mg daily in divided doses. *Maximum:* 30 mg daily.

Route	Onset	Steady State	Peak	Half-Life	Duration
P.O.	Unknown	Unknown	Several days to several wk	3 to 34 hr	Unknown
I.M.	Unknown	Unknown	1 to 6 hr	3 to 34 hr	Unknown

Mechanism of Action

Increases dopamine turnover by blocking postsynaptic dopamine receptors in the mesolimbic system. Eventually, dopamine neurotransmission decreases, resulting in antipsychotic effects.

Contraindications

Blood dyscrasias, coma, hypersensitivity to thiothixene or its components, Parkinson's disease, severe CNS depression, shock, use of quinidine

Interactions

DRUGS

amphetamines: Decreased effectiveness of either drug

antacids, antidiarrheals (adsorbent): Possibly reduced bioavailability of thiothixene

antihistamines, tricyclic antidepressants: Additive anticholinergic effects, causing severe constipation, ileus, or increased intraocular pressure

bromocriptine: Possibly increased serum prolactin level and decreased effectiveness of bromocriptine

carbamazepine: Possibly decreased blood thiothixene level

dopamine: Decreased vasoconstrictive effect of dopamine (in high doses)

ephedrine, phenylephrine: Possibly reduced vasopressor response

epinephrine: Possibly epinephrine reversal, leading to severe hypotension, tachycardia, and possibly an MI

erythromycin: Increased adverse effects of thiothixene

general anesthetics, opioid analgesics, tramadol: Additive CNS effects, increased risk of seizures

guanadrel, guanethidine: Possibly decreased antihypertensive effect of these drugs

hypotensive agents: Possibly excessive hypotension

levodopa: Possibly reduced effectiveness of levodopa

lithium: Possibly encephalopathic syndrome (with blood level exceeding 12 mEq/L)

MAO inhibitors: Possibly exaggerated extrapyramidal reactions

metaraminol, methoxamine, norepinephrine: Possibly reduced vasopressor response

pergolide: Possibly reduced effectiveness of pergolide

propranolol: Possibly seizures and increased hypotension

quinidine: Additive orthostatic hypotension, possibly prolonged QT interval

ACTIVITIES

alcohol use: Additive CNS effects, increased risk of seizures
smoking: Possibly decreased blood thiothixene level

Adverse Reactions

CNS: Agitation, akathisia, drowsiness, dystonia, fatigue, insomnia, light-headedness, neuroleptic malignant syndrome, paradoxical exacerbation of psychotic disorder, restlessness, seizures, syncope, tardive dyskinesia, weakness
CV: ECG changes, edema, hypotension, peripheral edema, tachycardia
EENT: Blurred vision, dry mouth, increased salivation, miosis, mydriasis, nasal congestion, retinopathy
ENDO: Amenorrhea, breast engorgement, galactorrhea, hyperglycemia, hypoglycemia
GI: Anorexia, constipation, diarrhea, elevated liver function test results, ileus, increased appetite, nausea, vomiting
GU: Glycosuria, impotence, priapism
HEME: Agranulocytosis, anemia, eosinophilia, hemolytic anemia, leukocytosis, leukopenia, pancytopenia, thrombocytopenia
SKIN: Contact dermatitis, decreased sweating, photosensitivity, pruritus, rash
Other: Hyperuricemia, weight gain

Overdose

Monitor patient for evidence of overdose, including coma; drowsiness; dyspnea; excitement; hypotension; myopia; muscle jerking, stiffness, tremor, or uncontrolled movements; seizures; tachycardia; tiredness; and weakness.

Maintain an open airway, monitor vital signs and be prepared to maintain temperature. Institute continuous ECG monitoring (up to 5 days) and seizure precautions according to facility protocol. Perform gastric lavage, and administer activated charcoal and a saline cathartic, as prescribed. Be aware that vomiting shouldn't be induced because of the potential for impaired consciousness or dystonic reactions of the head and neck.

Expect to administer phenytoin to control arrhythmias and norepinephrine or phenylephrine and I.V. fluids to treat hypotension, as prescribed. Epinephrine shouldn't be used because of risk of paradoxical hypotension. Anticipate digitalizing patient for heart failure, as prescribed.

Administer diazepam, followed by phenytoin, to manage seizures, as prescribed. To treat CNS depression, administer a stimulant, such as amphetamine or dextroamphetamine, as prescribed. Anticipate administering benztropine or diphenhydramine to manage acute dyskinetic effects. Dialysis is ineffective for treating thioxanthene overdose.

Institute suicide precautions according to facility policy, and anticipate psychiatric re-evaluation.

Nursing Considerations

- Administer thiothixene capsules with food or milk if needed to minimize GI distress.
- Don't administer drug within 1 hr of an antacid.
- Dilute oral solution with 2 to 4 oz (60 to 120 ml) of a carbonated beverage, fruit or tomato juice, milk, soup, or water before administering. Measure dose, and administer using a calibrated measuring device. Avoid spilling solution on skin because drug may cause contact dermatitis.
- Avoid inadvertent I.V. administration of thiothixene injection solution. It's intended for I.M. use only.
- Be aware that I.M. administration usually is reserved for acute, severe agitation or for patients who can't take oral preparations.
- Maintain patient in recumbent position for 30 minutes after I.M. injection to minimize orthostatic hypotension.
- Assess patient for early signs of potentially irreversible tardive dyskinesia, a syndrome of involuntary rhythmic movements of the face, jaw, mouth, or tongue.
- **WARNING** Be aware that drug can precipitate neuroleptic malignant syndrome, a serious condition characterized by altered mental status, arrhythmias, diaphoresis, hyperpyrexia, muscle rigidity, and tachycardia, especially in patients with hyperthyroidism or thyrotoxicosis. Signs and symptoms may be severe enough to cause life-threatening respiratory depression.
- Monitor patient's serum calcium level because hypocalcemia may lead to dystonic reactions.
- Keep in mind that hypotension from thiothixene may precipitate angina in patients with known cardiac disease.
- **WARNING** Be aware that drug-induced adverse CNS reactions may mimic or suppress neurologic signs and symptoms of CNS disorders, such as brain tumor, encephalitis, encephalopathy, meningitis, Reye's syndrome, and tetanus.
- If patient is a child with an acute illness—such as CNS infection, dehydration, gastroenteritis, measles, or varicella-zoster infection—monitor her for extrapyramidal symptoms, particularly dystonias.

- Observe patient for symptoms of adverse hematologic reactions, such as sore throat and other symptoms of infection. If they occur, be prepared to obtain CBC, as ordered, and discontinue thiothixene, as prescribed.
- If patient has a history of seizures or EEG abnormalities, take seizure precautions because drug can lower seizure threshold.
- Assess patient for eye pain because drug's anticholinergic effects may worsen angle-closure glaucoma. If male patient has benign prostatic hyperplasia, assess him for urine retention.

PATIENT TEACHING
- Fully inform patient facing long-term thiothixene therapy about risk of developing tardive dyskinesia.
- Advise patient to avoid exposure to sunlight and ultraviolet light and to apply sunscreen when outdoors.
- Urge patient to avoid smoking or to begin a smoking cessation program while taking thiothixene.
- Encourage patient to avoid extreme temperature changes during drug therapy to prevent hyperthermia or hypothermia caused by decreased sweating.
- Instruct patient to immediately report sore throat or other symptoms of infection to prescriber.

tiagabine hydrochloride
Gabitril

Class and Category
Chemical class: Nipecotic acid derivative
Therapeutic class: Anticonvulsant
Pregnancy category: C

Indications and Dosages
▶ *As adjunct to treat partial seizures*
TABLETS
Adults. *Initial:* 4 mg daily; increased by 4 mg daily every wk up to 16 mg daily, then dosage increased by 4 to 8 mg daily every wk until desired response occurs. *Usual:* 32 to 56 mg daily. *Maximum:* 56 mg daily in 2 to 4 divided doses.
Children ages 12 to 18. *Initial:* 4 mg daily for 1 wk, then increased by 4 to 8 mg daily every wk until desired response occurs. *Maximum:* 32 mg daily in 2 to 4 divided doses.
DOSAGE ADJUSTMENT For patients with impaired hepatic function, dosage individualized and reduced, or dosing interval extended if needed, because of reduced drug clearance.

Route	Onset	Steady State	Peak	Half-Life	Duration
P.O.	Unknown	Unknown	Unknown	4 to 9 hr	Unknown

Mechanism of Action
Appears to inhibit neuronal and glial uptake of gamma-aminobutyric acid (GABA), the major inhibitory neurotransmitter in the CNS. Tiagabine makes more GABA available in the CNS to open chloride channels in the post-synaptic membranes, thereby leading to membrane hyperpolarization and preventing transmission of nerve impulses.

Contraindications
Hypersensitivity to tiagabine or its components

Interactions
DRUGS
benzodiazepines, CNS depressants: Possibly additive CNS depression
carbamazepine, phenobarbital, phenytoin: Possibly decreased tiagabine effectiveness
ACTIVITIES
alcohol use: Possibly additive CNS depression

Adverse Reactions
CNS: Amnesia, anxiety, asthenia, ataxia, confusion, depression, dizziness, drowsiness, EEG abnormalities, hostility, impaired cognition, insomnia, light-headedness, paresthesia, seizures, status epilepticus, tremor, weakness
EENT: Pharyngitis, stomatitis
GI: Abdominal pain, diarrhea, increased appetite, nausea, vomiting
GU: UTI
MS: Dysarthria
SKIN: Ecchymosis, rash

Overdose
Monitor patient for evidence of overdose, including agitation, ataxia, coma, confusion, depression, dysarthria, hostility, lethargy, myoclonus, seizures, somnolence, and weakness.

Maintain an open airway, monitor vital signs, and institute seizure precautions according to facility protocol. To decrease drug absorption in a conscious patient not at risk for coma or seizures, be prepared to induce vomiting or perform gastric lavage. For an unconscious patient, anticipate assisting with insertion of an endotracheal tube and then performing gastric lavage. The tube's inflated cuff will help prevent aspiration of gastric contents. Dialysis is ineffective for treating tiagabine overdose because the drug is highly protein-bound and extensively metabolized in the liver.

Institute suicide precautions according to facility policy, and anticipate psychiatric re-evaluation.

Nursing Considerations
• Administer tiagabine with food.
• **WARNING** Expect to taper dosage gradually, as prescribed, because stopping abruptly may increase seizure frequency. Be prepared to implement seizure precautions, as needed.

PATIENT TEACHING
• Instruct patient to take tiagabine with food.
• Advise patient to avoid hazardous activities until she knows how the drug affects her and to avoid alcohol during therapy.
• Caution patient who also takes a CNS depressant that tiagabine may increase depressant effect.
• Instruct patient not to abruptly stop taking tiagabine. Explain that prescriber usually tapers drug over 4 weeks, to reduce the risk of withdrawal seizures.

timolol maleate
Apo-Timol (CAN), Blocadren, Novo-Timol (CAN)

Class and Category
Chemical class: Beta blocker
Therapeutic class: Vascular headache prophylactic
Pregnancy category: C

Indications and Dosages
▶ *To prevent migraine headache*
TABLETS
Adults. *Initial:* 10 mg b.i.d. *Maintenance:* 20 mg daily in divided doses. *Maximum:* 30 mg daily; discontinued after 8 wk, as prescribed, if maximum dose is ineffective.

Route	Onset	Steady State	Peak	Half-Life	Duration
P.O.	30 min	Unknown	1 to 2 hr	4 hr	4 to 8 hr

Mechanism of Action
Competitively blocks beta-adrenergic receptors in vascular smooth muscle, which prevents arterial dilation and reduces the frequency of migraines.

Contraindications

Acute bronchospasm; cardiogenic shock; children; heart failure; hypersensitivity to timolol, other beta blockers, or their components; second- or third-degree AV block; severe asthma, chronic bronchitis, or emphysema; severe sinus bradycardia

Interactions

DRUGS

allergen immunotherapy, allergenic extracts for skin testing: Increased risk of serious systemic adverse reactions or anaphylaxis

amiodarone: Additive depressant effect on cardiac conduction, negative inotropic effect

anesthetics (hydrocarbon inhalation): Increased risk of myocardial depression and hypotension

beta blockers: Additive beta blockade effects

calcium channel blockers, clonidine, diazoxide, guanabenz, reserpine, other hypotension-producing drugs: Additive hypotensive effect and, possibly, other beta blockade effects

cimetidine: Possibly interference with timolol clearance

estrogens: Decreased antihypertensive effect of timolol

fentanyl, fentanyl derivatives: Possibly increased risk of initial bradycardia after induction doses of fentanyl or derivative (with long-term timolol use)

glucagon: Possibly blunted hyperglycemic response

insulin, oral antidiabetic drugs: Possibly masking of tachycardia in response to hypoglycemia, impaired glucose control

lidocaine: Decreased lidocaine clearance, increased risk of lidocaine toxicity

MAO inhibitors: Increased risk of significant hypertension

neuromuscular blockers: Possibly potentiated and prolonged action of these drugs

NSAIDs: Possibly decreased hypotensive effect

phenothiazines: Increased blood levels of both drugs

phenytoin (parenteral): Additive cardiac depressant effect

sympathomimetics, xanthines: Possibly mutual inhibition of therapeutic effects

Adverse Reactions

CNS: Asthenia, CVA, decreased concentration, depression, dizziness, fatigue, fever, hallucinations, headache, insomnia, nervousness, nightmares, paresthesia, syncope, vertigo

CV: Angina, arrhythmias, bradycardia, cardiac arrest, chest pain, edema, palpitations, Raynaud's phenomenon, vasodilation

EENT: Diplopia, dry eyes, eye irritation, ptosis, tinnitus, vision changes
ENDO: Hyperglycemia, hypoglycemia
GI: Abdominal pain, diarrhea, hepatomegaly, indigestion, nausea, vomiting
GU: Decreased libido, impotence
MS: Arthralgia, decreased tolerance to exercise, extremity pain, muscle weakness
RESP: Bronchospasm, cough, crackles, dyspnea
SKIN: Alopecia, diaphoresis, hyperpigmentation, pruritus, purpura, rash
Other: Anaphylaxis, weight loss

Overdose

Monitor patient for signs and symptoms of overdose, including bluish discoloration of the nail beds and palms of the hands, bradycardia, dizziness, dyspnea, hypotension, irregular heartbeat, seizures, and syncope. Maintain open airway, and institute continuous ECG monitoring and seizure precautions according to facility protocol. Be prepared to perform gastric lavage, followed by the administration of activated charcoal.

To treat bradycardia that occurs with hypotension, administer atropine or glucagon, as prescribed. Expect to administer a catecholamine—such as dobutamine, dopamine, epinephrine, isoproterenol, or norepinephrine—to give chronotropic and inotropic support and to treat hypotension. Calcium chloride may be effective in improving myocardial contractility because overdose with timolol may cause hypocalcemia. Keep in mind that transvenous pacing may be needed to treat heart block.

If the patient develops cardiac failure or pulmonary edema, anticipate the use of digoxin, furosemide, or a beta$_2$ agonist, such as isoproterenol. To treat bronchospasm, anticipate the need for a theophylline derivative. Be prepared to treat seizures with diazepam or lorazepam, as prescribed.

Nursing Considerations

• **WARNING** If patient is diabetic, be aware that timolol may mask signs and symptoms of acute hypoglycemia. The drug also may mask certain signs of hyperthyroidism, such as tachycardia.
• Be aware that timolol may prolong hypoglycemia by interfering with glycogenolysis or may promote hyperglycemia by decreasing tissue sensitivity to insulin.
• If patient has a history of systolic heart failure or left ventricu-

lar dysfunction, monitor blood pressure and cardiac output, as appropriate, because timolol's negative inotropic effect can depress cardiac output.

- **WARNING** Be aware that timolol shouldn't be discontinued abruptly because doing so could cause an MI, myocardial ischemia, severe hypertension, or ventricular arrhythmias, particularly if patient has cardiovascular disease.
- Expect varied drug effectiveness in elderly patients; they may be less sensitive to drug's antihypertensive effect or more sensitive because of reduced drug clearance.
- If patient is elderly with age-related peripheral vascular disease or if patient has Raynaud's phenomenon, monitor her for impaired circulation. Such patients may experience exacerbated signs and symptoms from increased alpha stimulation. Elderly patients also are at increased risk for beta blocker–induced hypothermia.
- If timolol worsens a skin condition, such as psoriasis, notify prescriber.

PATIENT TEACHING
- Instruct patient taking timolol to inform prescriber of chest pain, fainting, light-headedness, or shortness of breath, which may indicate the need for dosage change.
- Encourage patient to lie down in a dark, quiet room to help relieve her migraine headache.
- Caution patient not to stop taking drug abruptly. Timolol dosage must be tapered gradually under prescriber's supervision.
- If patient has diabetes mellitus, instruct her to frequently monitor blood glucose level during therapy.
- Warn patient with psoriasis about possible flare-ups of skin condition.

Other Therapeutic Uses
Timolol maleate is also indicated for the following:
- To manage hypertension
- To provide long-term prophylaxis after an MI

tolcapone
Tasmar

Class and Category
Chemical class: Nitrobenzophenone
Therapeutic class: Antidyskinetic
Pregnancy category: C

Indications and Dosages

▶ *As adjunct (with levodopa and carbidopa) to treat Parkinson's disease*
TABLETS
Adults. *Initial:* 100 mg t.i.d. *Maximum:* 200 mg t.i.d.

Route	Onset	Steady State	Peak	Half-Life	Duration
P.O.	Unknown	Unknown	Unknown	2 to 3 hr	Unknown

Mechanism of Action

Prolongs plasma half-life of levodopa by inhibiting catechol-*O*-methyltransferase (COMT), an enzyme responsible for metabolizing catecholamines—including dopa, dopamine, epinephrine, norepinephrine, and their hydroxylated metabolites. COMT inhibition reduces the amount of metabolizing enzyme for levodopa, which results in a more sustained plasma levodopa level. This action makes more levodopa available for diffusion into the CNS, where it's converted to dopamine.

Contraindications

Confusion, hyperpyrexia, or rhabdomyolysis with previous use of tolcapone; hepatic dysfunction; hypersensitivity to tolcapone or its components

Interactions

DRUGS
desipramine: Possibly increased frequency of adverse effects
levodopa: Increased levodopa bioavailability, with increased risk of orthostatic hypotension and syncope
MAO inhibitors: Possibly inhibited catecholamine metabolism

Adverse Reactions

CNS: Confusion, dizziness, drowsiness, dyskinesia, fatigue, fever, hallucinations, headache, lethargy, loss of balance
CV: Chest pain, orthostatic hypotension
EENT: Dry mouth
GI: Abdominal pain, anorexia, cholestasis, constipation, diarrhea, elevated liver function test results, fulminant liver failure, hepatic impairment, vomiting
GU: Bright yellow urine, hematuria
MS: Muscle cramps, rhabdomyolysis
RESP: Dyspnea, upper respiratory tract infection
SKIN: Diaphoresis, jaundice

Overdose

Information about tolcapone overdose isn't available, although healthy volunteers who received high doses for 1 week had dizziness, nausea, and vomiting. Expect to give supportive, symptomatic care, as needed. Be aware that tolcapone is highly protein-bound, so hemodialysis is ineffective for treating overdose.

Institute suicide precautions according to facility policy, and anticipate psychiatric re-evaluation.

Nursing Considerations

• Determine status of liver function before starting tolcapone therapy; then monitor liver function test results every 2 to 4 weeks for the first 6 months and periodically thereafter, as ordered to detect hepatic impairment.
• Use tolcapone cautiously in patients with severe dyskinesia or dystonia because drug may cause rhabdomyolysis.
• Assess patient for hallucinations, especially if she's over age 75.
• Anticipate that drug may precipitate or worsen dyskinesia.
• Expect tolcapone to be discontinued if no improvement occurs after 3 weeks of use, if liver enzymes exceed twice the normal upper limit, or the patient has evidence of hepatic impairment, such as persistent nausea, fatigue, lethargy, anorexia, jaundice, dark urine, pruritus, or right upper quadrant tenderness.

PATIENT TEACHING

• Inform patient that urine may turn bright yellow during therapy.
• Advise patient to avoid potentially hazardous activities until she knows how the drug affects her.
• Urge patient to notify prescriber immediately about darkened urine, decreased appetite, fatigue, jaundice, lethargy, light-colored stools, and right-sided abdominal pain.
• Caution patient not to abruptly stop taking drug. Explain that prescriber will supervise tapering of drug dosage.
• Urge patient to have regular follow-up appointments and laboratory tests.

topiramate

Topamax

Class and Category

Chemical class: Sulfamate-substituted monosaccharide
Therapeutic class: Anticonvulsant
Pregnancy category: C

Indications and Dosages

▶ *As adjunct to treat partial seizures, primary generalized tonic-clonic seizures, and seizures in Lennox-Gastaut syndrome*
CAPSULES, TABLETS
Adults and adolescents age 17 and over. *Initial:* 25 to 50 mg daily in divided doses b.i.d. for 1 wk. Increased by 25 to 50 mg daily every wk. *Maintenance:* 200 to 400 mg daily in divided doses b.i.d. *Maximum:* 1,600 mg daily.
Children ages 2 to 16. *Initial:* 25 mg or less every day at bedtime for 1 wk. Increased every 1 to 2 wk by 1 to 3 mg/kg daily in divided doses every 12 hr, as prescribed. *Usual:* 5 to 9 mg/kg daily in divided doses every 12 hr.
▶ *To treat partial onset or primary generalized tonic-clonic seizures*
CAPSULES
Adults and children age 10 and over. *Initial:* 25 mg b.i.d. morning and evening. Increased by 50 mg daily q. wk. *Maintenance:* 200 mg b.i.d. morning and evening.
▶ *To prevent migraine headache*
CAPSULES, TABLETS
Adults. *Initial:* 25 mg daily in evening for 1 wk; then 25 mg b.i.d. for 1 wk; then 25 mg in morning and 50 mg in evening for 1 wk. *Maintenance:* 50 mg b.i.d.
DOSAGE ADJUSTMENT For patients with moderate to severe renal impairment, dosage possibly reduced by 50%.

Route	Onset	Steady State	Peak	Half-Life	Duration
P.O.	Unknown	4 days	Unknown	21 hr	Unknown

Mechanism of Action

May block the spread of seizures through its ability to reduce the length and frequency of excitatory transmission. Topiramate increases the availability of the inhibitory neurotransmitter gamma-aminobutyric acid (GABA) by blocking voltage-sensitive sodium channels. This action promotes the movement of chloride ions into neurons.

Contraindications

Hypersensitivity to topiramate or its components

Interactions

DRUGS
antihistamines, barbiturates, benzodiazepines, CNS depressants, opioid

analgesics, skeletal muscle relaxants, tricyclic antidepressants: Additive CNS depression

carbamazepine: Decreased blood topiramate level

carbonic anhydrase inhibitors: Increased risk of renal calculus formation

digoxin: Possibly decreased blood digoxin level

ethinyl estradiol: Increased risk of breakthrough bleeding

oral contraceptives: Increased risk of breakthrough bleeding, decreased contraceptive efficacy

phenobarbital: Altered blood phenobarbital level

phenytoin: Decreased blood topiramate level

probenecid: Possibly blocked renal tubular reabsorption of topiramate and decreased blood topiramate level

valproic acid: Decreased blood levels of both drugs

ACTIVITIES

alcohol use: Additive CNS depression

Adverse Reactions

CNS: Agitation, anxiety, asthenia, ataxia, confusion, decreased concentration, depression, dizziness, fatigue, fever, hallucinations, headache, hypoesthesia, insomnia, irritability, memory loss, mood changes, nervousness, paresthesia, psychomotor slowing, psychosis, slurred speech, somnolence, suicidal ideation, syncope, tremors

CV: Cardiac arrest, chest pain, hot flashes, hypertension, hypotension, palpitations, vasodilation

EENT: Blurred vision, diplopia, dry mouth, eye pain, gingivitis, hearing loss, nystagmus, pharyngitis, rhinitis, sinusitis, taste perversion, tinnitus, tongue edema, vision changes

ENDO: Breast pain, hyperglycemia

GI: Abdominal pain, anorexia, constipation, diarrhea, dyspepsia, flatulence, gastroenteritis, gastroesophageal reflux, hepatic failure, hepatitis, indigestion, nausea, pancreatitis, vomiting

GU: Cystitis, decreased libido, dysmenorrhea, dysuria, frequent urination, impotence, menstrual irregularities, renal calculi, renal tubular acidosis, UTI, vaginitis

HEME: Anemia, leukopenia

MS: Arthralgia, back pain, leg cramps or pain, muscle weakness

RESP: Bronchitis, cough, dyspnea, pulmonary embolism, upper respiratory tract infection

SKIN: Acne, alopecia, erythema multiforme, pemphigus, pruritus, rash, reduced sweating, Stevens-Johnson syndrome, toxic epidermal necrolysis

Other: Dehydration, metabolic acidosis, weight gain

Overdose

Limited information is available about topiramate overdose. Expect to provide supportive and symptomatic care, as needed and prescribed.

To decrease drug absorption, be prepared to induce vomiting or perform gastric lavage. Be aware that hemodialysis is effective in lowering the blood topiramate level.

Institute suicide precautions according to facility policy, and anticipate psychiatric re-evaluation.

Nursing Considerations

- Obtain a baseline serum bicarbonate level before topiramate therapy starts, and monitor it periodically throughout therapy, as ordered.
- Give capsule with water and have patient swallow it whole. If needed, open capsules and empty contents onto a spoonful of soft food. Discard unused portion.
- Never store food sprinkled with drug for use at a later time.
- Don't break topiramate tablets because they have a bitter taste.
- **WARNING** Monitor patient for acute myopia and secondary angle-closure glaucoma, which may occur in the first month of therapy. Assess patient for signs and symptoms such as decreased visual acuity and eye pain. Notify prescriber immediately if they occur, and expect to discontinue the drug.
- **WARNING** Anticipate an increase in seizure activity if therapy stops abruptly. Implement seizure precautions, as appropriate, according to facility protocol.
- If patient has a history of renal calculi, assess her for signs of recurrence.

PATIENT TEACHING

- Instruct patient to swallow topiramate tablets whole.
- Teach patient to sprinkle the contents of the capsule on a small amount (1 teaspoonful) of soft food, such as applesauce or pudding, and to swallow the contents without chewing.
- Encourage patient to maintain adequate hydration to minimize the risk of renal calculus formation.
- Urge patient to avoid potentially hazardous activities until she knows how the drug affects her.
- Inform patient to notify her prescriber immediately if she develops blurred vision or eye pain.
- Advise patient to watch for decreased sweating and significantly increased body temperature, especially during hot weather, and

to notify prescriber immediately if they occur.
- Tell patient to maintain an adequate fluid intake to minimize the risk of kidney stone formation.
- Advise female patient about possible breakthrough bleeding. If she takes an oral contraceptive, encourage her to use another form of contraception during therapy.

tranylcypromine sulfate
Parnate

Class and Category
Chemical class: Nonhydrazine derivative
Therapeutic class: Antidepressant
Pregnancy category: Not rated

Indications and Dosages
▶ *To treat major depressive episodes without melancholia*
TABLETS
Adults and adolescents over age 16. 30 mg daily in divided doses. After first 2 wk, increased by 10 mg daily every 1 to 3 wk, as prescribed. *Maintenance:* 10 to 40 mg daily. *Maximum:* 60 mg daily.
DOSAGE ADJUSTMENT For elderly patients, initial dosage possibly reduced to 2.5 to 5 mg daily and increased by 2.5 to 5 mg every 3 to 4 days, as prescribed; maximum dosage limited to 45 mg daily. Alternative therapies should be carefully considered for patients older than age 60. For patients receiving electroconvulsive therapy, dosage reduced to 10 mg b.i.d. during the series, then 10 mg daily for maintenance.

Route	Onset	Steady State	Peak	Half-Life	Duration
P.O.	7 to 10 days	Unknown	4 to 8 wk	Unknown	10 days

Mechanism of Action
Irreversibly binds to MAO, reducing its activity and resulting in increased levels of neurotransmitters, including dopamine, epinephrine, and norepinephrine. This regulation of CNS neurotransmitters helps ease depression.

Contraindications
Cardiovascular disease; cerebrovascular disease; heart failure; hepatic disease; history of headaches; hypersensitivity to tranyl-

cypromine or its components; hypertension; pheochromocytoma; severe renal impairment; use of anesthetics, antihypertensives, bupropion, buspirone, carbamazepine, CNS depressants, cyclobenzaprine, dextromethorphan, meperidine, other MAO inhibitors, selective serotonin reuptake inhibitors, sympathomimetics, or tricyclic antidepressants

Interactions

DRUGS

amoxapine, bupropion, maprotiline, selective serotonin reuptake inhibitors, trazodone, tricyclic antidepressants: Increased risk of severe hypertensive crisis, increased anticholinergic effects

anticonvulsants: Additive CNS depression

antihistamines: Possibly prolonged anticholinergic and CNS depressant effects

antipsychotics: Additive anticholinergic, hypotensive, and sedative effects

beta blockers: Possibly worsened bradycardia

bromocriptine: Increased blood prolactin level and interference with bromocriptine effects

buspirone: Increased blood pressure

dextroamphetamine, isometheptene, local anesthetics, naphazoline, oxymetazoline, psychostimulants, sympathomimetics, tetrahydrozoline, xylometazoline: Increased risk of severe hypertensive reaction

dextromethorphan, tryptophan: Increased risk of serotonin syndrome

diuretics: Additive hypotensive effects

doxapram: Increased vasopressor effects

furazolidone, procarbazine, selegiline: Increased risk of severe hyperpyretic or hypertensive crisis, seizures, or death

guanadrel, guanethidine: Increased risk of moderate to severe hypertension

insulin, oral antidiabetic drugs: Possibly prolonged hypoglycemic response

levodopa: Increased vasopressor effects, hypertension, adverse cardiovascular effects

meperidine: Increased risk of coma, diaphoresis, excitation, hypertension, rigidity, severe respiratory depression, shock and, possibly, death

methyldopa: Increased risk of hallucinations

metrizamide, tramadol: Increased risk of seizures

succinylcholine: Possibly prolonged succinylcholine effects

FOODS

aged cheese; avocados; bananas; broad or fava beans; cured sausage (bologna, pepperoni, and salami) or other meat; overripe fruit; pickled fish, meats, or poultry; protein extract; smoked fish, meats, or poultry; soy sauce; yeast extract; and other foods high in pressor amines, such as tyramine: Increased risk of sudden, severe hypertension

caffeine-containing beverages and foods: Increased risk of severe hypertensive crisis and dangerous arrhythmias

ACTIVITIES

alcohol-containing products that also may contain tyramine, such as beer (including reduced-alcohol and alcohol-free beer), hard liquor, liqueurs, sherry, wine (red and white): Increased risk of hypertensive crisis

Adverse Reactions

CNS: Anxiety, chills, dizziness, drowsiness, fever, headache, insomnia, intracranial hemorrhage, paresthesia, restlessness, suicidal ideation, tremor, weakness

CV: Bradycardia, chest pain, edema, hypertensive crisis, orthostatic hypotension, palpitations, tachycardia

EENT: Blurred vision, dry mouth, mydriasis, photophobia, tinnitus

GI: Abdominal pain, anorexia, constipation, diarrhea, nausea, vomiting

GU: Ejaculation disorders, impotence, urine retention

HEME: Agranulocytosis, anemia, leukopenia, thrombocytopenia

MS: Muscle spasms, myoclonus, neck stiffness

SKIN: Clammy skin, diaphoresis

Overdose

Monitor patient for signs and symptoms of overdose, including anxiety; confusion; cool, clammy skin; diaphoresis; dizziness; drowsiness; dyspnea; fever; hallucinations; headache; hyperreflexia or hyporeflexia; hypertension or hypotension; insomnia; irritability; muscle stiffness; respiratory depression; seizures; and tachycardia. Signs and symptoms may be minimal for the first 12 hours and reach a maximum by 24 to 48 hours, so frequently monitor patient during this time period.

Maintain an open airway, administer oxygen, as prescribed, and be prepared to assist with endotracheal intubation if the patient develops respiratory failure. Institute seizure precautions according to facility protocol. Monitor temperature, and expect to treat hyperpyrexia with an antipyretic and a cooling blanket, as prescribed. Be prepared to induce vomiting or perform gastric lavage, followed by administration of activated charcoal, as prescribed, to decrease tranylcypromine absorption. Protect patient's airway against aspiration. Hemodialysis, hemoperfusion, and peritoneal dialysis may be effective for treating tranylcypromine overdose. Be aware that treatment to induce urine acidification may also be prescribed to increase drug elimination.

Anticipate using I.V. fluids and a vasopressor, such as norepinephrine, to treat hypotension and an alpha blocker, such as phentolamine or phenoxybenzamine, to treat hypertension. Expect to treat seizures with diazepam and to avoid giving a phenothiazine because of possible hypotensive effects.

Expect to administer dantrolene, 2.5 mg/kg daily in divided doses, as prescribed, to treat signs and symptoms of a hypermetabolic state, including coma, hyperpyrexia, hyperreflexia, muscle rigidity, respiratory failure, tachycardia, and tremor. Monitor patient for hepatotoxicity and pleural and pericardial effusion.

Institute suicide precautions according to facility policy, and anticipate psychiatric re-evaluation.

Nursing Considerations

- Monitor patient's blood pressure during tranylcypromine therapy to detect hypertensive crisis and to decrease the risk of orthostatic hypotension.
- **WARNING** Notify prescriber immediately if patient has evidence of hypertensive crisis (drug's most serious adverse effect), such as chest pain, headache, neck stiffness, and palpitations. Expect to stop drug immediately if such signs occur.
- Anticipate that therapeutic response may take up to 4 weeks.
- Expect drug to aggravate signs and symptoms of Parkinson's disease, including muscle spasms, myoclonic movement, and tremor.
- Keep dietary restrictions in place for at least 2 weeks after stopping tranylcypromine because of the slow recovery from drug's enzyme-inhibiting effects.
- Ideally, expect to stop drug 10 days before elective surgery, as prescribed, to avoid hypotension.
- Be aware that abrupt cessation of drug can precipitate original signs and symptoms.
- If patient is diabetic, frequently assess her blood glucose level to detect possible loss of blood glucose control.
- Anticipate that coadministration with a selective serotonin reuptake inhibitor may cause confusion, seizures, severe hypertension, and other, less severe symptoms.
- If patient (especially a child or adolescent) is severely depressed, monitor her for suicidal tendencies. Take safety measures, and notify prescriber immediately.
- Assess patient for sudden insomnia. If it develops, notify pre-

scriber and be prepared to administer drug early in the day.

PATIENT TEACHING

• Instruct patient to avoid foods that contain cheese and that are high in tyramine—such as anchovies, avocados, bananas, beer, canned figs, caviar, chocolate, dried fruit, fava beans, liqueurs, meat tenderizers, overripe fruit, pickled herring, raspberries, sauerkraut, sherry, sour cream, soy sauce, wine, yeast extract, and yogurt—while taking tranylcypromine.

• Urge patient to continue dietary restrictions for at least 2 weeks after therapy stops.

• Advise patient to notify prescriber immediately about chest pain, dizziness, headache, nausea, neck stiffness, palpitations, rapid heart rate, sweating, and vomiting.

• Urge patient to avoid alcohol and excessive caffeine intake during therapy.

• **WARNING** Alert parents to watch their child or adolescent closely for abnormal thinking or behavior or an increase in aggression or hostility. If unusual changes occur, stress importance of notifying prescriber.

• Suggest that patient change position slowly to minimize effects of orthostatic hypotension.

• Advise patient to avoid potentially hazardous activities until she knows how the drug affects her.

• Advise patient not to take other prescription or OTC drugs without consulting prescriber.

• Caution patient not to stop taking drug abruptly to avoid recurrence of original signs and symptoms.

• Instruct woman to use effective contraception during tranylcypromine therapy to prevent fetal abnormalities and to notify prescriber immediately if she knows or suspects she's pregnant.

trazodone hydrochloride

Class and Category

Chemical class: Triazolopyridine derivative
Therapeutic class: Antidepressant
Pregnancy category: C

Indications and Dosages

▶ *To treat major depression, with or without generalized anxiety*

TABLETS

Adults. *Initial:* 150 mg daily in divided doses, increased by 50 mg daily every 3 to 4 days, p.r.n., as prescribed. *Maximum:* 400 mg daily for outpatients, 600 mg daily for inpatients.

Children ages 6 to 18. *Initial:* 1.5 to 2 mg/kg daily in divided doses, increased every 3 to 4 days, p.r.n., as prescribed. *Maximum:* 6 mg/kg daily in divided doses.

DOSAGE ADJUSTMENT For elderly patients, initial dosage possibly reduced to 75 mg daily in divided doses, increased every 3 to 4 days, p.r.n., as prescribed.

Route	Onset	Steady State	Peak	Half-Life	Duration
P.O.	1 to 2 wk	4 days	Unknown	3 to 9 hr	Unknown

Mechanism of Action

Blocks serotonin reuptake along the presynaptic neuronal membrane, causing an antidepressant effect. Trazodone exerts an alpha-adrenergic blocking action and produces modest histamine blockade, causing a sedative effect. It also inhibits the vasopressor response to norepinephrine, which reduces blood pressure.

Contraindications

Hypersensitivity to trazodone or its components, recovery from an acute MI

Interactions

DRUGS

amprenavir, erythromycin, indinavir, itraconazole, ketoconazole, nefazodone, protease inhibitors, ritonavir: Possibly increased blood trazodone level with increased risk of adverse reactions

anticonvulsants: Decreased seizure threshold

antihypertensives: Increased risk of excessive hypotension

anxiolytics, brompheniramine, carbinoxamine, chlorpheniramine, clemastine, dimenhydrinate, diphenhydramine, doxylamine, general anesthetics, methdilazine, opioid analgesics, phenothiazines, sedative-hypnotics, skeletal muscle relaxants: Increased CNS depression, increased risk of respiratory depression and hypotension

barbiturates: Decreased seizure threshold and barbiturate effectiveness, increased drowsiness

buspirone, selective serotonin reuptake inhibitors, tricyclic antidepressants: Possibly excessive serotonergic stimulation

carbamazepine: Decreased blood trazodone level

clonidine: Interference with clonidine's antihypertensive effect

digoxin: Possibly increased blood digoxin level and risk of digitalis toxicity
MAO inhibitors: Increased serotonin-related effects
warfarin: Decreased anticoagulation response
ACTIVITIES
alcohol use: Increased CNS depression, increased risk of respiratory depression and hypotension

Adverse Reactions

CNS: Dizziness, drowsiness, fatigue, headache, light-headedness, nervousness, suicidal ideation, syncope, tremor
CV: Arrhythmias, hypotension, orthostatic hypotension, palpitations
EENT: Blurred vision, dry mouth
GI: Constipation, indigestion, nausea, vomiting
GU: Anorgasmy, ejaculation disorders, increased libido, priapism
SKIN: Pruritus, rash

Overdose

Monitor patient for signs and symptoms of overdose, including coma, dizziness, drowsiness, dry mouth, dyspnea, headache, hypotension, incontinence, lack of coordination, myalgia, nausea, shivering, tachycardia, tinnitus, and vomiting.

Maintain an open airway, monitor cardiac function, and give supportive and symptomatic care, as needed and prescribed.

To decrease drug absorption in a conscious patient who isn't at risk for coma, be prepared to induce vomiting or perform gastric lavage. Expect that oral activated charcoal or a stimulant cathartic may also be prescribed. For an unconscious patient, anticipate assisting with the insertion of an endotracheal tube and then performing gastric lavage. The inflated cuff of the endotracheal tube will help prevent aspiration of gastric contents into the lungs. Forced diuresis may be prescribed to enhance drug elimination.

Institute suicide precautions according to facility policy, and anticipate psychiatric re-evaluation.

Nursing Considerations

• Administer trazodone shortly after a meal or light snack to reduce nausea.
• Give larger portion of daily dose at bedtime if drowsiness occurs.
• Because trazadone's mechanism of action is similar to that of selective serotonin reuptake inhibitors, expect high doses (6 to 8 mg/kg) to increase blood serotonin level and low doses (0.05 to 1 mg/kg) to decrease blood serotonin level.

- Expect most patients who respond to trazodone to do so by the end of the second week.
- Closely monitor depressed patient (esepcially a child or adolescent) for suicidal thoughts or tendencies.
- Be aware that adverse CNS reactions usually improve after a few weeks of therapy.
- **WARNING** Be aware that trazodone therapy may increase the risk of priapism.

PATIENT TEACHING
- Urge patient to avoid taking trazodone on an empty stomach because doing so may increase dizziness or light-headedness.
- **WARNING** Alert parents to watch their child or adolescent closely for abnormal thinking or behavior, such as an increase in aggression or hostility. If unusual changes occur, stress importance of notifying prescriber.
- Advise patient to avoid alcohol while taking drug.
- Caution patient to avoid hazardous activities during therapy.
- Advise patient not to fast during therapy because of the increased risk of adverse CNS reactions.
- Instruct male patient to notify prescriber immediately about priapism.

triazolam

Alti-Triazolam (CAN), Apo-Triazo (CAN), Gen-Triazolam (CAN), Halcion, Novo-Triolam (CAN)

Class, Category, and Schedule

Chemical class: Benzodiazepine
Therapeutic class: Sedative-hypnotic
Pregnancy category: X
Controlled substance schedule: IV

Indications and Dosages

▶ *To provide short-term management of insomnia*

TABLETS
Adults. 0.125 to 0.25 mg at bedtime. *Maximum:* 0.5 mg daily (for patients with inadequate response to usual dose).

DOSAGE ADJUSTMENT For elderly or debilitated patients, initial dosage reduced to 0.125 mg at bedtime and maximum dosage limited to 0.25 mg daily.

Route	Onset	Steady State	Peak	Half-Life	Duration
P.O.	15 to 30 min	Several days	Unknown	1.5 to 5.5 hr	Unknown

Mechanism of Action
Potentiates the effects of the inhibitory neurotransmitter gamma-aminobutyric acid (GABA), which increases the inhibition of the ascending reticular activating system and produces varying levels of CNS depression, including anticonvulsant activity, coma, hypnosis, sedation, and skeletal muscle relaxation.

Contraindications
Hypersensitivity to triazolam or its components, itraconazole or ketoconazole therapy, pregnancy

Interactions
DRUGS

anxiolytics, barbiturates, brompheniramine, carbinoxamine, cetirizine, chlorpheniramine, clemastine, cyproheptadine, dimenhydrinate, diphenhydramine, doxylamine, general anesthetics, methdilazine, opioid analgesics, sedative-hypnotics, phenothiazines, promethazine, tramadol, tricyclic antidepressants, trimeprazine: Increased sedation, respiratory depression

cimetidine, diltiazem, disulfiram, erythromycin, probenecid, verapamil: Increased sedation

fluconazole: Increased blood triazolam level and effects

flumazenil: Increased risk of withdrawal signs and symptoms

itraconazole, ketoconazole: Delayed triazolam elimination

oral contraceptives: Increased blood triazolam level

FOODS

grapefruit juice: Increased blood triazolam level and sedation

ACTIVITIES

alcohol use: Increased sedation, respiratory depression

Adverse Reactions
CNS: Anxiety, ataxia, confusion, depression, dizziness, drowsiness, fatigue, headache, insomnia, nightmares, syncope, talkativeness, tremor, vertigo

Other: Physical and psychological dependence

Overdose
Monitor patient for evidence of overdose, including bradycardia, coma, confusion, dyspnea, hyporeflexia, seizures, severe drowsiness, shakiness, slurred speech, staggering, and weakness.

Maintain an open airway and continuous ECG monitoring, and give I.V. fluids, as prescribed, to support blood pressure and diuresis. Take seizure precautions according to facility protocol.

To decrease drug absorption in a conscious patient who isn't at risk for coma or seizures, be prepared to induce vomiting or perform gastric lavage. Expect that oral activated charcoal may also be prescribed. For an unconscious patient, anticipate assisting with the insertion of an endotracheal tube and then performing gastric lavage. The inflated cuff of the endotracheal tube will help prevent aspiration of gastric contents into the lungs.

Anticipate the use of a benzodiazepine receptor antagonist such as flumazenil to reverse the sedative effects. Be aware that flumazenil may induce seizures, especially in a patient who has been taking benzodiazepines for a long time or who has also ingested a cyclic antidepressant. If excitation occurs, a barbiturate shouldn't be used because it may increase excitement and prolong CNS depression. Dialysis is ineffective for treating benzodiazepine overdose.

Institute suicide precautions according to facility policy, and anticipate psychiatric re-evaluation.

Nursing Considerations
- Be aware that triazolam shouldn't be discontinued abruptly, even after only 1 to 2 weeks of therapy. Doing so can cause withdrawal signs and symptoms, including abdominal cramps, confusion, depression, diaphoresis, hyperacusis, insomnia, irritability, nausea, nervousness, paresthesia, perceptual disturbances, photophobia, tachycardia, tremor, and vomiting.
- **WARNING** Assess patient for evidence of physical and psychological dependence, and notify prescriber if they occur.
- Monitor respiratory rate and depth and ABG results, as appropriate, because drug may worsen ventilatory failure in patient with pulmonary disease, such as respiratory depression, severe COPD, or sleep apnea. If patient has acute intermittent porphyria, myasthenia gravis, or severe renal impairment, use drug cautiously because it may aggravate these conditions.
- Take safety precautions for elderly patients because drug may impair cognitive and motor function and increase risk of falling.
- If patient has advanced Parkinson's disease, use drug cautiously because it may worsen cognition, coordination, and psychosis.

PATIENT TEACHING
- Instruct patient to take triazolam exactly as prescribed and not to abruptly stop taking it because of the risk of withdrawal signs and symptoms.
- Caution patient about possible drowsiness.
- Urge patient to avoid alcohol because it increases sedation.

• Advise patient to notify prescriber about excessive drowsiness, known or suspected pregnancy, or nausea.

trifluoperazine hydrochloride

Apo-Trifluoperazine (CAN), Novo-Trifluzine,
PMS Trifluoperazine (CAN), Stelazine Concentrate

Class and Category

Chemical class: Piperazine phenothiazine
Therapeutic class: Antianxiety drug, antipsychotic drug
Pregnancy category: Not rated

Indications and Dosages

▶ *To treat psychotic disorders*
SYRUP, TABLETS
Adults and adolescents. *Initial:* 2 to 5 mg b.i.d., increased gradually, as needed. *Maintenance:* 15 to 20 mg daily. *Maximum:* 40 mg daily.
Children age 6 and over. *Initial:* 1 mg once or twice daily, increased gradually, as needed. *Maximum:* 15 mg daily.
I.M. INJECTION
Adults and adolescents. 1 to 2 mg every 4 to 6 hr, as needed. *Maximum:* 10 mg daily.
Children age 6 and over. 1 mg once or twice daily, as needed.

▶ *To relieve anxiety*
SYRUP, TABLETS, I.M. INJECTION
Adults and adolescents. *Initial:* 1 to 2 mg b.i.d., increased gradually, as needed. *Maximum:* 6 mg daily for 12 wk.

Route	Onset	Steady State	Peak	Half-Life	Duration
P.O.	Up to several wk	4 to 7 days	6 wk to 6 mo	Unknown	Unknown

Mechanism of Action

Blocks postsynaptic dopamine receptors, increasing dopamine turnover and decreasing dopamine neurotransmission. This action may depress the areas of the brain that control activity and aggression, including the cerebral cortex, hypothalamus, and limbic system. Trifluoperazine may relieve anxiety by indirectly reducing arousal and increasing the filtering of internal stimuli to the reticular activating system.

Incompatibilities

Don't administer trifluoperazine concentrate with carbamazepine oral suspension because a rubbery, orange precipitate may form.

Contraindications

Blood dyscrasias; bone marrow depression; cerebral arteriosclerosis; coma; coronary artery disease; hepatic dysfunction; hypersensitivity to trifluoperazine, other phenothiazines, or their components; myeloproliferative disorders; severe hypertension or hypotension; significant CNS depression; subcortical brain damage; use of high doses of CNS depressants

Interactions

DRUGS

adsorbent antidiarrheals, antacids (aluminum- and magnesium-containing): Possibly inhibited absorption of oral trifluoperazine

amantadine, anticholinergics, antidyskinetics, antihistamines: Possibly intensified adverse anticholinergic effects, increased risk of trifluoperazine-induced hyperpyrexia

amphetamines: Decreased stimulant effect of amphetamines, decreased antipsychotic effect of trifluoperazine

anticonvulsants: Lowered seizure threshold

antithyroid drugs: Increased risk of agranulocytosis

apomorphine: Possibly decreased emetic response to apomorphine, additive CNS depression

appetite suppressants: Decreased effects of appetite suppressants

beta blockers: Increased blood levels of both drugs, possibly leading to additive hypotensive effect, arrhythmias, irreversible retinopathy, and tardive dyskinesia

bromocriptine: Impaired therapeutic effects of bromocriptine

cisapride, disopyramide, erythromycin, pimozide, probucol, procainamide, quinidine: Prolonged QT interval, increased risk of ventricular tachycardia

CNS depressants: Additive CNS depression

ephedrine, metaraminol: Decreased vasopressor response to ephedrine

epinephrine: Blocked alpha-adrenergic effects of epinephrine

extrapyramidal reaction–causing drugs (droperidol, haloperidol, metoclopramide, metyrosine, risperidone): Increased severity and frequency of extrapyramidal reactions

hepatotoxic drugs: Increased risk of hepatotoxicity

hypotension-producing drugs: Possibly severe hypotension with syncope

levodopa: Decreased antidyskinetic effect of levodopa
lithium: Reduced absorption of oral trifluoperazine, possibly encephalopathy and additive extrapyramidal effects
MAO inhibitors, maprotiline, tricyclic antidepressants: Possibly prolonged and intensified sedative and anticholinergic effects, increased blood level of antidepressants, impaired trifluoperazine metabolism, increased risk of neuroleptic malignant syndrome
mephentermine: Decreased antipsychotic effect of trifluoperazine and vasopressor effect of mephentermine
methoxamine, phenylephrine: Decreased vasopressor effect and shortened duration of action of these drugs
metrizamide: Increased risk of seizures
opioid analgesics: Increased risk of CNS and respiratory depression, orthostatic hypotension, severe constipation, and urine retention
ototoxic drugs: Possibly masking of some symptoms of ototoxicity, such as dizziness, tinnitus, and vertigo
phenytoin: Lowered seizure threshold; inhibited phenytoin metabolism, possibly leading to phenytoin toxicity
photosensitizing drugs: Possibly additive photosensitivity and intraocular photochemical damage to choroid, lens, or retina
thiazide diuretics: Possibly hyponatremia and water intoxication
ACTIVITIES
alcohol use: Increased CNS and respiratory depression, increased hypotensive effect

Adverse Reactions
CNS: Akathisia, altered temperature regulation, dizziness, drowsiness, extrapyramidal reactions (dystonia, pseudoparkinsonism, tardive dyskinesia)
CV: Hypotension, orthostatic hypotension, tachycardia
EENT: Blurred vision, dry mouth, nasal congestion, ocular changes (deposits of fine particles in cornea and lens), pigmentary retinopathy
ENDO: Galactorrhea, gynecomastia
GI: Constipation, epigastric pain, nausea, vomiting
GU: Ejaculation disorders, menstrual irregularities, urine retention
SKIN: Contact dermatitis, decreased sweating, photosensitivity, pruritus, rash
Other: Injection site irritation and sterile abscess, weight gain

Overdose
Monitor patient for signs and symptoms of overdose, including agitation, areflexia and hyperreflexia, arrhythmias, blurred vision,

cardiac arrest, coma, confusion, disorientation, drowsiness, dry mouth, dyspnea, heart failure, hyperpyrexia, hypotension, hypothermia, mydriasis, pulmonary edema, QRS complex changes, respiratory depression, seizures, shock, stupor, tachycardia, ventricular fibrillation, and vomiting.

Maintain an open airway, monitor patient for arrhythmias, and maintain temperature. Institute seizure precautions according to facility protocol. Perform gastric lavage and administer activated charcoal, as prescribed. Be aware that vomiting shouldn't be induced because of the potential for impaired consciousness or dystonic reactions of the head and neck.

Don't give drugs that may prolong the QT interval—such as disopyramide, procainamide, or quinidine—to treat arrhythmias because these drugs may have an additive effect with trifluoperazine. Expect to give phenytoin to control arrhythmias and norepinephrine or phenylephrine and I.V. fluids to treat hypotension, as prescribed. Epinephrine shouldn't be used because of a risk of paradoxical hypotension. Anticipate digitalizing patient for heart failure, as prescribed. Expect to treat electrolyte imbalance and maintain acid-base balance, as prescribed, and to give diazepam followed by phenytoin to manage seizures. Avoid giving a barbiturate because it may potentiate CNS and respiratory depression.

Anticipate administering benztropine or diphenhydramine, as prescribed, to manage acute dyskinetic effects. Dialysis is ineffective for treating phenothiazine overdose. Expect to continue ECG monitoring for at least 5 days. Be aware that phenothiazine tablets are visible on X-ray.

Institute suicide precautions according to facility policy, and anticipate psychiatric re-evaluation.

Nursing Considerations

- Use trifluoperazine cautiously in patients with glaucoma because of drug's anticholinergic effect.
- Protect concentrate from light. Refrigeration isn't required.
- Dilute concentrate in at least 2 oz (60 ml) of diluent just before giving it. Use carbonated beverage, coffee, fruit or tomato juice, milk, orange syrup or simple syrup, tea, water, or a semisolid food, such as pudding or soup.
- Before administration, examine parenteral solution. Although it may turn slightly yellow without altering its potency, don't use it if discoloration is pronounced or precipitate is present.
- For I.M. use, inject drug slowly, deep into upper outer quadrant of the buttocks. Keep patient in a supine position for 30 min-

utes after injection to minimize hypotensive effect.

• Rotate I.M. injection sites to avoid irritation and sterile abscesses.

• **WARNING** Monitor patient closely for tardive dyskinesia, which may continue after treatment stops. Signs include uncontrolled movements of arms, body, cheeks, jaw, legs, mouth, or tongue. Notify prescriber if such signs occur.

• Closely monitor elderly patients and severely ill or dehydrated children. They're at increased risk for adverse CNS reactions.

• **WARNING** Be aware that trifluoperazine can cause neuroleptic malignant syndrome. Monitor patient for such signs and symptoms as altered level of consciousness, autonomic instability (diaphoresis, hypertension or hypotension, sinus tachycardia), dyspnea, hyperthermia, and severe extrapyramidal dysfunction. Notify prescriber immediately if such signs and symptoms develop, and be prepared to discontinue therapy.

• To prevent contact dermatitis, avoid skin contact with oral or injection solution.

PATIENT TEACHING

• Instruct patient to take trifluoperazine exactly as prescribed and not to stop taking drug abruptly or without consulting prescriber.

• Advise patient to take drug with food or a full glass of milk or water to minimize adverse GI reactions.

• Urge patient to consult prescriber before using other drugs because of possible interactions.

• Instruct patient to notify prescriber immediately if she experiences difficulty swallowing or speaking and tongue protrusion.

• Caution patient to avoid alcohol during therapy.

• Advise patient to avoid potentially hazardous activities until she knows how the drug affects her.

• Instruct patient to change position slowly to minimize effects of orthostatic hypotension.

• Urge patient to avoid exposure to the sun and extreme heat because drug may cause photosensitivity and interfere with thermoregulation. Encourage her to wear sunscreen when outdoors.

triflupromazine hydrochloride
Vesprin

Class and Category
Chemical class: Phenothiazine
Therapeutic class: Antipsychotic drug
Pregnancy category: Not rated

Indications and Dosages

▶ *To treat psychotic disorders*

I.M. INJECTION

Adults and adolescents. 60 mg, as needed. *Maximum:* 150 mg daily.

Children age 30 months and over. 0.2 to 0.25 mg/kg, as needed. *Maximum:* 10 mg daily.

Mechanism of Action

Blocks postsynaptic dopamine receptors, increasing dopamine turnover and decreasing dopamine neurotransmission. This action may depress the areas of the brain that control activity and aggression, including the cerebral cortex, hypothalamus, and limbic system.

Contraindications

Blood dyscrasias, bone marrow depression, cerebral arteriosclerosis, coma or severe CNS depression, concurrent use of large amount of CNS depressants, coronary artery disease, hepatic dysfunction, hypersensitivity to phenothiazines, severe hypertension or hypotension, subcortical brain damage

Interactions

DRUGS

amantadine, anticholinergics, antidyskinetics, antihistamines: Possibly intensified adverse anticholinergic effects, increased risk of trifluopromazine-induced hyperpyrexia

amphetamines: Decreased stimulant effect of amphetamines, decreased antipsychotic effect of trifluopromazine

anticonvulsants: Lowered seizure threshold

antithyroid drugs: Increased risk of agranulocytosis

apomorphine: Possibly decreased emetic response to apomorphine, additive CNS depression

appetite suppressants: Decreased anorectic effect of appetite suppressants

beta blockers: Increased blood levels of both drugs, possibly leading to additive hypotensive effect, arrhythmias, irreversible retinopathy, and tardive dyskinesia

bromocriptine: Impaired therapeutic effects of bromocriptine

cisapride, disopyramide, erythromycin, pimozide, probucol, procainamide, quinidine: Prolonged QT interval, increased risk of ventricular tachycardia

CNS depressants: Additive CNS depression

ephedrine: Decreased vasopressor response to ephedrine

epinephrine: Blocked alpha-adrenergic effects of epinephrine

extrapyramidal reaction–causing drugs (droperidol, haloperidol, metoclopramide, metyrosine, risperidone): Increased severity and frequency of extrapyramidal reactions

hepatotoxic drugs: Increased risk of hepatotoxicity

hypotension-producing drugs: Possibly severe hypotension with syncope

levodopa: Decreased antidyskinetic effect of levodopa

lithium: Possibly encephalopathy and additive extrapyramidal effects

MAO inhibitors, maprotiline, tricyclic antidepressants: Increased CNS depression, impaired triflupromazine metabolism, increased risk of neuroleptic malignant syndrome

mephentermine: Possibly antagonized antipsychotic effect of triflupromazine and vasopressor effect of mephentermine

metaraminol: Decreased vasopressor effect of metaraminol

methoxamine, phenylephrine: Decreased vasopressor effect and shortened duration of action of these drugs

metrizamide: Increased risk of seizures

opioid analgesics: Increased risk of CNS and respiratory depression, orthostatic hypotension, severe constipation, and urine retention

ototoxic drugs: Possibly masking of symptoms of ototoxicity, such as dizziness, tinnitus, and vertigo

phenytoin: Lowered seizure threshold; inhibited phenytoin metabolism, possibly leading to phenytoin toxicity

photosensitizing drugs: Possibly additive photosensitivity and intraocular photochemical damage to choroid, lens, or retina

thiazide diuretics: Possibly hyponatremia and water intoxication

ACTIVITIES

alcohol use: Increased CNS and respiratory depression, increased hypotensive effect

Adverse Reactions

CNS: Akathisia, altered temperature regulation, dizziness, drowsiness, extrapyramidal reactions (dystonia, pseudoparkinsonism, tardive dyskinesia)

CV: Hypotension, orthostatic hypotension, tachycardia

EENT: Blurred vision, dry mouth, nasal congestion, ocular changes (deposits of fine particles in cornea and lens), pigmentary retinopathy

ENDO: Galactorrhea, gynecomastia

GI: Constipation, epigastric pain, nausea, vomiting
GU: Ejaculation disorders, menstrual irregularities, urine retention
SKIN: Decreased sweating, photosensitivity, pruritus, rash
Other: Injection site irritation and sterile abscess, weight gain

Overdose

Monitor patient for signs and symptoms of overdose, including agitation, areflexia and hyperreflexia, arrhythmias, blurred vision, cardiac arrest, coma, confusion, disorientation, drowsiness, dry mouth, dyspnea, heart failure, hyperpyrexia, hypotension, hypothermia, mydriasis, pulmonary edema, QRS complex changes, respiratory depression, seizures, shock, stupor, tachycardia, ventricular fibrillation, and vomiting.

Maintain am open airway, monitor patient for arrhythmias, and maintain temperature. Institute seizure precautions according to facility protocol. When treating arrhythmias, don't give any drug that may prolong the QT interval—such as disopyramide, procainamide, or quinidine—because these drugs may have an additive effect with triflupromazine. Expect to give phenytoin to control arrhythmias and norepinephrine or phenylephrine and I.V. fluids to treat hypotension, as prescribed. Epinephrine shouldn't be used because of a risk of paradoxical hypotension. Anticipate digitalizing patient for heart failure, as prescribed. Expect to treat electrolyte imbalance and maintain acid-base balance, as prescribed, and to give diazepam, followed by phenytoin to manage seizures. Avoid giving a barbiturate because it may potentiate CNS and respiratory depression.

Anticipate giving benztropine or diphenhydramine, as prescribed, to manage acute dyskinetic effects. Dialysis is ineffective for treating phenothiazine overdose. Expect to continue ECG monitoring for at least 5 days.

Institute suicide precautions according to facility policy, and anticipate psychiatric re-evaluation.

Nursing Considerations

- Use triflupromazine cautiously in patients with glaucoma because of drug's anticholinergic effects.
- Before administration, examine parenteral solution, which may turn slightly yellow without altering potency. Don't use solution if discoloration is pronounced or precipitate is present.
- For I.M. administration, inject drug slowly and deep into upper outer quadrant of buttocks. Keep patient in a supine position for 30 minutes afterward to minimize hypotensive effect.
- Rotate I.M. injection sites to avoid irritation and sterile abscesses.

- **WARNING** Monitor patient closely for tardive dyskinesia, which may continue after treatment stops. Signs include uncontrolled movements of arms, body, cheeks, jaw, legs, mouth, or tongue. Notify prescriber if such signs occur.
- Closely monitor elderly patients and severely ill or dehydrated children; they're at increased risk for adverse CNS reactions.
- To prevent contact dermatitis, avoid skin contact with injection solution.

PATIENT TEACHING
- Instruct patient to change position slowly to minimize effects of orthostatic hypotension.
- Urge patient to avoid potentially hazardous activities until she knows how the drug affects her.
- Instruct patient to notify prescriber immediately if she experiences difficulty swallowing or speaking and tongue protrusion.
- Caution patient to avoid alcohol during therapy.
- Urge patient to avoid exposure to the sun and extreme heat because drug may cause photosensitivity and interfere with thermoregulation. Encourage her to wear sunscreen when outdoors.

Other Therapeutic Uses
Triflupromazine hydrochloride is also indicated for the following:
•To treat nausea and vomiting

trihexyphenidyl hydrochloride
Apo-Trihex (CAN), Artane, Artane Sequels, PMS Trihexyphenidyl (CAN), Trihexane, Trihexy

Class and Category
Chemical class: Tertiary amine
Therapeutic class: Antidyskinetic
Pregnancy category: C

Indications and Dosages
▶ *To treat parkinsonism*
ELIXIR, TABLETS
Adults. *Initial:* 1 to 2 mg on day 1, divided into 3 equal doses and given with meals. Total daily dose increased by 2 mg every 3 to 5 days until desired response or maximum dose is reached. *Maximum:* 15 mg daily.
E.R. CAPSULES
Adults. 5 mg after breakfast; additional 5 mg 12 hr later, if needed. *Maximum:* 15 mg daily.

▶ *To treat drug-induced extrapyramidal signs and symptoms*
TABLETS
Adults. 1 mg daily, increased to 5 to 15 mg daily, as prescribed, to control signs and symptoms.

Route	Onset	Steady State	Peak	Half-Life	Duration
P.O.	1 hr	Unknown	Unknown	5.5 to 10 hr	6 to 12 hr

Mechanism of Action

Blocks acetylcholine action at cholinergic receptor sites, restoring the brain's normal dopamine and acetylcholine balance, which relaxes muscle movement and decreases drooling, rigidity, and tremor. Trihexyphenidyl also may inhibit dopamine reuptake and storage, which prolongs dopamine's action.

Contraindications

Achalasia, bladder neck or prostatic obstruction, narrow-angle glaucoma, hypersensitivity to trihexyphenidyl or its components, megacolon, myasthenia gravis, pyloric or duodenal obstruction, stenosing peptic ulcer

Interactions

DRUGS
amantadine, anticholinergics, MAO inhibitors, tricyclic antidepressants: Increased anticholinergic effects
antidiarrheals (adsorbent): Possibly decreased therapeutic effects of trihexyphenidyl
chlorpromazine: Decreased blood chlorpromazine level
CNS depressants: Increased sedative effect
levodopa: Increased efficacy of levodopa
ACTIVITIES
alcohol use: Increased sedation

Adverse Reactions

CNS: Confusion, dizziness, drowsiness, excitement, nervousness
EENT: Blurred vision; dry eyes, mouth, nose, or throat; mydriasis
GI: Constipation, nausea, vomiting
GU: Dysuria, urine retention
SKIN: Decreased sweating

Overdose

Monitor patient for evidence of overdose, including clumsiness; dyspnea; hallucinations; insomnia; seizures; severe drowsiness; severe dryness of mouth, nose, or throat; tachycardia; toxic psychoses; unsteadiness; and unusually dry, flushed, warm skin.

Maintain open airway, monitor vital signs, and institute seizure precautions according to facility protocol, as needed. Expect to induce vomiting or perform gastric lavage to decrease absorption of drug, as prescribed, except in patients who may be convulsive, precomatose, or psychotic. If the patient is an adult, expect to administer physostigmine salicylate, 1 to 2 mg I.M. or I.V., repeated in 2 hours, as needed, to reverse cardiovascular and CNS toxic effects. Be prepared to administer a short-acting barbiturate or diazepam, as prescribed, to control excitement. Pilocarpine 0.5% may be prescribed to treat mydriasis.

Institute suicide precautionary measures according to facility policy, and anticipate psychiatric re-evaluation.

Nursing Considerations

- Use trihexyphenidyl cautiously in patients with cardiovascular, hepatic, or renal disorders. Patients with cardiovascular disorders—such as atherosclerosis, hypertension, and ischemic heart disease—are at risk for tachycardia and coronary ischemia from drug's positive chronotropic effects. Hepatic and renal dysfunction increase the risk of adverse reactions.
- Before therapy begins, assess patient's muscle rigidity and tremor to establish a baseline. During therapy, reassess patient to detect improvement and to evaluate drug effectiveness.
- Also before therapy begins, obtain baseline evaluation of the patient's intraocular pressure; check it periodically throughout trihexyphenidyl therapy, as ordered, because drug can precipitate incipient glaucoma.

PATIENT TEACHING
- Instruct patient to take trihexyphenidyl after meals.
- Teach patient not to break or chew E.R. capsules.
- Instruct patient to use calibrated device to measure elixir.
- Advise patient to avoid potentially hazardous activities until she knows how the drug affects her.
- Caution patient to avoid alcohol during therapy.
- Advise patient with dry eyes or increased contact lens awareness to use lubricating drops or stop wearing contact lenses during drug therapy.
- Warn patient with parkinsonism not to stop taking trihexyphenidyl abruptly because symptoms may increase suddenly.
- Advise patient to maintain hydration and avoid exercise during hot weather because drug may increase risk of heatstroke.

trimipramine maleate

Apo-Trimip (CAN), Novo-Tripramine (CAN), Rhotrimine (CAN), Surmontil

Class and Category

Chemical class: Dibenzazepine derivative
Therapeutic class: Antidepressant
Pregnancy category: C

Indications and Dosages

▶ *To treat depression*

CAPSULES

Adults in inpatient settings. *Initial:* 100 mg daily in divided doses, increased gradually in a few days to 200 mg daily. *Maximum:* 300 mg daily in 2 to 3 wk.

Adolescents in inpatient settings. *Initial:* 50 mg daily in divided doses, increased as needed. *Maximum:* 100 mg daily.

Adults in outpatient settings. *Initial:* 75 mg daily in divided doses, increased gradually up to 150 mg daily, as needed. *Maintenance:* 50 to 150 mg daily. *Maximum:* 200 mg daily.

Adolescents in outpatient settings. *Initial:* 50 mg daily in divided doses, increased as needed. *Maximum:* 100 mg daily.

DOSAGE ADJUSTMENT For elderly patients, initial dosage reduced to 50 mg daily in divided doses, and maximum dosage limited to 100 mg daily.

Route	Onset	Steady State	Peak	Half-Life	Duration
P.O.	2 to 3 wk	2 to 6 days	Unknown	7 to 30 hr	Unknown

Mechanism of Action

Inhibits the reuptake of norepinephrine at presynaptic neurons, thus increasing its concentration in synapses. The action of this tricyclic antidepressant may elevate mood and relieve depression.

Contraindications

Hypersensitivity to trimipramine, other dibenzazepine tricyclic antidepressants, or their components; recovery period after an MI; use within 14 days of therapy with an MAO inhibitor or other tricyclic antidepressant

Interactions

DRUGS

amantadine, anticholinergics, antidyskinetics, antihistamines: Increased anticholinergic effects, especially confusion, hallucinations, and nightmares

anticonvulsants: Increased CNS depression, lowered seizure threshold (high doses of trimipramine), decreased anticonvulsant effect

antithyroid drugs: Increased risk of agranulocytosis

barbiturates, carbamazepine: Decreased blood level and therapeutic effects of trimipramine

bupropion, clozapine, cyclobenzaprine, haloperidol, loxapine, maprotiline, molindone, phenothiazines, thioxanthenes: Intensified and prolonged sedative and anticholinergic effects of both drugs, increased risk of seizures

cimetidine: Decreased trimipramine metabolism, possibly leading to trimipramine toxicity

clonidine: Decreased hypotensive effect and increased CNS depressant effect of clonidine

CNS depressants: Increased hypotension and CNS and respiratory depression

disulfiram, ethchlorvynol: Transient delirium, increased risk of CNS depression (with ethchlorvynol)

fluoxetine: Increased blood trimipramine level

guanadrel, guanethidine: Decreased hypotensive effect

MAO inhibitors: Increased risk of death, hyperpyrexia, hypertensive crisis, and severe seizures

methylphenidate: Decreased methylphenidate effects, increased blood trimipramine level

metrizamide: Increased risk of seizures

naphazoline (ophthalmic), oxymetazoline (nasal or ophthalmic), phenylephrine (nasal or ophthalmic), xylometazoline (nasal): Increased vasopressor effect of these drugs

oral anticoagulants: Increased anticoagulant activity

phenothiazines: Increased blood trimipramine level, decreased phenothiazine metabolism

pimozide, probucol: Increased risk of arrhythmias, possibly prolonged QT interval

sympathomimetics: Increased risk of arrhythmias, hyperpyrexia, and severe hypertension

thyroid hormones: Increased intended and toxic effects of both drugs

ACTIVITIES

alcohol use: Increased hypotension and CNS and respiratory depression

Adverse Reactions

CNS: Anxiety, ataxia, confusion, CVA, delirium, dizziness, drowsiness, excitement, extrapyramidal reactions, hallucinations, headache, insomnia, nervousness, nightmares, parkinsonism, seizures, suicidal ideation, tremor

CV: Arrhythmias, orthostatic hypotension
EENT: Blurred vision, dry mouth, increased intraocular pressure, taste perversion, tinnitus, tongue swelling
ENDO: Gynecomastia, syndrome of inappropriate ADH secretion
GI: Constipation, diarrhea, heartburn, ileus, increased appetite, nausea, vomiting
GU: Sexual dysfunction, testicular swelling, urine retention
HEME: Agranulocytosis, bone marrow depression
RESP: Wheezing
SKIN: Alopecia, diaphoresis, jaundice, photosensitivity, pruritus, rash, urticaria
Other: Facial edema, weight gain

Overdose

Monitor patient for evidence of overdose, including agitation, arrhythmias, confusion, disturbed concentration, drowsiness, dyspnea, fever, hallucinations, irregular heartbeat, mydriasis, restlessness, seizures, unusual fatigue, vomiting, and weakness.

Maintain an open airway, institute continuous ECG monitoring for at least 5 days, and closely observe patient's blood pressure, respiratory rate, and temperature. Be prepared to treat arrhythmias with lidocaine and sodium bicarbonate, as prescribed. Anticipate possible digitalization to prevent heart failure. Institute seizure precautions according to facility protocol, and administer anticonvulsant therapy, as prescribed.

Be prepared to perform gastric lavage to decrease drug absorption. Expect to administer activated charcoal followed by a bowel stimulant to enhance drug elimination. Because tricyclic antidepressants are highly protein bound, dialysis, exchange transfusions, and forced diuresis are ineffective for treating overdose.

Although I.V. physostigmine isn't routinely recommended, it may be prescribed to reverse the anticholinergic effects of trimipramine in comatose patients with respiratory depression, serious arrhythmias, severe hypertension, or uncontrollable seizures.

Institute suicide precautions according to facility policy, and anticipate psychiatric re-evaluation.

Nursing Considerations

- **WARNING** Monitor children and adolescents closely for suicidal thinking and behavior because trimipramine increases the risk in these age-groups, particularly when therapy starts or dosage changes because depression may worsen temporarily during these times.

- During the initial and stabilization intervals, expect to monitor the ECG of patients who are receiving a high dose of trimipramine .
- Expect to gradually reduce dosage, as prescribed, before electroconvulsive therapy.

PATIENT TEACHING

- Instruct patient to take the last dose of trimipramine early in the evening to avoid insomnia.
- **WARNING** Alert parents to watch their child or adolescent closely for abnormal thinking or behavior, an increase in aggression or hostility, and any suicidal tendencies, especially when therapy starts or dosage changes. If unusual changes occur, stress the importance of notifying prescriber.
- Advise patient to avoid potentially hazardous activities until she knows how the drug affects her.
- Encourage patient to change position slowly to minimize effects of orthostatic hypotension.
- Urge patient to avoid alcohol during therapy.
- Advise patient to avoid excessive exposure to sunlight and to wear sunscreen when she's outdoors.
- Instruct patient to notify prescriber about unusual bruising and signs and symptoms of infection.
- Suggest that patient use sugarless gum or hard candy to relieve dry mouth.
- Inform patient that she may need to continue maintenance therapy for about 3 months to maintain remission.

tubocurarine chloride

Class and Category

Chemical class: Isoquinoline derivative
Therapeutic class: Anticonvulsant
Pregnancy category: C

Indications and Dosages

▶ *To manage muscle contractions from seizures in electroconvulsive therapy*

I.V. INJECTION

Adults. 157 mcg/kg (0.157 mg/kg) over 30 to 90 sec, given just before electroconvulsive therapy. Expect the initial dose to be 3 mg less than the calculated total dose.

Route	Onset	Steady State	Peak	Half-Life	Duration
I.V.	1 min	Unknown	2 to 5 min	84 to 120 min	20 to 40 min

Mechanism of Action

Reduces the intensity of skeletal muscle contractions caused by electrically induced seizures. Normally, when a nerve impulse arrives at a somatic motor nerve terminal, it triggers acetylcholine (ACh) stored in synaptic vesicles to be released into the neuromuscular junction. The released ACh binds with nicotinic receptors embedded in the skeletal muscle motor endplate, as shown top right, triggering muscle cell depolarization and contraction.

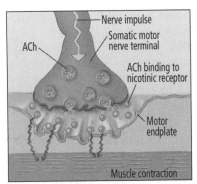

Tubocurarine is a nondepolarizing neuromuscular blocker that acts as a competitive antagonist of ACh. By binding to the nicotinic receptors, as shown bottom right, it prevents transmission of the action potential at the neuromuscular junction, thereby

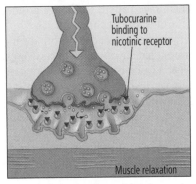

sustaining skeletal muscle relaxation and eliminating the peripheral muscular manifestations of seizures. The drug has no effect on the CNS processes involved with seizures because it doesn't cross the blood-brain barrier.

Incompatibilities

Don't mix tubocurarine with barbiturates, such as methohexital or thiopental, because a precipitate may form.

Contraindications

Hypersensitivity to tubocurarine or its components, patients in whom histamine release may be dangerous

Interactions
DRUG

alfentanil, fentanyl, sufentanil: Prevented or reversed muscle rigidity caused by these drugs

aminoglycosides, anesthetics, capreomycin, citrate-anticoagulated blood, clindamycin, lidocaine (I.V.), lincomycin, polymyxins, procaine (I.V.), trimethaphan: Additive neuromuscular blocking effects

beta blockers, calcium salts: Prolonged and enhanced effects of tubocurarine

magnesium salts, procainamide, quinidine: Enhanced blockade effects

opioid analgesics: Additive histamine release effects, additive respiratory depressant effects, and worsened bradycardia and hypotension

Adverse Reactions
CV: Arrhythmias, bradycardia, edema, hypotension, shock, tachycardia
RESP: Bronchospasm
SKIN: Erythema, flushing, itching, rash
Other: Anaphylaxis

Overdose
Monitor patient for signs and symptoms of overdose, including apnea, hypotension, paralysis, and shock.

Maintain open airway, and assist with manual or mechanical ventilation until patient resumes normal respiratory function. Monitor vital signs, and plan to assess neuromuscular blockade effects with a peripheral nerve stimulator. Treat hypotension with I.V. fluids and a vasopressor, as needed and prescribed.

To antagonize the effects of tubocurarine, expect to administer a cholinesterase inhibitor, such as edrophonium, neostigmine, or pyridostigmine. Expect that an anticholinergic drug, such as atropine, will also be prescribed to counteract the cholinergic adverse effects of the cholinesterase inhibitor. Plan to observe the patient for at least 1 hour after reversal for the return of muscle relaxation.

Nursing Considerations
- If patient has a history of cardiovascular disease or is hypotensive, monitor her for further decrease in blood pressure.
- Monitor patient for bronchospasm and hypotension because tubocurarine may cause increased histamine release.

- Keep emergency equipment and drugs nearby in case respiratory depression occurs.

PATIENT TEACHING
- Explain the need for frequent hemodynamic monitoring.

Other Therapeutic Uses

Tubocurarine chloride is also indicated for the following:
- To produce skeletal muscle paralysis during anesthesia or mechanical ventilation
- As diagnostic aid for myasthenia gravis

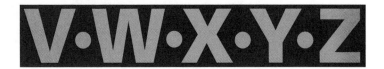

valproic acid

Alti-Valproic (CAN), Depakene, Deproic (CAN), Dom-Valproic (CAN), Med Valproic (CAN), Novo-Valproic (CAN), Nu-Valproic (CAN), PMS-Valproic Acid (CAN), pms-Valproic Acid E.C. (CAN)

valproate sodium

Depacon

divalproex sodium

Depakote, Depakote ER, Depakote Sprinkle, Epival (CAN)

Class and Category

Chemical class: Carboxylic acid derivative
Therapeutic class: Anticonvulsant, antimanic drug, antimigraine drug
Pregnancy category: D

Indications and Dosages

▶ *To treat simple or complex absence seizures, complex partial seizures, myoclonic seizures, and generalized tonic-clonic seizures as monotherapy*
CAPSULES, DELAYED-RELEASE SPRINKLE CAPSULES, DELAYED-RELEASE TABLETS, SYRUP, I.V. INFUSION (VALPROIC ACID, VALPROATE SODIUM, DIVALPROEX SODIUM)

Adults and adolescents. *Initial:* 10 to 15 mg/kg daily in divided doses b.i.d. or t.i.d., increased by 5 to 10 mg/kg daily every wk, as needed and as prescribed. *Maximum:* 60 mg/kg daily.
Children. *Initial:* 15 to 45 mg/kg daily in divided doses b.i.d. or t.i.d., increased by 5 to 10 mg/kg daily every wk, as needed and as prescribed.

▶ *As adjunct to treat simple or complex absence seizures, complex partial seizures, myoclonic seizures, and generalized tonic-clonic seizures*
CAPSULES, DELAYED-RELEASE SPRINKLE CAPSULES, DELAYED-RELEASE TABLETS, SYRUP, I.V. INFUSION (VALPROIC ACID, VALPROATE SODIUM, DIVALPROEX SODIUM)

Adults and adolescents. 10 to 30 mg/kg daily in divided doses, increased by 5 to 10 mg/kg daily every wk, as needed and as prescribed.
Children. 30 to 100 mg/kg daily in divided doses, as prescribed.

DOSAGE ADJUSTMENT For adults being converted from immediate-release divalproex tablets to delayed-release tablets, dosage increased to 8% to 20% more than total daily dose of immediate-release tablets and given once daily.

▶ *To treat acute manic phase of bipolar disorder*
DELAYED-RELEASE TABLETS (DIVALPROEX SODIUM)
Adults. *Initial:* 750 mg daily in divided doses. *Maximum:* 60 mg/kg daily.

▶ *To treat acute mania or mixed episodes in bipolar disorder*
EXTENDED-RELEASE TABLETS (VALPROIC ACID)
Adults. *Initial:* 25 mg/kg daily as a single dose and then increased rapidly to achieve therapeutic effect. *Maximum:* 60 mg/kg daily with duration of therapy limited to 3 wk.

▶ *To prevent migraine headache*
DELAYED-RELEASE TABLETS (DIVALPROEX SODIUM)
Adults. 250 mg every 12 hr, increased p.r.n. *Maximum:* 1 g daily.
EXTENDED-RELEASE TABLETS
Adults. 500 mg daily, increased, as needed and prescribed, up to 1 g daily. *Maximum:* 1 g daily.

Route	Onset	Steady State	Peak	Half-Life	Duration
P.O., I.V.	Unknown	Unknown	Unknown	6 to 16 hr	Unknown

Mechanism of Action

May decrease seizure activity by blocking reuptake of gamma-aminobutyric acid (GABA), the most common inhibitory neurotransmitter in the brain. GABA is known to suppress the rapid firing of neurons by inhibiting voltage-sensitive sodium channels. The antimanic and antimigraine actions of divalproex sodium are unknown, but they are believed to be related to the drug's ability to increase GABA, mimic GABA, or enhance GABA's inhibitory effect.

Contraindications

Hepatic dysfunction; hypersensitivity to valproic acid, valproate sodium, divalproex sodium, or their components

Interactions

DRUGS
aspirin, heparin, NSAIDs, oral anticoagulants, thrombolytics: Increased inhibition of platelet aggregation and risk of bleeding
barbiturates, primidone: Increased blood levels of both drugs, additive CNS effects

carbamazepine: Possibly decreased valproic acid effectiveness
cholestyramine: Decreased bioavailability of valproic acid
clonazepam: Increased risk of absence seizures
CNS depressants: Increased CNS depression
diazepam: Inhibited diazepam metabolism
ethosuximide: Unpredictable blood ethosuximide level
felbamate: Impaired valproic acid metabolism and increased blood drug level
haloperidol, loxapine, MAO inhibitors, maprotiline, phenothiazines, thioxanthenes, tricyclic antidepressants: Increased CNS depression, lowered seizure threshold
lamotrigine: Decreased lamotrigine clearance
mefloquine: Decreased blood levels of valproic acid, divalproex sodium, and valproate sodium; increased risk of seizures
phenytoin: Increased risk of phenytoin toxicity, loss of seizure control
topiramate: Increased risk of hyperammonemia and encephalopathy
ACTIVITIES
alcohol use: Additive CNS depression

Adverse Reactions

CNS: Agitation, ataxia, confusion, depression, dizziness, drowsiness, euphoria, hallucinations, headache, hyperesthesia, lack of coordination, lethargy, loss of seizure control, paresthesia, psychosis, sedation, tremor, vertigo, weakness
EENT: Diplopia, nystagmus, pharyngitis, spots before eyes
ENDO: Galactorrhea, hyperglycemia
GI: Abdominal pain, anorexia, constipation, diarrhea, elevated liver function test results, hepatitis, hepato-renal syndrome, hepatotoxicity, increased appetite, indigestion, nausea, pancreatitis, vomiting
GU: Menstrual irregularities, nephritis, oliguria
HEME: Eosinophilia, hematoma, leukopenia, neutropenia, prolonged bleeding time, thrombocytopenia
MS: Arthralgia, dysarthria
SKIN: Alopecia, diaphoresis, erythema multiforme, jaundice, petechiae, photosensitivity, pruritus, rash, Stevens-Johnson syndrome
Other: Facial edema, hyperammonemia, injection site pain, lymphadenopathy, multi-organ hypersensitivity reaction, weight gain or loss

Overdose

Monitor patient for signs and symptoms of overdose, including asterixis, coma, hallucinations, heart block, restlessness, and somnolence.

Maintain an open airway, assess patient for arrhythmias, and monitor vital signs and urine output.

To decrease drug absorption, be prepared to induce vomiting or perform gastric lavage; be aware that drug absorption depends on the drug form involved in the overdose and that the enteric-coated tablets may take 1 to 4 hours to be absorbed. Hemodialysis may be effective in reducing the blood valproate level.

Anticipate the use of naloxone to treat CNS depression; be prepared to treat seizures because naloxone may reverse the anticonvulsant effect of valproate.

Institute suicide precautions according to facility policy, and anticipate psychiatric re-evaluation.

Nursing Considerations

- Give oral valproic acid or divalproex with food to minimize GI irritation, if necessary.
- Administer drug at least 2 hours before or 6 hours after cholestyramine.
- Don't mix syrup with carbonated beverages; doing so may produce an unpleasant-tasting mixture and irritate the mouth and throat.
- Don't break or allow patient to chew delayed-release tablets.
- As needed, mix contents of delayed-release sprinkle capsules in small amount of semisolid food just before administration. Instruct patient not to chew contents of delayed-release sprinkle capsules.
- For I.V. administration, dilute prescribed dose with at least 50 ml of compatible diluent, and infuse over 60 minutes.
- Be aware that patient should be switched from I.V. to P.O. form of valproic acid as soon as possible.
- Be aware that patient with hypoalbuminemia or another protein-binding deficiency is at increased risk for valproic acid toxicity.
- **WARNING** Although rare, life-threatening multi-organ hypersensitivity reaction may occur during initiation of valproic acid therapy. Monitor patient closely for fever, rash, and such organ involvement as lymphadenopathy, hepatitis, liver function test abnormalities, eosinophilia, thrombocytopenia, neutropenia, nephritis, pruritis, oliguria, hepato-renal syndrome,

arthralgia, and asthenia. Notify prescriber immediately, discontinue drug, as ordered, and be prepared to provide supportive care.

- Assess patient for signs and symptoms of decreased hepatic function, including anorexia, facial edema, jaundice, lethargy, loss of seizure control, malaise, vomiting, and weakness.
- Monitor liver function test results, as ordered. Assess patient for signs and symptoms of hepatotoxicity during first 6 months of treatment, especially in children younger than age 2. Notify prescriber immediately if you suspect hepatotoxicity.
- Monitor platelet count, as ordered, for signs of thrombocytopenia, and notify prescriber if they appear.
- **WARNING** Be aware that hyperammonemia may occur even if patient's liver function test results are normal. Monitor ammonia levels, as ordered. If patient develops unexplained lethargy, vomiting, or changes in mental status with an increase in ammonia level, or if asymptomatic ammonia elevations are detected and persist, expect valproic acid to be discontinued.

PATIENT TEACHING

- Instruct patient to swallow capsules whole to prevent irritation to mouth and throat. However, delayed-release sprinkle capsules may be opened and contents mixed with food for easier swallowing. Instruct patient not to chew contents of delayed-release sprinkle capsules.
- Advise patient to avoid potentially hazardous activities during therapy because drug may affect mental and motor performance.
- Caution patient to avoid alcohol during therapy.
- If patient is female, urge her to notify prescriber immediately if she suspects or knows she's pregnant.
- Advise patient to notify prescriber if tremor develops during therapy; occurrence of tremor may be dose-related.
- Instruct patient to report any unusual, persistent, or severe signs and symptoms to prescriber, especially unexplained fever and rash accompanied by other complaints.

vardenafil hydrochloride
Levitra

Class and Category
Chemical class: Phosphodiesterase type 5 inhibitor

Therapeutic class: Anti-impotence drug
Pregnancy category: B

Indications and Dosages

▶ *To treat erectile dysfunction*
TABLETS
Adult men. 10 mg taken 1 hr before sexual activity; increased to 20 mg or decreased to 5 mg, as needed. *Maximum:* 20 mg. Drug may be taken only once daily regardless of dosage used.
DOSAGE ADJUSTMENT If patient takes ritonavir, dosage of vardenfil shouldn't exceed 2.5 mg in 72 hr. If patient takes indinavir, saquinavir, atazanavir, clarithromycin, ketoconazole (400 mg daily), itraconazole (400 mg daily), or another potent CYP3A4 inhibitor, dosage of vardenafil shouldn't exceed 2.5 mg in 24 hr. If patient takes ketoconazole 200 mg and itraconazole 200 mg daily, dosage of vardenafil shouldn't exceed 5 mg in 24 hr.

Route	Onset	Peak	Duration
P.O.	30 min	30 min to 2 hr	4 to 5 hr

Mechanism of Action

Enhances effect of nitric oxide (released in the penis by sexual stimulation) and inhibits phosphodiesterase type 5, which increases cGMP level, relaxes smooth muscle, and increases blood flow into the corpus cavernosum, producing an erection.

Contraindications

Concurrent use of an alpha blocker, concurrent continuous or intermittent nitrate therapy, hypersensitivity to vardenafil or its components

Interactions

DRUGS
alpha blockers, nitrates: Profound hypotension
atazanavir, clarithromycin, erythromycin, indinavir, itraconazole, ketoconazole, ritonavir, saquinavir: Increased vardenafil effects
class IA (procainamide, quinidine) and class III (amiodarone, sotalol) antiarrhythmics: Possibly increased QT-interval prolongation
indinavir, ritonavir: Reduced blood levels of indinavir and ritonavir
FOODS
grapefruit juice: Possibly increased vardenafil effect

Adverse Reactions

CNS: Dizziness, headache
CV: Hypotension
EENT: Nonarteritic anterior ischemic optic neuropathy, rhinitis, sinusitis
GI: Indigestion, nausea
MS: Back pain
SKIN: Flushing
Other: Flulike symptoms, increased creatine kinase level

Overdose

Vardenafil overdose hasn't been reported, and no antidote is known. Monitor patient for exaggerated adverse reactions.

Be prepared to give supportive and symptomatic care, as needed and prescribed. Dialysis is ineffective because vardenafil is highly protein bound and not eliminated by the kidneys.

Institute suicide precautions according to facility policy, and anticipate psychiatric re-evaluation.

Nursing Considerations

• Be aware that vardenafil shouldn't be used by men taking class IA (procainamide, quinidine) or class III (amiodarone, sotalol) antiarrhythmics or by men with congenital QT-interval prolongation because drug may potentiate QT-interval prolongation.
• Use vardenafil cautiously in men with renal or hepatic dysfunction, elderly men, and men with penile abnormalities that may predispose them to priapism.
• Also use cautiously in patients with left ventricular outflow obstruction, such as aortic stenosis, and those with severely impaired autonomic control of blood pressure because these conditions increase sensitivity to vasodilators, such as vardenafil.
• Monitor blood pressure and heart rate before and after giving drug, especially if patient takes an alpha blocker, because of increased risk of symptomatic hypotension.
• Monitor patient's vision, especially if he is over age 50; has diabetes, hypertension, coronary artery disease, or hyperlipidemia; or smokes, because vardenafil rarely leads to nonarteritic ischemic optic neuropathy and decreased vision, possibly permanent.

PATIENT TEACHING
• Explain that vardenafil should be taken 1 hour before sexual activity for best results.
• **WARNING** Warn patient not to take vardenafil if he also takes an organic nitrate (continuously or intermittently) or

within 4 hours of taking an alpha blocker because profound hypotension and death could result.
- Caution against taking vardenafil more than once daily or exceeding 20 mg daily.
- Tell patient to stop taking vardenafil and notify prescriber if he has sudden reeduction of vision in one or both eyes.
- Advise patient to seek sexual counseling to enhance drug's effects.
- To avoid possible penile damage and permanent loss of erectile function, urge patient to notify prescriber immediately if erection is painful or lasts longer than 4 hours.

varenicline
Chantix

Class and Category
Chemical class: Tartrate salt
Therapeutic class: Nicotinic blocker
Pregnancy category: C

▶ *As adjunct to smoking cessation treatment*
TABLETS
Adults. *Initial:* 0.5 mg daily for 3 days; then increased to 0.5 mg b.i.d. for 4 days; then increased to 1 mg b.i.d. for a total of 12 wk. If effective, an additional 12 wk of therapy may be given.
DOSAGE ADJUSTMENT If patient has severe renal impairment, dosage shouldn't exceed 0.5 mg b.i.d. If patient is undergoing hemodialysis for end-stage renal disease, dosage shouldn't exceed 0.5 mg daily.

Mechanism of Action
Binds to $alpha_4beta_2$ receptors, preventing nicotine from binding to and activating them. This inhibits nicotine from stimulating the central nervous mesolimbic dopamine system, thought to be the area that provides underlying reinforcement for and pleasure from smoking.

Contraindications
Hypersensitivity to varenicline or its components

Interactions
DRUG
nicotine (transdermal): Increased adverse reactions

Adverse Reactions

CNS: Abnormal dreams, agitation, anxiety, asthenia, attention difficulties, behavior changes, CVA, depression, dizziness, dysgeusia, fatigue, headache, insomnia, irritability, lethargy, malaise, mental impairment, restlessness, sensory disturbances, seizures, somnolence, suicidal ideation, thirst
CV: Angina, chest pain, edema, hypertension, MI, peripheral ischemia, thrombosis, ventricular extrasystoles
EENT: Dry mouth, epistaxis, gingivitis, rhinorrhea
ENDO: Hot flashes
GI: Abdominal pain, acute pancreatitis, anorexia, constipation, diarrhea, dyspepsia, flatuence, gastroesophageal reflux disease, GI hemorrhage, increased appetite, liver enzyme abnormalities, nausea, vomiting
GU: Acute renal failure, polyuria, urine retention
HEME: Leukocytosis, lymphadenopathy, splenomegaly, thrombocytopenia
RESP: Asthma, dyspnea, pulmonary embolism
MS: Arthralgia, back pain, muscle cramps, musculoskeletal pain, myalgia
SKIN: Diaphoresis, pruritus, rash, urticaria
Other: Flulike syndrome, hyperkalemia, hypersensitivity, hypokalemia

Overdose

Provide standard supportive measures for overdose. Varenicline is removed by dialysis in patients with end-stage renal disease, but there's no experience with dialysis following overdose.

Nursing Considerations

- Use cautiously in patients with renal disease because varenicline is excreted substantially by the kidneys.
- Review patient's medication history before starting varenicline therapy because smoking cessation may require adjustment to dosages of such drugs as theophylline, warfarin, and insulin.
- If patient develops nausea, the most common adverse reaction to varenicline, notify the prescriber because a dosage reduction may be helpful.
- Monitor patient closely for changes in behavior, agitation, depression, and suicidal thoughts or worsening of psychiatric conditions while patient is taking varenicline.

PATIENT TEACHING
- Alert patient that simultaneous use of nicotine patches won't

increase varenicline's effectiveness and may increase such adverse reactions as dizziness, nausea, and vomiting.
- Instruct patient to set a date to quit smoking and to start taking varenicline one week before that date.
- Tell patient to take drug after eating and with a full glass of water.
- Encourage patient to continue trying to quit smoking even if an early relapse occurs during varenicline therapy.
- Explain that the most common adverse reactions to varenicline therapy are nausea and insomnia and that they usually are transient. Urge patient to notify prescriber if they persist because dosage may need to be reduced.
- Instruct patient to avoid activities that require alertness until effects of smoking cessation with varenicline are known.
- Urge caregivers to monitor patient for evidence of suicidal tendencies or worsened psychiatric conditions and, if present, to notify prescriber.

venlafaxine hydrochloride
Effexor, Effexor XR

Class and Category
Chemical class: Phenylethylamine derivative
Therapeutic class: Antianxiety drug, antidepressant
Pregnancy category: C

Indications and Dosages
▶ *To treat generalized anxiety disorder or social anxiety disorder*
E.R. CAPSULES
Adults. *Initial:* 75 mg daily with a meal at same time each day, morning or evening (for some patients, 37.5 mg daily for 4 to 7 days before increasing to 75 mg daily), then increased by 75 mg daily every 4 days, as prescribed. *Maximum:* 225 mg daily.
▶ *To treat and prevent relapse of major depression*
E.R. CAPSULES
Adults. 75 mg daily with a meal at same time each day, morning or evening (for some patients, 37.5 mg daily for 4 to 7 days before increasing to 75 mg daily), then increased by 75 mg daily every 4 days, as prescribed. *Maximum:* 225 mg daily.
TABLETS
Adults. 75 mg daily in divided doses b.i.d. to t.i.d., increased by 75 mg daily every 4 days, as prescribed. *Maximum:* 375 mg daily (225 mg daily for outpatients).

▶ *To treat panic disorder*
E.R. CAPSULES
Adults. *Initial:* 37.5 mg daily for 7 days followed by weekly dosage increases of 75 mg daily, as needed. *Maximum:* 225 mg daily.
DOSAGE ADJUSTMENT Initial daily dose decreased by 25% to 50% for patients with mild to moderate renal impairment and by 50% for patients with hepatic impairment.

Route	Onset	Steady State	Peak	Half-Life	Duration
P.O.	2 wk	3 days	Unknown	3 to 7 hr*	Unknown

Mechanism of Action

Inhibits neuronal reuptake of serotonin and norepinephrine, along with its active metabolite, *O*-desmethylvenlafaxine. These actions raise serotonin and norepinephrine levels at nerve synapses, elevating mood and reducing depression.

Contraindications

Hypersensitivity to venlafaxine or its components, use within 14 days of MAO inhibitor therapy

Interactions

DRUGS

amitriptyline, clomipramine, desipramine, doxepin, haloperidol, imipramine, linezolid, lithium, nortriptyline, protriptyline, St. John's Wort, tramadol, trazodone, triptans, tryptophan supplements: Possibly serotonin syndrome
cimetidine: Decreased clearance and increased blood level of venlafaxine
clozapine: Possibly increased blood clozapine level leading to serious adverse effects such as seizures
ketoconazole: Increased plasma venlafaxine level
MAO inhibitors: Increased risk of hypertension; hyperthermia; mental status changes, including coma and delirium; muscle rigidity; and severe myoclonus
metoprolol: Increased plasma metoprolol level but decreased effectiveness in lowering blood pressure
warfarin: Possibly increased prothrombin time, partial thromboplastin time and INR

---

* 9 to 13 hr for the active metabolite, *O*-desmethylvenlafaxine.

Adverse Reactions

CNS: Agitation, anxiety, asthenia, chills, confusion, delusions, depression, dizziness, dream disturbances, drowsiness, dyskinesia, headache, homicidal or suicidal ideation, insomnia, mood changes, nervousness, paresthesia, seizures, serotonin syndrome, tremor

CV: Chest pain, hypertension, orthostatic hypotension, palpitations, sinus tachycardia, thrombophlebitis

EENT: Angle-closure glaucoma, blurred vision, dry mouth, mydriasis, pharyngitis, rhinitis, tinnitus

ENDO: Hot flashes, hypoglycemia, syndrome of inappropriate ADH secretion

GI: Abdominal pain, anorexia, constipation, diarrhea, flatulence, indigestion, nausea, vomiting

GU: Anorgasmia (women), decreased libido, ejaculation disorders, impotence

MS: Rhabdomyolysis

RESP: Eosinophilic pneumonia, interstitial lung disease

SKIN: Diaphoresis

Other: Hyponatremia, weight loss

Overdose

Monitor patient for signs and symptoms of overdose, including agitation, ECG changes (especially a prolonged QT interval), lethargy, paresthesia, seizures, serotonin syndrome, somnolence, tachycardia, and tremor.

Maintain an open airway, and institute continuous ECG monitoring and seizure precautions according to facility protocol.

To decrease drug absorption, be prepared to perform gastric lavage and administer activated charcoal, as prescribed. Hemodialysis is ineffective because venlafaxine has a large volume of distribution in the body.

Institute suicide precautions according to facility policy, and anticipate psychiatric re-evaluation.

Nursing Considerations

• Use cautiously in patients with increased intraocular pressure and those at risk for angle-closure glaucoma because venlafaxine may cause prolonged dilation of pupils.

• **WARNING** Monitor patient for signs and symptoms of serotonin syndrome (agitation, hallucinations, coma, tachycardia, labile blood pressure, hyperthermia, hyperreflexia, incoordination, nausea, vomiting, or diarrhea), especially in patients taking serotonergic drugs. If present, expect to withhold venlafaxine and provide supportive care.

• Monitor blood pressure frequently during venlafaxine therapy because drug may cause dose-related increase in supine diastolic pressure. Expect to reduce or stop drug, as prescribed, if increase develops.

• Monitor patient taking venlafaxine for depression closely for suicidal tendencies, especially when therapy starts and dosage changes because depression may worsen during these times.

• Weigh patient daily because drug may produce dose-dependent weight loss.

• Monitor patient's electrolytes, as ordered, because venlafaxine can cause hyponatremia, especially in elderly patients and those who are taking diuretics or are volume depleted. If patient develops evidence of hyponatremia, such as headache, difficulty concentrating, confusion, weakness, and unsteadiness, notify prescriber and be prepared to intervene as prescribed. Expect drug to be discontinued.

• **WARNING** Be aware that drug shouldn't be discontinued abruptly because doing so may cause asthenia, dizziness, headache, insomnia, and nervousness.

PATIENT TEACHING

• Instruct patient not to crush or chew E.R. capsules. However, if he has trouble swallowing capsules, tell him to open capsule, sprinkle contents on a spoonful of applesauce, and swallow immediately without chewing, followed by a glass of water.

• Instruct patient to take drug with food to reduce adverse GI effects.

• Alert caregivers and parents to monitor patient's behavior closely for suicidal thinking or behavior, especially when therapy starts or dosage changes.

• Caution patient to avoid potentially hazardous activities until he knows how the drug affects him.

• Advise patient to avoid alcohol during venlafaxine therapy.

• Advise patient to weigh himself daily and to notify prescriber about significant weight loss.

• Inform the patient that he may require several months of antidepressant therapy beyond the acute phase. Urge him to follow up with his prescriber to determine the need for continued therapy and the proper dose.

• Advise patient not to abruptly stop taking drug.

• Caution female patient to alert prescriber if she becomes preg-

nant because she'll need a different antidepressant. Taking venlafaxine during the third trimester increases the risk of harm to
the fetus.
- Advise patient to consult prescriber before taking any other prescribed or OTC product because of risk of drug interactions.
- Urge caregivers to monitor patient closely for suicidal tendencies, especially when therapy starts or dosage changes.

zaleplon
Sonata

Class, Category, and Schedule
Chemical class: Pyrazolopyrimidine derivative
Therapeutic class: Sedative-hypnotic
Pregnancy category: C
Controlled substance schedule: IV

Indications and Dosages
▶ *To provide short-term treatment of insomnia*
TABLETS
Adults up to age 65. 10 mg daily at bedtime., as prescribed, for
7 to 10 days. *Maximum:* 20 mg daily.
DOSAGE ADJUSTMENT For elderly patients and those who
have hepatic impairment or take cimetidine, dosage possibly
reduced to 5 mg daily.

Route	Onset	Steady State	Peak	Half-Life	Duration
P.O.	30 min	Unknown	Unknown	1 hr	4 hr

Mechanism of Action
Selectively binds with type 1 benzodiazepine (BZ_1 or $omega_1$) receptors on
the gamma-aminobutyric acid-A receptor complex. This binding produces
muscle relaxation and sedation as well as antianxiety and anticonvulsant
effects.

Contraindications
Hypersensitivity to zaleplon or its components

Interactions
DRUGS
*amitriptyline; amoxapine; azatadine; benzodiazepines; brompheniramine;
chlorpheniramine; clemastine; clomipramine; clozapine; cyproheptadine;*

dexchlorpheniramine; diphenhydramine; doxepin; entacapone; haloperidol; hydroxyzine; imipramine; maprotiline; mirtazapine; molindone; nefazodone; nortriptyline; olanzapine; opioid analgesics; other anxiolytics, sedatives, and hypnotics; phenindamine; phenothiazines; pimozide; pramipexole; promethazine; quetiapine; risperidone; ropinirole; thioridazine; trazodone; trimipramine; tripelennamine: Possibly additive CNS depression
carbamazepine, phenobarbital, phenytoin, rifampin: Reduced zaleplon effects
cimetidine: Increased blood zaleplon level
flumazenil: Reversal of zaleplon's sedative effect
FOODS
high-fat foods: Prolonged absorption time and reduced effectiveness of zaleplon
ACTIVITIES
alcohol use: Increased CNS depression

Adverse Reactions
CNS: Amnesia, anxiety, depression, dizziness, drowsiness, fever, hallucinations, hypertonia, insomnia, paresthesia, seizures, sleep-driving, tremor, vertigo
EENT: Dry mouth, gingivitis, glossitis, mouth ulcers, stomatitis
GI: Anorexia, colitis, constipation, eructation, esophagitis, flatulence, gastritis, gastroenteritis, increased appetite, indigestion, melena, nausea, rectal bleeding, vomiting
MS: Back pain
SKIN: Photosensitivity, pruritus, rash
Other: Anaphylaxis, angioedema, physical and psychological dependence

Overdose
Monitor patient for signs and symptoms of overdose, including ataxia, coma, confusion, drowsiness, dyspnea, hypotension, hypotonia, and lethargy.

Maintain an open airway, and monitor cardiac and CNS status. To decrease drug absorption in a conscious patient who isn't at risk for coma, be prepared to perform gastric lavage. For an unconscious patient, anticipate assisting with the insertion of an endotracheal tube and then performing gastric lavage. The inflated cuff of the endotracheal tube will help prevent aspiration of gastric contents into the lungs.

Anticipate the use of flumazenil to reverse the sedative and respiratory depressant effects of zaleplon. Expect to treat hypotension with I.V. fluids, as prescribed.

Institute suicide precautions according to facility policy, and anticipate psychiatric re-evaluation.

Nursing Considerations

- Administer zaleplon just before bedtime because its onset of action is rapid.
- Avoid giving drug with or after a heavy, high-fat meal because decreased absorption may reduce drug's effects.
- **WARNING** If patient has major depression, anticipate an increased risk of suicidal ideation. Implement suicide precautions, as appropriate, according to facility policy, especially when therapy starts or dosage changes.
- **WARNING** Monitor patient closely after he receives zaleplon because anaphylaxis or angioedema, although rare, may occur with the first dose or with later doses. Notify prescriber immediately, and be prepared to provide supportive emergency care.
- Monitor patient for signs of drug abuse, including increased frequency of drug use or repeated drug-seeking behaviors, because zaleplon has an abuse potential similar to that of benzodiazepines and benzodiazepine-like hypnotics.

PATIENT TEACHING

- Inform patient that zaleplon is for short-term use only. Advise him not to use drug for anything other than insomnia.
- Caution patient not to exceed prescribed dosage.
- Instruct patient to take zaleplon immediately before bedtime or right after experiencing difficulty falling asleep because of rapid onset of action.
- Teach patient alternative measures for relaxation and sleep induction.
- Advise patient to consult prescriber before taking other CNS depressants.
- Urge patient to avoid alcohol during zaleplon therapy.
- Instruct patient to notify prescriber if inability to sleep continues. Dosage may need to be adjusted.
- Tell family to report sleep-driving episodes, in which patient drives while not fully awake and usually has no recall of the event.
- Urge caregivers to monitor patient closely for suicidal tendencies, especially when therapy starts or dosage changes.
- Instruct patient to seek immediate medical attention for possible allergic reaction, such as skin reaction, throat tightening, or difficulty breathing.

ziprasidone hydrochloride
Geodon

Class and Category
Chemical class: Benzisoxazole derivative
Therapeutic class: Antipsychotic drug
Pregnancy category: C

Indications and Dosages
▶ *To treat schizophrenia*
CAPSULES
Adults. *Initial:* 20 mg b.i.d. Dosage increased as indicated every 2 or more days. *Usual:* 20 to 80 mg b.i.d. *Maximum:* 100 mg b.i.d.
▶ *To treat acute manic or mixed episodes in bipolar disorder*
CAPSULES
Adults. *Initial:* 40 mg b.i.d. with food on day 1, increased to 60 mg or 80 mg on day 2, followed by individualized adjustments, as needed.

Route	Onset	Steady State	Peak	Half-Life	Duration
P.O.	Unknown	1 to 3 days	Unknown	Unknown	Unknown

Mechanism of Action
Selectively blocks serotonin and dopamine receptors in the mesocortical tract of the CNS, thereby suppressing psychotic signs and symptoms.

Contraindications
Concomitant use of other drugs that prolong QT interval, history of arrhythmia or of prolonged QT interval, hypersensitivity to ziprasidone or its components, recent acute MI, uncompensated heart failure

Interactions
DRUGS
antihypertensives: Additive antihypertensive effects
carbamazepine: Possibly decreased blood ziprasidone level
CNS depressants: Increased CNS depressant effects
dopamine agonists, levodopa: Decreased therapeutic effects of these drugs
drugs that prolong QT interval (including dofetilide, pimozide, quinidine, sotalol, sparfloxacin, and thioridazine): Increased risk of prolonged QT or QTc interval, torsades de pointes, and sudden death

ketoconazole: Possibly increased blood ziprasidone level
FOODS
all foods: Increased ziprasidone absorption

Adverse Reactions

CNS: Akathisia, amnesia, anxiety, asthenia, CVA, depression, dizziness, dystonia, extrapyramidal reactions, hypertonia, neuroleptic malignant syndrome, serotonin syndrome, somnolence, tardive dyskinesia, tremor
CV: Chest pain, hypercholesterolemia, orthostatic hypotension, prolonged QT or QTc interval, tachycardia, thrombophlebitis
EENT: Abnormal vision, dry mouth, increased salivation, rhinitis, tongue edema
ENDO: Hyperglycemia
GI: Anorexia, constipation, diarrhea, dysphagia, indigestion, nausea
GU: Priapism, urinary incontinence
MS: Arthralgia, dysarthria, myalgia
RESP: Cough, pulmonary embolus, upper respiratory tract infection
SKIN: Allergic dermatitis, rash, urticaria
Other: Angioedema, weight gain

Overdose

Monitor patient for signs and symptoms of overdose, including arrhythmias, hypertension, sedation, and slurred speech.

Maintain an open airway, monitor vital signs, and institute continuous ECG monitoring to assess patient for arrhythmias. Consider the possibility that patient ingested multiple drugs. Expect to perform gastric lavage and administer activated charcoal, as prescribed. Be aware that vomiting shouldn't be induced because of the potential for impaired consciousness or dystonic reactions of the head and neck.

When treating arrhythmias, don't administer any drug that may prolong the QT interval—such as disopyramide, procainamide, or quinidine—because these drugs may have an additive effect with ziprasidone. Expect to administer I.V. fluids to treat hypotension, as prescribed. Dopamine or epinephrine shouldn't be used because of risk of paradoxical hypotension.

Anticipate giving an anticholinergic, as prescribed, to treat acute dyskinetic effects. Dialysis is ineffective for ziprasidone overdose.

Institute suicide precautions according to facility policy, and anticipate psychiatric re-evaluation.

Nursing Considerations

- Use caution in elderly patients with dementia-related psychosis; they have increased risk of serious or fatal adverse reactions.
- **WARNING** If patient has hypokalemia or hypomagnesemia, assess him for abnormal cardiac rhythm. Be aware that such symptoms as dizziness, palpitations, and syncope may indicate life-threatening torsades de pointes in this patient. Be prepared to discontinue ziprasidone if patient's QTc interval is greater than 500 msec.
- Monitor patient, especially if elderly and female, for involuntary dyskinetic movements, which may progress to irreversible tardive dyskinesia. If signs and symptoms develop, notify prescriber immediately, and be prepared to discontinue drug.
- Watch for evidence of neuroleptic malignant syndrome, a rare but potentially fatal adverse reaction. Signs and symptoms include acute renal failure, altered mental status, arrhythmia, blood pressure changes, diaphoresis, hyperpyrexia, irregular pulse, muscle rigidity, myoglobinuria (rhabdomyolysis), and tachycardia. Notify prescriber immediately if patient develops any of these signs or symptoms.
- Check patient's blood glucose and lipid levels routinely, as ordered, because the risk of developing hyperglycemia and hypercholesterolemia increases during risperidone therapy.
- Monitor patient closely for suicidal tendencies because patients with psychotic illness or bipolar disorder are at increased risk.

PATIENT TEACHING
- Tell patient to take drug with food to increase its absorption.
- Tell patient to notify his prescriber immediately if he feels faint or notices a change in the way his heart is beating.
- Advise patient to avoid potentially hazardous activities until he knows how the drug affects him.
- Instruct patient to rise slowly from seated or lying position to minimize effects of orthostatic hypotension.
- Instruct patient to tell other prescribers that he is taking ziprasidone before he takes any new drug.

zolmitriptan
Zomig, Zomig-ZMT

Class and Category
Chemical class: Selective 5-hydroxytryptamine$_1$ (5-HT$_1$) receptor agonist

Therapeutic class: Antimigraine drug
Pregnancy category: C

Indications and Dosages

▶ *To treat acute migraine headache*
TABLETS
Adults. 2.5 mg or less, repeated every 2 hr p.r.n. *Maximum:* 10 mg in 24 hr or 3 migraine treatments/mo.
DISINTEGRATING TABLETS
Adults. 2.5 mg, repeated every 2 hr p.r.n. *Maximum:* 10 mg in 24 hr or 3 migraine treatments/mo.
NASAL SPRAY
Adults. 5 mg (1 single-spray unit), repeated in 2 hr, if needed. *Maximum:* 10 mg/24 hr.
DOSAGE ADJUSTMENT Dosage reduced for patients with hepatic impairment.

Route	Onset	Steady State	Peak	Half-Life	Duration
P.O.	Unknown	Unknown	Unknown	3 hr	Unknown

Mechanism of Action

Binds to receptors on intracranial blood vessels and sensory nerves in the trigeminal-vascular system to stimulate negative feedback, which halts the release of serotonin. In this way, zolmitriptan selectively constricts inflamed and dilated cranial blood vessels in the carotid circulation and inhibits the production of proinflammatory neuropeptides.

Contraindications

Basilar or hemiplegic migraine, cardiovascular disease, concurrent use of ergotamine-containing drugs, hypersensitivity to zolmitriptan or its components, ischemic heart disease, Prinzmetal's angina, symptomatic Wolff-Parkinson-White syndrome or other accessory pathway conduction disorder, use of another 5-HT$_1$ agonist within past 24 hours, use within 14 days of MAO inhibitor therapy

Interactions

DRUGS
acetaminophen: Delayed peak effect of acetaminophen (by 1 hour)
cimetidine: Prolonged zolmitriptan half-life
ergot alkaloids: Prolonged vasoconstriction
fluoxetine, fluvoxamine, paroxetine, sertraline: Hyperreflexia, lack of coordination, and weakness

MAO inhibitors: Increased zolmitriptan effects
naratriptan, rizatriptan, sumatriptan: Prolonged zolmitriptan effects
oral contraceptives, propranolol: Increased blood zolmitriptan level

Adverse Reactions

CNS: Asthenia, dizziness, hyperesthesia, paresthesia, somnolence, vertigo

CV: Angina; coronary artery vasospasm; hypertension; MI; pain, pressure, or tightness in jaw, neck, or throat; palpitations; transient myocardial ischemia; ventricular fibrillation or tachycardia

EENT: Dry mouth

GI: Abdominal pain, bloody diarrhea, dysphagia, GI or splenic infarction, indigestion, ischemic colitis, nausea, vomiting

MS: Myalgia, myasthenia

SKIN: Diaphoresis, flushing

Other: Anaphylaxis, angioedema

Overdose

Overdose with zolmitriptan hasn't been reported; the most common adverse reaction that volunteers experienced during clinical studies was sedation.

Maintain an open airway, monitor vital signs, and initiate continuous ECG monitoring to assess patient for ischemia (for at least 15 hr). Expect to give symptomatic and supportive care, as needed and prescribed.

Institute suicide precautions according to facility policy, and anticipate psychiatric re-evaluation.

Nursing Considerations

- **WARNING** Expect an increased risk of vasoconstriction, which may lead to vascular and colonic ischemia with abdominal pain and bloody diarrhea, especially if patient has peripheral vascular disease (including Raynaud's phenomenon) or ischemic bowel disease.
- Monitor elderly patients and those with hepatic impairment for hypertension. If blood pressure rises significantly, notify prescriber immediately.

PATIENT TEACHING

- Instruct patient to consult prescriber before using zolmitriptan to treat more than three migraine headaches in 30 days.
- Advise patient not to remove disintegrating tablet from blister pack until just before use. Instruct him to peel open pack, place disintegrating tablet on his tongue to dissolve it, and then swallow it with saliva.

- Encourage patient to lie down in a dark, quiet room after taking drug to help relieve migraine.
- Instruct patient to seek emergency care for chest, jaw, or neck tightness after using drug because it may cause coronary artery vasospasm. Inform him that, if this occurs, subsequent doses may require ECG monitoring.
- Urge patient to report palpitations or rash to prescriber.

zolpidem tartrate

Ambien, Ambien CR, Tovalt

Class, Category, and Schedule

Chemical class: Imidazopyridine derivative
Therapeutic class: Sedative-hypnotic
Pregnancy category: B
Controlled substance schedule: IV

Indications and Dosages

▶ *To provide short-term treatment of insomnia*

TABLETS, ORALLY DISINTEGRATING TABLETS

Adults. 10 mg at bedtime for 7 to 10 days. *Maximum:* 10 mg daily.

DOSAGE ADJUSTMENT For elderly or debilitated patients and those with hepatic impairment, dosage possibly reduced to 5 mg at bedtime, with a maximum of 5 mg daily for nursing facility residents.

E.R. TABLETS

Adults. 12.5 mg immediately before bedtime.

DOSAGE ADJUSTMENT For elderly or debilitated patients and those with hepatic impairment, dosage reduced to 6.25 mg immediately before bedtime.

Route	Onset	Steady State	Peak	Half-Life	Duration
P.O.	Unknown	Unknown	Unknown	1.4 to 4.5 hr	Unknown

Mechanism of Action

May potentiate the effects of GABA and other inhibitory neurotransmitters. Zolpidem binds to specific benzodiazepine receptor sites in the limbic and cortical areas of the CNS. By binding to these receptor sites, zolpidem increases GABA's inhibitory effects and blocks cortical and limbic arousal and preserves deep sleep (stages 3 and 4).

Contraindications
Hypersensitivity to zolpidem or its components, ritonavir therapy

Interactions
DRUGS

azole antifungals: Increased CNS activity and additive adverse effects of zolpidem

barbiturates, chlorpromazine, general anesthetics, opioid agonists, other CNS depressants, phenothiazines, tramadol, tricyclic antidepressants: Possibly increased CNS depression and reduced psychomotor function

bupropion: Increased blood zolpidem level, possibly visual hallucinations and loss of alertness

desipramine, imipramine: Increased risk of visual hallucinations and reduced alertness

flumazenil: Antagonized sedative effect of zolpidem

haloperidol: Increased CNS depression

ketoconazole: Increased sedative effects of zolpidem

nevirapine: Decreased blood zolpidem level

rifabutin, rifampin: Increased zolpidem clearance

selective serotonin reuptake inhibitors: Increased risk of delusions, disorientation, and hallucinations

FOODS

all foods: Increased time to peak blood zolpidem level, decreased effects of zolpidem

ACTIVITIES

alcohol use: Increased CNS depression

Adverse Reactions
CNS: Amnesia, dizziness, drowsiness, headache, lethargy, paradoxical CNS stimulation (including agitation, euphoria, hallucinations, hyperactivity, and nightmares), sleep-driving

GI: Constipation, diarrhea, indigestion, nausea, vomiting

Other: Anaphylaxis, angioedema, withdrawal signs and symptoms

Overdose
Monitor patient for signs and symptoms of overdose, including ataxia, bradycardia, coma, diplopia, dizziness, drowsiness, dyspnea, and nausea.

Maintain an open airway, and monitor cardiac and CNS status. To decrease drug absorption in a conscious patient who isn't at risk for coma, be prepared to perform gastric lavage followed by administration of activated charcoal, as prescribed. For an unconscious patient, anticipate assisting with the insertion of an endotracheal tube and then performing gastric lavage. The inflated cuff of the endotracheal tube will help prevent aspiration of gastric contents into the lungs. Anticipate the use of flumazenil to reverse the sedative and respiratory depressant effects. Hemodialysis is ineffective for treating zolpidem overdose.

Institute suicide precautions according to facility policy, and anticipate psychiatric re-evaluation.

Nursing Considerations

- Administer zolpidem just before bedtime because drug has a rapid onset of action.
- Expect patient to receive no more than a 1-month supply of drug for outpatient therapy.
- **WARNING** If zolpidem is withdrawn abruptly (especially after prolonged therapy), monitor patient for withdrawal signs and symptoms, such as abdominal cramps or discomfort, fatigue, flushing, inconsolable crying, light-headedness, nausea, nervousness, panic attack, rebound insomnia, and vomiting.
- Expect drug to produce anticonvulsant and muscle relaxant effects at high doses.
- If patient receives another CNS depressant, expect to administer reduced zolpidem dosage, as prescribed.

PATIENT TEACHING

- Caution patient to take drug exactly as prescribed and not to increase dosage unless directed by prescriber.
- Tell patient taking the extended-release form of zolpidem to swallow the tablets whole and not to break, crush, or chew them.
- Instruct patient taking orally disintegrating form of zolpidem to place the tablet on his tongue, where it will dissolve and can then be swallowed with saliva. It may be taken with or without water.
- Instruct patient to take zolpidem immediately before bedtime on an empty stomach.
- Advise patient to notify prescriber immediately about abdominal cramps or discomfort, fatigue, flushing, inconsolable crying, light-headedness, nausea, nervousness, panic attack, and vomiting.
- Tell family to report sleep-driving episodes, in which patient drives while not fully awake and usually has no recall of doing so.

zonisamide

Zonegran

Class and Category

Chemical class: Benzisoxazole derivative, sulfonamide
Therapeutic class: Anticonvulsant
Pregnancy category: C

Indications and Dosages

▶ *As adjunct to treat partial seizures*

CAPSULES

Adults and adolescents age 16 and over. *Initial:* 100 mg daily.
Dosage increased by 100 mg daily every 2 wk, as needed. *Usual:*
200 to 400 mg daily. *Maximum:* 600 mg daily.

Route	Onset	Steady State	Peak	Half-Life	Duration
P.O.	Unknown	14 days	Unknown	63 hr	Unknown

Mechanism of Action

May stop the spread of seizures and suppress their foci by blocking sodium
channels and reducing voltage-dependent, inward currents from calcium
channels. This action stabilizes neuronal membranes and suppresses synchro-
nized neuronal hyperactivity.

Contraindications

Hypersensitivity to sulfonamides, zonisamide, or their components

Interactions

DRUGS

carbamazepine, phenobarbital, phenytoin, valproate: Possibly decreased
blood zonisamide level
CNS depressants: Additive CNS depressant effects

FOODS

grapefruit juice: Possibly decreased metabolism of zonisamide

Adverse Reactions

CNS: Agitation, ataxia, dizziness, irritability, somnolence
GI: Anorexia

Overdose

Monitor patient for signs and symptoms of overdose, including
bradycardia, coma, hypotension, and respiratory depression.

Maintain open airway, monitor vital signs, and institute continuous ECG monitoring. Expect to give symptomatic and sup-

portive care, as needed and prescribed.

To decrease drug absorption in a conscious patient who isn't at risk for coma, be prepared to induce vomiting or perform gastric lavage. For an unconscious patient, anticipate assisting with the insertion of an endotracheal tube and then performing gastric lavage. The inflated cuff of the endotracheal tube will help prevent aspiration of gastric contents into the lungs. Dialysis is ineffective for treating zonisamide overdose.

Institute suicide precautionary measures according to facility policy, and anticipate psychiatric re-evaluation.

Nursing Considerations

- **WARNING** Monitor results of CBC and other laboratory tests for signs of blood dyscrasias because zonisamide is a sulfonamide and can be absorbed systemically. Systemic absorption may result in life-threatening reactions, including agranulocytosis, aplastic anemia, fulminant hepatic necrosis, Stevens-Johnson syndrome, toxic epidermal necrolysis, and other blood dyscrasias.
- Be aware that patients receiving doses of 300 mg daily or more are at increased risk for adverse CNS reactions, including decreased concentration, drowsiness, fatigue, and impaired speech.
- Monitor serum creatinine and BUN levels for signs of abnormally decreased GFR. Expect some decrease in GFR during first 4 weeks of treatment and a return to baseline within 2 to 3 weeks after drug is discontinued.
- Monitor patient for signs and symptoms of renal calculi.
- Be aware that zonisamide shouldn't be discontinued abruptly because doing so may increase the frequency of seizures.

PATIENT TEACHING

- Inform patient that zonisamide is usually prescribed with other anticonvulsants and that he should continue to take all drugs as prescribed.
- Instruct patient to swallow capsules whole and not to chew them or break them open.
- Inform patient that prescriber may have to adjust dosage over several weeks or months before maintenance dosage is achieved.
- Advise patient to use caution when driving or performing other activities that require mental alertness because zonisamide commonly causes decreased concentration, dizziness, and somnolence, particularly during first month of therapy.

- Advise patient to wear a medical identification bracelet or necklace with information about his seizure disorder.
- Unless contraindicated, encourage patient to drink 6 to 8 glasses of water each day to prevent kidney stones.
- Advise patient to rise slowly from a lying or seated position to reduce the risk of dizziness.

APPENDICES

SEIZURE CLASSIFICATION

Drug therapy for seizures is highly individualized and depends, in part, on the type of seizure. The various types of seizures are grouped into three categories: generalized, partial, and unclassified.

Generalized seizures involve both hemispheres of the brain and cause bilateral, symmetrical signs and symptoms. These seizures usually involve some type of physical or sensory impairment with or without loss of consciousness.

Partial seizures involve one hemisphere of the brain and cause signs and symptoms specific to the functioning of the affected hemisphere. These seizures may not involve physical or sensory impairment or loss of consciousness.

Unclassified seizures exhibit none of the characteristics of generalized or partial seizures.

The following table lists the types of seizures by category, their characteristics, and the drugs that may be used to treat them. Be aware that a variety of drugs may be used to treat seizures, either alone or in combination with other drugs.

Type of Seizure	Characteristics	Drug Therapy
Generalized seizures		
Absence (petit mal)	• No aura • Sudden loss of awareness; patient may appear to be staring or daydreaming • Patient maintains muscle tone with no loss of postural control • No postictal confusion • May be accompanied by subtle, bilateral motor signs and symptoms, such as rapid blinking, chewing movements, or mild clonic hand movements • May occur frequently over the course of a day, and patient may be unaware of recurrence and unable to account for lapses in memory • Usually begins in childhood and may resolve in adolescence, continue through adolescence, or convert to tonic-clonic seizures in adulthood	clonazepam ethosuximide lamotrigine valproic acid

(continued)

SEIZURE CLASSIFICATION *(continued)*

Type of Seizure	Characteristics	Drug Therapy
Generalized seizures *(continued)*		
Atonic	• Sudden loss of body tone lasting 1 to 2 seconds • May cause a quick head drop or nodding movements; if prolonged, patient may collapse • No loss of consciousness, but may cause postictal confusion	clonazepam felbamate lamotrigine topiramate* valproic acid
Clonic	• Brief generalized spasm, followed by asymmetric bilateral jerks • Lasts several minutes • Usually occurs in patients age 4 to 8	carbamazepine felbamate lamotrigine phenobarbital phenytoin primidone topiramate valproic acid
Myoclonic	• Sudden, brief muscle contractions in arms, legs, or trunk • Minimal or no loss of consciousness	clonazepam felbamate lamotrigine topiramate* valproic acid
Tonic	• Sudden rigidity of muscles • Loss of consciousness • Flushing • Increased heart rate • Pupil changes	carbamazepine felbamate lamotrigine phenobarbital phenytoin primidone topiramate valproic acid
Tonic-clonic (grand mal)	• Begins abruptly and has four phases: *Preictal:* Aura (may not present) *Tonic (15–60 seconds):* Loud cry at onset, rigid muscle activity, loss of consciousness, impaired breathing with cyanosis, increased heart rate and blood pressure, dilated pupils *Clonic (2–5 minutes):* Rapid breathing; rapid, violent, bilateral jerking *Postictal:* Muscle flaccidity, return to consciousness with drowsiness and confusion, incontinence, excessive salivation, headache, muscle fatigue	carbamazepine felbamate lamotrigine phenobarbital phenytoin primidone topiramate valproic acid

*Used as adjunctive therapy.

SEIZURE CLASSIFICATION *(continued)*

Type of Seizure	Characteristics	Drug Therapy
Partial seizures		
Complex partial	• Aura usually present, consisting of auditory, olfactory, or visual alterations; déjà vu; fear or feeling of impending doom; or a sense of detachment • Impairment of consciousness that may progress to a loss of consciousness • Automatisms, such as lip smacking, picking at clothes, repeating phrases, or running	carbamazepine gabapentin* lamotrigine phenobarbital phenytoin primidone tiagabine* topiramate* valproic acid
Partial seizures with secondary generalization	• May start as a simple partial seizure and progress to a generalized seizure • May start as a complex partial seizure and progress to a generalized seizure • May start as a simple partial seizure, progress to a complex partial seizure, and then to a generalized seizure	carbamazepine gabapentin* lamotrigine phenobarbital phenytoin primidone tiagabine* topiramate* valproic acid
Simple partial	• Autonomic, motor, psychic or psychologic, or somatosensory signs and symptoms (such as paresthesias or auditory, olfactory, or visual alterations) • Loss of control of affected area for 5 to 15 seconds • No impairment or loss of consciousness	carbamazepine gabapentin* lamotrigine phenobarbital phenytoin pregabalin* primidone tiagabine* topiramate* valproic acid
Unclassified seizures		
Neonatal spasms; infantile seizures	• Often present in neonates and infants; may be caused by an immature central nervous system	prednisone vigabatrin

*Used as adjunctive therapy.

CYTOCHROME P450 ENZYME SYSTEM

Drugs are metabolized primarily by the cytochrome P450 enzyme system, which consists of isoenzymes found mostly in the liver. For a patient taking a combination of drugs, an interaction may occur when a drug or molecule affects the metabolism of another drug.

Use the following chart to identify potential drug interactions and related nursing considerations. The items in the chart are grouped by cytochrome P450 isoenzymes and the substrates, inducers, and inhibitors with which they interact.

Substrates	Inducers	
CYP1A2 isoenzyme		
acetaminophen, alosetron, aminophylline, amitriptyline, betaxolol, caffeine, chlorpromazine, clomipramine, clozapine, cyclobenzaprine, desipramine, diazepam, duloxetine, estradiol, fluvoxamine, haloperidol, imipramine, maprotiline, methadone, metoclopramide, mirtazapine, nortriptyline, olanzapine, ondansetron, phenothiazines, pimozide, propafenone, propranolol, ramelteon, riluzole, ritonavir, ropinirole, tacrine, tamoxifen, theophylline, thioridazine, thiothixene, trifluoperazine, verapamil, warfarin, zileuton, zolpidem	carbamazepine, charbroiled foods, cigarette smoke, cruciferous vegetables (such as cabbage and turnips), moricizine, nicotine, omeprazole, phenobarbital, phenytoin, primidone, rifampin, ritonavir	
CYP2A6 isoenzyme		
dexmedetomidine, letrozole, montelukast, nicotine, ritonavir, tamoxifen	barbiturates	

Substrates are drugs metabolized by a particular cytochrome P450 isoenzyme.

Inducers are drugs, foods, or environmental factors that increase the metabolic activity of an isoenzyme, which may decrease the therapeutic effect of a substrate.

Inhibitors are drugs, foods, or environmental factors that decrease the metabolic activity of an isoenzyme, which may increase accumulation of the substrate to toxic levels.

Nursing Considerations	Inhibitors	Nursing Considerations
• Be aware that increased substrate metabolism may take days to weeks to occur. • Monitor patient for signs and symptoms of reduced therapeutic effect of substrate. • Monitor patient for reduced blood level of substrate. • Anticipate that substrate dosage may be increased. • Expect that inducer may be discontinued or dosage reduced; then monitor patient for increased blood level of substrate and possible toxicity.	amitriptyline, anastrozole, cimetidine, ciprofloxacin, citalopram, clarithromycin, clomipramine, diethyl-dithiocarbamate, diltiazem, doxepin, enoxacin, entacapone, erythromycin, ethinyl estradiol, fluoxetine, fluvoxamine, grapefruit juice, imipramine, isoniazid, ketoconazole, levofloxacin, mexiletine, norfloxacin, paroxetine, ritonavir, sertraline, tacrine, trimipramine, zileuton	• Be aware that decreased substrate metabolism may occur immediately or within 24 hr. • Monitor patient for adverse reactions. • Monitor patient for increased blood level of substrate and for signs and symptoms of toxicity.
• Be aware that increased substrate metabolism may take days to weeks to occur. • Monitor patient for signs and symptoms of reduced therapeutic effect of substrate. • Monitor patient for reduced blood level of substrate. • Anticipate that substrate dosage may be increased. • Expect that inducer may be discontinued or dosage reduced; then monitor patient for increased blood level of substrate and possible toxicity.	diethyldithiocarbamate, entacapone, ketoconazole, letrozole, miconazole, ritonavir, tranylcypromine	• Be aware that decreased substrate metabolism may occur immediately or within 24 hr. • Monitor patient for adverse reactions. • Monitor patient for increased blood level of substrate and for signs and symptoms of toxicity.

(continued)

CYTOCHROME P450 ENZYME SYSTEM *(continued)*

Substrates	Inducers
CYP2C isoenzyme	
antipyrine, carvedilol, clozapine, mephobarbital, mestranol, tamoxifen	carbamazepine, phenobarbital, phenytoin, primidone, rifampin
CYP2C8 isoenzyme	
benzphetamine, carbamazepine, diazepam, diclofenac, ibuprofen, mephobarbital, naproxen, omeprazole, paclitaxel, pioglitazone, retinoic acid, rosiglitazone, tolbutamide, warfarin	carbamazepine, phenobarbital, phenytoin, primidone, rifampin
CYP2C9 isoenzyme	
alosetron, amitriptyline, celecoxib, dapsone, diclofenac, flurbiprofen, fluvastatin, glimepiride, ibuprofen, imipramine, indomethacin, irbesartan, losartan, metronidazole, mirtazapine, montelukast, naproxen, phenytoin, piroxicam, quetiapine, ramelteon, ritonavir, rosiglitazone, sildenafil, tetrahydrocannabinol (THC), tolbutamide, torsemide, warfarin, zafirlukast, zileuton	carbamazepine, fluconazole, fluoxetine, phenobarbital, phenytoin, rifampin,

Nursing Considerations	Inhibitors	Nursing Considerations
• Be aware that increased substrate metabolism may take days to weeks to occur. • Monitor patient for signs and symptoms of reduced therapeutic effect of substrate. • Monitor patient for reduced blood level of substrate. • Anticipate that substrate dosage may be increased. • Expect that inducer may be discontinued or dosage reduced; then monitor patient for increased blood level of substrate and possible toxicity.	isoniazid, ketoconazole, ketoprofen	• Be aware that decreased substrate metabolism may occur immediately or within 24 hr. • Monitor patient for adverse reactions. • Monitor patient for increased blood level of substrate and for signs and symptoms of toxicity.
• Be aware that increased substrate metabolism may take days to weeks to occur. • Monitor patient for signs and symptoms of reduced therapeutic effect of substrate. • Monitor patient for reduced blood level of substrate. • Anticipate that substrate dosage may be increased. • Expect that inducer may be discontinued or dosage reduced; then monitor patient for increased blood level of substrate and possible toxicity.	anastrozole, omeprazole	• Be aware that decreased substrate metabolism may occur immediately or within 24 hr. • Monitor patient for adverse reactions. • Monitor patient for increased blood level of substrate and for signs and symptoms of toxicity.
• Be aware that increased substrate metabolism may take days to weeks to occur. • Monitor patient for signs and symptoms of reduced therapeutic effect of substrate.	amiodarone, anastrozole, cimetidine, diclofenac, disulfiram, entacapone, fluoxetine, flurbiprofen, fluvastatin, fluvoxamine, isoniazid, ketoconazole, ketoprofen, metronidazole,	• Be aware that decreased substrate metabolism may occur immediately or within 24 hr. • Monitor patient for adverse reactions. *(continued)*

CYTOCHROME P450 ENZYME SYSTEM *(continued)*

Substrates	Inducers	
CYP2C9 isoenzyme *(continued)*		
CYP2C18 isoenzyme		
dronabinol, naproxen, omeprazole, piroxicam, proguanil, propranolol, retinoic acid, warfarin	carbamazepine, phenobarbital, phenytoin, rifampin	
CYP2C19 isoenzyme		
amitriptyline, carisoprodol, citalopram, clomipramine, diazepam, divalproex sodium, hexobarbital, imipramine, lansoprazole, mephenytoin, mephobarbital, olanzapine, omeprazole, pantoprazole, pentamidine, phenytoin, propranolol, ritonavir, tolbutamide, topiramate, valproic acid, warfarin	carbamazepine, phenobarbital, phenytoin, rifampin	

Nursing Considerations	Inhibitors	Nursing Considerations
• Monitor patient for reduced blood level of substrate. • Anticipate that substrate dosage may be increased. • Expect that inducer may be discontinued or dosage reduced; then monitor patient for increased blood level of substrate and possible toxicity.	omeprazole, phenylbutazone, ritonavir, sertraline, trimethoprim/sulfamethoxazole, valproic acid, warfarin, zafirlukast	• Monitor patient for increased blood level of substrate and for signs and symptoms of toxicity.
• Be aware that increased substrate metabolism may take days to weeks to occur. • Monitor patient for signs and symptoms of reduced therapeutic effect of substrate. • Monitor patient for reduced blood level of substrate. • Anticipate that substrate dosage may be increased. • Expect that inducer may be discontinued or dosage reduced; then monitor patient for increased blood level of substrate and possible toxicity.	cimetidine	• Be aware that decreased substrate metabolism may occur immediately or within 24 hr. • Monitor patient for adverse reactions. • Monitor patient for increased blood level of substrate and for signs and symptoms of toxicity.
• Be aware that increased substrate metabolism may take days to weeks to occur. • Monitor patient for signs and symptoms of reduced therapeutic effect of substrate. • Monitor patient for reduced blood level of substrate. • Anticipate that substrate dosage may be increased. • Expect that inducer may be discontinued or dosage reduced; then monitor patient for increased blood level of substrate and possible toxicity.	cimetidine, citalopram, entacapone, felbamate, fluconazole, fluoxetine, fluvoxamine, isoniazid, ketoconazole, letrozole, omeprazole, oxcarbazepine, ritonavir, sertraline, tolbutamide, topiramate, tranylcypromine	• Be aware that decreased substrate metabolism may occur immediately or within 24 hr. • Monitor patient for adverse reactions. • Monitor patient for increased blood level of substrate and for signs and symptoms of toxicity.

(continued)

CYTOCHROME P450 ENZYME SYSTEM *(continued)*

Substrates	Inducers	
CYP2D6 isoenzyme		
amitriptyline, amphetamine, aripiprazole, atomoxetine, bupropion, captopril, carvedilol, chlorpheniramine, chlorpromazine, clomipramine, clozapine, codeine, cyclobenzaprine, delavirdine, desipramine, dextromethorphan, diphenhydramine, dolasetron, donepezil, doxepin, duloxetine, encainide, flecainide, fluoxetine, fluphenazine, haloperidol, hydrocodone, hydrocortisone, imipramine, labetalol, loratidine, maprotiline, meperidine, methadone, methamphetamine, metoclopramide, metoprolol, mexiletine, mirtazapine, molindone, morphine, nortriptyline, olanzapine, oxycodone, paroxetine, pentazocine, perphenazine, pindolol, promethazine, propafenone, propranolol, quetiapine, risperidone, ritonavir, selegiline, sertraline, tamoxifen, thioridazine, timolol, trazodone, trimipramine, venlafaxine, yohimba, zolpidem	None known	
CYP2E1 isoenzyme		
acetaminophen, caffeine, clozapine, dapsone, dextromethorphan, eszopiclone, ethanol, isoniazid, ondansetron, ritonavir, tamoxifen, theophylline, venlafaxine	ethanol, isoniazid	
CYP3A3/4 isoenzyme		
acetaminophen, alprazolam, amiodarone, amitriptyline, amlodipine, anastrozole, aripiprazole, atorvastatin, benzphetamine, bromocriptine, budesonide, bupropion, buspirone, caffeine, cannabinoids, carbamazepine, chlorpromazine, cimetidine, citalopram, clarithromycin, clindamycin, clomipramine, clonazepam, cocaine, codeine, cortisol, cortisone, cyclobenzaprine, cyclosporine, dapsone, delavirdine, dexamethasone, dextromethorphan, diazepam, digoxin, diltiazem, disopyramide, dolasetron, donepezil, doxycycline, dronabinol, eletriptan, enalapril, erythromycin, estradiol, eszopiclone, ethinyl estradiol, ethosuximide, felodipine, fentanyl, fexofenadine, fluoxetine, glyburide, granisetron, hydrocortisone,	carbamazepine, dexamethasone, ethosuximide, glucocorticoids, griseofulvin, nafcillin, nelfinavir, nevirapine, oxcarbazepine, phenobarbital, phenylbutazone, phenytoin, primidone, progesterone, rifabutin, rifampin, St. John's wort, sulfinpyrazone	

Nursing Considerations	Inhibitors	Nursing Considerations
None	amiodarone, celecoxib, chlorpromazine, cimetidine, citalopram, clomipramine, codeine, delavirdine, desipramine, diltiazem, entacapone, fluoxetine, fluphenazine, fluvoxamine, haloperidol, labetalol, methadone, paroxetine, perphenazine, propafenone, quinidine, ranitidine, risperidone, ritonavir, sertraline, thioridazine, valproic acid, venlafaxine, yohimba	• Be aware that decreased substrate metabolism may occur immediately or within 24 hr. • Monitor patient for adverse reactions. • Monitor patient for increased blood level of substrate and for signs and symptoms of toxicity.
• Be aware that increased substrate metabolism may take days to weeks to occur. • Monitor patient for signs and symptoms of reduced therapeutic effect of substrate. • Monitor patient for reduced blood level of substrate. • Anticipate that substrate dosage may be increased. • Expect that inducer may be discontinued or dosage reduced; then monitor patient for increased blood level of substrate and possible toxicity.	disulfiram and its metabolites, entacapone, ritonavir	• Be aware that decreased substrate metabolism may occur immediately or within 24 hr. • Monitor patient for adverse reactions. • Monitor patient for increased blood level of substrate and for signs and symptoms of toxicity.
• Be aware that increased substrate metabolism may take days to weeks to occur. • Monitor patient for signs and symptoms of reduced therapeutic effect of substrate. • Monitor patient for reduced blood level of substrate. • Anticipate that substrate dosage may be increased.	amiodarone, anastrozole, azithromycin, cannabinoids, cimetidine, clarithromycin, clotrimazole, cyclosporine, danazol, delavirdine, dexamethasone, diethyldithiocarbamate, diltiazem, disulfiram, entacapone, erythromycin, ethinyl estradiol, fluconazole, fluoxetine,	• Be aware that decreased substrate metabolism may occur immediately or within 24 hr. • Monitor patient for adverse reactions. • Monitor patient for increased blood level of substrate and for signs and symptoms of toxicity. *(continued)*

CYTOCHROME P450 ENZYME SYSTEM *(continued)*

Substrates	Inducers
CYP3A3/4 isoenzyme *(continued)*	
imipramine, indinavir, isradipine, itraconazole, ketoconazole, letrozole, lidocaine, loratadine, losartan, lovastatin, methadone, miconazole, midazolam, mifepristone, mirtazapine, montelukast, nefazodone, nelfinivir, nevirapine, nicardipine, nifedipine, nimodipine, nisoldipine, omeprazole, ondansetron, oral contraceptives, orphenadrine, paclitaxel, pantoprazole, pimozide, pioglitazone, pravastatin, prednisone, progesterone, propafenone, quetiapine, quinidine, quinine, ramelteon, repaglinide, retinoic acid, rifampin, risperidone, ritonavir, salmeterol, saquinavir, sertraline, sibutramine, sildenafil, simvastatin, sirolimus, tacrolimus, tadalafil, tamoxifen, temazepam, tetrahydrocannabinol (THC), theophylline, tolterodine, trazodone, tretinoin, triazolam, venlafaxine, verapamil, warfarin, yohimba, zaleplon, zileuton, ziprasidone, zolpidem	
CYP3A5-7 isoenzyme	
cortisol, ethinyl estradiol, lovastatin, midazolam, nifedipine, quinidine, triazolam	phenobarbital, phenytoin, primidone, rifampin

Nursing Considerations	Inhibitors	Nursing Considerations
• Expect that inducer may be discontinued or dosage reduced; then monitor patient for increased blood level of substrate and possible toxicity.	fluvoxamine, grapefruit juice, indinavir, isoniazid, itraconazole, ketoconazole, metronidazole, miconazole, nefazodone, nelfinavir, nevirapine, norfloxacin, omeprazole, paroxetine, propoxyphene, quinidine, quinine, quinupristin and dalfopristin, ranitidine, ritonavir, saquinavir, sertraline, valproic acid, verapamil, zafirlukast, zileuton	
• Be aware that increased substrate metabolism may take days to weeks to occur. • Monitor patient for signs and symptoms of reduced therapeutic effect of substrate. • Monitor patient for reduced blood level of substrate. • Anticipate that substrate dosage may be increased. • Expect that inducer may be discontinued or dosage reduced; then monitor patient for increased blood level of substrate and possible toxicity.	clotrimazole, ketoconazole, metronidazole, miconazole	• Be aware that decreased substrate metabolism may occur immediately or within 24 hr. • Monitor patient for adverse reactions. • Monitor patient for increased blood level of substrate and for signs and symptoms of toxicity.

COMMONLY ABUSED DRUGS

Treatment for a behavioral or mental health disorder may involve therapy for drug addiction. For your reference, the chart below lists commonly abused drugs, facts and statistics about their use, possible reasons for drug use, the signs and symptoms of abuse, and nursing considerations.

Generic and Trade Names (Street Names)	Facts and Statistics	Reasons for Use	
alcohol	• Over 14 million Americans may abuse alcohol. • More than 100,000 Americans die from alcohol-related causes annually. • Lost productivity and health expenses related to alcoholism may cost $100 billion annually. • Alcoholism is the second most common preventable cause of death among Americans.	• Sedative, calming effects • Relaxation • Reduces inhibitions • Variable effects that the user may control • Social acceptance • Legal above a certain age	
amphetamines **amphetamine and dextroamphetamine** Adderall **amphetamine sulfate dextroamphetamine sulfate** Dexedrine, Dexedrine Spansule, DextroStat (beans, bennies, Christmas trees, dexies, double trouble, pep pills, speed, uppers) **methamphetamine hydrochloride** Desoxyn (chalk, crank, crystal, crystal meth, fire, glass, ice, meth, quartz, speed)	• Amphetamines were used in the 1930s in OTC inhalers to treat nasal congestion. • In the past, these drugs were prescribed for weight loss, but this practice has been discontinued because of the high potential for abuse. • Amphetamines are available in capsule, liquid, powder, and tablet form; they may be orally ingested, injected, smoked, or snorted. • Recreational use is prevalent among adolescents and young adults attending nightclubs or rave gatherings. • They can be manufactured in illegal laboratories from OTC ingredients.	• Appetite suppressant effects • Euphoria • Increases alertness and energy • Increases sexuality	

Signs and Symptoms of Abuse	Nursing Considerations
• Loss of memory about significant events, such as commitments • Drinking alone or in secret • Gulping alcoholic beverages; ordering doubles • Intentionally becoming intoxicated • Irritability • Storing alcohol in unlikely places • Loss of interest in daily life and hobbies • Ritualized drinking habits; annoyance when ritual is disturbed or questioned • Malnutrition • Unpredictable or violent mood swings • Relationship problems • Tremors	• Assess patient for CNS effects of alcoholism, such as dementia, disordered thinking, and numbness in the hands and feet. • Monitor patient for signs and symptoms of alcohol-related conditions, such as cirrhosis, gastritis, heart failure, hypertension, pancreatitis, sexual dysfunction, and stroke. • Be aware that alcoholism may result in domestic abuse, poor performance at work or school, and accidental injuries; it may also increase the patient's risk of harm to himself or others. • Warn pregnant patient that alcohol can cause birth defects if taken in excess. • Teach patient that alcoholism is a chronic, progressive, and often fatal disease and that its cause may be genetic, psychological, or social.
• Agitation • Anxiousness and nervousness • Delusions of grandeur; severe depression or suicidal tendencies • Diarrhea • Dyspnea • Excited speech • Itching • Moodiness and irritability • Nausea • Sweating • Uncontrollable body movements (twitching fingers or facial and body muscles, lip-smacking, tongue protrusion, grimacing) • Visual and auditory hallucinations • Vomiting • Welts on skin	• Monitor patient who abuses amphetamines for aggressive or violent behavior, cardiac and neurologic dysfunction, memory loss, and psychosis. Be aware that long-term abuse of these drugs may cause brain damage, fatal kidney and lung disorders, liver damage, stroke, permanent and psychological problems. • Be aware that your patient with a behavioral or mental health disorder may be prescribed an amphetamine to treat attention deficit hyperactivity disorder (ADHD) or narcolepsy. • Inform patient that amphetamine abuse may increase her risk of infectious disease, especially hepatitis and HIV.

(continued)

COMMONLY ABUSED DRUGS (continued)

Generic and Trade Names (Street Names)	Facts and Statistics	Reasons for Use
benzodiazepines **alprazolam** Xanax **chlordiazepoxide hydrochloride** Librium **diazepam** Valium **lorazepam** Ativan (downers, nerve pills, tranks)	• Benzodiazepines, prescribed to treat anxiety, insomnia, and seizures, are the most commonly prescribed drugs in the U.S. and are frequently abused. • These drugs may be used as a replacement for heroin or to lessen the effects of other drugs, such as amphetamines, cocaine, or ecstasy. • Benzodiazepines are available in capsule and tablet form.	• Decreases anxiety • Decreases awareness: escape from reality • Reduces inhibitions
cannabinoids **dronabinol** Marinol **marijuana** (blunt, buds, chronic, doobie, dope, 420, ganja, grass, green, herb, joint, kryptonite, nail, Phillie, pot, reefer, sinsemilla, weed) **hashish, hashish oil** (hash, hash oil)	• Medicinal use of cannabinoids dates to 2700 B.C. in China. • Marijuana is obtained from the hemp plant, *Cannabis sativa;* dronabinol is a synthetic form of THC. • Hashish is marijuana processed in brick form; hashish oil is marijuana processed in a liquid form. • Marijuana is usually smoked in a pipe, water pipe, rolled into a cigarette, or packed into an empty cigar wrapper. It may also be mixed into food or brewed as tea.	• Short-term effects can occur rapidly after a single dose and disappear within a few hours • Effects can vary with amount taken, past use, circumstances of use, and user's frame of mind • Causes a feeling of euphoria
cocaine (blow, coke, flake, nose candy, powder, rock, shale, snow) **crack cocaine** (crack, free-base, rock)	• Cocaine is both a CNS stimulant and an anesthetic. • It is derived from the leaves of the *Erythroxylon coca* plant. • Cocaine may be injected, smoked, or snorted.	• Increases alertness and wakefulness • Elevates mood • Increases athletic performance • Decreases fatigue

Signs and Symptoms of Abuse	Nursing Considerations
• Altered mental status, such as confusion, insomnia, and irritability • Nystagmus • Slurred speech • Unsteady gait	• Monitor patient who has overdosed on benzodiazepines for CNS depression, which could be fatal if she has also ingested alcohol or another CNS depressant. • Be prepared to taper drug slowly to prevent signs and symptoms of withdrawal, such as altered perception, headache, paresthesias, and weight loss. • Warn pregnant patient that drug may cause fetal abnormalities and withdrawal symptoms in newborns. • Tell patient that tolerance to the drug develops quickly, leading to physical dependence.
• Slowed reaction time; decreased depth perception and peripheral vision. • Impairment of short-term memory, logical thinking, and ability to perform complex tasks. • Increased pulse and respiratory rate • Misjudgment of time • Reddened eyes • Sleepiness • Excessive talking or laughing	• Be aware that dronabinol may be prescribed to stimulate appetite in AIDS patients and to manage nausea and vomiting in cancer patients. • If patient uses hashish oil, monitor him for very high blood levels of THC. • Warn pregnant patient that drug may adversely affect fetal development. • Tell patient that marijuana use may cause physical and psychological dependence, leading to cravings that are the focus of the user's thoughts, feelings, and actions. • Inform patient that smoking marijuana may cause chronic lung disorders because the tar content is at least 50% higher than tobacco's.
• Anxiety • Dilated pupils • Dry mouth or nose • Euphoria • Excessive talking • Hyperactivity followed by depression • Irritability • Lack of appetite; insomnia • Weight loss	• Be aware that cocaine overdose may be fatal. Monitor patient for convulsions, heart attack, high fever, and stroke. • Inform patient that cocaine use may cause extreme antisocial and aggressive behavior and that high doses may cause psychosis with confusion, disorganized behavior, fear, hallucinations, and paranoia. *(continued)*

COMMONLY ABUSED DRUGS *(continued)*

Generic and Trade Names (Street Names)	Facts and Statistics	Reasons for Use
flunitrazepam Rohypnol (circles, forget-me pill, Mexican Valium, rib, roach-2, roaches, roche, roofies, roopies, rope, rophies, ropies, ruffies)	• In non-U.S. settings, flunitrazepam may be prescribed as a sedative or pre-anesthetic. • It may be used as a recreational psychoactive by adolescents and young adults attending nightclubs or rave gatherings. • It became known in the early 1990s as the date rape drug. • Flunitrazepam was banned by the U.S. Treasury Department in 1996, and its illegal use has declined since then.	• Initial effects can begin within 30 minutes and can last up to 12 hours • Sedative qualities may be 10 times more potent than diazepam's • Can cause anterograde amnesia
gamma hydroxybutyrate (blue verve, EZLay, G, gamma-oh, GBD, Georgia home boy, GHB, goop, grievous bodily harm, liquid X, liquid E)	• Gamma hydroxybutyrate is a naturally occurring component of human cells. • It was developed in early 1960s for use as an anesthetic but discontinued because of its adverse effects. • This drug is used as a recreational intoxicant, an agent to induce sleep, or a date rape drug.	• Onset of effect is fast (within 20 minutes) • Duration of effect may be short (1 hour) or longer if sipped slowly over an evening rather than drunk all at once • An effect similar to that of alcohol
heroin (H, junk, skag, smack, or names referring to specific geographical area such as *Mexican black tar*)	• Heroin is an opium derivative once manufactured as a safe, non-addictive substitute for morphine. • Heroin was used to treat many types of ailments until it became regulated in 1920 after the dangers of its use were recognized. • It is the most abused of the opiates. • It is usually injected but can be sniffed, snorted, or smoked. • The most common heroin user is over age 30, but use among younger adults and adolescents is increasing.	• Causes a feeling of euphoria • Rapid onset of effects (8 seconds when injected I.V.; 5 to 8 minutes when injected I.M.; 10 to 15 minutes when smoked or snorted) • Provides rapid pain relief

Signs and Symptoms of Abuse	Nursing Considerations
• Confusion • Decreased blood pressure • Dizziness • Drowsiness • Feelings similar to alcohol intoxication but without hangover • Gastrointestinal disturbances • Profound anterograde amnesia • Urine retention • Visual disturbances	• Be aware that long-term use of fluni-trazepam may cause tolerance, as well as psychological and physical dependence. • Instruct patient that flunitrazepam's sedative and toxic effects increase with concurrent use of alcohol.
• Decreased social inhibitions and motor skills, elevated mood, and feelings of relaxation (with moderate dose) • Difficulty focusing, dizziness, grogginess, mood changes, nausea, and slurred speech (with high dose) • Disorientation, respiratory depression, seizures, unconsciousness, and vomiting (with overdose)	• Monitor patient who has overdosed on gamma hydroxybutyrate for unconsciousness, which can lead to aspiration and suffocation. • Warn patient that drug may be both physically and psychologically addictive. • Inform patient that drug has a narrow margin between the amount required to produce euphoria and unconsciousness.
• Clouded mental functioning • Nausea • Respiratory depression • Dry mouth; heavy feeling of extremities; and warm, flushed skin • Severe itching • Spontaneous abortion • Vomiting	• Be aware that a heroin user has an increased risk of overdose because she rarely knows the actual strength of the drug or its true contents. She also has an increased risk of infectious disease, especially HIV, if she shares needles. • Monitor patient for long-term effects of heroin use, including arthritis, bacterial infections (including abscesses and infections of the heart lining and valves), collapsed veins, hepatitis B and C, and other rheumatologic problems. • Inform patient that the drug may be both physically and psychologically addictive. • Instruct patient that cravings for the drug can occur months after withdrawal is complete. *(continued)*

COMMONLY ABUSED DRUGS *(continued)*

Generic and Trade Names (Street Names)	Facts and Statistics	Reasons for Use
ketamine hydrochloride Ketalar (cat tranquilizer, K, ket, ketaset, lady K, special K, vitamin K)	• Ketamine was first synthesized in 1962 and used primarily for veterinary anesthesiology. • In 1965, it was found to be a useful anesthetic in humans, although patients reported adverse effects. • Ketamine has since became popular as a date rape drug and may be used recreationally by adolescents and young adults attending nightclubs or rave gatherings. • The drug has had a recent surge in popularity, leading to increased hospitalizations because of overdose.	• Causes a dream-like state and hallucinations • May have long duration of effects (up to 2 hours when snorted)
lysergic acid diethylamide (acid, blotter, cid, doses, L, LAD, LSD, microdots, paper, tabs, trips, window panes)	• Lysergic acid is a synthetic chemical derived from ergot, a fungus that grows on rye; it was first synthesized in 1938. • It gained popularity as a recreational drug in the 1960s and was made illegal in 1967. • It is typically taken orally as small, drug-laced paper squares, drug-laced sugar cubes, or powder.	• Fast onset of effects (20 to 60 minutes); effects depend on the amount ingested, the user's mood and personality, the surroundings, and when the user last ate • Long duration of full effects (up to 8 hrs), with up to 6 hours more before recovering complete sense of reality
methylenedioxymethamphetamine (Adam, beans, clarity, ecstasy, lover's speed, MDMA, rolls, X, XTC)	• Methylenedioxymethamphetamine was patented in early 1900s as appetite suppressant but was never tested in humans. • Its effects are similar to those of amphetamines and the hallucinogen mescaline. • It is usually taken orally as a tablet or capsule.	• Long duration of effects (usually 3 to 6 hours, but may continue for several weeks) • Stimulant and psychedelic effects • Stimulant effects may lead to excessive activity, such as prolonged dancing • Sense of thoughtfulness and contemplative mood

Signs and Symptoms of Abuse	Nursing Considerations
• Delayed or reduced sensations • Mental state ranging from dreamlike thoughts to compelling visions, complete dissociation, blackouts, and classic near-death experiences • Dry mouth • Dyspnea • Erotic feelings • Increased sociability • Nausea • Nervousness • Racing heart • Vertigo • Vomiting	• Monitor patient who has used ketamine for vomiting and unconsciousness, which can lead to aspiration and suffocation. • Be aware that the drug is more physically and psychologically addictive than other hallucinogens; users often take it once or more daily. • Inform patient that regular use may cause paranoia and egocentrism.
• Altered thought patterns • Feelings of insight, confusion, or paranoia • Labile emotional state • Mental and physical stimulation • Pupil dilation	• Assess patient on lysergic acid for frightened mental state that could lead to dangerous behavior. • Monitor patient for signs and symptoms of latent psychological and mental problems, such as schizophrenia. • Tell patient that recent use of the drug can have an additive effect on subsequent use and that recent physical or psychological traumas can increase distress while under the drug's influence. • Inform patient that the drug doesn't cause withdrawal symptoms even after heavy use.
• Altered mood • Anxiety • Dilated pupils • Hallucinations • Hot-and-cold flashes • Insomnia • Irrational behavior • Jaw clenching • Multiple thought pattern changes, such as paranoia or panic attacks	• Assess patient on methylenedioxymethamphetamine for dehydration, hypertension, and heart and kidney failure, which can result from excessive physical activity. • Monitor patient for heart attack, malignant hyperthermia, seizure, and stroke, which can result from high drug doses. • Warn patient of the drug's neurotoxic effects, including memory loss and permanent damage to serotonin-releasing neurons.

(continued)

COMMONLY ABUSED DRUGS (continued)

Generic and Trade Names (Street Names)	Facts and Statistics	Reasons for Use	
methylenedioxy-methamphetamine (continued)		• Smooth "comedown" effects that may last up to 24 hours	
nicotine	• Nicotine use is the leading preventable cause of death in the U.S. • It causes over 400,000 deaths at a cost of more than $50 billion in medical expenses annually. • About 80% of adults begin using nicotine before age 18. • Each day, nearly 3,000 children under age 18 become regular users.	• Calming, relaxing effects • Acceptance among peers • Pleasurable sensation • Effort to emulate people portrayed in nicotine advertisements	
nicotine oxide (hippy crack, laughing gas, N2O, nitrous)	• Nitrous oxide is a naturally occurring gas that's produced synthetically for sale and is used in dentistry as an analgesic. • It may be purchased for illegal use in the form of whipped cream chargers that the user opens inside a balloon and then inhales.	• Rapid onset of effects (within seconds) and short duration (several minutes) • Feeling of euphoria • Mild sedation • Rapid pain relief • May cause psychedelic dissociation	
oxycodone hydrochloride OxyContin (hillbilly heroin, oxy, oxycotton)	• Oxycodone is a synthetic form of morphine that was developed in 1995 as an analgesic to treat cancer pain and chronic pain. • It has become a commonly prescribed drug because its effects are released slowly over 12 hours.	• Feeling of euphoria • Heroin-like high	

Signs and Symptoms of Abuse	Nursing Considerations
• Nausea • Poor concentration • Skin tingling • Sweating • Teeth grinding • Unsteadiness • Vomiting	• Inform patient that withdrawal may cause permanent depression.
• Withdrawal symptoms when nicotine use is denied, such as difficulty concentrating, feelings of sadness or depression, hunger, irritability, and restlessness • Strong urge or need to smoke • Presence of nicotine stains on teeth or nails	• Assess patient for nicotine-related cardiovascular disorders, pulmonary disorders, and cancer, especially lung cancer. • Warn pregnant patient that nicotine use is harmful to fetal development. • Inform patient that smoking increases carbon monoxide content in the blood, causes shortness of breath, and exacerbates asthma. It also may cause impotence and infertility. • Tell patient that smoking may increase his spouse's risk of lung cancer and heart disease.
• Brief change in state of consciousness • Uncontrollable or inappropriate laughter	• Assess chronic nitrous oxide user for vitamin B_{12} deficiency, which may cause numbness in the fingers and toes and potentially long-term damage. • Be aware that an addicted user may require the drug many times a day every day. • Warn patient that she could suffocate if the plastic inhalation device remains on her face as consciousness decreases or if the valve of a nitrous oxide tank is left open in a confined space.
• Respiratory depression	• Assess long-term oxycodone user for signs and symptoms of damage to the liver and kidneys. • Be prepared to taper drug slowly to prevent signs and symptoms of withdrawal, such as flulike symptoms and pain. • Warn patient that breaking, chewing, or crushing an oxycodone tablet may result in a fatal dose. • Inform patient that use may cause physical dependence.

COMMON SOURCES OF CAFFEINE

Patients who take a CNS stimulant, such as amphetamine sulfate, should avoid products that contain caffeine because of a risk of additive CNS stimulant effects. Use the chart below as a quick-reference guide to common sources of caffeine and their caffeine content. Remember to advise your patient that the amount of caffeine in these products may change, so she should always read the product label or check with the manufacturer to verify caffeine content.

Beverages and Foods

Coffee (5 oz)
- brewed, drip method: 115 mg
- brewed, percolator: 80 mg
- espresso (2 oz): 100 mg
- instant: 65 mg
- brewed, decaffeinated: 3 mg
- instant, decaffeinated: 2 mg

Tea (5 oz)
- brewed (U.S. brands): 40 mg
- brewed (imported brands): 60 mg
- green: 15 mg
- instant: 30 mg

Bottled iced tea (12 oz)
- Lipton Brisk, all varieties: 9 mg
- Nestea Sweet Iced Tea: 26.5 mg
- Nestea Unsweetened Iced Tea: 26 mg
- Snapple Peach Tea (regular & diet): 31.5 mg

Soda (12 oz)
- A & W Cream Soda: 29 mg
- Barq's Root Beer: 23 mg
- Coca-Cola Classic, Cherry Coke: 34 mg
- Diet Coke: 45.6 mg
- Diet Pepsi: 36 mg
- Diet Sunkist Orange: 41 mg
- Dr. Pepper: 41 mg
- Jolt: 71.2 mg
- Mountain Dew: 55 mg
- Pepsi Cola: 38 mg
- Shasta Cola, Shasta Diet Cola: 44.4 mg
- Sunkist Orange: 40 mg
- Surge: 51 mg

Chocolate
- cocoa beverage (5 oz): 4 mg
- chocolate milk (8 oz): 5 mg
- milk chocolate (1 oz): 15 mg
- dark semisweet chocolate (1 oz): 20 mg
- baker's chocolate (1 oz): 26 mg

Over-the-Counter Drugs*

Cough and cold preparations
- Dristan Formula P (CAN): 16 mg
- Fendol: 32 mg
- Histosal: 30 mg
- Oradrine-2 (CAN): 32.4 mg
- Scot-Tussin Original 5-Action Cold Formula: 25 mg
- Sinapils: 32.5 mg

Diuretics
- Aqua-Ban: 100 mg

*Amount of caffeine in 1 caplet or tablet.

COMMON SOURCES OF CAFFEINE *(continued)*

Over-the-Counter Drugs* *(continued)*

Pain relievers
- Actamin Super: 65 mg
- Anacin Caplets/Tablets; Anacin Maximum Strength: 32 mg
- Aspirin-Free Excedrin Caplets: 65 mg
- Bayer Select Maximum Strength Headache Pain Relief Formula: 65 mg
- Cope: 32 mg
- Excedrin Caplets (CAN): 65 mg
- Excedrin Extra Strength Caplets/Tablets: 65 mg
- Excedrin Migraine: 65 mg
- Gelpirin: 32 mg
- Goody's Extra Strength Tablets: 16.25 mg
- Vanquish Caplets: 33 mg

Stimulants
- Caffedrine Caplets: 200 mg
- Dexitac Stay Alert Stimulant: 200 mg
- Enerjets: 75 mg
- Keep Alert: 200 mg
- NoDoz Maximum Strength Caplets: 200 mg
- Pep-Back: 100 mg
- Quick Pep: 150 mg
- Ultra Pep-Back: 200 mg
- Vivarin: 200 mg
- Wake-Up (CAN): 100 mg

*Amount of caffeine in 1 caplet or tablet.

COMMON SOURCES OF TYRAMINE

Tyramine is an amino acid released from proteins during aging, fermenting, pickling, smoking, and spoiling. In the body, tyramine triggers the release of norepinephrine from adrenergic nerve endings and is then deactivated by monoamine oxidase (MAO) in the liver and intestine. However, in a patient taking an MAO inhibitor, tyramine levels may increase and cause large amounts of norepinephrine to be released, which could lead to a hypertensive reaction.

The following chart lists common sources of tyramine. Use it as a guide to instruct your patient about the foods and beverages she should avoid during MAO inhibitor therapy.

Aged cheeses
- Blue
- Camembert
- Cheddar
- Gouda
- Parmesan
- Provolone
- Romano
- Stilton
- Swiss

Alcoholic beverages
- Beer (including non-alcoholic beer)
- Cognac
- Liqueurs
- Sherry
- Wine

Fish
- Caviar
- Cured or dried fish
- Fermented, smoked, or otherwise aged fish
- Pickled herring
- Shrimp paste
- Spoiled fish

Fruits
- Bananas (in large quantities)
- Figs
- Prunes
- Raisins

Meats
- Beef or chicken liver
- Corned beef
- Smoked and processed meats (such as bologna, pepperoni, salami)

Vegetables
- Avocados (especially if overripe)
- Chinese pea pods
- Fava beans
- Fermented bean curd
- Flat Italian beans
- Olives
- Pickles
- Sauerkraut
- Soybean paste

Other sources
- Beverages containing caffeine
- Cheese-filled desserts
- Monosodium glutamate (MSG)
- Protein supplements
- Soups containing protein extract
- Soy sauce
- Yeast extracts

DRUGS THAT CAUSE SEROTONIN SYNDROME

Serotonin syndrome occurs when serotonin accumulates to a toxic level in the central nervous system. This may occur within a day after the following:

- Therapeutic use of a drug known to inhibit serotonin reuptake, such as clomipramine, or a selective serotonin reuptake inhibitor (SSRI), such as citalopram, fluoxetine, fluvoxamine, paroxetine, or sertraline
- Therapeutic use of two drugs that increase the level of serotonin when combined
- Illegal use of methylenedioxymethamphetamine (MDMA or ecstasy)
- A drug overdose.

The signs and symptoms of serotonin syndrome may be mild to severe, such as agitation, ataxia, diaphoresis, fever, hyperreflexia, or tremor. Because serotonin syndrome can be fatal, focus your assessment on finding the cause of your patient's signs and symptoms. Be aware that this condition may be caused by an agent, such as electroconvulsive therapy or lithium, or by one of the drugs listed in the chart below.

Drugs that act as serotonin receptor agonists
- buspirone
- sumatriptan

Drugs that decrease serotonin metabolism
- isocarboxazid
- monoamine oxidase (MAO) inhibitors
- phenelzine
- selegiline
- tranylcypromine

Drugs that increase serotonin release
- amphetamine
- cocaine
- reserpine

Drugs that increase serotonin synthesis
- L-tryptophan

Drugs that inhibit serotonin reuptake
- amitriptyline
- amphetamine
- citalopram
- clomipramine
- cocaine
- desipramine
- dextromethorphan
- doxepin
- duloxepine
- escitalopram
- fluoxetine
- fluvoxamine
- imipramine
- meperidine
- nefazodone
- nortriptyline
- paroxetine
- protriptyline
- sertraline
- trazodone
- venlafaxine

Drug combinations taken within two weeks of each other
- dextromethorphan and an SSRI
- dihydroergotamine and an SSRI
- lithium and an SSRI
- L-tryptophan and an SSRI
- an MAO inhibitor and an SSRI
- sumatriptan and an SSRI

PSYCHOTROPIC HERBAL REMEDIES

Patients today are more aware of the potential benefits of alternative therapies, such as herbal remedies, which may be purchased as OTC preparations from supermarkets and health food stores, and even over the Internet. Your patient with a behavioral or mental health disorder may be taking such a remedy for its potential psychotropic effects.

Herbal Remedy	Indications	Usual Adult Dosages	
Black cohosh	• To treat anxiety	**Caplets, capsules:** 500 to 600 mg t.i.d. (standardized to 1 mg triterpenes/caplet or capsule). **Extract:** 3 to 4 ml t.i.d. (1:1 dilution). **Powdered rhizome:** 1 to 2 g. **Solid dry powdered extract:** 250 to 500 mg (4:1 dilution). **Tincture:** 4 to 6 ml b.i.d. or t.i.d. (1:5 dilution).	
Chamomile	• To alleviate anxiety • To treat insomnia	**Capsules:** 300 to 400 mg up to 6 times/day (standardized to 1% apigenin and 0.5% essential oil). **Extract:** 1 to 2 ml t.i.d. (1:1 dilution with 45% ethanol). **Tea:** 2 to 4 oz p.r.n. **Tincture:** 3 to 10 ml t.i.d. (1:5 dilution with 45% ethanol).	
Ephedra	• For CNS stimulation • For weight reduction	**Capsules, tablets (crude herb):** 500 to 1,000 mg b.i.d. or t.i.d. **Extract:** 12 to 25 mg total alkaloids b.i.d. or t.i.d. (standardized to ephedrine). **Tea:** 1.5 to 9 g herb in 1 pint boiling water, let stand for 5 min, drink in divided doses. **Tincture:** 15 to 30 drops b.i.d. or t.i.d.	

The following chart lists some common herbal remedies with psychotropic effects, their indications, usual adult dosages, adverse reactions, and nursing considerations for treating a patient taking an herbal remedy, including possible interactions with prescribed drug therapies.

Adverse Reactions	Nursing Considerations
CV: Hypotension **GI:** Anorexia, nausea, vomiting **GU:** Uterine stimulation	• Be aware that black cohosh is contraindicated in pregnant patients because it may cause uterine stimulation. **Drug–Herb Interactions** *antihypertensives:* Possibly increased hypotensive effect *hormone replacement drugs:* Possibly altered therapeutic effects of these drugs
Other: Hypersensitivity	•WARNING Be aware that chamomile is contraindicated in pregnant patients because it may cause spontaneous abortion. • Warn a patient with asthma or allergies not to use chamomile because it may cause a sensitivity reaction if he's allergic to sunflowers, ragweed, or members of the aster family.
CNS: Anxiety, confusion, dizziness, hallucinations, headache, insomnia, nervousness, poor concentration, seizures, tremor **CV:** Angina, arrhythmias, hypertension, MI, palpitations, stroke **GI:** Anorexia, constipation, diarrhea, nausea, vomiting **GU:** Dysuria, urine retention, uterine contractions **RESP:** Dyspnea **SKIN:** Exfoliative dermatitis **Other:** Hypersensitivity	• Be aware that ephedra has been banned by the FDA and is contraindicated in patients with a history of angina; arrhythmias, including heart block and tachycardia; diabetes; hypersensitivity to ephedra or sympathomimetics; hypertension; hyperthyroidism; narrow-angle glaucoma; prostatic hyperplasia; psychosis; or seizure disorder. •WARNING Instruct patient to inform all health care providers that he's taking the herb because it has many possible drug interactions. • Tell patient to avoid caffeinated beverages because they may increase the herb's stimulating effects. • Inform patient taking herb to avoid bitter orange, ginseng, green tea, guarana, Indian sida, kola nut, malvaceae, Siberian ginseng, soapwort, and yerba maté because of increased risk of hypertension and CNS stimulation. *(continued)*

PSYCHOTROPIC HERBAL REMEDIES *(continued)*

Herbal Remedy	Indications	Usual Adult Dosages	
Evening primrose oil	• To treat depression • To alleviate stress	**Capsules containing 320 to 480 mg *cis*-gamma linoleic acid (GLA)/capsule:** 3 to 12 capsules q.d.	
Ginkgo biloba	• To increase alertness • To improve short-term memory • To treat cerebrovascular insufficiency • To treat depression	*To increase alertness and improve short-term memory* **Capsules, tablets:** 60 mg t.i.d. (standardized to 24% flavonoid glycosides). *To treat cerebrovascular insufficiency* **Capsules, tablets:** 80 mg t.i.d. (standardized to 24% flavonoid glycosides). *To treat depression* **Capsules, tablets:** 40 mg t.i.d.	
Ginseng	• To improve cognitive functioning • To improve concentration • To lessen fatigue • To alleviate stress	**Capsules:** 200 to 500 mg extract q.d. **Infusion:** 3 g herb in boiling water, let stand 10 min, strain; may be taken t.i.d. for 3 to 4 wk. **Powdered root:** 1 to 4 g q.d. **Standardized extract:** 200 to 500 mg extract q.d. **Tincture:** 1 to 2 ml extract q.d. (1:1 dilution).	
Gotu kola	• For CNS stimulation	**Capsules:** 450 mg q.d. **Dried leaf:** 0.3 to 0.6 g t.i.d.	

Adverse Reactions	Nursing Considerations
CNS: Headache, temporal lobe seizures (in schizophrenia) **GI:** Anorexia, diarrhea, nausea, vomiting **SKIN:** Rash **Other:** Hypersensitivity, immunosuppression, inflammation	• Be aware that evening primrose oil is contraindicated in patients with hypersensitivity to the herb or a seizure disorder. • Tell patient to store herb in a sealed container away from heat and moisture. **Drug–Herb Interactions** *phenothiazine:* Possibly increased risk of seizures
CNS: Anxiety, headache, restlessness **GI:** Anorexia, diarrhea, nausea, vomiting **Other:** Hypersensitivity	• Be aware that ginkgo biloba is contraindicated in patients with a history of a coagulation or platelet disorder, including hemophilia, and those with hypersensitivity to the herb. • Inform patient that it may take 6 months of continuous use for herb to be effective. **Drug–Herb Interactions** *anticoagulants, platelet inhibitors:* Possibly increased risk of bleeding *MAO inhibitors:* Possibly increased MAO inhibition
CNS: Anxiety, insomnia, restlessness (high doses) **CV:** Chest pain, hypertension, palpitations **GI:** Anorexia, diarrhea (high doses), nausea, vomiting **SKIN:** Rash **Other:** Ginseng abuse syndrome (edema, hypertonia, insomnia), hypersensitivity	• Be aware that ginseng is contraindicated in patients with a history of a cardiac disorder, hypersensitivity to ginseng, or hypertension. • Tell patient to avoid concurrent use of ginseng and ephedra because of risk of hypertension and CNS stimulation. • Inform diabetic patient that herb may cause hypoglycemia. • Advise patient to avoid caffeine and other stimulants because overstimulation may occur. • Inform patient that herb shouldn't be used continuously for more than 3 months. **Drug–Herb Interactions** *anticoagulants:* Possibly decreased anticoagulant effects *antidiabetic drugs:* Possibly decreased serum glucose level *MAO inhibitors:* Possibly increased risk of maniclike syndrome
CNS: Sedation **ENDO:** Increased serum glucose level **SKIN:** Contact dermatitis, pruritus, rash **Other:** Hypercholesterolemia, hypersensitivity	• Be aware that gotu kola is contraindicated in patients with hypersensitivity to the herb or to celery. • Inform patient that herb isn't the same as other cola products and should not be confused as such. **Drug–Herb Interactions** *antidiabetic drugs, antilipemics:* Possibly decreased effectiveness of these drugs *(continued)*

PSYCHOTROPIC HERBAL REMEDIES *(continued)*

Herbal Remedy	Indications	Usual Adult Dosages	
Hops	• As an analgesic • To treat depression • To treat insomnia	**Infusion:** 0.4 g (1 tsp) ground hops cone in 8 oz boiling water, let stand 15 min. **Extract:** 0.5 to 1 ml t.i.d. **Cut herb:** 0.5 g as a single dose.	
Kava	• To alleviate anxiety • To treat depression • To treat insomnia • To treat psychosis	*To treat anxiety and depression* **Extract:** 45 to 70 kava lactones t.i.d. (standardized). *To treat insomnia* **Extract:** 190 to 200 mg kava lactones 1 hr h.s. (standardized). *To treat psychosis* **Capsules, tablets:** 400 to 500 mg up to 6 times/day. **Extract:** 70 mg kava lactones t.i.d. (standardized). **Tincture:** 15 to 30 drops t.i.d. in water (1:2 dilution).	
Kudzu	• To treat alcoholism	**P.O. decoction:** Cut root into 0.4 to 0.7 cm slices, place in water 12 to 15 times the weight of the root; decoct 30 min.	
Lemon balm	• To alleviate anxiety • To treat depression • To treat hysteria • To treat insomnia	**Infusion:** 1.5 to 4.5 g herb in boiling water, let set 10 min, strain; may take 8 to 10 g/day.	

Adverse Reactions	Nursing Considerations
CNS: Decreased reaction time, dizziness, sedation **GI:** Anorexia, nausea, vomiting **Other:** Anaphylaxis, hypersensitivity	• Be aware that hops are contraindicated in women with breast, uterine, or cervical cancer because herb may have estrogenic effects. • Monitor patient for altered therapeutic effect of other drug therapies because herb inhibits the function of cytochrome P450 isoenzymes. • Warn patient to avoid alcohol and OTC CNS depressants because of a risk of increased CNS depression. **Drug–Herb Interactions** *antidepressants, antihistamines, antipsychotic drugs, CNS depressants:* Possibly increased CNS depressant effects *estrogens:* Possibly increased hormone levels
CNS: Hyperreflexia **EENT:** Blurred vision, red eyes **GI:** Anorexia, hepatotoxicity, nausea, vomiting **GU:** Hematuria **HEME:** Decreased serum albumin, bilirubin, and protein levels; decreased lymphocyte and platelet counts; increased RBC count **RESP:** Dyspnea, pulmonary hypertension **SKIN:** Jaundice, scaling (high doses) **Other:** Hypersensitivity, weight loss	• Be aware that kava is contraindicated in patients with a history of hypersensitivity to the herb, major depressive disorder, or Parkinson's disease. •**WARNING** Be aware that kava may cause liver toxicity. Adivse patient to his notify health care provider of abdominal pain, darkened urine, jaundice, or light-colored stools. • Warn patient that herb may be habit forming and shouldn't be used for longer than 3 months. **Drug–Herb Interactions** *antiparkinsonian drugs:* Possibly decreased effectiveness of these drugs *CNS depressants:* Possibly increased risk of sedation
GI: Anorexia, nausea, vomiting **Other:** Hypersensitivity	• Be aware that kudzu is contraindicated in patients with hypersensitivity to the herb. • Tell patient to avoid alcohol because it could cause a disulfiram-like reaction. **Drug–Herb Interactions** *antiarrhythmics, digoxin:* Possibly enhanced cardiac effects
GI: Anorexia, nausea **Other:** Hypersensitivity	• Be aware that lemon balm is contraindicated in patients with hypersensitivity to the herb or hypothyroidism. • Tell patient to store herb in a sealed container away from heat and moisture and that, with proper storage, herb may be kept for up to 1 year.

(continued)

PSYCHOTROPIC HERBAL REMEDIES *(continued)*

Herbal Remedy	Indications	Usual Adult Dosages	
Melatonin	• To treat insomnia	**Tablets:** 75 mg h.s.	
Passion flower	• To alleviate anxiety • To treat insomnia	*To treat anxiety* **Dried herb:** 0.25 to 1 g t.i.d. **Fluid extract:** 0.5 to 1 ml t.i.d. **Drops:** 10 to 30 drops t.i.d. (0.7% flavonoids). **Tea:** 4 to 6 tsp of herb in 3 divided doses. **Tincture:** 0.5 to 2 ml t.i.d. *To treat insomnia* **Dried herb tea:** 4 to 8 g h.s. **Dry powdered extract:** 300 to 450 mg h.s. (2.6% flavonoids). **Fluid extract:** 2 to 4 ml ($\frac{1}{2}$ to 1 tsp) h.s. (1:1 dilution). **Tincture:** 6 to 8 ml (1 to 2 tsp) h.s. (1:5 dilution).	
Skullcap	• To treat insomnia • To prevent seizures	**Dried herb tea:** 2 g t.i.d. **Fluid extract:** 2 to 4 ml t.i.d. (1:1 dilution in 25% alcohol). **Tincture:** 1 to 2 ml t.i.d. (1:5 dilution in 45% alcohol).	

Adverse Reactions	Nursing Considerations
CNS: Altered sleep pattern, confusion, headache, hypothermia, sedation **CV:** Tachycardia **GI:** Anorexia, nausea, vomiting **Other:** Decreased serum estradiol, LH, and progesterone levels, hypersensitivity	• Be aware that melatonin is contraindicated in patients with a history of cardiovascular or hepatic disease, CNS disorders, depression, or hypersensitivity to melatonin. • Advise patient to avoid CNS stimulants, such as caffeine, because of synergistic effect that could exacerbate insomnia. • Tell patient to store herb in sealed container away from heat and moisture. **Drug–Herb Interactions** *benzodiazepines:* Possibly increased antianxiety effects *CNS stimulants:* Possibly exacerbation of insomnia
CNS: CNS depression (high doses) **GI:** Anorexia, nausea, vomiting **Other:** Hypersensitivity	• Be aware that passion flower is contraindicated in patients with hypersensitivity to the herb and in pregnant patients because it may cause uterine stimulation. • If patient is taking high doses or has used herb for prolonged period, monitor him for signs and symptoms of toxicity, including drowsiness, nonsustained ventricular tachycardia, prolonged QT interval, severe nausea, and vomiting. **Drug–Herb Interactions** *CNS depressants, MAO inhibitors:* Possibly increased risk of sedation
CNS: Confusion, euphoria, seizures, stupor (overdose of tincture form), tremors **CV:** Arrhythmias (overdose of tincture form) **GI:** Anorexia, hepatotoxicity, nausea, vomiting **Other:** Hypersensitivity	• Be aware that skullcap is contraindicated in patients with hypersensitivity to the herb. **Drug–Herb Interactions** *immunosuppressants:* Possibly decreased effects of these drugs *(continued)*

PSYCHOTROPIC HERBAL REMEDIES *(continued)*

Herbal Remedy	Indications	Usual Adult Dosages	
St. John's wort	• To alleviate anxiety • To treat depression	**Capsules, extract, solid forms, tincture:** 300 mg t.i.d. (standardized to 0.3% hypericin).	
Valerian	• To alleviate anxiety • To treat insomnia	**Extract:** 400 to 900 mg 1 hr h.s. (standardized). **Tea (crude herb):** 1 tsp crude herb q.i.d. **Tincture:** 3 to 5 ml q.i.d. (standardized).	
Yohimba	• To treat depression • To treat erectile dysfunction	**Tincture:** 5 to 10 drops t.i.d. **Tablets:** 15 to 30 mg q.d.	

Adverse Reactions	Nursing Considerations
CNS: Dizziness, insomnia, restlessness **GI:** Abdominal cramps, constipation **SKIN:** Photosensitivity, rash **Other:** Hypersensitivity	• Be aware that St. John's wort is contraindicated in patients with hypersensitivity to the herb. • Advise patient to avoid alcohol and tyramine-rich foods because herb may increase MAO inhibition. • Monitor patient taking an amphetamine, MAO inhibitor, selective serotonin reuptake inhibitor, trazodone, or a tricyclic antidepressant for signs and symptoms of serotonin syndrome, such as altered mental status, hyperpyrexia, and tremor. • Inform patient that the herb's therapeutic effect may take up to 6 weeks of continuous use. **Drug–Herb Interactions** *amphetamines, MAO inhibitors, selective serotonin reuptake inhibitors, trazodone, tricyclic antidepressants:* Possibly increased risk of serotonin syndrome *cyclosporine:* Possibly decreased drug effectiveness *indinavir:* Possibly decreased antiretroviral effect *paroxetine:* Possibly increased sedation
CNS: Headache, insomnia, restlessness **CV:** Palpitations **EENT:** Vision changes **GI:** Anorexia, hepatotoxicity, nausea, vomiting **Other:** Hypersensitivity	• Be aware that valerian is contraindicated in patients with hepatic disease or hypersensitivity to the herb. **Drug–Herb Interactions** *CNS depressants:* Possibly increased CNS depression *MAO inhibitors, phenytoin, warfarin:* Possibly decreased therapeutic effects of these drugs
CNS: Anxiety, dizziness, headache, manic reaction (psychiatric patient), restlessness, tremor **CV:** Hypertension, tachycardia **GI:** Anorexia, diarrhea, nausea, vomiting **GU:** Dysuria, nephrotoxicity **SKIN:** Flushing **Other:** Hypersensitivity	• Be aware that yohimba is contraindicated in patients with a history of angina pectoris, anxiety disorder, bipolar disorder, gastric or duodenal ulcers, hepatic or renal disease, hypertension, hypersensitivity to yohimba, prostatitis, schizophrenia, or suicidal tendencies. • Caution patient that long-term effects greater than 10 weeks aren't known. • Urge patient to avoid CNS stimulants, such as caffeine, because of a risk of increased CNS stimulation. • Tell patient to avoid foods high in tyramine while taking herb because of a risk of hypertension. **Drug–Herb Interactions** *alpha-adrenergic receptor blockers, sympathomimetics:* Possibly increased risk of yohimba toxicity *CNS stimulants, selective serotonin reuptake inhibitors:* Possibly increased CNS stimulation *MAO inhibitors:* Possibly increased MAO inhibition *tricyclic antidepressants:* Possibly increased risk of hypertension

TREATING DRUG OVERDOSE

Early recognition and fast medical treatment are essential when treating a suspected drug overdose. An overdose may be intentional, such as with a severely depressed or psychotic patient who wishes to end her life, or accidental, such as with someone who is seeking the mind-altering effects of the drug. Patients can overdose on many types of substances, including herbal remedies, illegal or street drugs, OTC products, and prescription drugs. Some psychotropic drugs—especially amphetamines, barbiturates, benzodiazepines, opiates, and tricyclic antidepressants—are commonly involved in an overdose.

If the onset of a patient's signs and symptoms is abrupt and multiple organ systems are involved, then suspect that she may have overdosed on a drug. Focus your assessment on finding out the following information:

- the drug or drugs involved in the overdose
- the amounts of the drugs involved
- the time when the drugs were taken
- the patient's current signs and symptoms
- pertinent health history, including the patient's age, allergies, drug history, present illnesses, and weight
- the first-aid measures she may already have received.

Treatment

Treatment for a drug overdose involves support of your patient's vital functions, removing the toxin from her body, managing her signs and symptoms, and preventing further complications.

Supportive Treatment

Expect to establish and maintain an open airway, assess your patient's breathing, monitor her level of consciousness, and maintain her circulation. Be prepared to establish I.V. access, frequently monitor her vital signs, and initiate continuous ECG monitoring. Also, check the patient's serum glucose level to rule out hypoglycemia.

Drug Removal

After giving supportive treatment, expect to reduce absorption and enhance drug elimination by giving activated charcoal or a cathartic or by performing gastric lavage. Ipecac syrup, once standard treatment to induce vomiting, is rarely used today because activated charcoal acts more quickly and is more effective.

Activated charcoal is a fine, odorless, tasteless, black powder that adsorbs a variety of drugs and chemicals on the surfaces of the charcoal particles. Mix activated charcoal with water to the consistency of a milkshake and administer it orally or by lavage tube. Activated charcoal isn't effective for adsorbing caustic alkalis, cyanide, ethanol, methanol, and mineral acids. Because activated charcoal can adsorb ipecac syrup, avoid giving these substances together.

Cathartics may be used to speed the passage of gastric contents through the GI system to help decrease absorption of the overdosed

TREATING DRUG OVERDOSE (continued)

drug. A cathartic may also be used with activated charcoal to decrease drug absorption. Common cathartics include magnesium sulfate and magnesium citrate (saline cathartics) and sorbitol (a hyperosmotic cathartic). A cathartic may be given orally or by lavage tube. Monitor the patient's fluid and electrolyte status because of the loss of GI contents. Be aware that a magnesium-containing cathartic shouldn't be given to a patient with decreased renal function because of the risk of magnesium toxicity.

Ipecac syrup is used rarely and only after consulting a regional poison control center or medical toxicologist. It acts as a GI irritant and causes vomiting. To induce vomiting, give ipecac syrup with at least 8 oz (240 ml) of water in an adult or 4 to 8 oz (120 to 240 ml) of water in a child. It's contraindicated if the patient has CNS depression, is having a seizure (because of the risk of aspiration), or has ingested a caustic substance or a petroleum product (because the vomited substance may damage the esophagus or cause aspiration pneumonia). Don't administer ipecac syrup to a patient who will be treated with activated charcoal because of the possibility of vomiting and then aspirating the activated charcoal.

Gastric lavage may be used when the overdose drug isn't adsorbed by activated charcoal. A large-bore lavage tube (36-F for adults and 24-F for children) is inserted orally and may be more effective than a smaller tube inserted nasally. The solution used for lavage is either tap water or NS, but NS may reduce the risk of water intoxication in children. Gastric lavage may be used in a comatose patient as long as her airway is protected by the insertion of a cuffed endotracheal tube to prevent aspiration of stomach contents into the lungs. Be aware that seizures should be brought under control before performing gastric lavage. Gastric lavage is contraindicated in patients who have ingested a caustic agent. Expect to use 200 to 300 ml of fluid per wash in an adult and 50 to 100 ml of fluid per wash in a child, as prescribed. Multiple, small washings may be used so that the drug isn't forced into the intestine. Expect to continue lavage until the stomach contents are clear.

Nursing Considerations for Treating Overdose

- To prevent future overdose attempts, teach the patient and her caregiver about the proper use of all her drugs.
- Be aware that you may need to limit your patient's access to her drugs if she overdosed intentionally.
- Notify all health care providers involved in the care of the patient about her overdose, and expect the patient to be referred for psychiatric re-evaluation.
- Urge your patient to schedule follow-up visits with her health care provider to monitor her compliance and response to drug therapy.
- Contact your local poison control center if you need specific information about treating an overdose.

BODY MASS INDEX CALCULATION

Body mass index (BMI) is a formula used to determine obesity; it's calculated by dividing a person's weight in kilograms by his height in meters squared (kg/m^2). A BMI of 25 or higher increases your patient's risk of developing hypertension, cardiovascular disease, type 2 diabetes mellitus, and stroke. It also increases the risk that he won't respond effectively to the usual drug dosages. If your patient has an abnormal BMI, be prepared to make dosage adjustments that are individualized based on body weight, as prescribed.

WEIGHT (POUNDS)

HEIGHT (INCHES)

Height																		
58	91	96	100	105	110	115	119	124	129	134	138	143	148	153	158	162	167	172
59	94	99	104	109	114	119	124	128	133	138	143	148	153	158	163	168	173	178
60	97	102	107	112	118	123	128	133	138	143	148	153	158	163	168	174	179	184
61	100	106	111	116	122	127	132	137	143	148	153	158	164	169	174	180	185	190
62	104	109	115	120	126	131	136	142	147	153	158	164	169	175	180	186	191	196
63	107	113	118	124	130	135	141	146	152	158	163	169	175	180	186	191	197	203
64	110	116	122	128	134	140	145	151	157	163	169	174	180	186	192	197	204	209
65	114	120	126	132	138	144	150	156	162	168	174	180	186	192	198	204	210	216
66	118	124	130	136	142	148	155	161	167	173	179	186	192	198	204	210	216	223
67	121	127	134	140	146	153	159	166	172	178	185	191	198	204	211	217	223	230
68	125	131	138	144	151	158	164	171	177	184	190	197	203	210	216	223	230	236
69	128	135	142	149	155	162	169	176	182	189	196	203	209	216	223	230	236	243
70	132	139	146	153	160	167	174	181	188	195	202	209	216	222	229	236	243	250
71	136	143	150	157	165	172	179	186	193	200	208	215	222	229	236	243	250	257
72	140	147	154	162	169	177	184	191	199	206	213	221	228	235	242	250	258	265
73	144	151	159	166	174	182	189	197	204	212	219	227	235	242	250	257	265	272
74	148	155	163	171	179	186	194	202	210	218	225	233	241	249	256	264	272	280
75	152	160	168	176	184	192	200	208	216	224	232	240	248	256	264	272	279	287
76	156	164	172	180	189	197	205	213	221	230	238	246	254	263	271	279	287	295
	19	20	21	22	23	24	25	26	27	28	29	30	31	32	33	34	35	36

BODY MASS INDEX

The table below will help you find your patient's BMI easily. It converts pounds to kilograms and inches to meters, and then it shows the BMI. To use it, simply find the patient's height on either side of the table; then move across the row to the weight that most closely matches your patient's. At the bottom of the column containing the weight, you'll find the BMI for that patient. For example, the BMI for a patient who is 70" tall and weighs 208 lb is 30.

WEIGHT (POUNDS)

																		HEIGHT (INCHES)
177	181	186	191	196	201	205	210	215	220	224	229	234	239	244	248	253	258	58
183	188	193	198	203	208	212	217	222	227	232	237	242	247	252	257	262	267	59
189	194	199	204	209	215	220	225	230	235	240	245	250	255	261	266	271	276	60
195	201	206	211	217	222	227	232	238	243	248	254	259	264	269	275	280	285	61
202	207	213	218	224	229	235	240	246	251	256	262	267	273	278	284	289	295	62
208	214	220	225	231	237	242	248	254	259	265	270	278	282	287	293	299	304	63
215	221	227	232	238	244	250	256	262	267	273	279	285	291	296	302	308	314	64
222	228	234	240	246	252	258	264	270	276	282	288	294	300	306	312	318	324	65
229	235	241	247	253	260	266	272	278	284	291	297	303	309	315	322	328	334	66
236	242	249	255	261	268	274	280	287	293	299	306	312	319	325	331	338	344	67
243	249	256	262	269	276	282	289	295	302	308	315	322	328	335	341	348	354	68
250	257	263	270	277	284	291	297	304	311	318	324	331	338	345	351	358	365	69
257	264	271	278	285	292	299	306	313	320	327	334	341	348	355	362	369	376	70
265	272	279	286	293	301	308	315	322	329	338	343	351	358	365	372	379	386	71
272	279	287	294	302	309	316	324	331	338	346	353	361	368	375	383	390	397	72
280	288	295	302	310	318	325	333	340	348	355	363	371	378	386	393	401	408	73
287	295	303	311	319	326	334	342	350	358	365	373	381	389	396	404	412	420	74
295	303	311	319	327	335	343	351	359	367	375	383	391	399	407	415	423	431	75
304	312	320	328	336	344	353	361	369	377	385	394	402	410	418	426	435	443	76
37	38	39	40	41	42	43	44	45	46	47	48	49	50	51	52	53	54	

BODY MASS INDEX

MECHANISM OF ACTION ILLUSTRATIONS TABLE

This table lists all drugs whose mechanisms of action are illustrated in this book, along with drugs that have a mechanism of action that is similar to the illustrated ones.

Drugs with illustrations	Drugs with a similar mechanism of action
acamprosate	none
alprostadil	none
amitriptyline hydrochloride	amoxapine, clomipramine hydrochloride, desip-ramine hydrochloride, doxepin hydrochloride, imipramine hydrochloride, imipramine pamoate, nortriptyline hydrochloride, protriptyline hydrochloride, trimipramine maleate
carbamazepine	ethotoin, fosphenytoin sodium, lamotrigine, mephenytoin, phenytoin, phenytoin sodium
disulfiram	none
entecapone	tolcapone
levodopa	none
lorazepam	alprazolam, chlordiazepoxide hydrochloride, clonazepam, clorazepate dipotassium, diazepam, estazolam, flurazepam hydrochloride, halazepam, oxazepam, quazepam, temazepam, triazolam
orlistat	none
perphenazine	chlorpromazine, chlorpromazine hydrochloride, fluphenazine decanoate, fluphenazine enanthate, fluphenazine hydrochloride, haloperidol, haloperidol decanoate, haloperidol lactate, mesoridazine besylate, mol-indone hydrochloride, pimozide, prochlorperazine, prochlorperazine edisylate, prochlorperazine maleate, thioridazine, thioridazine hydrochloride, thiothixene, thiothixene hydrochloride, trifluoperazine hydrochloride, triflupromazine hydrochloride
phenelzine sulfate	isocarboxazid, tranylcypromine sulfate
tacrine	donepezil hydrochloride, rivastigmine tartrate
tubocurarine	none

WEIGHTS AND EQUIVALENTS

The following three charts show approximate equivalents among the various systems of measurement.

Liquid Equivalents Among Household, Apothecaries', and Metric Systems

HOUSEHOLD	APOTHECARIES'	METRIC
1 teaspoon (tsp)	1 fluid dram	5 milliliters (ml)
1 tablespoon (tbs)	0.5 fluid ounce	15 ml
2 tbs (1 ounce [1 oz])	1 fluid ounce	30 ml
1 cupful	8 fluid ounces	240 ml
1 pint (pt)	16 fluid ounces	473 ml
1 quart (qt)	32 fluid ounces	946 ml (1 liter)

Solid Equivalents Among Apothecaries' and Metric Systems

APOTHECARIES'	METRIC
15 grains (gr)	1 gram (g) (1,000 milligrams [mg])
10 gr	0.6 g (600 mg)
7.5 gr	0.5 g (500 mg)
5 gr	0.3 g (300 mg)
3 gr	0.2 g (200 mg)
1.5 gr	0.1 g (100 mg)
1 gr	0.06 g (60 mg) or 0.065 g (65 mg)
0.75 gr	0.05 g (50 mg)
0.5 gr	0.03 g (30 mg)
0.25 gr	0.015 g (15 mg)
1/60 gr	0.001 g (1 mg)
1/100 gr	0.6 mg
1/120 gr	0.5 mg
1/150 gr	0.4 mg

(continued)

WEIGHTS AND EQUIVALENTS *(continued)*

Solid Equivalents Among Avoirdupois, Apothecaries', and Metric Systems

AVOIRDUPOIS	APOTHECARIES'	METRIC
1 gr	1 gr	0.065 g
15.4 gr	15 gr	1 g
1 ounce (1 oz)	480 gr	28.35 g
437.5 gr	1 oz	31 g
1 pound (lb)	1.33 lb	454 g
0.75 lb	1 lb	373 g
2.2 lb	2.7 lb	1 kilogram (kg)

ABBREVIATIONS

The following abbreviations, which are common to nursing practice, are used throughout the book.

ABG	arterial blood gas
a.c.	before meals
ACE	angiotensin-converting enzyme
ADH	antidiuretic hormone
AIDS	acquired immunodeficiency syndrome
ALT	alanine aminotransferase
ANA	antinuclear antibodies
APTT	activated partial thromboplastin time
AST	aspartate aminotransferase
ATP	adenosine triphosphate
AV	atrioventricular
b.i.d.	twice a day
BUN	blood urea nitrogen
°C	degrees Celsius
cAMP	cyclic adenosine monophosphate
(CAN)	Canadian drug trade name
cap	capsule
CBC	complete blood count
cGMP	cyclic guanosine monophosphate
CK	creatine kinase
Cl	chloride
cm	centimeter
CMV	cytomegalovirus
CNS	central nervous system
COPD	chronic obstructive pulmonary disease
C.R.	controlled-release
CSF	cerebrospinal fluid
CV	cardiovascular
CVA	cerebrovascular accident
D_5LR	dextrose 5% in lactated Ringer's solution
D_5NS	dextrose 5% in normal saline solution
$D_5/0.2NS$	dextrose 5% in quarter-normal saline solution
$D_5/0.45NS$	dextrose 5% in half-normal saline solution
D_5W	dextrose 5% in water
$D_{10}W$	dextrose 10% in water
$D_{50}W$	dextrose 50% in water
dl	deciliter
DNA	deoxyribonucleic acid
DS	double-strength *(continued)*

ABBREVIATIONS *(continued)*

EC	enteric-coated
ECG	electrocardiogram
EEG	electroencephalogram
EENT	eyes, ears, nose, and throat
ENDO	endocrine
E.R.	extended-release
°F	degrees Fahrenheit
FDA	Food and Drug Administration
g	gram
GFR	glomerular filtration rate
GI	gastrointestinal
gtt	drop
GU	genitourinary
H_1	histamine$_1$
H_2	histamine$_2$
HDL	high-density lipoprotein
HEME	hematologic
HIV	human immunodeficiency virus
HPV	human papilloma virus
hr	hour
h.s.	at bedtime
HSV	herpes simplex virus
HZV	herpes zoster virus
I.D.	intradermal
IgA	immunoglobulin A
IgE	immunoglobulin E
I.M.	intramuscular
INR	international normalized ratio
I.V.	intravenous
IVPB	intravenous piggyback
kg	kilogram
KIU	kallikrein inactivator units
L	liter
LA	long-acting
LD	lactate dehydrogenase
LDL	low-density lipoprotein
LR	lactated Ringer's solution
M	molar
m^2	square meter
MAO	monoamine oxidase
mcg	microgram

ABBREVIATIONS *(continued)*

mEq	milliequivalent
mg	milligram
MI	myocardial infarction
min	minute
ml	milliliter
mm	millimeter
mm^3	cubic millimeter
mmol	millimole
mo	month
MS	musculoskeletal
msec	millisecond
Na	sodium
NaCl	sodium chloride
NG	nasogastric
ng	nanogram
NPH	human isophane insulin
NPO	nothing by mouth
NS	normal saline solution
0.225NS	quarter-normal saline (0.225%) solution
0.45NS	half-normal saline (0.45%) solution
NSAID	nonsteroidal anti-inflammatory drug
OTC	over the counter
p.c.	after meals
PCA	patient-controlled analgesia
P.O.	by mouth
P.R.	by rectum
p.r.n.	as needed
PSVT	paroxysmal supraventricular tachycardia
PT	prothrombin time
PTCA	percutaneous transluminal coronary angioplasty
PVC	premature ventricular contraction
q	every
q.i.d.	four times a day
RBC	red blood cell
REM	rapid eye movement
RESP	respiratory
RNA	ribonucleic acid
RSV	respiratory syncytial virus
SA	sinoatrial
S.C.	subcutaneous

(continued)

ABBREVIATIONS *(continued)*

sec	second
S.L.	sublingual
S.R.	sustained-release
stat	immediately
supp	suppository
tab	tablet
T_3	triiodothyronine
T_4	thyroxine
t.i.d.	three times a day
tsp	teaspoon
USP	United States Pharmacopeia
UTI	urinary tract infection
VLDL	very low-density lipoprotein
WBC	white blood cell
wk	week

INDEX

INDEX

- **Generic and alternate names:** lowercase initial letter
- **Trade names:** uppercase initial letter
- **Illustrations:** *i* after page number
- **Tables:** *t* after page number